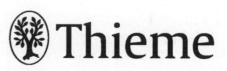

Textbook of Otorhinolaryngology—Head and Neck Surgery

A Competency-Based Approach for Undergraduates

Suresh Pillai, DLO, DNB (ORL)
Professor
Department of Otorhinolaryngology;
Head of Unit III
Division of Head and Neck Surgery
Kasturba Medical College
Manipal Academy of Higher Education
Manipal, Karnataka, India

Kailesh Pujary, MS (ORL), DNB, MBA-HCS, MNAMS
Professor and Head
Department of Otorhinolaryngology;
Head of Unit I
Division of Otology and Lateral Skull Base Surgery
Kasturba Medical College
Manipal Academy of Higher Education
Manipal, Karnataka, India

Thieme
Delhi • Stuttgart • New York • Rio de Janeiro

Publishing Director: Ritu Sharma
Senior Development Editor: Dr. Nidhi Srivastava
Director-Editorial Services: Rachna Sinha
Project Manager: Shipra Sehgal
Managing Director & CEO: Ajit Kohli

Thieme Medical and Scientific Publishers Private Limited.
A - 12, Second Floor, Sector - 2, Noida - 201 301,
Uttar Pradesh, India, +911204556600
Email: customerservice@thieme.in
www.thieme.in

Cover design: © Thieme
Cover image source: © Thieme
Page make-up by RECTO Graphics, India

Printed in India by Magic International Pvt. Ltd.

5 4 3 2 1

ISBN: 978-93-95390-20-0
Also available as an e-book:
eISBN (PDF): 978-93-95390-21-7
eISBN (ePub): 978-93-95390-23-1

Contents

Section G: General ENT

Videos

Preface

Otolaryngology is a blend of art and science—art in the way incisions are shaped, in patient communication, and in the elegance of the surgical procedure; and science because of an unwavering reliance on evidence in all our decision-making. That is why Michelangelo's David has been chosen for the cover; a sculpture at the peak of human aesthetic achievement but grounded in a deep, pioneering understanding of human anatomy.

The idea for this book germinated during two major recent events. The revamping of the MBBS curriculum and the onset of the pandemic, which gave us time to formulate a novel approach to ear, nose, and throat (ENT) education in the country.

Dr. Kailesh Pujary and I have assembled a knowledgeable team of authors for this textbook from India, Nepal, Malaysia, and the United States. Their contributions have greatly enhanced the quality of the book, and we sincerely thank them for their efforts.

We tried to make this book informative and stimulating. As far as possible, we have worked within the framework of the newly prescribed Competency-Based Medical Education curriculum. We have approached this task by dividing the textbook into seven sections based on conventional anatomical categorization. These sections have relevant surgical procedures and video explanations and are supplemented by additional readings.

Many talented people were involved in helping us bring out the first edition of this textbook. We would like to express our gratitude to the development editors and project managers at Thieme India as well as the interns, residents, and faculty who helped shape the book.

The hours were long, and sleep was short. I must thank my wife, Dr. Manna Valiathan, for her constant support and encouragement and for tolerating me as I spent long hours closeted in the library. Special thanks to my sons, Aditya and Pranav, who provided valuable inputs from time to time. We hope you will enjoy reading the book as much as we enjoyed writing it.

We would like to place on record our sincere thanks to Abhinaya Swaminathan, Aishwarya Kulkarni, Alisha Lizbeth Mathew, Anjali Pujary, Arun Kumar J.S., Donna Cardoza, Farnaz Nasrin Islam, H. Vijayendra, Hari Prakash P., Kishan Madikeri Mohan, Mihika Sinha, and Pallavi Pavithran for their help in drawing diagrams and sharing images for this textbook.

Suresh Pillai, DLO, DNB (ORL)

Preface

Where we have reached in life is often defined by the years of hard work and the faith we have in what we do.

Being in the field of otolaryngology–head and neck surgery has been an enriching experience. There has been rapid growth in this field over the past three decades, which gives the younger generation more to look forward to. Over the years, teaching has become a passion which has culminated in this book.

Dr. Suresh Pillai and I along with quite a few colleagues of medical colleges in India felt the need for a good book on otorhinolaryngology for the undergraduate students, especially with the new guidelines being laid down in the Competency-Based Medical Education (CBME) curriculum. Having friends and good colleagues in the field has helped us in bringing out this book with shared enthusiasm. We will remain grateful to the chapter authors and to those who have contributed photos and diagrams (including my daughter Anjali). I have been immensely encouraged by my wife (also an otolaryngologist!) and my friends (Prashanth Prabhu, Sanjay Bhalla, and Prashant Bhatia) in the field, whose excitement about the book spurred me on.

My gratitude to Prof. Jaspal for my initiation, to Dr. Arun Kumar for support in my career, and to Prof. Hazarika, Prof. Dipak Nayak, and Prof. Balakrishnan for my formative years.

I am blessed to have the support of my family—Parul (wife), Arjun (son), Anjali (daughter), Harish (brother), Kritish (brother), and Jyoti (sister)—and the vision of my parents.

I wish this book provides a good foundation for students in their journey in the medical field.

Kailesh Pujary, MS (ORL), DNB, MBA-HCS, MNAMS

Contributors

Afraz Jahan
Assistant Professor
Department of Community Medicine
Kasturba Medical College
Manipal Academy of Higher Education
Manipal, Karnataka, India

Ajay Bhandarkar
Associate Professor
Department of ENT and Head and Neck Surgery
Kasturba Medical College
Manipal Academy of Higher Education
Manipal, Karnataka, India

Ajoy Mathew Varghese
Professor and Head
Department of ENT
Christian Medical College
Vellore, Tamil Nadu, India

Amit Kumar Sharma
Senior Consultant (Formerly Professor and Head)
Department of ENT
Artemis Hospital
Gurgaon, Haryana, India

Andrews C. Joseph
Professor
Department of ENT
Amala Institute of Medical Sciences
Thrissur, Kerala, India

Anil Kumar R.
Professor
Department of ENT
Bangalore Medical College and Research Institute
Bangalore, Karnataka, India

Anusha Shashidhara Shetty
Assistant Professor
Department of Otolaryngology and Head and Neck Surgery
Kasturba Medical College
Manipal Academy of Higher Education
Manipal, Karnataka, India

A. Rajeshwary
Professor
Department of Otorhinolaryngology and Head Neck Surgery
KS Hegde Medical Academy
Mangalore, Karnataka, India

Arun Alexander
Professor
Department of ENT
Jawaharlal Institute of Postgraduate Medical Education and
  Research
Pondicherry, India

Ashish Chandra Agarwal
Associate Professor
Department of ENT
Dr. Ram Manohar Lohia Institute of Medical Sciences
Lucknow, Uttar Pradesh, India

Ashok S. Naik
Professor
Department of ENT
SDM College of Medical Sciences and Hospital
Dharwad, Karnataka, India

Avinash Mohan
Senior Resident
Department of ENT
Dr. Somervel Memorial CSI Medical College
Thiruvananthapuram, Kerala, India

Bini Faizal
Professor and Head
Department of ENT
Amrita Institute of Medical Sciences and Research Centre
Amrita Vishwapeedham University
Kochi, Kerala, India

B. Vishwanath
Professor and Head
Department of ENT
Bangalore Medical College and Research Institute
Bangalore, Karnataka, India

Chandrakiran C.
Professor and Head
Department of ENT and Head and Neck Surgery
M S Ramaiah Medical College
Bangalore, Karnataka, India

Chantal Barbot
Fellow
Department of Pediatric Otolaryngology
Texas Children's Hospital
Houston, Texas, USA

Cimona Dsouza
Senior Resident
Department of Otorhinolaryngology and Head and Neck Surgery
Father Muller Medical College and Hospital
Mangalore, Karnataka, India

D. Deviprasad
Professor and Head
Department of Otorhinolaryngology and Head and Neck Surgery
Kasturba Medical College
Manipal Academy of Higher Education
Mangalore, Karnataka, India

Deepa R.
Professor
Department of ENT
Government Medical College
Kannur, Kerala, India

Deepak K. Mehta
Director
Pediatric Aerodigestive Center;
Associate Professor of Otolaryngology
Division of Pediatric Otolaryngology
Baylor College of Medicine
Texas Children's Hospital
Houston, Texas, USA

Deepak Nayak M.
Associate Professor
Department of Pathology
Kasturba Medical College
Manipal Academy of Higher Education
Manipal, Karnataka, India

Deepalakshmi Tanthry
Assistant Professor
Department of ENT
A.J. Institute of Medical Sciences and Research Center
Mangalore, Karnataka, India

Devaraja K.
Associate Professor
Department of Otorhinolaryngology
Kasturba Medical College
Manipal Academy of Higher Education
Manipal, Karnataka, India

Harsh Ajay Suri
Senior Resident
Department of Otorhinolaryngology and Head and Neck Surgery
Yenepoya Medical College
Mangalore, Karnataka, India

Inku Shrestha Basnet
Professor
Department of ENT and Head and Neck Surgery
Kathmandu Medical College
Sinamangal, Kathmandu, Nepal

Jaspal Singh Sahota
Vice-Chancellor
Manipal University College Malaysia
Melaka, Malaysia

Jonathan Chiao
Pediatric Otolaryngology Fellow
Division of Pediatric Otolaryngology
Baylor College of Medicine
Texas Children's Hospital
Houston, Texas, USA

Kailesh Pujary
Professor and Head
Department of Otorhinolaryngology;
Head of Unit I
Division of Otology and Lateral Skull Base Surgery
Kasturba Medical College
Manipal Academy of Higher Education
Manipal, Karnataka, India

Kamlesh Dubey
Professor
Department of ENT
Manipal University College Malaysia
Melaka, Malaysia

Kartik Herkal
Assistant Professor
Department of Otorhinolaryngology and Head and Neck Surgery
JJM Medical College
Davanagere, Karnataka, India

Kiran Chawla
Professor
Department of Microbiology
Kasturba Medical College
Manipal Academy of Higher Education
Manipal, Karnataka, India

Kirthinath Ballal
Associate Professor
Department of Community Medicine
Kasturba Medical College
Manipal Academy of Higher Education
Manipal, Karnataka, India

K.P. Basavaraju
Professor and Head of Department
Department of Otorhinolaryngology and Head and Neck Surgery
JJM Medical College
Davanagere, Karnataka, India

Krishna Koirala
Professor and Head
Department of ENT and Head Neck Surgery
Manipal College of Medical Sciences
Pokhara, Nepal

K.S. Gangadhara Somayaji
Professor
Department of Otorhinolaryngology and Head Neck Surgery
Yenepoya Medical College
Mangalore, Karnataka, India

Kshithi K.
Senior Resident
Department of ENT and Head and Neck Surgery
Kasturba Medical College
Manipal Academy of Higher Education
Mangalore, Karnataka, India

Kuldeep Moras
Professor and Head
Department of Otorhinolaryngology
Father Muller Medical College
Mangalore, Karnataka, India

L. Sudarshan Reddy
Professor and Head of Department
Department of ENT
Osmania Medical College
Hyderabad, Telangana, India

Mahesh Bhat T.
Professor
Department of Otorhinolaryngology and Head and Neck Surgery
Father Muller Medical College and Hospital
Mangalore, Karnataka, India

Mahesh Santhraya G.
Professor and Head
Department of ENT and Head and Neck Surgery
A.J. Medical College
Mangalore, Karnataka, India

Mary Kurien
Professor
Department of ENT
Pondicherry Institute of Medical Sciences
Puducherry, India

Meera Niranjan Khadilkar
Assistant Professor
Department of Otorhinolaryngology and Head and Neck Surgery
Kasturba Medical College
Manipal Academy of Higher Education
Mangalore, Karnataka, India

Monika Pokharel
Associate Professor and Head of Department
Department of Otorhinolaryngology and Head and Neck Surgery
Kathmandu University School of Medical Sciences
Dhulikhel, Nepal

Nagaraj Maradi
Assistant Professor
Department of ENT and Head and Neck Surgery
SS Institute of Medical Sciences and Research Center
Davangere, Karnataka, India

Navneet Kumar
Professor
Department of ENT
Christian Medical College
Ludhiana, Punjab, India

Navneeta Gangwar
Professor and Head
Department of ENT
Jaipur National University Institute of Medical Sciences and
    Research Centre
Jaipur, Rajasthan, India

Poorvi V. Sharma
Assistant Professor
Department of Otorhinolaryngology and Head and Neck Surgery
Kasturba Medical College
Manipal Academy of Higher Education
Manipal, Karnataka, India

Prerit Rao
Senior Resident
Department of Otorhinolaryngology and Head and Neck Surgery
Kasturba Medical College
Manipal Academy of Higher Education
Manipal, Karnataka, India

P. Thirunavukarasu
Professor
Department of ENT
Sri Ramachandra Medical College
Chennai, Tamil Nadu, India

R. Archana Pillai
Associate Professor
Department of ENT and Head and Neck Surgery
Sree Gokulam Medical College and Research Foundation
Thiruvananthapuram, Kerala, India

Rejee Ebenezer R.
Professor and Head
Department of ENT
Dr. Somervel Memorial CSI Medical College
Thiruvananthapuram, Kerala, India

Rukma Bhandary
Associate Professor
Department of ENT
AJ Institute of Medical, Sciences and Research Centre
Mangalore, Karnataka, India

Sajilal M.
Associate Professor
Department of ENT
Dr. SMCSI Medical College
Thiruvananthapuram, Kerala, India

Sanchit Bajpai
Fellow (Head and Neck Oncology)
Department of ENT and Head Neck Surgery
Kasturba Medical College
Manipal Academy of Higher Education
Mangalore, Karnataka, India

Sathappan Subramanian
Consultant ENT Surgeon;
Deputy Dean
Faculty of Medicine
University of Cyberjaya
Kuala Lumpur, Malaysia

Shama Shetty
Assistant Professor
Department of Otorhinolaryngology
Kasturba Medical College
Manipal Academy of Higher Education
Manipal, Karnataka, India

Shrinath D. Kamath P.
Additional Professor
Department of ENT
K.S. Hegde Medical Academy
Mangalore, Karnataka, India

Soorya Pradeep
Senior Resident
Department of ENT
Christian Medical College
Vellore, Tamil Nadu, India

Sreenivas Kamath K.
Senior Resident
Department of ENT and Head and Neck Surgery
Kasturba Medical College
Manipal Academy of Higher Education
Mangalore, Karnataka, India

Suja Sreedharan
Professor
Department of Otolaryngology
Kasturba Medical College
Manipal Academy of Higher Education
Mangalore, Karnataka, India

Sunil Varghese
Assistant Professor
Department of ENT
Christian Medical College
Ludhiana, Punjab, India

Suresh Pillai
Professor
Department of Otorhinolaryngology;
Head of Unit III
Division of Head and Neck Surgery
Kasturba Medical College
Manipal Academy of Higher Education
Manipal, Karnataka, India

Sushmitha Kabekkodu
Assistant Professor
Department of Otorhinolaryngology and Head and Neck Surgery
Kasturba Medical College
Manipal Academy of Higher Education
Mangalore, Karnataka, India

Sweekritha N. Bhat
Fellow (Head and Neck Oncology)
Department of ENT and Head-Neck Surgery
Kasturba Medical College
Manipal Academy of Higher Education
Mangalore, Karnataka, India

Thripthi Rai
Associate Professor
Department of Otorhinolaryngology and Head and Neck Surgery
Kasturba Medical College
Manipal Academy of Higher Education
Mangalore, Karnataka, India

Tulasi Karanth
ENT – HNS Specialist
Bikaner, Rajasthan, India

Udayabhanu H.N.
Associate Professor
Department of Otorhinolaryngology and Head and Neck Surgery
Akash Institute of Medical Sciences and Research Centre
Bangalore, Karnataka, India

Vadisha Bhat
Professor and Head
Department of ENT
K.S. Hegde Medical Academy
NITTE (Deemed to be University)
Mangalore, Karnataka, India

Venkatesha B.K.
Professor
Department of ENT and Head and Neck Surgery
SS Institute of Medical Sciences and Research Center
Davangere, Karnataka, India

Vijayalakshmi Subramaniam
Professor and Head
Department of Otorhinolaryngology and Head and Neck Surgery
Yenepoya Medical College
Mangalore, Karnataka, India

Vijendra Shenoy S.
Professor
Department of ENT and Head and Neck Surgery
Kasturba Medical College
Manipal Academy of Higher Education
Mangalore, Karnataka, India

Vinay V. Rao
Associate Professor
Department of ENT
Father Muller Medical College
Mangalore, Karnataka, India

Vishwas K. Pai
Assistant Professor
Department of ENT
A.J. Institute of Medical Sciences
Mangalore, Karnataka, India

Yogeesha B.S.
Professor and Head
Department of ENT and Head and Neck Surgery
SS Institute of Medical Sciences and Research Center
Davangere, Karnataka, India

Competency Mapping Chart

Competency Code	COMPETENCY The student should be able to	Page no.
Anatomy and Physiology of Ear, Nose, and Throat (ENT) and Head and Neck		
EN1.1	Describe the anatomy and physiology of ENT and head and neck	1, 14, 196, 205, 321, 328, 334, 416 426, 519, 548
EN1.2	Describe the pathophysiology of common diseases in ENT	603
Clinical Skills		
EN2.1	Elicit, document, and present an appropriate history in a patient presenting with an ENT complaint	430, 603
EN2.2	Demonstrate the correct use of a headlamp in the examination of the ENT	23
EN2.3	Demonstrate the correct technique of examination of the ear including otoscopy	23
EN2.4	Demonstrate the correct technique of performance and interpret tuning fork tests	36
EN2.5	Demonstrate the correct technique of examination of the nose and paranasal sinuses including the use of nasal speculum	211
EN2.6	Demonstrate the correct technique of examining the throat including the use of a tongue depressor	337
EN2.7	Demonstrate the correct technique of examination of neck including elicitation of laryngeal crepitus	553
EN2.8	Demonstrate the correct technique to perform and interpret pure tone audiogram and impedance audiogram	36
EN2.9	Choose correctly and interpret radiological, microbiological, and histological investigations relevant to the ENT disorders	626, 647
EN2.10	Identify and describe the use of common instruments used in ENT surgery	504, 513, 657
EN2.11	Describe and identify by clinical examination malignant and premalignant ENT diseases	187, 301, 373, 597, 603
EN2.12	Counsel and administer informed consent to patients and their families in a simulated environment	621
EN2.13	Identify, resuscitate, and manage ENT emergencies in a simulated environment (including tracheostomy, anterior nasal packing, removal of foreign bodies in ENT and upper respiratory tract)	409, 486, 495, 543
EN2.14	Demonstrate the correct technique to instilling topical medications into the ENT in a simulated environment	23
EN2.15	Describe the national programs for prevention of deafness, cancer, and noise and environmental pollution	640
Diagnostic and Therapeutic Procedures in ENT		
EN3.1	Observe and describe the indications for and steps involved in the performance of otomicroscopic examination in a simulated environment	23
EN3.2	Observe and describe the indications for and steps involved in the performance of diagnostic nasal endoscopy	220
EN3.3	Observe and describe the indications for and steps involved in the performance of rigid/flexible laryngoscopy	434, 501
EN3.4	Observe and describe the indications for and steps involved in the removal of foreign bodies from ENT	79, 297, 409, 504, 513, 543

Competency Code	COMPETENCY The student should be able to	Page no.
EN3.5	Observe and describe the indications for and steps involved in the surgical procedures in ENT	178, 316, 509
EN3.6	Observe and describe the indications for and steps involved in the skills of emergency procedures in ENT	486, 504
Management of Diseases of ENT		
EN4.1	Elicit, document, and present a correct history; demonstrate and describe the clinical features; choose the correct investigations; and describe the principles of management of otalgia	76
EN4.2	Elicit, document, and present a correct history; demonstrate and describe the clinical features; choose the correct investigations; and describe the principles of management of diseases of the external ear	79
EN4.3	Elicit, document, and present a correct history; demonstrate and describe the clinical features; choose the correct investigations; and describe the principles of management of ASOM	95
EN4.4	Demonstrate the correct technique to hold visualize and assess the mobility of the tympanic membrane and its mobility and interpret and diagrammatically represent the findings	23
EN4.5	Elicit, document, and present a correct history; demonstrate and describe the clinical features; choose the correct investigations; and describe the principles of management of OME	95
EN4.6	Elicit, document, and present a correct history; demonstrate and describe the clinical features; choose the correct investigations; and describe the principles of management of discharging ear	95
EN4.7	Elicit, document, and present a correct history; demonstrate and describe the clinical features; choose the correct investigations; and describe the principles of management of CSOM	95
EN4.8	Elicit, document, and present a correct history; demonstrate and describe the clinical features; choose the correct investigations; and describe the principles of management of squamosal type of CSOM	95
EN4.9	Demonstrate the correct technique for syringing wax from the ear in a simulated environment	23
EN4.10	Observe and describe the indications for and steps involved in myringotomy and myringoplasty	166, 168
EN4.11	Enumerate the indications, describe the steps, and observe a mastoidectomy	174
EN4.12	Elicit, document, and present a correct history; demonstrate and describe the clinical features; choose the correct investigations; and describe the principles of management of hearing loss	53
EN4.13	Describe the clinical features, investigations, and principles of management of otosclerosis	128
EN4.14	Describe the clinical features, investigations, and principles of management of sudden sensorineural hearing loss	53
EN4.15	Describe the clinical features, investigations, and principles of management of noise-induced hearing loss	53
EN4.16	Observe and describe the indications for and steps involved in the performance of pure tone audiometry	36
EN4.17	Enumerate the indications and interpret the results of an audiogram	36
EN4.18	Describe the clinical features, investigations, and principles of management of facial nerve palsy	134
EN4.19	Describe the clinical features, investigations, and principles of management of vertigo	143
EN4.20	Describe the clinical features, investigations, and principles of management of Meniere's disease	153
EN4.21	Describe the clinical features, investigations, and principles of management of tinnitus	160
EN4.22	Elicit, document, and present a correct history; demonstrate and describe the clinical features; choose the correct investigations; and describe the principles of management of squamosal type of nasal obstruction	235
EN4.23	Describe the clinical features, investigations, and principles of management of deviated nasal septum	235
EN4.24	Enumerate the indications, observe, and describe steps in the septoplasty	310
EN4.25	Elicit, document, and present a correct history; demonstrate and describe the clinical features; choose the correct investigations; and describe the principles of management of squamosal type of nasal polyps	281, 316
EN4.26	Elicit, document, and present a correct history; demonstrate and describe the clinical features; choose the correct investigations; and describe the principles of management of squamosal type of adenoids	344
EN4.27	Elicit, document, and present a correct history; demonstrate and describe the clinical features; choose the correct investigations; and describe the principles of management of squamosal type of allergic rhinitis	258

Competency Code	COMPETENCY The student should be able to	Page no.
EN4.28	Elicit, document, and present a correct history; demonstrate and describe the clinical features; choose the correct investigations; and describe the principles of management of squamosal type of vasomotor rhinitis	264
EN4.29	Elicit, document, and present a correct history; demonstrate and describe the clinical features; choose the correct investigations; and describe the principles of management of squamosal type of acute and chronic rhinitis	245
EN4.30	Elicit, document, and present a correct history; demonstrate and describe the clinical features; choose the correct investigations; and describe the principles of management of squamosal type of epistaxis	289
EN4.31	Describe the clinical features, investigations, and principles of management of trauma to the face and neck	566
EN4.32	Describe the clinical features, investigations, and principles of management of nasopharyngeal angiofibroma	386
EN4.33	Elicit, document, and present a correct history; demonstrate and describe the clinical features; choose the correct investigations; and describe the principles of management of squamosal type of acute and chronic sinusitis	267, 316
EN4.34	Describe the clinical features, investigations, and principles of management of tumors of maxilla	301
EN4.35	Describe the clinical features, investigations, and principles of management of tumors of nasopharynx	386
EN4.36	Describe the clinical features, investigations, and principles of management of diseases of the salivary glands	556
EN4.37	Describe the clinical features, investigations, and principles of management of Ludwig's angina	583
EN4.38	Elicit, document, and present a correct history; demonstrate and describe the clinical features; choose the correct investigations; and describe the principles of management of type of dysphagia	535
EN4.39	Elicit, document, and present a correct history; demonstrate and describe the clinical features; choose the correct investigations; and describe the principles of management of squamosal type of acute and chronic tonsillitis	358
EN4.40	Observe and describe the indications for and steps involved in a tonsillectomy/adenoidectomy	344, 358
EN4.41	Describe the clinical features, investigations, and principles of management of acute and chronic abscesses in relation to pharynx	583
EN4.42	Elicit, document, and present a correct history; demonstrate and describe the clinical features; choose the correct investigations; and describe the principles of management of hoarseness of voice	430, 434, 509
EN4.43	Describe the clinical features, investigations, and principles of management of acute and chronic laryngitis	440
EN4.44	Describe the clinical features, investigations, and principles of management of benign lesions of the vocal cord	460
EN4.45	Describe the clinical features, investigations, and principles of management of vocal cord palsy	448
EN4.46	Describe the clinical features, investigations, and principles of management of malignancy of the larynx and hypopharynx	402, 470
EN4.47	Describe the clinical features, investigations, and principles of management of stridor	477
EN4.48	Elicit, document, and present a correct history; demonstrate and describe the clinical features; choose the correct investigations; and describe the principles of management of airway emergencies	486
EN4.49	Elicit, document, and present a correct history; demonstrate and describe the clinical features; choose the correct investigations; and describe the principles of management of foreign bodies in the air and food passages	495, 539
EN4.50	Observe and describe the indications for and steps involved in tracheostomy	486
EN4.51	Observe and describe the care of the patient with a tracheostomy	486
EN4.52	Describe the clinical features, investigations, and principles of management of diseases of esophagus	524
EN4.53	Describe the clinical features, investigations, and principles of management of HIV manifestations of the ENT	613

Competency Code	COMPETENCY The student should be able to	Page no.
	Integration	
	Human Anatomy	
AN36.1	Describe the (1) morphology, relations, blood supply, and applied anatomy of palatine tonsil and (2) composition of soft palate	328, 358
AN36.2	Describe the components and functions of Waldeyer's lymphatic ring	328
AN36.3	Describe the boundaries and clinical significance of pyriform fossa	328
AN36.4	Describe the anatomical basis of tonsilitis, tonsillectomy, adenoids, and peritonsillar abscess	583
AN36.5	Describe the clinical significance of Killian's dehiscence	328
AN37.1	Describe and demonstrate features of nasal septum, lateral wall of nose, their blood supply, and nerve supply	196
AN37.2	Describe location and functional anatomy of paranasal sinuses	196
AN37.3	Describe anatomical basis of sinusitis and maxillary sinus tumors	196, 267, 301
AN38.1	Describe the morphology, identify structure of the wall, nerve supply, blood supply, and actions of intrinsic and extrinsic muscles of the larynx	416
AN38.2	Describe the anatomical aspects of laryngitis	440
AN38.3	Describe anatomical basis of recurrent laryngeal nerve injury	448
AN39.2	Explain the anatomical basis of hypoglossal nerve palsy	321, 548
AN40.1	Describe and identify the parts, blood supply, and nerve supply of external ear	1
AN40.2	Describe and demonstrate the boundaries, contents, relations, and functional anatomy of middle ear and auditory tube	1, 181
AN40.3	Describe the features of internal ear	1
AN40.4	Explain anatomical basis of otitis externa and otitis media	1
AN40.5	Explain anatomical basis of myringotomy	166
	Physiology	
PY10.15	Describe and discuss functional anatomy of ear and auditory pathways and physiology of hearing	14
PY10.16	Describe and discuss pathophysiology of deafness. Describe hearing tests	36, 53
PY10.20	Demonstrate (i) hearing, (ii) testing for smell, and (iii) taste sensation in volunteer/simulated environment	23
	Dentistry	
DE4.1	Discuss the prevalence of oral cancer and enumerate the common types of cancer that can affect tissues of the oral cavity	373
DE4.2	Discuss the role of etiological factors in the formation of precancerous/cancerous lesions	373
DE4.3	Identify potential precancerous/cancerous lesions	373
DE4.4	Counsel patients to risks of oral cancer with respect to tobacco, smoking, alcohol, and other causative factors	621
	General Medicine	
IM24.17	Describe and discuss the etiopathogenesis, clinical presentation, identification, functional changes, acute care, stabilization, management, and rehabilitation of hearing loss in the elderly	53
	Pediatrics	
PE14.2	Discuss the risk factors, clinical features, diagnosis, and management of kerosene ingestion	524
PE28.1	Discuss the etiopathogenesis, clinical features, and management of nasopharyngitis	344
PE28.2	Discuss the etiopathogenesis of pharyngotonsillitis	352, 358
PE28.3	Discuss the clinical features and management of pharyngotonsillitis	352, 358

Competency Code	COMPETENCY The student should be able to	Page no.
PE28.4	Discuss the etiopathogenesis, clinical features, and management of acute otitis media (AOM)	95
PE28.5	Discuss the etiopathogenesis, clinical features, and management of epiglottitis	440
PE28.6	Discuss the etiopathogenesis, clinical features, and management of acute laryngo-tracheo-bronchitis	440
PE28.7	Discuss the etiology, clinical features, and management of stridor in children	477
PE28.8	Discuss the types, clinical presentation, and management of foreign body aspiration in infants and children	495
PE28.9	Elicit, document, and present age-appropriate history of a child with upper respiratory problem including stridor	477
PE28.10	Perform otoscopic examination of the ear	23
PE28.11	Perform throat examination using tongue depressor	337
PE28.12	Perform examination of the nose	211
PE28.17	Interpret X-ray of the paranasal sinuses and mastoid; and/or use written report in case of management. Interpret CXR in foreign body aspiration and lower respiratory tract infection, understand the significance of thymic shadow in pediatric chest X-rays	647
PE31.1	Describe the etiopathogenesis, management, and prevention of allergic rhinitis in children	258
General Surgery		
SU20.1	Describe etiopathogenesis of oral cancer, symptoms, and signs of pharyngeal cancer. Enumerate the appropriate investigations and discuss the principles of treatment	373, 393, 597

1 Anatomy of the Ear

Rukma Bhandary

The competencies covered in this chapter are as follows:

EN1.1 Describe the anatomy of the ear.

AN40.1 Describe and identify the parts, blood supply, and nerve supply of the external ear.

AN40.2 Describe and demonstrate the boundaries, contents, relations, and functional anatomy of the middle ear and the auditory tube.

AN40.3 Describe the features of the internal ear.

AN40.4 Explain the anatomical basis of the otitis externa and the otitis media.

Introduction

The ear is a special sense organ responsible for hearing and equilibrium. It is divided into three parts (**Fig. 1.1**):
- External ear.
- Middle ear.
- Inner ear.

External Ear

The external ear is made up of the following:
- Pinna (auricle).
- External auditory canal.

■ Pinna

Development

The pinna develops from six tubercles of His around the first branchial cleft (**Fig. 1.2**).

Anatomy

The pinna is made up of a single sheet of yellow elastic cartilage covered by the perichondrium and skin, and the ear lobule, which comprises the areolar and adipose connective tissue. It has two surfaces: medial and lateral. The lateral surface is concave and has folds. The skin is thin and adherent to the perichondrium (in the medial aspect, the skin is slightly thicker with some subcutaneous tissue). The most prominent outer fold is the *helix* and the fold anterior to it is the *antihelix*. The antihelical fold divides superiorly into two crura, enclosing a space called the fossa triangularis. The boat-shaped space behind the fossa triangularis is known as the scaphoid fossa. Below the lower crus of the antihelix and the root of the helix is the region called the *cymba concha*. This is the surface landmark for the mastoid antrum.

In the center of the auricle, there is a hollow depression called the concha. The concha helps direct the sound into the external auditory canal. Immediately anterior to the beginning of the external acoustic meatus is a cartilaginous elevation called the *tragus*. The antitragus is opposite the tragus separated from it by the intertragic notch. The incisura terminalis is an area between the superior part of the tragus and the root of the helix, which has fibrous tissue but is devoid of cartilage. This is the site for performing an endaural incision of the middle ear.

Nerve Supply

- The greater auricular nerve (C2, C3) supplies most of the medial surface of the pinna and the posterior part of the lateral surface.
- The lesser occipital nerve (C2) supplies the upper part of the medial surface.
- The auriculotemporal nerve (V3) supplies the tragus, crus of helix, and the adjacent part of the helix.
- The auricular branch of the vagus nerve (cranial nerve [CN] X), also called Arnold's nerve, supplies the concha and the corresponding eminence on the medial surface.
- The facial nerve, which is distributed with fibers of the auricular branch of the vagus, supplies the concha and the retroauricular groove.

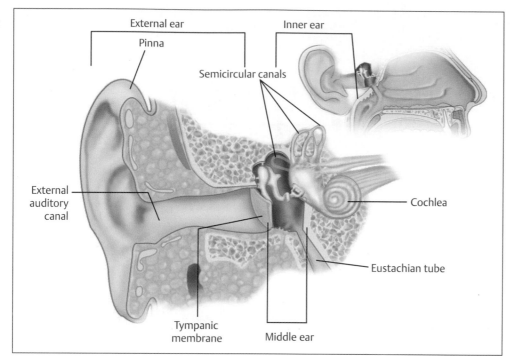

Fig. 1.1 Anatomical division of the ear.

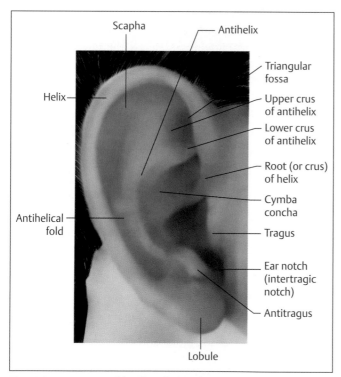

Fig. 1.2 Anatomical landmarks on the pinna.

Clinical Importance

Auricular hematoma: It is the collection of blood between the cartilage and its overlying perichondrium which is usually due to direct trauma to the area. This leads to disruption of blood flow to the cartilage and its necrosis and finally a deformity called the "cauliflower ear." Hence, it needs prompt diagnosis and treatment with drainage.

■ External Auditory Meatus

Development

The *external auditory meatus* develops from the first branchial cleft.

Anatomy

The external auditory meatus is "*S*"-shaped and approximately 2.4 cm in length. It extends from the deep part of the concha to the tympanic membrane. The external auditory canal is divided into two parts: the lateral one-third formed by cartilage and the medial two-third formed by bone.

The lateral one-third of the canal is directed upward, backward, and medially. The medial two-third is directed downward, forward, and medially. Therefore, to visualize the tympanic membrane, the pinna has to be pulled upward, backward, and laterally. In infants, the bony part is shorter and, therefore, the pinna has to be pulled downward and outward during examination.

The cartilaginous part is a continuation of the cartilage of the pinna. The *fissures of Santorini* are defects in the cartilage anteriorly. Through these defects, infection and neoplasms from the parotid reach the canal or vice versa. The skin covering the cartilaginous part is thick and is composed of ceruminous and pilosebaceous glands, which secrete wax. The outer part of the canal has fine hair. The hair follicles are prone to staphylococcal bacterial infection when underlying factors are present.

The bony part is formed by the tympanic and squamous parts of the temporal bone. It is lined by thin skin adherent to the periosteum. There is a narrowing called the isthmus about 6 mm lateral to the tympanic membrane. Anteroinferiorly, in the deep bony meatus, there may be a deficiency called *foramen of Huschke* (foramen tympanicum), which communicates with the temporomandibular joint. This permits spread of infection from the canal to the joint and from a fistula from the parotid into the canal.

Relations

Superiorly: Middle cranial fossa.
Posteriorly: Mastoid air cells and facial nerve.
Inferiorly: Parotid gland.
Anteriorly: Temporomandibular joint.

Nerve Supply

- Anterior wall and roof: Auriculotemporal nerve (V3).
- Posterior wall and floor: Auricular branch of the vagus nerve (CN X).

- Posterior wall of the auditory canal also receives sensory fibers of CN VII through the auricular branch of the vagus nerve.

> **Pearl**
>
> In herpes zoster oticus, lesions are seen along the distribution of the facial nerve, that is, the concha, the posterior part of the tympanic membrane, and the postauricular region.

Tympanic Membrane

■ Development

The tympanic membrane develops from the ectoderm, mesoderm, and the endoderm of the first pharyngeal arch.

■ Anatomy

The tympanic membrane forms a partition between the external auditory meatus and the middle ear (**Fig. 1.3a, b**). It is set at an angle wherein the posterosuperior portion is more lateral than the anteroinferior portion. The tympanic membrane forms an angle of 55 degrees with the floor. Its dimensions are 9 to 10 mm superoinferiorly, 8 to 9 mm anteroposteriorly, and 0.1 mm in thickness.

It has two parts:
- Pars tensa.
- Pars flaccida.

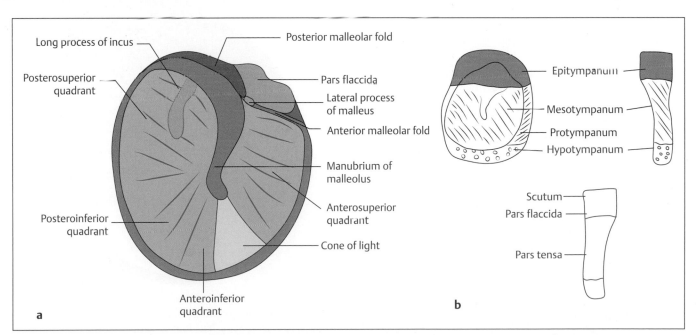

Fig. 1.3 **(a)** Tympanic membrane. **(b)** Diagram representing the lateral view and coronal view of the tympanic membrane, demonstrating the division of the middle ear space into the epitympanum, mesotympanum, and hypotympanum.

Pars Tensa

This is the part of the tympanic membrane that lies below the anterior and posterior malleolar folds.

It forms most of the membrane. It is thickened at the periphery to form a fibrous annulus, which is attached at the tympanic sulcus of the tympanic part of temporal bone. The central part of the pars tensa is tented inward at the tip of the malleus called the umbo. A bright cone of light can be seen radiating from the tip of the malleus to the periphery in the anteroinferior quadrant due to the angulation of the tympanic membrane.

Pearl

A cone of light is visualized on a normal tympanic membrane due to reflection of light.

Reasons:

- Angulation of 55 degrees of the tympanic membrane with the floor of the external auditory canal.
- The tympanic membrane is obliquely placed so that the length of the anterior canal wall is longer than the length of the posterior canal wall.
- The membrane is not flat but tented with the apex at the umbo.

Pars Flaccida

It is also called Shrapnell's membrane. It is situated above the anterior and posterior malleolar folds, above the level of the lateral process of the malleus and attaches at the notch of Rivinus.

The tympanic membrane has three layers:

- The outer epithelial layer (three to four layers of keratinizing squamous cells), which is continuous with the external canal.
- The middle fibrous layer, which encloses the handle of malleus and has three types of fibers: Radial, circular, and parabolic.
- Inner mucosal layer (single layer of simple squamous or cuboidal cells), which is continuous with the middle ear mucosa.

The fibrous layer in the pars flaccida is thin and is not arranged into various fibers as in the pars tensa.

The pars tensa can be divided into four quadrants by drawing two imaginary lines at right angles to each other. The first is a vertical line along the handle of the malleus and the second is a horizontal line at the level of the umbo. The four quadrants thus created are anterosuperior, anteroinferior, posterosuperior, and posteroinferior (**Fig. 1.4**).

■ Nerve Supply

- Anterior half of the lateral surface: Auriculotemporal nerve (V3).
- Posterior half of the lateral surface: Auricular branch of the vagus nerve (CN X).
- Medial surface: Tympanic branch of CN IX (Jacobson's nerve).

The Middle Ear Cleft

■ Development

The tympanic cavity and eustachian tube develop from the tubotympanic recess.

■ Anatomy

The middle ear cleft comprises the eustachian tube, tympanic cavity, aditus ad antrum, and mastoid air cells.

■ Tympanic Cavity

The tympanic cavity, also called the middle ear, lies in between the external and inner ear. It is biconcave in shape. The vertical and anteroposterior diameters are 15 mm, while the transverse diameter is 6 mm at the upper part, 2 mm at the center, and 4 mm at the lower part.

The tympanic cavity is further divided into three parts:

- *Epitympanum or attic*: This region is situated above the malleolar folds of the tympanic membrane (medial to

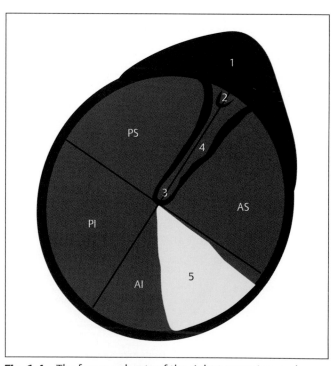

Fig. 1.4 The four quadrants of the right tympanic membrane. Abbreviations: 1, Pars flaccida; 2, lateral process of malleus; 3, umbo; 4, handle of malleus; 5, cone of light; AI, anteroinferior; AS, anterosuperior; PI, posteroinferior; PS, posterosuperior.

the pars flaccida and the scutum). It contains the head of the malleus, incudomalleolar joint, and body and short process of the incus. It links to the mastoid antrum through the aditus, posterosuperiorly.

- *Mesotympanum*: It is situated medial to the pars tensa; *protympanum* refers to the anterior part of the meso-tympanum around the eustachian tube opening.
- *Hypotympanum*: This is the region below the level of the mesotympanum.

The tympanic cavity is a box-shaped six-sided cavity. The following are the boundaries:

- *Lateral wall*: This is formed by the tympanic membrane and partly by a portion of the squamous part of the temporal bone (scutum) above and the lateral wall of the hypotympanum below. This separates the external ear from the middle ear.
- *Medial wall*: This separates the middle ear from the inner ear (**Fig. 1.5**). The *promontory* is the most prominent structure and produces a bulge on the medial wall, which is formed by the underlying basal turn of the cochlea. The *tympanic plexus* lies on the surface of the promontory. The *processus cochleariformis* is a bony

projection above the promontory, around which the tensor tympani hooks before getting attached to the neck of the malleus. The *oval window* (fenestra vestibuli) is located posterosuperior to the promontory. It is closed by the footplate of the stapes and the annular ligament. The *round window* membrane (membrana fenestrae cochleae) lies posteroinferior to the promontory. The niche of the round window is directed posteriorly and closed by the secondary tympanic membrane, separating the middle ear from the scala tympani of the cochlea. The tympanic segment of the facial nerve is located immediately posterior to the processus cochleariformis (first genu), travels posteriorly above the promontory, and posterosuperior to the stapes footplate up to the second genu on the medial wall. The part of the tympanic segment, just above the oval window, is the commonest site of dehiscence of the fallopian canal. The *bony lateral semicircular canal* lies posterosuperior to the second genu of the facial nerve.

- *Anterior wall*: This is a bony wall that separates the middle ear from the internal carotid artery (**Fig 1.6**). The important structures passing through the anterior wall

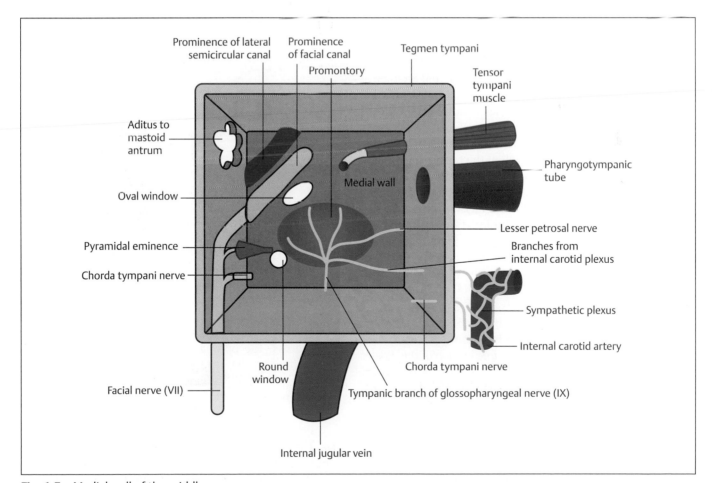

Fig. 1.5   Medial wall of the middle ear.

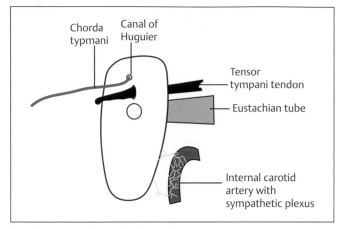

Fig. 1.6 Anterior wall of middle ear.

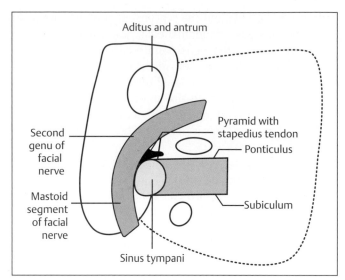

Fig. 1.7 Diagram depicting the key structures and areas in relation to the posterior wall of the middle ear.

to the tympanic cavity are the chorda tympani nerve, tensor tympani muscle, eustachian tube, anterior malleolar ligament, and anterior tympanic artery.

- *Posterior wall*: This part is situated close to the mastoid air cells (**Figs. 1.7** and **1.8**). The upper part has an opening called the aditus leading backward from the posterior epitympanum to the mastoid antrum. Below the aditus, there is a triangular bony projection called the pyramid through which the stapedius tendon is transmitted to be attached to the neck of the stapes. The vertical portion of the facial nerve (from the second genu) courses down the posterior wall to exit through the stylomastoid foramen. The facial nerve lies antero-infero-medial to the lateral semicircular canal. Two recesses extend posteriorly from the mesotympanum, that is, the facial recess and the sinus tympani. The sinus tympani lies between the facial nerve and the medial wall of the mesotympanum. The niche of two labyrinthine windows communicates at the posterior extremity with the deep recess. It is separated from the facial recess laterally by the pyramid. The facial recess is lateral to the facial nerve, bounded by the fossa incudis superiorly and chorda tympani inferiorly, the posterosuperior meatal wall laterally, and the pyramid medially. It may be directly accessed via the posterior tympanotomy approach.
- *Floor*: A thin plate of bone that separates the middle ear from the bulb of the internal jugular vein lodges in the jugular fossa forms the floor. It has a tympanic canaliculus for the passage of the tympanic branch of the glossopharyngeal nerve.
- *Roof*: The tegmen tympani separates the tympanic cavity from the middle cranial fossa. It is formed by the petrous and squamous parts of the temporal bone with the petrosquamous suture.

■ Contents of the Middle Ear

- *Ossicles*: These are three tiny bones that conduct sound from the eardrum to the oval window:

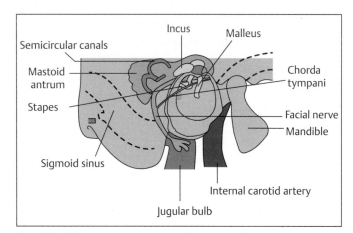

Fig. 1.8 The mastoid region and the middle ear cavity.

- The *malleus* (hammer) is the largest and the most lateral ossicle measuring 8 mm in length (**Fig. 1.9**). The parts include the head, neck, handle, and anterior and lateral processes. The head is situated in the epitympanum. A lateral (short) process projects laterally from the neck, whereas the handle is firmly fixed to the pars tensa.
- The *incus* (anvil) has a body, short process, and long process. The body articulates with the head of the malleus in the attic and the short process projects into the attic. The long process projects downward behind the handle of the malleus, running parallel, and articulates with the stapes head via the lenticular process.
- The *stapes* (stirrup) is the smallest ossicle measuring 3.5 mm. It consists of a head, neck, footplate, and anterior and posterior crura. The footplate of the stapes is held to the oval window by the annular ligament.

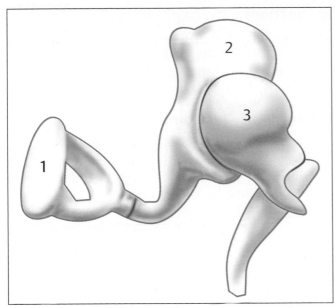

Fig. 1.9 Middle ear ossicles. 1, Stapes; 2, incus; 3, malleus.

- *Muscles*: There are two muscles in the middle ear, the tensor tympani and stapedius muscles. They decrease the movement of the ossicles. The tensor tympani is inserted into the neck of the malleus. It is the first arch muscle supplied by the mandibular branch of the trigeminal nerve. The stapedius is a second arch muscle, inserted into the neck of the stapes and supplied by the nerve to the stapedius, which is a branch of the facial nerve.
- *Mucosal folds and ligaments* support and supply blood to the ossicles, divide the tympanic cavity into compartments, and may limit or direct spread of cholesteatoma.
- *Nerves*: The chorda tympani is a branch of the facial nerve and carries the sense of taste. It enters the middle ear from the posterior wall and runs forward and lateral to the incus, and medial to the malleus, exiting through the anterior wall. The tympanic plexus lies on the promontory. It is formed by the tympanic branch of the glossopharyngeal nerve, and sympathetic fibers from the plexus around the internal carotid artery. The tympanic plexus innervates the medial surface of the tympanic membrane, tympanic cavity, mastoid air cells, and the bony eustachian tube. It also carries the secretomotor fibers to the parotid gland. Tympanic neurectomy, that is, resection of the tympanic branch of the glossopharyngeal nerve in the middle ear had been used in the treatment of Frey's syndrome.
- *Vessels*: A plexus of vessels is formed by the stylomastoid and caroticotympanic arteries.

■ Blood Supply of the Middle Ear Cavity

Blood supply to the middle ear cavity is through the branches of the middle meningeal artery, maxillary artery,

ascending pharyngeal artery, and the stylomastoid branch of the posterior auricular artery. Venous drainage is through the pterygoid venous plexus and superior petrosal sinus.

■ Nerve Supply

The nerve supply of the middle ear cavity is through the tympanic plexus.

■ Lymphatic Drainage

Lymphatic drainage of the middle ear cavity is through the preauricular and retropharyngeal lymph nodes.

■ Epithelial Lining of the Middle Ear Cavity

The lining mucosa is the ciliated columnar epithelium in the anteroinferior part (eustachian tube, anterior mesotympanum, and hypotympanum), low cuboidal epithelium in the posterior mesotympanum, and pavement (flat nonciliated) epithelium in the epitympanum and mastoid. There is an abundance of mucosal glands and goblet cells toward the eustachian tube which gradually reduces and is absent toward the posterior and superior parts of the tympanic cavity.

Eustachian Tube

The eustachian tube and its relation to the middle ear is shown in **Fig. 1.10**.

■ Development

The eustachian tube develops from the tubotympanic recess.

■ Anatomy

The eustachian tube connects the middle ear to the nasopharynx. It is approximately 36-mm long in an adult. It runs upward, backward, and laterally from the nasopharynx. The nasopharyngeal opening lies 1.25 cm behind and below the posterior end of the inferior turbinate.

The eustachian tube has two parts: a lateral bony part, which is 12-mm long, and a medial cartilaginous part, which is 24-mm long. The medial cartilaginous part forms a prominence in the nasopharynx called the torus tubarius. The tympanic opening of the eustachian tube is higher than the pharyngeal opening.

In infants and young children, the tube is more horizontal and shorter, and the bony part is relatively wider. This anatomical variation allows infections from the nasopharynx to reach the middle ear more easily.

The tubal tonsils (Gerlach's tonsils) are seen near the pharyngeal end of the eustachian tube, which may be enlarged leading to eustachian tube obstruction. There is

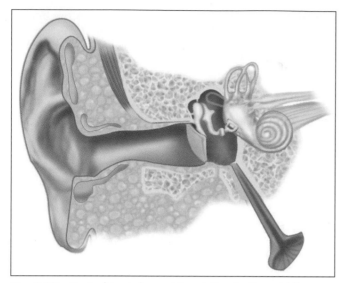

Fig. 1.10 Eustachian tube and its relation to the middle ear.

also a layer of fibrofatty tissue related to the membranous part of the cartilaginous portion, known as the Ostmann pad of fat. This keeps the eustachian tube closed, thereby protecting from nasopharyngeal reflux through the tube. The fossa of Rosenmuller is a lateral pharyngeal recess behind the torus tubarius. It is a common site for nasopharyngeal malignancy.

Muscles attached to the eustachian tube are as follows:
- Levator veli palatini.
- Tensor veli palatini.
- Salpingopharyngeus.
- Tensor tympani.

> **Pearl**
>
> The tensor tympani muscle plays a role in protection of the tympanic membrane and the middle ear in response to loud sounds.
>
> The levator veli palatini, tensor veli palatini, and salpingopharyngeus muscles play a vital role in ventilation of the middle ear by active opening and closing of the eustachian tube due to palatal movements.

The tensor veli palatini and tensor tympani muscles are innervated by the mandibular branch of the trigeminal nerve, whereas the salpingopharyngeus and levator veli palatini muscles are innervated by the pharyngeal plexus.

■ Blood Supply

Blood supply to the Eustachian tube is through the ascending pharyngeal artery, middle meningeal artery, and artery of the pterygoid canal.

■ Venous Drainage

Venous drainage is through the pterygoid plexus.

■ Functions

- Ventilation of the middle ear cleft equalizes the middle ear pressure with the atmospheric pressure.
- It prevents nasopharyngeal reflux.
- It helps in clearance of the middle ear secretions.

■ Ventilatory Anatomy

The middle ear cleft is normally well ventilated. The air comes from the nasopharynx via the eustachian tube into the anterior mesotympanum. From here, the air column goes up to the anterior epitympanum via the isthmus tympani anticus and then backward into the posterior epitympanum. A part of this air passes through the aditus to ventilate the mastoid, and a part of it comes via the isthmus tympani posticus to ventilate the posterior mesotympanum. From the posterior mesotympanum, the air percolates to the hypotympanum. Abnormalities of this ventilatory anatomy lead to inflammatory disorders of the middle ear.

Mastoid

■ Development

Development of the mastoid is from the squamous and petrous bone. The persistent petrosquamosal lamina, the Korner septum, is surgically important, as it may hinder the identification of the antrum. It divides the air cells into medial and lateral groups. Its development depends on the development of the sternocleidomastoid muscle. It begins after the first year of life when the child holds up his or her head. It forms a definite elevation at the end of the second year. Pneumatization completes by the age of 6 years. The facial nerve lies superficially up to the age of 2 years.

■ Anatomy

The mastoid consists of three parts:
- *Aditus ad antrum*: It is a short canal connecting the epitympanum with the mastoid antrum. The short process of the incus lies on the floor. The facial nerve (fallopian canal) also runs along the floor. The lateral semicircular canal lies on the medial wall. The bone lateral to the aditus appears like a bridge during ear surgeries.
- *Mastoid antrum*: It is the largest air cell in the mastoid bone. The antrum serves as an important landmark in mastoid surgeries. Anteriorly, the antrum receives the aditus. Medially, it is related to the horizontal semicircular canal. The roof is formed by the tegmen antri. The sinodural or Citelli's angle is the angle between the tegmen antri and the sigmoid sinus. The lateral wall is formed by the cortex of the mastoid bone that lies medial to the suprameatal triangle. The mastoid

antrum lies approximately 12 to 15 mm from the outer mastoid cortex.

- *MacEwen's triangle* is the bony surface marking for the mastoid antrum. It is bounded by the temporal line of the supramastoid crest, the posterosuperior bony meatal wall, and a line drawn at a tangent to the posterior canal wall. Posteroinferiorly, the antrum communicates with numerous mastoid air cells.
- *Mastoid air cells*: These are variable in number, size, and distribution, and communicate with the mastoid antrum.

The mastoid air cell system has been classified by Allam into the following:

- Mastoid: Mastoid antrum, periantral cells, dural, sinudural, perisinus, central, tip, and perifacial.
- Labyrinthine: Supralabyrinthine and infralabyrinthine groups.
- Petrous: Peritubular and apical cells.
- Accessory: Squamous, occipital, zygomatic, and styloid cells.

There are three types of mastoid processes:

- Cellular (pneumatized): It has large and numerous air cells. About 80% are cellular mastoids in the normal population. This is considered normal.
- Diploic: This comprises small and lesser number of air cells.
- Sclerotic (eburnated): Air cells are almost absent in this. The primary sclerotic mastoid is present since birth. The secondary sclerotic mastoid is due to chronic middle ear disease.
- The diploic and sclerotic types are due to eustachian tube obstruction. The air cells are mainly located in the petromastoid and squamous parts of the temporal bone.

Inner Ear

The inner ear, also known as the labyrinth, serves as an important organ for hearing and balance.

■ Development

The development of the inner ear starts in the 3rd week of intrauterine life, and it is completed by the 16th week of intrauterine life. The membranous labyrinth develops from the otic capsule, differentiating into various parts like sensory end organ of hearing and balance. The bony labyrinth also develops from the otic capsule. It is a mesenchymal condensation around the membranous labyrinth, which is converted into cartilage. Between this cartilage and labyrinth is loose periodic tissue that disappears around the utricle and saccule to form the vestibule. This tissue around the semicircular duct also disappears, forming the semicircular canal.

■ Anatomy

The inner ear is well protected, lying in the petrous temporal bone (**Fig. 1.11**). It consists of two parts: (1) the bony labyrinth and (2) the membranous labyrinth.

- *The bony labyrinth* has a central part called the vestibule with an anteriorly placed cochlea and posteriorly placed semicircular canals.

It is divided into three parts:

- *Vestibule*: It is the central part of the bony labyrinth, measuring around 5 mm. It lies between the medial wall of the middle ear and the internal acoustic meatus. The landmarks on the vestibule are the following:
  - *Lateral wall*: The fenestra vestibuli (oval window) is a bean-shaped opening in the lateral wall, occupied by the footplate of the stapes and the surrounding annular ligament.
  - *Medial wall*: The medial wall of the vestibule has a prominent crest in the midline called the

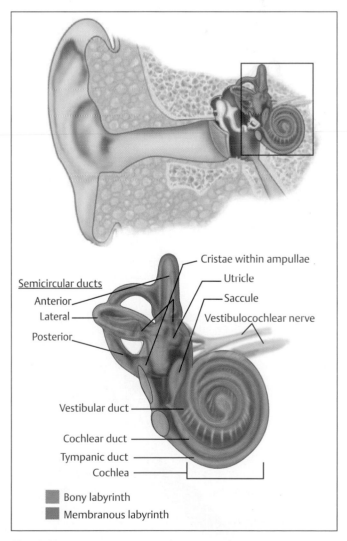

Semicircular ducts
Anterior
Lateral
Posterior

Cristae within ampullae
Utricle
Saccule
Vestibulocochlear nerve

Vestibular duct
Cochlear duct
Tympanic duct
Cochlea

■ Bony labyrinth
■ Membranous labyrinth

Fig. 1.11   Inner ear anatomy.

vestibular crest. This crest divides the anteriorly placed depression called the spherical recess from the posteriorly placed depression called the elliptical recess. The spherical recess houses the saccule and has multiple apertures called the macula cribrosa media for the passage of the inferior vestibular nerve filaments. The elliptical recess houses the utricle and has multiple apertures called the macula cribrosa superior (Mike's dot) for the passage of the superior vestibular nerve filaments. The vestibular crest splits anteriorly to enclose the cochlear recess, which has multiple apertures for cochlear nerve filaments. The elliptical recess is inferiorly related to the opening of the vestibular aqueduct, which opens outside the dura. The anterior aspect of the vestibule has one opening, which communicates with the cochlea. The posterior aspect of the vestibule has five openings for the ampullated and nonampullated ends of the semicircular canals.

– *Semicircular canal*: There are three semicircular canals located posterior to the vestibule: (1) superior (anterior), (2) posterior (vertical), and (3) lateral (horizontal) semicircular canals. Each forms two-thirds of a circle. These are unequal in length. The diameter of each of the three semicircular canals is 0.8 mm. All the semicircular canals have an ampullated end that houses the sensory organ of the canals and a nonampullated end. The ampullated ends of the three semicircular canals open separately into the vestibule. The nonampullated ends of the superior and the posterior semicircular canals combine to form a common nonampullated end called the crus commune, whereas the nonampullated end of the posterior canal opens separately into the vestibule.

Unique features of the semicircular canals are the following:

○ *Superior semicircular canal*: It is 15 to 20 mm in length. It lies transverse to the bony axis of the petrous part of the temporal bone. The ampulla is in the anterolateral end and opens in the upper lateral part of the vestibule. The other end fuses with the superior limb of the posterior canal to form the crus commune, which is 4 mm in length and opens in the medial part of the vestibule.

○ *Lateral semicircular canal*: It projects as a rounded bulge in the aditus ad antrum of the middle ear cleft. It is 12 to 15 mm in length and lies at an angle of 30 degrees to the horizontal plane. The ampullary end opens into the upper part of the vestibule, whereas the posterior part opens into the lower part below the orifice of the crus commune.

○ *Posterior semicircular canal*: It is 18 to 22 mm in length. It lies parallel and close to the posterior portion of the temporal bone. The lower ampullated limb opens into the lower part of the vestibule and the upper limb joins the crus commune.

The angle formed by the three semicircular canals is called the solid angle. The triangle is bounded anteriorly by the bony labyrinth, posteriorly by the sigmoid sinus, and superiorly by the superior sagittal sinus and the dura is called Trautmann's triangle. It is a weak area through which infection can spread to the posterior fossa. It is also used as an approach to the posterior fossa.

– *Cochlea*: The anterior portion of the labyrinth is formed by a snail-like structure called the cochlea (**Fig. 1.12**). The height from the base to the apex is 5 mm and the diameter at the base is 9 mm. The length of the tube is 30 mm. It is a hollow structure

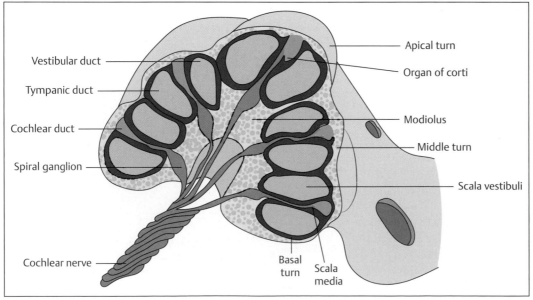

Vestibular duct
Tympanic duct
Cochlear duct
Spiral ganglion
Cochlear nerve
Apical turn
Organ of corti
Modiolus
Middle turn
Scala vestibuli
Basal turn
Scala media

Fig. 1.12 Section of the bony cochlea showing the membranous structures inside.

with two and three-fourths turns around a conical central axis called the modiolus. The base of the modiolus is directed toward the internal acoustic meatus and is perforated for the passage of the cochlear nerve. It is divided into two parts: (1) osseous spiral lamina and (2) membranous spiral lamina (basilar membrane). The osseous spiral laminae are projections from the modiolus.

The cochlea is divided into three longitudinal channels: the scala vestibuli or vestibular duct above, the scala tympani or tympanic duct below, and the scala media, cochlear duct, in between. The site where the scala vestibuli and the scala tympani communicate at the apex of the cochlea is called helicotrema. The scala vestibuli is in continuity with the vestibule at the oval window and is closed by the footplate of the stapes. The secondary tympanic membrane at the fenestra cochleae separates the scala tympani from the tympanic cavity. The cochlear duct (scala media) is separated from the scala vestibule by the Reissner membrane and from the scala tympani by the basilar membrane.

The osseous spiral lamina houses the spiral ganglion, which contains the nerve fibers from the organ of Corti and direct the nerve fibers toward the internal acoustic meatus as the cochlear nerve.

- Membranous labyrinth: The membranous labyrinth contains the endolymph and the specialized vestibular and cochlear receptors (**Fig. 1.13**). The vestibular receptor organs are the macula (utricle and saccule) and the cristae (ampulla of the semicircular canals). Physiologically, the membranous labyrinth is divided into three parts:
  – Membranous vestibular labyrinth: It is made up of the saccule, utricle, and the endolymphatic duct and sac. The saccule is connected to the cochlear labyrinth by the membranous cochlear reuniens. The saccule and utricle are connected to each other by the utriculosaccular duct, which continues as the endolymphatic duct. The endolymphatic duct opens into the endolymphatic sac, which lies outside the posterior cranial fossa dura. The saccule occupies the spherical recess containing specialized vestibular epithelium. The utricle occupies the elliptical recess of the bony vestibule. The three semicircular ducts open into the posterior wall of the utricle. The vestibular receptor organs of the utricle and the saccule are called the macula. The macula of the saccule lies vertically in the medial surface of the saccule, whereas the macula of the utricle lies in the horizontal plane. These organs are composed of hair cells, supporting cells, and a gelatinous mass/statoconial membrane. The statoconial membrane is composed of mucopolysaccharides, secreted by supporting cells. It also contains calcium carbonate crystals called otolith or statoconia.

  – Membranous semicircular canal (cristae ampullaris): These are suspended within the bony semicircular canal. It opens through five openings into the posterior wall of the utricle. The crista is a saddle-shaped ridge within each membranous ampulla. It is a sensory end organ covered by the neuroepithelium with hair cells and sensory cells, and a dome-shaped gelatinous mass called the cupula.

  The hair cells are of two types:
  - Type I: These are flask-shaped cells enclosed with a nerve chalice, seen in the summit of the cristae.
  - Type II: These are cylindrical with no nerve chalice, located in the periphery of the cristae.

  The hair cells contain a kinocilium, which is prominent, tall, and not uniformly arranged in the macula with many small cilia (60–110) known as the stereocilia. A curved line called the striola divides each macula into medial and lateral halves.

  The three semicircular canals open into the posterior wall of the utricle via five openings.

  – Membranous cochlea: The cochlear duct or the scala media occupies the middle portion of the cochlear canal and is triangular in cross section (**Fig. 1.14**). The floor is formed by the basilar membrane, which has a thin inner part called the zona arcuata (supports the organ of Corti) and a thick outer portion called the zona pectinate. The roof of the cochlear duct is formed by Reissner's membrane, and the lateral wall by the stria vascularis and the bony wall of the cochlea.

  The organ of Corti (**Fig. 1.15**) is spread like a ribbon along the basilar membrane in the scala media. It contains the following:
  - The tunnel of Corti composed of two rows of rods (pillar cells) separates the inner hair cells and outer hair cells. It forms a triangle with the basilar membrane and contains the cortilymph. There is one row of inner hair cells and three to four rows of outer hair cells. These hair cells are supported by pillar cells, Deiters' cells, and Hensen's cells. The tips of the outer hair cells are attached to the undersurface of the tectorial membrane.

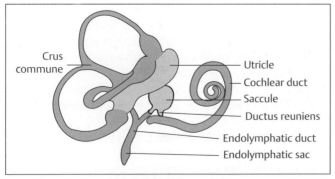

Fig. 1.13 Membranous labyrinth.

Crus commune — Utricle — Cochlear duct — Saccule — Ductus reuniens — Endolymphatic duct — Endolymphatic sac

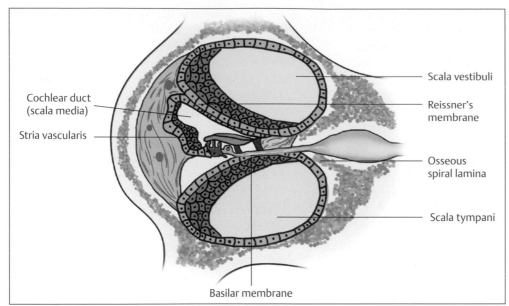

Fig. 1.14 Cross section of the cochlea.

Cochlear duct (scala media)

Stria vascularis

Scala vestibuli

Reissner's membrane

Osseous spiral lamina

Scala tympani

Basilar membrane

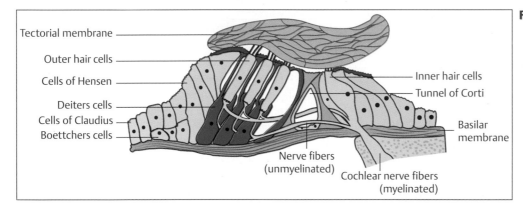

Fig. 1.15 Organ of Corti.

Tectorial membrane

Outer hair cells

Cells of Hensen

Deiters cells

Cells of Claudius

Boettchers cells

Inner hair cells

Tunnel of Corti

Basilar membrane

Nerve fibers (unmyelinated)

Cochlear nerve fibers (myelinated)

○ The tectorial membrane consists of a gelatinous material with delicate fibers, overlying the organ of Corti. The shearing force between the hair cells and the tectorial membrane provides stimulus to the hair cells.

○ The stria vascularis on the lateral wall of the organ of corti plays a vital role in maintaining ionic composition and electric potential of the endolymph.

Inner Ear Fluids and Their Circulation

• The perilymph resembles extracellular fluid, rich in sodium ions. It fills the space between the bony and membranous labyrinths. It communicates with the cerebrospinal fluid (CSF) through the aqueduct of the cochlea, which opens into the scala tympani near the round window. This duct contains connective tissue resembling the arachnoid, through which the perilymph percolates. The perilymph is formed either by the filtrate of blood serum from the capillaries of the spiral ligament or by a direct continuation of the CSF.

• The endolymph fills the entire membranous labyrinth. It resembles an intracellular fluid and is rich in potassium ions. It is secreted by the secretory cells of the stria vascularis, and dark cells (of the utricle and ampulla of the semicircular canal). There are two theories of flow: (1) longitudinal (cochlea, utricle, saccule, endolymphatic duct, and endolymphatic sac) and (2) radial (secreted and absorbed by the stria vascularis).

Blood Supply of Inner Ear

The labyrinthine artery arises from the anteroinferior cerebellar artery and accompanies the facial and vestibulocochlear nerves in the internal acoustic meatus. It divides into three branches to supply the inner ear:

• The anterior vestibular artery (supplies the macula of the utricle and the crista of the superior and lateral semicircular canals).

• The vestibulocochlear branch (supplies the posterior semicircular canal).

• The cochlear branch (supplies the cochlea).

Points to Ponder

- The external ear protrudes out and has a cartilaginous framework to absorb shock and trauma.
- Perichondritis is inflammation of the outer perichondrium of the pinna and is usually due to trauma, infections, ear piercings, or ear surgery.
- The cymba concha is an important landmark as it denotes the surface marking for the mastoid antrum.
- The mastoid antrum is the largest air cell within the mastoid bone and is always present.
- The external auditory canal is formed by a lateral cartilaginous part and a medial bony part. Wax is produced in the cartilaginous part.
- The normal tympanic membrane has a cone of light in the anteroinferior quadrant.
- There are two muscles in the middle ear, the tensor tympani and the stapedius, which help dampen the transmission of loud sounds into the inner ear. This protects the ear from acoustic trauma.
- The mastoid bone is classified as being cellular, diploic, or sclerotic. The normal mastoid bone is cellular.
- The eustachian tube equalizes the middle ear pressure with atmospheric pressure. Dysfunction can lead to middle ear disease.
- The organ of Corti is responsible for the transduction of sound. It converts sound vibrations to electrical signals.

Case-Based Questions

1. **A 36-year-old man comes to the ear, nose, and throat (ENT) clinic complaining of right-sided ear block. What are the important anatomical points that should be taken into account during the clinical examination of this patient?**

Answer

The pinna must be pulled backward, upward, and laterally to straighten the external auditory canal so that the tympanic membrane can be visualized.

The tympanic membrane is normally pearly gray, shiny, and translucent with a cone of light in the anteroinferior quadrant.

The mastoid bone behind the pinna has a rough outer surface for the attachment of the muscles and is nontender.

2. **A 25-year-old man presented with pain behind the ear after an upper respiratory tract infection.**

   a. If you are suspecting mastoiditis, which region would you like to elicit tenderness?

   b. What is MacEwen's triangle?

Answers

a. The cymba concha is the surface landmark for the mastoid antrum.

b. MacEwen's triangle is the landmark to identify the mastoid antrum during surgery.

   The mastoid antrum is the largest air cell in the mastoid bone. The boundaries of the triangle are as follows:

   - Superiorly, the horizontal temporal line.
   - Anteroinferiorly, the posterosuperior boundary of the external auditory canal.
   - Posteriorly, a line drawn tangent to the posterior boundary of the external auditory canal meeting the temporal line above.

   The mastoid antrum lies at a depth of 15 mm from the surface of the temporal bone.

Frequently Asked Questions

1. What is the length of the external auditory canal?
2. What is the cone of light?
3. What are the parts of the stapes?
4. What is a solid angle?
5. What is the stria vascularis?
6. What are the functions of the eustachian tube?

Endnote

Antonio Scarpa (1752–1832) was an Italian anatomist. His achievements in medicine were extraordinary. He was the first person to describe the membranous labyrinth. He also described the vestibular ganglion, Scarpa's ganglion, and the nasopalatine nerve or Scarpa's nerve. He laid the foundation for the study of the physiology of hearing.

2 Physiology of the Ear

Vishwas K. Pai

The competencies covered in this chapter are as follows:

EN1.1 Describe the anatomy and physiology of the ear, nose, throat, and head and neck.

PY10.15 Describe and discuss the functional anatomy of the ear and auditory pathways and physiology of hearing.

Introduction

The ear is a complex organ responsible for hearing and balance.

Physiology of Hearing

Hearing occurs when sound vibrations from the outside are conducted through the external ear and the middle ear and reach the inner ear where, by a process of transduction, nerve impulses are generated. These impulses are then transmitted to the brain and are interpreted as sound.

Pitch is the perception of different frequencies of sound. *Frequency* is documented as cycles per second, or hertz. Although the audible range of sound extends from about 20 Hz to 20 kHz, the human ear is most sensitive to frequencies from 1 to 4 kHz. *Loudness* is the intensity of sound, noted in decibels (dB).

The hearing process broadly involves three major transformations of sound energy before it is transmitted to the central nervous system as nerve impulses:
- Transmission by mechanical conduction of sound through the external and middle ear.
- Transduction of sound is where mechanical sound energy is converted to electrical impulses.
- Conduction of electrical impulses to the brain through nerves.

■ Transmission of Sound through the External and Middle Ear

Role of the Pinna and External Auditory Canal

- *Head shadow effect*: A sound source at one side will produce a more intense stimulus of the ear nearest to it and the sound will arrive sooner, thus providing a mechanism for *sound localization.*
- The shape of the pinna navigates higher-frequency sounds and funnels them into the ear canal (*sound concentration*).
- The auditory canal acts as a resonating tube and amplifies sound by 15 to 22 dB between 3,000 and 4,000 Hz. This adds to the sensitivity (and susceptibility to damage) of the ear at these frequencies. The external canal also protects the tympanic membrane.

Role of the Middle Ear

The eustachian tube helps maintain pressure on either side of the tympanic membrane, which is important for sound transmission. Equal pressure, on either side, allows for maximum vibration and better hearing.

Impedance Matching

When sound travels from one medium (air in the middle ear) to another (fluid in the cochlea), there is resistance (or impedance) to the transmission of sound. Only 3% is transmitted; the rest is reflected. This amounts to a loss of 30 dB. The tympanic membrane and the ossicles function to overcome the *impedance mismatch* between the air and the inner ear fluids, and thus the middle ear serves as a transformer, or *impedance matching* device.

Transformer Action of the Middle Ear

The impedance matching mechanism of the ear works through three mechanisms:
- *Catenary lever action*: This is also known as the curved membrane effect. This was originally pointed out by Helmholtz in 1868. The tympanic membrane is firmly attached to the annulus laterally. The membrane then curves medially toward the umbo. The movement of

the tympanic membrane between the annulus and the umbo is greater than at the umbo. This creates a lever action, which increases the force acting on the umbo by two times.

- *Hydraulic lever*: Approximately 55 mm² is the vibrating surface of the tympanic membrane, which is connected to the stapes footplate via the ossicular chain. The area of the footplate is 3.2 mm². This differential in surface area between these structures helps produce a 17:1 increase in sound energy that is transmitted across the middle ear.
- *Ossicular lever*: The handle of the malleus and the long process of the incus move simultaneously. Since the handle of the malleus is 1.3 times longer, the *ossicular lever ratio* amounts to about 1.3:1, which gives a mechanical advantage.

The above actions of the *hydraulic lever* and the *ossicular lever* together give a transformer ratio of 1.3 × 17, which is equal to 22:1. This gives a 27-dB gain (**Fig. 2.1**).

Overall Sound Transformation of the Impedance Matching System

It is to be noted that if you calculate the value of all three impedance matching mechanisms (catenary lever + hydraulic lever + ossicular lever), then the sound pressure impinging on the tympanic membrane is increased by 44 times by the time it reaches the footplate of the stapes, which translates to a 33-dB gain in sound (catenary lever = two times; hydraulic lever =17 times; and ossicular lever = 1.3 times).

Note: The ossicular chain, on vibration, conducts sound to the oval window. A movement of the oval window inward allows the round window to move outward. This is called the phase difference. There is very little sound vibration

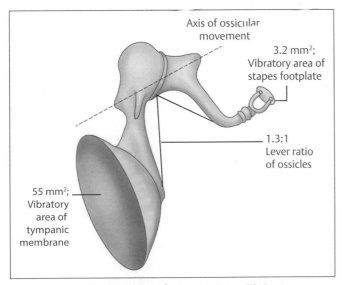

Fig. 2.1 Transformer ratio of 17:1 × 1.3:1 = 22:1.

Axis of ossicular movement

3.2 mm²; Vibratory area of stapes footplate

1.3:1 Lever ratio of ossicles

55 mm²; Vibratory area of tympanic membrane

being conducted through the air in the middle ear. This is preferentially carried by the ossicles.

> ### Pearl
> The round window reflex of light is noted during middle ear surgery when assessing the integrity of the ossicular chain. When the handle of the malleus is moved, the transmitted movement moves the round window outward. This is appreciated as light reflecting when saline or blood is placed over the round window.

Function of the Muscles of the Middle Ear

- When the tensor tympani contracts, it pulls the handle of the malleus medially, tensing the tympanic membrane.
- When the stapedius contracts, it pulls the stapes footplate outward from the oval window, which reduces the intensity of sound reaching the cochlea. In high-intensity sound, the stapedius contracts in the same ear and the contralateral ear (*acoustic reflex*).
- The contractions of the middle ear muscles are not instantaneous. When activated, these contractions dampen the sound waves reaching the inner ear by reducing the vibration of the ossicular chain.

Transmission of Sound by Bone Conduction

Conduction of sound through bone is not very well understood. But there is clear transmission of vibration through bone. When the footplate of a tuning fork is placed over the mastoid bone, after being struck and set into vibration, sound can be heard.

Sound vibrations cause the skull to vibrate, and these are transmitted to the fluids in the cochlea. This is by direct compression of the otic capsule. This will cause vibration of the perilymph in both the scala vestibuli and the scala tympani. This simultaneous vibration of the perilymph of the scala vestibuli and tympani does not cancel each other out as would be expected because the round window membrane is more freely mobile than the footplate of the stapes. This allows the basilar membrane to move leading to stimulation of the organ of Corti. This is called compression bone conduction.

Transmission of Sound in a Diseased Ear

- In eustachian tube dysfunction and with minimal effusion, there is increased stiffness in the middle ear transformation resulting in low-frequency conductive hearing loss.
- In middle ear effusion, due to mass effect, there is low- and high-frequency loss.
- In small central perforation, due to reduced surface area, there is minimal conductive hearing loss (15 dB) in low frequencies.

- In large central perforation, due to a larger loss of surface area and sound passage to the round window, there is mild conductive hearing loss (30 dB).
- In perforation with ossicular discontinuity, due to loss of surface area and lever action (some direct passage of sound to the footplate), there is moderate conductive hearing loss (45 dB).
- In an intact tympanic membrane with ossicular discontinuity where there is no transmission of sound to the oval window, there is moderately severe conductive hearing loss (60 dB).
- In pars flaccida perforation with an intact vibrating surface, there will be normal hearing (hearing gets affected only if the ossicles are involved).

Transmission of Sound within the Inner Ear

Transmission of Sound Waves in the Cochlea

Sound waves delivered to the stapes footplate lead to the creation of pressure waves within the perilymph of the scala vestibuli of the cochlea (**Fig. 2.2**).

This traveling wave moves from the base of the cochlea to the tip of the cochlea through the helicotrema into the scala tympani. A traveling wave, with a certain frequency, grows in amplitude as it moves toward the apex of the cochlea till maximum displacement has occurred at the site in the cochlea aimed for that particular frequency. The basal turn of the cochlea is tuned to high frequencies, whereas the apex is more for the low frequencies. The wave is transmitted to the endolymph inside the cochlear duct due to which displacement of the basilar membrane occurs. This causes the organ of Corti to move against the tectorial membrane, stimulating the generation of electrical nerve impulses to the brain. The stiffness of the basilar membrane is responsible for its tonotopic specificity.

Loudness is perceived by the degree of movement of the basilar membrane. When sound increases, the amplitude of vibration of the basilar membrane also increases. This will lead to an increase in the number of hair cells stimulated and the rate at which they fire the nerve impulses. The outer hair cells act as a cochlear modifier, enhancing the basilar membrane movement at a particular frequency.

Theories of Hearing

Helmholtz's place theory: High-frequency sounds stimulate the basal turn and low-frequency sounds stimulate the apical region.

Rutherford's frequency theory: The entire length of the basilar membrane is stimulated, and its frequency of movement determines the type of sound.

Wever's volley resonance theory: This theory states that neurons in the auditory nerve respond to sound by firing action potentials at different times, out of phase with each other. When these action potentials are combined, they produce sound of higher frequency.

Von Bekesy's traveling wave theory: The transmitted wave starts from the basal turn of the cochlea and moves toward the apex; the extent of displacement of the basilar membrane varies with frequency, which determines the pitch.

■ Transduction of Mechanical Vibrations

Because of a difference in the potassium content between the endolymph and the perilymph, an *endocochlear potential* develops. The endolymph has a high positive potential due to high potassium concentration and low sodium

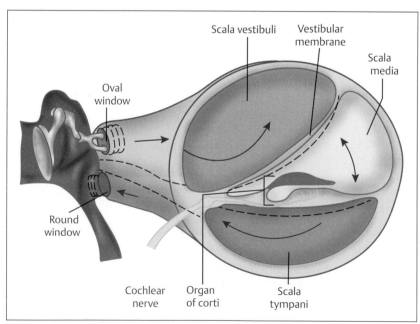

Fig. 2.2 Movement of sound waves through the scala vestibuli to the scala media and then to the scala tympani.

Scala vestibuli

Vestibular membrane

Scala media

Oval window

Round window

Cochlear nerve

Organ of corti

Scala tympani

content when compared to the perilymph. The difference in ion concentration between the perilymph and endolymph is maintained and stabilized by Reissner's membrane.

Sound waves traveling through the perilymph in the scala vestibuli pass through Reissner's membrane and into the cochlear duct. This will eventually lead to vibration of the organ of Corti, which is found on the basilar membrane. The organ of Corti has hair cells arranged as inner hair cells and outer hair cells and they have stereocilia, which brush against the tectorial membrane (**Fig. 2.3**).

Stereocilia displacement against the tectorial membrane during vibrations of the basilar membrane leads to depolarization of the hair cells. When the stereocilia are bent in the direction of the longer stereocilia, ion channels open up and potassium ions move into the cell. When the stereocilia are bent in the opposite direction, ion channels are closed.

Depolarization of the hair cells leads to the release of neurotransmitters, which are absorbed by the distal cochlear nerve fibers leading to the transmission of impulses along the nerve (**Figs. 2.4** and **2.5**).

The conversion of the mechanical sound energy into electrical impulses is known as transduction of sound.

Roles of Various Structures in the Cochlea

Flowchart 2.1 explains the functions of the various anatomical structures of the inner ear.

■ Cochlear Nerve and Central Auditory Pathways

Auditory Nerve Fibers

The eighth cranial nerve or vestibulocochlear nerve consists of the cochlear nerve, which innervates the cochlea and the vestibular nerve, which innervates the utricle, saccule, and the semicircular canals. The neurons of the spiral ganglion are called bipolar cells as fibers extend from the opposite ends of the cell body. The longer central fibers

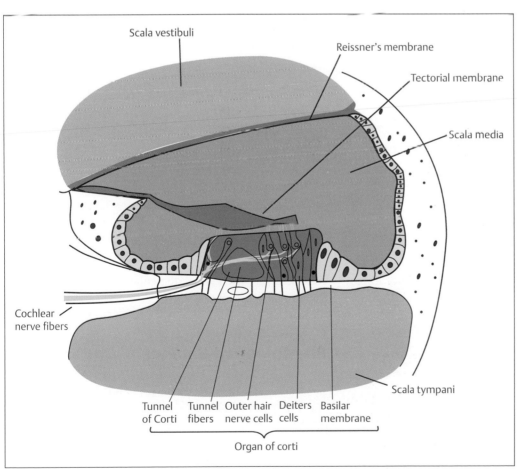

Fig. 2.3 Structure of the cochlea. The endolymph is present in the scala media or the cochlear duct, whereas the perilymph is present in the scala vestibuli and the scala tympani.

Scala vestibuli

Reissner's membrane

Tectorial membrane

Scala media

Cochlear nerve fibers

Scala tympani

Tunnel of Corti | Tunnel fibers | Outer hair nerve cells | Deiters cells | Basilar membrane

Organ of corti

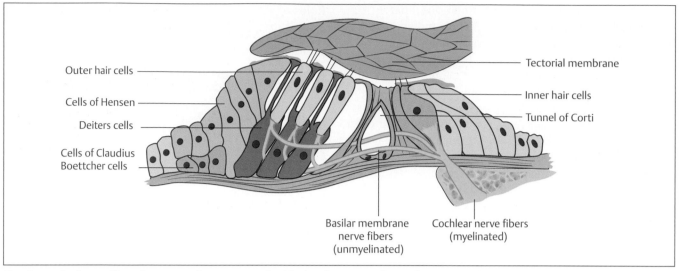

Fig. 2.4 The hair cells in the organ of Corti are embedded in the tectorial membrane. The shearing force will bend the stereocilia.

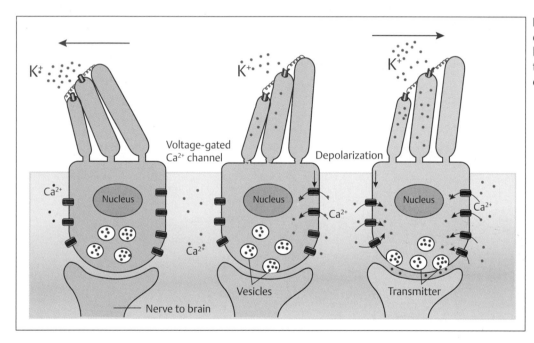

Fig. 2.5 When the stereocilia are deflected toward the kinocilium, ion channels open, there is potassium influx, and depolarization occurs.

form the cochlear nerve and the shorter peripheral fibers innervate the inner and outer hair cells. The cochlear nerve exits through the modiolus, passes through the internal auditory canal, and then enters the medulla oblongata.

Auditory Pathway

In the medulla oblongata, the fibers of the cochlear nerve terminate at the dorsal and ventral cochlear nuclei (**Fig. 2.6**). Each cochlear nerve fiber branches at the cochlear nucleus, sending one branch to the dorsal and the other branch to the ventral cochlear nucleus.

From the cochlear nuclei, nerve fibers pass through the superior olivary complex, lateral lemniscus, inferior colliculus, and the medial geniculate body, eventually terminating in the auditory cortex.

Physiology of Balance

The inner ear receptors, namely, the macula of the saccule and utricle, and the crista ampullaris of the semicircular canals sense the static and dynamic positional status of the human body and play a major role in maintenance of balance. In short, we need gaze and posture stabilization and correct perception of verticality to maintain balance, which is mainly dependent on the inner ear labyrinth (**Fig. 2.7**).

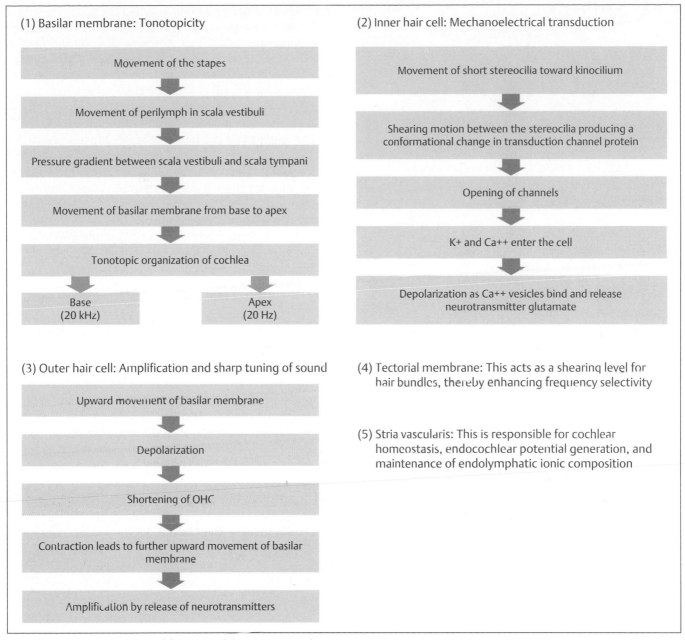

Flowchart 2.1   Structure and function of the inner ear in hearing.

■ Principles of Maintenance of Balance

Maintenance of balance in a human being follows the simple physiological principle of a reflex arc. The reflex arc includes a sensory component, a relay center or a nucleus, motor response supported by the central nervous system.

The sensory components involved in maintenance of balance include the eyes, vestibular labyrinth, and the proprioceptors (**Flowchart 2.2**). The vestibular labyrinth is responsible in the detection of static movement of an individual (head movements and spatial orientation), whereas the eyes and the proprioceptors are responsible for the detection of dynamic movement of the individual (visual

movement or body movement with respect to surroundings). Information from these sensory receptors relays in the vestibular nucleus. The vestibular nucleus informs the brain that a particular sensory input has been received. The brain searches its memory to ascertain whether such inputs have been received in the past to generate a motor response through the motor pathway. The speediness of the motor response is dependent on the past vestibular memory. The efferent motor system includes the muscular movements of the eyes, limbs, neck, and trunk to maintain a stable body in the environment. The extrapyramidal system also provides critical input and helps in the modulation of motor responses. The response generated by the

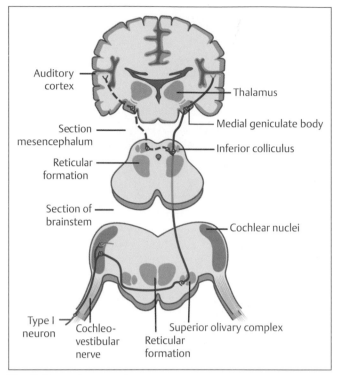

Fig. 2.6 Auditory pathway.

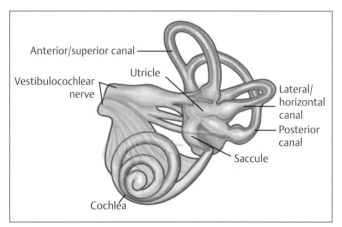

Fig. 2.7 Membranous labyrinth of the inner ear.

eyes to a vestibular stimulus is called the vestibulo-ocular reflex, that generated by the limbs and trunk is called the vestibulospinal reflex, and that generated by the neck is called the vestibulocollic reflex (**Flowchart 2.3**). Any conflict in the sensory information relayed by the various sensory components will produce vertigo.

The concepts required for understanding sensory stimulation of the vestibular system are the following:

- The longest hair cell on the receptor organ is called the kinocilium and the rest of the hair cells are called the stereocilia. The movement of the stereocilia toward the kinocilium causes depolarization of the cell and hence stimulation of the nerve endings.
- The kinocilium is placed toward the utricle in the lateral semicircular canal and away from the utricle in the superior and posterior semicircular canal. Hence, an ampullopetal movement in the lateral semicircular canal causes stimulation of the ipsilateral labyrinthine nerve endings, and an ampullofugal movement in the superior and posterior semicircular canals causes stimulation of the ipsilateral labyrinthine nerve endings. Movements of the head stimulates the semicircular canals depending on the plane of movement.
- The sensory organ is located in the horizontal plane in the utricle and in the vertical plane in the saccule. Hence, a forward–backward movement and a side-to-side movement of the body stimulate the utricle and an up–down movement stimulates the saccule to generate an appropriate balance and stable motor response.

Pearl

Unterberger's test is performed in patients with vertigo to determine if there is a peripheral cause. There are three ways to maintain balance: (1) visual, (2) through proprioceptive impulses from the limbs, and (3) from an intact labyrinthine system. If a patient has vertigo due to a peripheral cause, then during the performance of Unterberger's test, the patient will sway toward the side of the lesion.

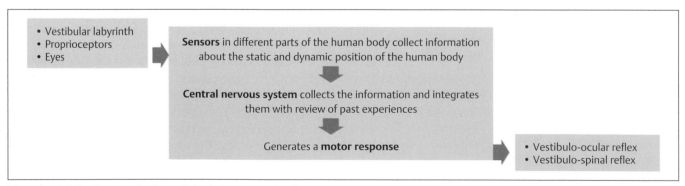

Flowchart 2.2 Demonstration of the balance mechanism.

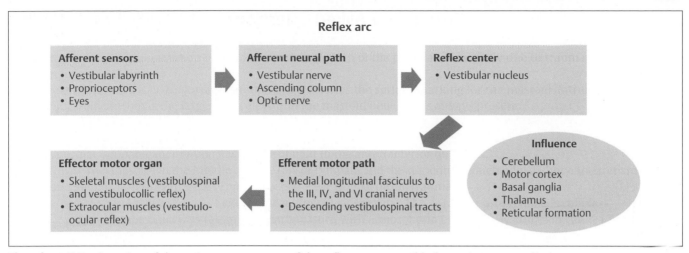

Flowchart 2.3 Overview of the various components of the reflex arc responsible for maintenance of balance.

Points to Ponder

- The pinna helps collect and localize sound. It also helps concentrate the sound toward the opening of the external auditory canal.
- The acoustic properties of the external ear are one of the reasons why noise-induced hearing losses occur first and most prominently at the 4-kHz region (boiler's notch).
- Impedance matching is achieved by the following:
  - Effective vibratory area of the tympanic membrane, which is 17 to 20 times greater than that of the stapes footplate.
  - Lever action of the ossicular chain: The long process of the incus is shorter by a factor of 1.3 than the length of the manubrium and the neck of the malleus.
  - Shape of the tympanic membrane.
- Sound transmission and transduction: The stapes footplate → oval window → perilymph of scala vestibuli → helico-trema (opening at the apex of the cochlea) → perilymph of the scala tympani.
- Release of neurotransmitters following movements of the stereocilia stimulates the nerve fibers at the base of the hair cells. These are transmitted as electrical impulses to the cochlear nuclei via the cochlear nerve.
- Because about half of the fibers of the auditory pathways cross the midline, while the others ascend on the same side of the brain, each ear is represented in both the right and left cortices. When the auditory cortical area of one side is injured by trauma or stroke, binaural hearing may not be affected.

Case-Based Questions

1. **In order to determine whether a newborn baby was able to hear, the doctor ordered a test on the second day after birth. This was part of the newborn screening program for deafness implemented by the hospital to pick up deafness among children early.**

   a. What is the name of the test?

   b. What is the principle behind the test?

Answers

a. The test is called the otoacoustic emission (OAE) test.

b. The normal cochlear not only receives sound waves but also produces its own sounds called OAE. Soft clicking sounds are used to stimulate the cochlea in a newborn as part of the screening program to pick up early deafness. The clicks stimulate the cochlear hair cells to produce sounds, which are then picked up by a microphone in the external auditory canal. If OAE is present, the newborn infant is presumed to have normal hearing.

Frequently Asked Questions

1. What is the role of the pinna and external auditory canal in sound transmission?

2. What is an impedance mismatch in sound transmission in the ear and how is it overcome?

3. What is the role of the middle ear muscles during sound transmission?

4. What is phase difference in inner ear sound transmission?

5. Trace the auditory pathway.

Endnote

Georg von Bekesy (1899–1972) was a Hungarian biophysicist. He conducted experiments and determined that the basilar membrane moved like a surface wave when stimulated by sound. And the maximum amplitude of the waves depended on the frequency of the sound. High frequencies cause waves at the basal turn of the cochlea, whereas low frequencies produce waves of maximum amplitude toward the apex of the cochlea. This is called the place theory of hearing or traveling wave theory for which he was awarded the Nobel prize in Physiology or Medicine in 1961.

3 History Taking and Examination of the Ear

Meera Niranjan Khadilkar and Sushmitha Kabekkodu

> **The competencies covered in this chapter are as follows:**
>
> EN2.3 Demonstrate the correct technique of examination of the ear including otoscopy.
>
> EN3.1 Observe and describe the indications for and steps involved in the performance of otomicroscopic examination in a simulated environment.
>
> EN4.4 Demonstrate the correct technique to hold, visualize and assess the mobility of the tympanic membrane, and interpret and diagrammatically represent the findings.
>
> PE28.10 Perform an otoscopic examination of the ear.
>
> EN2.2 Demonstrate the correct use of a headlamp in the examination of the ear, nose, and throat.
>
> PY10.20 Demonstrate hearing (tuning fork test) in a volunteer or a simulated environment.
>
> EN4.9 Demonstrate the correct technique for syringing wax from the ear in a simulated environment.
>
> EN2.14 Demonstrate the correct technique to instilling topical medications into the ear.

History Taking in the Ear

■ Patient Details

- **Name:** The full name of the patient addressed with the title (Master, Ms, Mr, Mrs, Shri, Smt) will help identify the patient and maintain a rapport.
- **Age:** The age of the patient helps narrow down the diagnosis. Acute otitis media is more common in children. Presbycusis is seen in the elderly.
- **Sex:** The gender of the patient also helps narrow down the diagnosis. Keloids are common in women with a history of ear piercing.
- **Socioeconomic status:** Chronic otitis media is more common in the lower socioeconomic groups.
- **Occupation:** Noise-induced hearing loss is more frequent in patients working in noisy conditions.
- **Address:** It is essential for patient identification and tracing.

■ History

Chief Complaints

Complaints must be documented in the patient's own words, in the chronological order, based on the duration or severity. The common complaints related to the ear are the following:

- Ear pain.
- Ear discharge.
- Decreased hearing.
- Blocked sensation/fullness in the ear.
- Itching in the ear.
- Ringing sensation in the ear or tinnitus.
- Growth in the ear.
- Swelling in or around the ear.
- Foreign body in the ear.
- Giddiness/vertigo.
- Facial weakness or paralysis.

History of Presenting Illness

A detailed description of the chief complaints must be recorded. The mode of onset (sudden/gradual), laterality (unilateral/bilateral), duration, severity, nature (intermittent/continuous), progress, aggravating and relieving factors, and associated complaints are noted.

- **Ear pain (otalgia):** Ear pain can be primary (local cause) or referred (from other regions in the head and neck due to a common nerve supply).
  - *Primary otalgia* may be due to conditions in the following:
    - ○ *Auricle*: Trauma or perichondritis.

○ *External auditory canal*: Impacted wax, furuncle, acute otitis externa, impacted foreign body, malignant otitis externa, and malignancy.

○ *Middle ear/mastoid*: Acute otitis media, chronic otitis media with cholesteatoma, complications of chronic otitis media, acute mastoiditis, malignancy, and barotrauma.

- *Referred otalgia* may occur due to conditions in other parts of the head and neck, referred to the ear via the following:

○ *Fifth cranial nerve (auriculotemporal branch of mandibular nerve)*: Dental causes like caries tooth, periapical abscess, impacted teeth, ill-fitting dentures, temporomandibular joint disorders, and oral ulcers/malignancy.

○ *Ninth cranial nerve (Jacobson's nerve)*: Oropharyngeal causes like acute tonsillitis, post-tonsillectomy, peritonsillar abscess, elongated styloid process, ulcers or malignancy of the tonsil, the base of the tongue, and soft palate,

○ *Tenth cranial nerve (Arnold's nerve)*: Ulcer/malignancy in the vallecula, epiglottis, larynx, and hypopharynx.

○ *C2 and C3 spinal nerves (greater auricular nerve, lesser occipital nerve)*: Cervical spine diseases like spondylosis, tuberculosis, and injury.

- **Ear discharge (otorrhea):** A discharging ear can be due to infection or trauma. It should be documented as profuse or scanty, intermittent or continuous, type of discharge (mucoid, purulent, serous, or watery), foul smelling or not, blood stained or not. Aggravating factors like upper respiratory tract infection or swimming and whether it is relieved with medication or not should be noted. The causes of ear discharge may be the following:
  - *External auditory canal*: Otitis externa, malignancy, and otomycosis.
  - *Middle ear/mastoid*: Acute otitis media, chronic otitis media, and cholesteatoma.

Ear discharge may be *scanty* in the atticoantral (squamosal) type of chronic otitis media and otitis externa, and *profuse* in the tubotympanic (mucosal) type of chronic otitis media.

Purulent ear discharge is seen in the furuncle, squamosal type of chronic otitis media, acute mastoiditis, and malignant otitis externa. *Mucoid/mucopurulent* ear discharge is seen in the tubotympanic type of chronic otitis media and later stages of acute otitis media. *Watery* ear discharge is seen in cerebrospinal fluid (CSF) leak, atopic dermatitis/eczema of the external auditory canal. *Blood-tinged* ear discharge is seen in the initial stages of acute otitis media, posttrauma, granulations, and malignancy. Foul-smelling ear discharge is seen in the squamosal type of chronic otitis media and some forms of otitis externa.

- **Hearing loss:** It can be unilateral or bilateral and sudden or insidious in onset. Sudden-onset hearing loss can be seen in acute otitis media, posttrauma, and labyrinthitis. Hearing loss is insidious in onset in chronic otitis media, otitis media with effusion, otosclerosis, presbycusis, and acoustic neuroma. Hearing loss can be conductive (external or middle ear causes), sensorineural (inner ear or cochlear nerve causes), or mixed. The progression should be documented. The degree of hearing loss may be mild, moderate, or severe. Family history of hearing loss may point toward Ménière's disease or otosclerosis. Drug history for intake of ototoxic drugs (salicylates, cytotoxic drugs, quinine, and aminoglycosides) should be elicited. Enquire about sudden or long-term (occupational) exposure to loud sounds like acoustic trauma and noise-induced hearing loss, respectively.

Pearl

Hearing loss and difficulty in hearing speech:
- 0–25 dB (normal): No significant difficulty with faint speech.
- 26–40 dB (mild loss): Difficulty with faint speech.
- 41–55 dB (moderate loss): Frequent difficulty with normal speech.
- 56–70 dB (moderately severe loss): Frequent difficulty even with loud speech.
- 71–91 dB (severe loss): Only shouted or amplified speech can be understood.
- >91 dB (profound loss): Usually even amplified speech cannot be understood.

Pearl

- *Paracusis of Willis*: The patient hears better in noisy environment (otosclerosis).
- *Autophony*: The patient hears their own voice louder (patulous eustachian tube).
- *Diplacusis*: The patient perceives different pitches in both ears (Ménière's disease).
- *Hyperacusis*: The patient experiences increased sensitivity to normal sound (stapedius muscle paralysis, congenital syphilis).
- *Recruitment*: The patient cannot hear at normal intensity, but a slight increase in intensity causes discomfort (cochlear pathology).

- **Tinnitus:** It is the perception or sensation of sound in the ear with no external stimulus. It may be subjective or objective and pulsatile or nonpulsatile. A note should be made regarding laterality, duration, and severity and nature of tinnitus.

Subjective tinnitus is perceived only by the patient.

Objective tinnitus is perceived by the patient and the examiner. It is seen in vascular tumors, patulous eustachian tube, arteriovenous malformations, palatal myoclonus, and temporomandibular joint dysfunction.

Pulsatile tinnitus is intermittent. It may be idiopathic or due to causes such as hypertension, anemia, pregnancy, and exercise. *Nonpulsatile tinnitus* is continuous, usually associated with hearing loss. *Isolated tinnitus* without hearing loss may be seen in migraine or may be psychogenic.

- **Vertigo:** It is the sensation of rotation of the surrounding with respect to the person or person with respect to the surroundings. Onset, duration, progression, severity, associated features, aggravating factors, and relieving factors should be documented. Vertigo lasting for a few seconds to minutes is seen in benign positional paroxysmal vertigo (BPPV). Vertigo lasting more than 20 minutes is typically seen in Ménière's disease. Vertigo lasting for a longer duration may be seen in labyrinthitis or vestibular neuronitis.

Pearl

The Tullio phenomenon is a condition where very loud sound causes vertigo. This is seen in a labyrinthine fistula.

- **Blocked sensation or fullness in the ear:** It may occur due to wax, foreign body, eustachian tube dysfunction, or Ménière's disease.
- **Itching in the ear:** It is commonly seen in otomycosis. It may also be seen in atopic dermatitis, allergy, and with cerumen.

Past History

A history of similar complaints in the past has to be noted along with the treatment received. Previous history of surgery should be noted. Any comorbidities like diabetes, hypertension, asthma, tuberculosis (can involve the middle ear or the medications for tuberculosis can affect hearing and balance), and allergy should be documented.

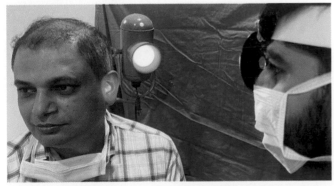

Fig. 3.1   Bull's eye lamp in use with light focused on the ear.

Personal History

Diet, lifestyle, sleep, bowel and bladder habits, and menstrual history should be documented in this section. Any habits (smoking, drinking, tobacco chewing) also should be noted. Aural hygiene, that is, the use of ear buds and water entering the ear during bathing or swimming especially in chronic otitis media and certain forms of otitis externa, can be documented here or in the history of presenting illness.

Family History

History of similar complaints in the family and history of contact (in case of infectious diseases) should be noted in this section. Certain types of hearing loss can be hereditary.

Birth/Obstetric History

In children, an additional note should be made regarding any significant events during the pre-, peri-, and postnatal period. History of infection and drug use during gestation should be noted. This would be important for possible early screening for hearing loss.

Examination of the Ear

The patient is seated upright in front of the examiner.

■ Light Sources for Examination

A head mirror and a Bull's eye lamp can be used for examination. Other light sources include headlamps, headlights, and otoscopes.

Bull's Eye Lamp

It consists of a cylindrical metal container with vents. A 100-W bulb is inside and is the source of light. The front has an opening that has a biconvex mirror (**Fig. 3.1**). The lamp is kept 30 cm behind the patient's left ear. When switched on, the light is focused onto a head mirror, which is concave. The diameter of the mirror is 89 mm and it has a circular opening in the center, which is 19 mm in diameter. The focal length of the mirror is 25 cm. The plastic head band helps adjust and fit to the size of the head. The head mirror is placed over the right eye such that it touches the nose. To focus, one needs to close the left eye and see with the right eye through the opening in the mirror. Once focused, both eyes are used for visualization (**Fig. 3.2**).

Headlamp

The headlamp is easy to use, mobile, and provides adequate illumination (**Fig. 3.3**). A 9-W bulb placed in front of a flexible concave mirror, supported by a plastic headband. The patient is seated in front of the examiner. The headlamp is

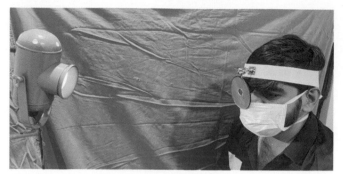

Fig. 3.2 Head mirror for light reflection.

worn such that the bulb and the mirror lie in the midline. The position is adjusted to focus on the area of interest.

Headlight

A headlight is preferred. It is attached to a cold light source, which may be halogen or light-emitting diode (LED). The headlight that can be recharged is easily portable and convenient to use (**Fig. 3.4**).

In addition, an otoscope is also used for visualization of the external auditory canal and tympanic membrane (**Fig. 3.5**).

There are seven aspects to be examined in the ear. These include the following:

- Examination of the pinna, preauricular area, and postauricular area.
- Examination of the external auditory canal.
- Examination of the tympanic membrane.
- Assessment of hearing.
- Assessment of equilibrium.
- Facial nerve examination.
- Examination of the eustachian tube.

■ Examination of the Pinna, Preauricular Area, and Postauricular Area

- **Pinna or auricle:**
  - *Size*: Note whether the pinna is normal, large (macrotia), or small (microtia).
  - *Shape*: Look for congenital abnormalities or acquired conditions like cauliflower ear.
  - *Position*: Developmentally, the ear can be more anteriorly rotated or this can occur following a surgery.
  - The presence of swelling or discoloration should be documented. A reddish swollen tender pinna is noted in hematoma auris and perichondritis. A non-inflamed fluctuant swelling in the upper part of the pinna may be suggestive of a pseudocyst. A sebaceous cyst typically has a punctum. Keloids are firm lesions that appear over ear-piercing sites. Malignant tumors such as squamous cell carcinoma, basal cell carcinoma, and malignant melanoma may involve the pinna.

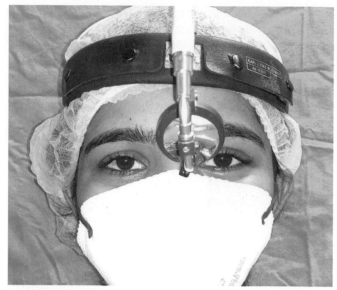

Fig. 3.3 Technique of donning the headlamp.

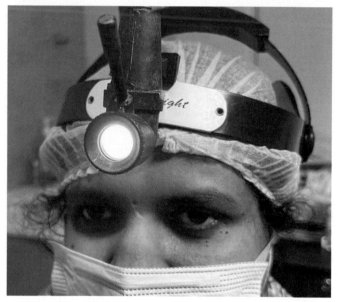

Fig. 3.4 Headlight.

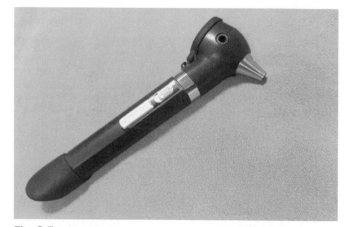

Fig. 3.5 Otoscope.

– *Tragal tenderness:* Digital pressure is applied over the tragus. Tenderness is pathognomonic of acute localized otitis externa (furuncle), involving the anterior canal wall or roof. In a furuncle involving the posterior canal wall, pulling the pinna during examination would be painful (**Fig. 3.6**).

Pearl

- Macrotia: Larger than an average pinna.
- Microtia: Smaller than an average pinna.
- Anotia: Absence of the pinna.
- Polyotia: Accessory pinnae.
- Cryptotia: The upper part of the pinna is hidden.
- Lop ear: Upper helix folded over the lower part of the pinna.
- Bat ear: Abnormally protruded pinna.

- **Preauricular area:**
  - Scars in this region may be due to an endaural incision, an incision for parotidectomy, or prior removal of lesions like preauricular sinus.
  - Preauricular tags are nonfunctional appendages.
  - Failure of fusion of hillocks of His during development may result in preauricular, sinus, or fistula, with or without discharge.
  - Preauricular lymph nodes may be enlarged due to infection of the conjunctiva, eyelids, scalp, and skin of the cheek.
  - One should also check for tenderness in the temporomandibular joint and also note any painful movements on making the patient open and close the mouth.
  - If there is a swelling in this region, examination should include inspection and palpation.
- **Postauricular area:**
  - Lymphadenopathy may occur due to scalp infection or otitis externa.
  - The normal mastoid on palpation is not smooth but rough or bosselated. The mastoid becomes smooth with ironed feel in mastoiditis.
  - Scar may be indicative of previous ear surgery.
  - Postauricular fistula (mastoid cutaneous) may occur as a consequence of mastoiditis.
  - *Mastoid tenderness* is elicited by applying pressure at three points, that is, the cymba concha, midpoint of the posterior border of the mastoid, and mastoid tip. Mastoid tenderness is a sign of mastoiditis (**Fig. 3.7**).
  - A swelling seen in the mastoid area should be described under the heading of inspection and palpation.
  - Note the condition of the postauricular groove. It can get obliterated in the mastoid abscess.

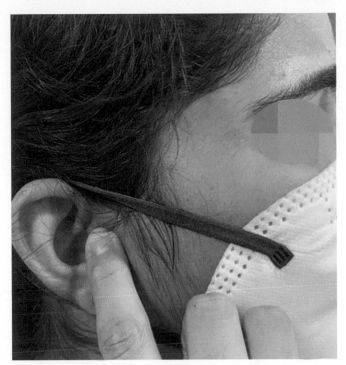

Fig. 3.6 Demonstration of tragal tenderness.

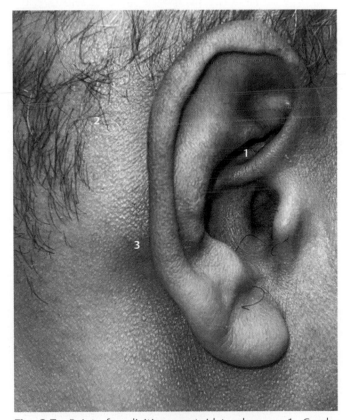

Fig. 3.7 Points for eliciting mastoid tenderness. 1. Cymba concha. 2. Along the midpoint of the posterior border of the mastoid bone. 3. The tip of the mastoid.

■ Examination of the External Auditory Canal

- As the external auditory canal has a sigmoid curvature, complete visualization requires retraction of the pinna in an *upward*, *backward*, and *lateral* direction. In children, the direction is downward and laterally.
- Examination should be initially without the speculum and then with the speculum.
- The speculum should snugly fit the canal. A small speculum would go deeper causing pain, and also the field of view is narrow. A larger speculum may press on the skin, which may fold into the view of the speculum, reducing visualization.
- Earwax (cerumen) appears as a brownish to black, dry or wet blob in the external auditory canal. It may be soft or hard.
- Otitis externa causes swelling of the canal, with or without discharge.
- In otomycosis or fungal infection of the external auditory canal, the discharge appears as gray, black, or white masses of spores or hyphae (depending on the type of fungus).
- Foreign bodies such as cotton balls, beads, and insects may be noted in the canal.
- Granulation tissue appears as pinkish to red masses as a result of chronic infection or trauma.

■ Examination of the Tympanic Membrane

- The tympanic membrane (eardrum) appears as a pearly while structure at the medial aspect of the ear canal (**Fig. 3.8**).
- The lower three-fourths is called *pars tensa*, and the upper one-fourth is called *pars flaccida* (Shrapnell's membrane).
- It is divided into four quadrants by an imaginary vertical line drawn through the handle of the malleus and another line perpendicular to it at the umbo level.
- *Cone of light* is a standard feature observed in the antero-inferior quadrant due to the reflection of light coming from the headlamp or the otoscope.
- Fluid-filled blebs (myringitis bullosa) or granulation tissue (myringitis granulosa) may be seen on the tympanic membrane.
- The tympanic membrane is initially congested in acute otitis media. It then starts bulging outward, and a perforation with pulsatile discharge appears.
- Tympanic membrane perforation or retraction pocket occurs in chronic otitis media.
- Tympanic membrane perforation involving the pars tensa may be *central* when it does not involve the annulus or *marginal* when the annulus is involved. Central perforation is seen in the tubotympanic (mucosal) type of chronic otitis media, whereas marginal perforation

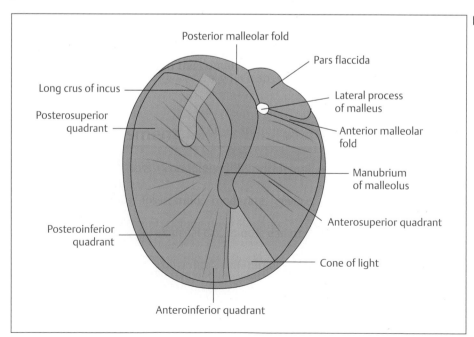

Fig. 3.8 Normal tympanic membrane.

is seen in the atticoantral (squamosal) type of chronic otitis media.

- Attic retraction or perforation occurs in the atticoantral type of chronic otitis media.
- Fluid levels may be noted behind the intact tympanic membrane or retraction may be seen in serous otitis media.
- A thickened whitish plaque may be seen medial to the tympanic membrane in tympanosclerosis.
- The mobility of the tympanic membrane should be checked especially in a retracted tympanic membrane, that is, by Valsalva maneuver, Toynbee maneuver, or Siegelization. It should be avoided, although in a recently healed perforation or in a thinned-out membrane.

Differential diagnosis of white patch on the tympanic membrane includes the following:
- Tympanosclerosis.
- Otomycosis.
- Dried ear drops.
- Prior surgery with placement of cartilage.
- Underlying congenital cholesteatoma.

■ Assessment of Hearing

The examiner must pay close attention to the patient's response during the introduction, that is, whether the patient raises the voice or speaks softly, and the use of hearing aid (**Figs. 3.9, 3.10, 3.11,** and **3.12**). The commonly performed tuning fork tests are Rinne, Weber, and absolute

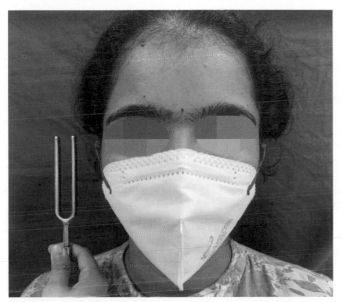

Fig. 3.9　Rinne's test: Testing air conduction.

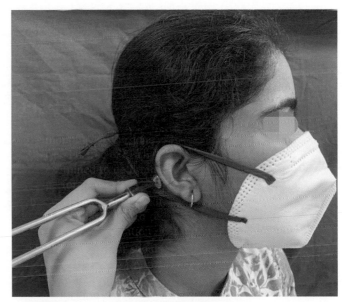

Fig. 3.10　Rinne's test: Testing bone conduction.

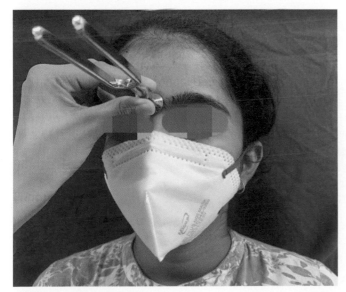

Fig. 3.11　Weber's test.

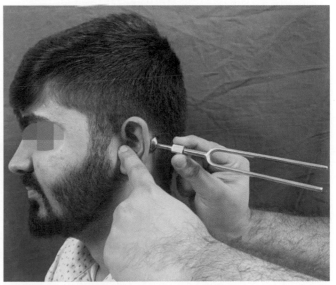

Fig. 3.12　Absolute bone conduction (ABC) test.

bone conduction or ABC. These are described in detail in Chapter 4 "Assessment of Hearing."

The interpretations of the tuning fork tests are outlined in **Tables 3.1** and **3.2**.

■ Assessment of Equilibrium

Spontaneous Nystagmus

The patient is seated facing the examiner. The examiner holds the index finger 45 cm away from the patient in the central position and moves the finger in vertical and horizontal directions, not exceeding 30 degrees from the center, to evade gaze nystagmus. Spontaneous nystagmus is suggestive of organic pathology. Nystagmus due to vestibular lesion can be suppressed by optic fixation, that is, by fixing gaze at a particular point. It may be further heightened by testing in a dark room or by using Frenzel glasses.

Fistula Test

The ear canal is subjected to pressure changes, stimulating the labyrinth, inducing nystagmus or vertigo. Alternating tragal pressure toward the canal is applied, or a Siegel speculum is used. Normally, the labyrinth is not stimulated. This is a *negative fistula test*. In cases of cholesteatoma eroding the lateral semicircular canal, fenestration surgery, post-stapedotomy fistula, or round window membrane rupture, the labyrinth is stimulated. This is a *positive fistula test*.

False-Positive Fistula Test

This may occur in Ménière's disease and congenital syphilis. Fibrous bands connect the footplate of the stapes and the macula of the utricle in Ménière's disease. The footplate of the stapes is hypermobile in congenital syphilis. When the footplate moves, the macula is stimulated, leading to a false-positive test.

False-Negative Fistula Test

The patient does not develop vertigo or nystagmus despite a labyrinthine fistula as a cholesteatoma is covering it. It can also occur when the labyrinth is not functioning, that is, dead labyrinth (end stage of labyrinthitis).

Other Tests

Tests like Romberg's test, Unterberger's test, gait, dysdiadochokinesia, and dysmetria are done when complications are suspected.

■ Facial Nerve Examination

Facial nerve function may be affected in diseases of the ear such as chronic otitis media, malignant otitis externa, herpes zoster oticus, fracture of the temporal bone, and benign and malignant tumors of the external or middle ear.

Testing the Peripheral Branches of the Facial Nerve

The facial nerve has five peripheral branches that supply muscles of facial expression (**Table 3.3**).

Figs. 3.13, 3.14, 3.15, 3.16, and **3.17** demonstrate the testing of the various muscles of facial expression.

Otoscopy

- The external auditory canal and tympanic membrane are better visualized using an otoscope, which magnifies two times.

Table 3.1 Tuning fork tests and degree of hearing loss

Tuning fork	Degree of conductive hearing loss	Air–bone gap
At 256 Hz, Rinne negative	Mild	15–30 dB
At 512 Hz, Rinne negative	Moderate	30–45 dB
At 1,024 Hz, Rinne negative	Severe	45–60 dB

Table 3.2 Interpretation of the various tests and the types of hearing loss

Tuning fork test	Normal	Conductive hearing loss	Sensorineural hearing loss
Rinne	Positive	Negative	Positive
Weber	Not lateralized	Lateralized to the poorer ear	Lateralized to the better ear
Absolute bone conduction (ABC)	Same as the examiner	Same as the examiner	Shortened
Schwabach	Same as the examiner	Lengthened	Shortened
Bing	Positive	Negative	Positive
Gelle	Positive	Negative	Positive

Table 3.3 Action of individual muscles supplied by the facial nerve

Peripheral branch	Muscle	How to test	Signs of facial nerve palsy
Temporal	Frontalis	Looking up or raising the eyebrows	Asymmetry during forehead wrinkling
Zygomatic	Orbicularis oculi	Close eyes tightly	Incomplete eyelid closure
Buccal	Buccinator	Blowing out the cheeks with the mouth closed	Inability to blow out the cheeks due to air escape from the affected side
Mandibular	Zygomaticus major	Smiling	Deviation of the angle of the mouth to the unaffected side
Cervical	Platysma	Clenching the teeth and depressing the angles of the mouth	Folds of the platysma seen in the neck

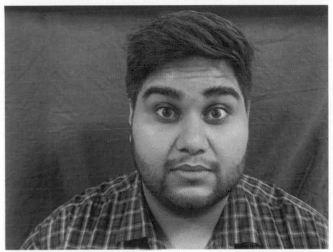

Fig. 3.13 Testing the temporal branch of the facial nerve.

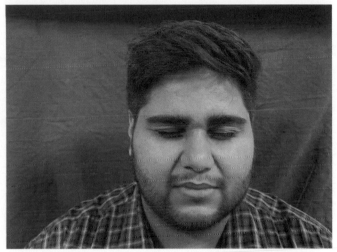

Fig. 3.14 Testing the zygomatic branch of the facial nerve.

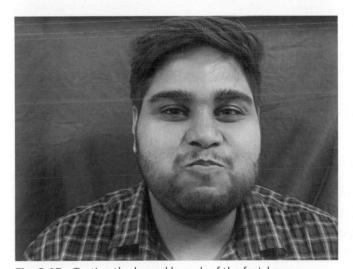

Fig. 3.15 Testing the buccal branch of the facial nerve.

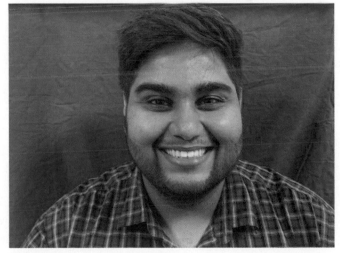

Fig. 3.16 Testing the mandibular branch of the facial nerve.

- The patient is seated in front of the examiner, with the affected ear facing the examiner.
- An appropriately sized aural speculum is attached to the otoscope before insertion.
- The pinna is retracted upward, backward, and outward.

- The otoscope is held like a pen, using the little finger as the pivot in front of the ear (zygoma) to prevent trauma if the patient turns/moves abruptly (**Fig. 3.18**).
- The external auditory canal and tympanic membrane are examined.

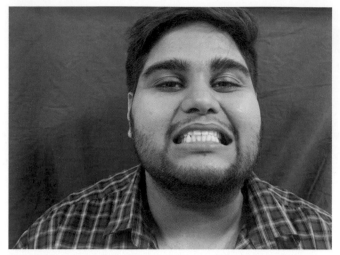

Fig. 3.17 Testing the cervical branch of the facial nerve.

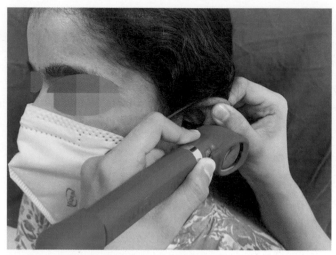

Fig. 3.18 Otoscopic examination of the ear.

- Pneumatic otoscopy may be performed to assess the mobility of the tympanic membrane.
- In addition, the otoscope may be used in infants or children for examination of the nasal cavities.

■ Pneumatic Otoscopy for Examination of the Eustachian Tube

- This technique is used to assess the mobility of the tympanic membrane.
- It may be performed either using an otoscope with pneumatic attachment or by using Siegel's speculum attached to an aural speculum.
- Alternatively, Valsalva maneuver may be employed to assess the mobility of the tympanic membrane (**Fig. 3.19**).

Indications

- Suspected serous otitis media.
- Adhesive otitis media.
- Atelectasis.

Contraindications

- The presuppurative stage of acute otitis media.

Technique

- No anesthesia is required.
- The otoscope with an appropriate-sized aural speculum is held focusing on the tympanic membrane, ensuring a good seal in the external auditory canal.
- The bulb of the pneumatic attachment is pressed to create positive pressure over the tympanic membrane. A mobile tympanic membrane moves *inward* with *positive* pressure.

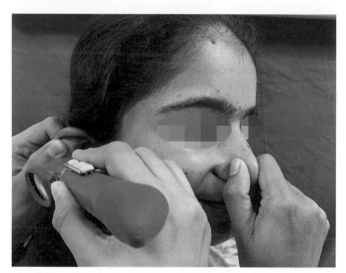

Fig. 3.19 Pneumatic otoscopy by Valsalva maneuver.

- The bulb of the pneumatic attachment is released to create negative pressure over the tympanic membrane. A mobile tympanic membrane moves *outward* with *negative* pressure.
- Mobility may be restricted in thickened tympanic membrane and serous otitis media.
- An air-fluid level may also be noted medial to the tympanic membrane, suggestive of serous otitis media.

Complications

- Ear discomfort.
- Giddiness, nausea, and vomiting (due to vestibular stimulation).
- Tympanic membrane perforation, especially in a thinned-out membrane.
- Ossicular discontinuity (**Video 3.1**).

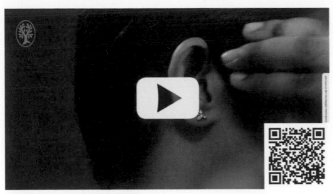

Video 3.1 Examination of ear.

Otomicroscopy

The external auditory canal and tympanic membrane may also be visualized in the outpatient setup using an operating microscope. With good illumination and magnification for visualization, procedures can be done with both hands for diagnostic and therapeutic purposes (**Fig. 3.20**).

Indications

- Earwax removal.
- Foreign body extraction.
- Removal of debris or epithelial flakes.
- Aural toilet.
- To confirm the presence or absence of perforation.
- For taking discharge samples for culture and sensitivity.

Technique

- The patient lies supine with the affected ear upward.
- The microscope is maneuvered into position to visualize and focus the ear canal and tympanic membrane.
- An appropriate-sized aural speculum is used for an unobstructed view.
- The required diagnostic examination or therapeutic intervention is performed.

Complications

- Injury to the external auditory canal or tympanic membrane due to instrumentation.
- Giddiness during suction cleaning.
- Syncopal attack.

Syringing

Syringing is a technique used to clear the external auditory canal of debris, cerumen, discharge, or foreign body (**Figs. 3.21** and **3.22**).

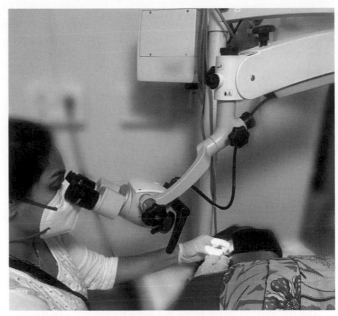

Fig. 3.20 Technique of otomicroscopy.

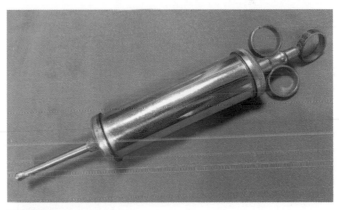

Fig. 3.21 Aural syringe.

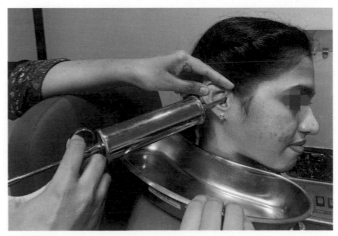

Fig. 3.22 Demonstration of syringing of the ear.

Indications

- Earwax (cerumen).
- Inorganic foreign body.
- Otomycosis.
- Any other debris.

Contraindications

- Acute or chronic otitis media.
- Otitis externa.
- Organic foreign body.
- Thinned out tympanic membrane.
- Tympanic membrane perforation.

Technique

- The patient is seated in front of the examiner with the head tilted to the opposite side.
- A protective apron is worn by the patient.
- The patient is asked to hold a kidney tray below the ear to be syringed to collect the fluid returning from the ear and to tilt the ear over the kidney tray (**Video 3.2**).
- The pinna is retracted upward, backward, and outward.
- Normal saline at room temperature is used for syringing. The syringe is directed toward the posterosuperior part of the ear canal.
- The jet of saline dislodges the contents of the ear canal and is flushed out into the kidney tray.
- The ear canal and tympanic membrane are inspected. Once the contents are out, dry mopping of the canal is done using cotton swab.

Complications

- Injury to the external auditory canal.
- Injury to the tympanic membrane.
- Bleeding.
- Vertigo.
- Syncope.

■ Topical Medication Instillation

Instillation of medications into the external auditory canal is performed for conditions such as impacted cerumen, otitis media, and otitis externa.

Indications

- Impacted hard earwax (cerumen).
- Chronic otitis media.
- Otomycosis.
- Otitis externa.
- Topical anesthesia.
- Immobilization of live insect (foreign body).

Contraindications

In a perforated tympanic membrane, antibiotic with steroid ear drops may be used. Other drops may cause discomfort or infection.

Types of Topical Ear Medications

- Antibiotics with/without steroids.
- Analgesics.
- Antifungals.
- Wax solvents.
- Turpentine oil.
- Steroids.

Technique

- The patient is either seated in front of the examiner with the affected ear facing upward or supine with the affected ear upward (**Fig. 3.23**).
- Following hand hygiene, the pinna is retracted upward, backward, and outward.
- The dropper of the bottle is held just above the opening of the external auditory canal, avoiding contact of the tip of the bottle with canal skin.

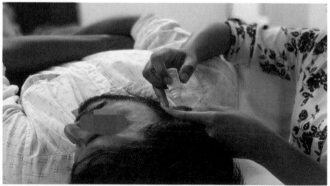

Video 3.2 Examination under microscope and ear syringing.

Fig. 3.23 Demonstration of instillation of ear drops.

- The bottle is squeezed to instil the prescribed number of drops.
- The pinna is released and the patient remains in the same position for 3 to 5 minutes.
- The tragus is inermittently rubbed against the opening of the canal (*tragal pumping*). In doing so, it facilitates the inward movement of the ear drops.
- The patient returns to the normal position; excess medicine dripping out of the ear is wiped away.
- The bottle is recapped ensuring that the bottle tip is untouched.

Complications

- Ototoxicity.
- Dependency.
- Chronic dermatitis of ear canal.
- Long-term use of steroid or quinolones drops can cause otomycosis.

Points to Ponder

- A clear, concise history is essential to arrive at a provisional diagnosis in most ear conditions.
- A good light source is necessary to examine the ear. It can be in the form of a Bull's eye lamp and mirror, headlamp, or headlight.
- Examination of the ear should follow the correct sequence of examination, which is as follows: pinna, preauricular region, postauricular region, external auditory canal, tympanic membrane, tuning fork tests, facial nerve function, and vestibular testing when necessary.
- Otomicroscopy is performed to confirm the otoscopic findings and also to carry out various procedures in the ear.
- Syringing is commonly performed to remove wax.
- During ear drop instillation, the tragus is pushed inward to allow the drops to enter the deeper parts of the meatus.

Case-Based Question

1. **An elderly woman presented with a 2-month history of left ear discharge. It was intermittent but profuse in quantity. Otoscopic ear examination revealed mucopurulent discharge in the external auditory canal. The tympanic membrane could not be visualized.**

   a. What is the next step in the examination if there is profuse discharge?

   b. Can syringing be carried out to remove the discharge?

   c. How will you explain the instillation of ear drops to the patient?

   Answers

   a. Otomicroscopic examination of the ear to remove the discharge by suction. If a microscope is not available, dry mopping can be done with a cotton wool carrier. Once the canal is free of discharge, the tympanic membrane can be examined to determine the presence, site, and size of the perforation.

   b. Syringing is contraindicated in patients with perforation. In this case, due to the mucopurulent nature of the discharge, a perforation can be suspected.

   c. The affected ear should be up. The patient lies on one side and the drops are instilled without the tip touching the canal. The drops are then pushed into the canal by applying pressure on the tragus (tragal pumping). The patient then lies in that position for 3 to 5 minutes.

Frequently Asked Questions

1. What are the light sources available for examination of the ear?

2. What are the points to be noted during the postauricular examination?

3. Describe Rinne's test. How do you interpret it?

4. What is Weber's test? How do you perform this?

5. What is the fistula test?

6. What is the correct technique of instilling ear drops?

7. What are the contraindications for syringing of the ear?

Endnote

Since ancient times, a syringe with a piston was regarded as an ideal tool for removing discharge from the ear. Celsus (first century AD) mentioned that ear discharge and foreign bodies can be removed from the ear canal with syringe and water. Gradually, it fell into disrepute for cleaning the ear. It was recommended by barber surgeons only for irrigating wounds and giving enemas. It was only in the early 19th century that Itard (1821), in France, started describing ear syringing for removal of hard wax. Then, Schmalz, in 1827, in Germany described the use of a kidney-shaped bowl for catching the fluid from the ear.

4 Assessment of Hearing

Deepalakshmi Tanthry

The competencies covered in this chapter are as follows:

EN2.4 Demonstrate the correct technique of performance and interpret the tuning fork tests.

EN2.8 Demonstrate the correct technique to perform and interpret pure tone audiogram and impedance audiogram.

EN4.16 Observe and describe the indications for and steps involved in the performance of pure tone audiometry.

EN4.17 Enumerate the indications and interpret the results of an audiogram.

PY10.16 Describe the hearing tests.

Introduction

Hearing loss refers to total or partial inability to hear sounds. It can be of three types:

- **Conductive hearing loss:** Any disease affecting the traveling of sound waves through the external ear, tympanic membrane, or ossicular chain leads to conductive type of hearing loss. The etiology may be in the external ear (cerumen, infections, exostoses, and tumors) and/or the middle ear (fluid, chronic otitis media, tympanosclerosis, trauma, and tumors).
- **Sensorineural hearing loss:** Any disease affecting the cochlea (sensory), and the auditory nerve and its connections (neural) type. Retrocochlear type of hearing loss is sensorineural involving the auditory nerve.
- **Mixed type of hearing loss:** It refers to hearing loss caused by a defect in both the conductive and sensorineural components.

Aims of Assessment

- Type of hearing loss: conductive, sensorineural, or mixed.
- Degree of hearing loss: mild, moderate, severe, or profound.
- Localization of disease: external ear, middle ear, or inner ear.
- Cause of hearing loss: congenital, inflammatory, traumatic, and tumors.

Hearing loss can be assessed clinically or by audiometric tests.

The intensity of sound in decibels for various environmental noise is given in **Box 4.1**.

Clinical Tests of Hearing

■ Speech Test

It is a simple, nonstandardized screening test to check the ability of a person to hear words without any visual assistance. The subject is asked to repeat five words spoken loudly at a distance of around 5 m. The *whisper (whispered voice) test* involves the occlusion of the patient's nontest ear and whispering sounds at different levels of loudness (soft, medium, and loud voices) from a distance of 2 feet from the test ear. It may indicate a hearing loss of 20 dB if not perceived. Finger friction test, watch test, and ballpoint click tests are few other clinical tests (**Fig. 4.1**).

■ Tuning Fork Tests

The tuning fork (**Fig. 4.2**), a two-pronged fork made of steel or aluminum, is widely used to clinically quantify and qualify hearing loss. When set into vibration by striking against

Box 4.1 Intensity of sound in decibels for various environmental noise	
Leaves fluttering:	20 dB
Normal speech:	60 dB
Traffic:	60 to 100 dB
Airplane:	120 dB
Pain threshold:	120 to 140 dB

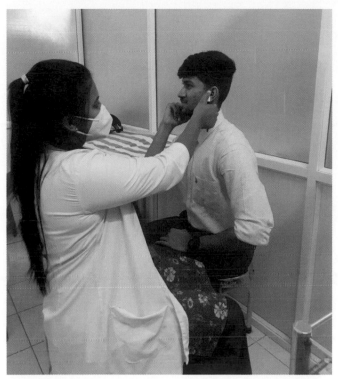

Fig. 4.1 Ballpoint click test.

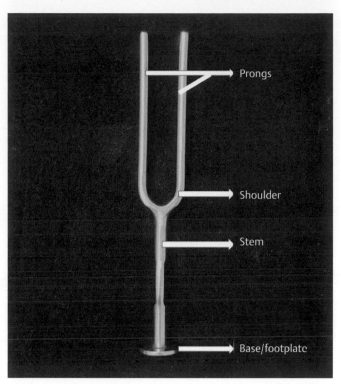

Fig. 4.2 Tuning fork and parts.

a firm or resilient surface, it emits a pure tone, a stimulus that is of a single frequency, the pitch of which depends on the length and mass of the two prongs. The tuning fork consists of two prongs (or tines), a stem, and a foot piece. It is used to differentiate between conductive and sensorineural hearing loss. The different frequencies are 128, 256, 512, 1,024, and 2,048 Hz. Routinely, 256, 512, and 1,024 Hz are used in ear, nose, and throat (ENT) practice.

Pearl

The tuning fork was invented by a British musician John Shore in 1711. It was introduced in the field of otology by E. Schmalz.

The prerequisites for conducting tuning fork tests are essentially a quiet room, tuning forks (256, 512, and 1,024 Hz), and a stool. After the initial examination of the ear, the patient is informed about the procedure.

Rinne's Test

Principle

It is a highly sensitive test. It compares air conduction (AC) and bone conduction (BC). AC is the sound transmitted through the tympanic membrane and middle ear ossicles to the cochlea. In conductive hearing loss sounds, AC will be decreased. BC is when the cochlea is directly stimulated

by the vibrations conducted through the skull bypassing the external and middle ear. BC measures only the cochlear function. In sensory hearing loss, sounds delivered via BC will be decreased.

Method

Threshold method: The vibrating end of the tuning fork is set into motion by striking the prongs at the junction of the upper one-third and lower two-thirds against a firm surface (**Figs. 4.3** and **4.4**). The vibrating tuning fork's foot piece is then placed on the mastoid process just above and behind the external auditory canal. The foot piece should be placed on the skin with no intervening hair. The examiner's fingers or the patient's pinna should not be in contact with the prongs. The patient is asked to indicate when the sound disappears. The tuning fork is then held 2 cm away from the external auditory canal such that both the prongs vibrate parallel to the acoustic axis. If the patient still perceives sound, it means AC is better than BC.

Loudness method: Alternatively, the vibrating tuning fork is kept on the mastoid and then in front of the ear canal. The patient is asked which is louder, that is, over the mastoid or in front of the pinna.

Interpretation

Rinne's test is positive when AC is better than BC. It is negative when BC is greater than AC.

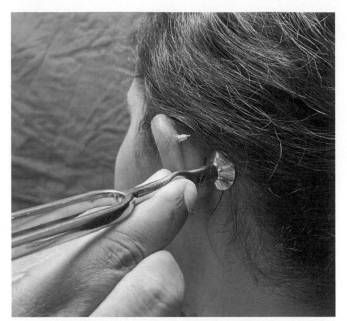

Fig. 4.3 Rinne's test for bone conduction (BC).

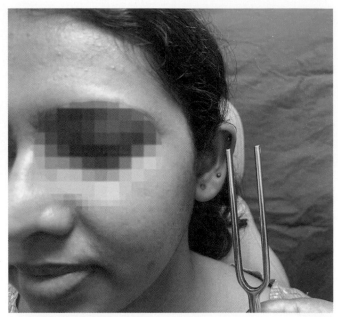

Fig. 4.4 Rinne's test for air conduction (AC).

False-negative Rinne's test is seen in severe unilateral sensorineural hearing loss due to sound being transmitted from the test ear to the nontest ear by BC. The patient perceives this BC and presumes it as being heard in the test ear. The AC is absent and response of BC is due to transcranial transmission from the opposite ear.

Reduced positive Rinne's test is when AC is better than BC but both are reduced. This is seen in sensorineural hearing loss.

Equivocal Rinne's test is when AC and BC are the same and is seen in mild conductive hearing loss.

Weber's Test

Principle

In purely unilateral, conductive hearing loss, there is increased ability to hear BC sounds better because of two reasons: Masking effect and occlusion effect.

Method

A vibrating tuning fork of 512 Hz is placed in the middle of the forehead or the vertex. The patient is asked whether sound is heard louder in one ear, not heard in either ear, or heard equally, that is, whether there is lateralization to one ear or it is central. Sound travels directly via the bone to the cochlea. Normally, sound is heard equally in both ears (**Fig. 4.5**).

Inference

Tone is lateralized to the affected ear in conductive hearing loss. This occurs due to reduced ambient sound in the

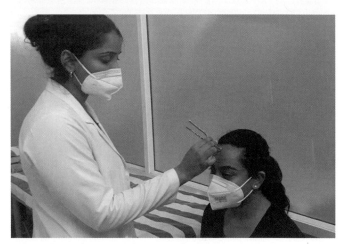

Fig. 4.5 Weber's test being performed.

affected ear, which is known as the *masking effect*. There is also less or absent dissipation of low-frequency sounds through the ear canal that usually occurs in normal ears. This is called the *occlusion effect*. The tone is heard better in the normal ear when there is sensorineural loss in the affected ear.

The tone is heard better in the worse ear in bilateral conductive hearing loss. The tone is heard better in the normal ear when there is mixed hearing loss in the affected ear.

Pearl

An ideal tuning fork for Weber's test is one that has a long tone decay (maintains its tone for a long time after being struck) and does not cause bone vibration. So a tuning fork of 512 Hz is used.

Schwabach's Test

Principle

The test compares the patient's hearing with that of the examiner, provided the examiner's hearing is normal.

Procedure

The vibrating tuning fork is placed over the mastoid of the patient. Once he or she indicates that sound is not heard, the examiner places the tuning fork on his or her mastoid (without occlusion of the meatus). Vibratory energy of the tones of the fork decreases overtime, making the tones softer. The patient should indicate whether the tone is heard or not each time. When the patient no longer hears the tone, the examiner immediately places the stem behind his or her own ear and, using a watch, notes the number of seconds the tone is audible after the patient stops hearing it.

Inference

In normal Schwabach, both the patient and examiner stop hearing the tone emitted by the fork at the same time, which means the patient has normal BC. Diminished Schwabach is when the patient stops hearing the sound before the examiner. The patient's BC is impaired in that ear, that is, the patient has sensorineural hearing loss. Prolonged Schwabach is when the patient hears the sound longer than the examiner. Due to conductive hearing loss in that ear, the ambient sound is not heard, which allows for the longer duration of perception of the sound.

Absolute Bone Conduction (Modified Schwabach Test)

The patient's BC is compared with that of the examiner (assuming that he or she has a normal hearing). The vibrating tuning fork is placed on the mastoid. The external auditory canal occluded by pressing the tragus inward, to prevent ambient noise entering through the AC route. Once the patient indicates that the sound is not heard, the tuning fork is placed on the examiner's mastoid with occlusion of the ear canal by pressing the tragus inward (**Fig. 4.6**).

Inference

In normal conditions, the BC of the patient is equal to that of the examiner. It is reduced in sensorineural hearing loss, that is, BC of the patient is reduced when compared to the examiner. (The examiner will hear the sound after the patient stops hearing it.)

Pearl

The interpretation as to the type and side of hearing loss is better when Weber's test, Rinne's test, and absolute bone conduction (ABC) are done. Weber's test can detect a difference of 3 to 5 dB between the two ears.

Gelle's Test

This test examines the effect of increased air pressure in the ear canal. It is performed by placing a vibrating tuning fork over the mastoid. The pressure in the external auditory canal is increased using a Siegel speculum, which pushes the tympanic membrane and ossicles inward. This raises the intralabyrinthine pressure and causes immobility of the basilar membrane. Due to relative fixity, hearing is reduced. No change in hearing is noted when the ossicles are fixed as in otosclerosis.

Inference

Gelle's test is positive in normal hearing and sensorineural hearing loss. The test is negative when there is fixity of the ossicular chain.

Bing Test

Procedure

The vibrating tuning fork is placed on the mastoid of the patient while the examiner alternatively closes and opens the ear canal by pressing the tragus inward.

Inference

The test is positive in normal hearing or sensorineural hearing loss. The individual will hear louder when the canal is occluded, and softer when the canal is open. The test is negative in conductive hearing loss where there will be no change.

■ Tuning Fork Tests for Malingering

Synonyms of malingering include functional hearing loss, nonorganic disease, pseudohypoacusis, and feigning deafness.

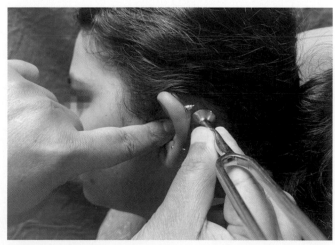

Fig. 4.6 Modified Schwabach's test being performed with finger pressing the tragus inward.

Malingering should be considered when the person suddenly presents with no relevant history, shows a sense of urgency, or shows behavioral exaggeration. There will be discrepancy in the hearing evaluation and observed behavior of the person. It is usually done for benefits like compensation or change of place or occupation.

Stenger's Test

Principle

The test is based on Stenger's (fused image) phenomenon. When a person is presented with the same intensity of sound in both ears, he will hear a single sound. The sound will be heard in the ear in which the intensity is more or when the sound is closer to the ear.

Procedure

Two tuning forks with a frequency of 512 Hz are kept equidistantly from both ears. The patient should be able to hear equally well on either side. In malingering, when the tuning fork is moved closer to the affected ear, the patient denies hearing on the normal side too.

Teal's Test

Procedure

A vibrating tuning fork is placed over the mastoid process of the "affected" ear. The patient accepts to hear it. Then the patient is blindfolded, and a nonvibrating tuning fork is placed on the mastoid process. The malingering patient claims to hear the sound.

Chimani–Moos Test

It is a variation of Weber's test. In Weber's test, the patient hears better in the occluded ear. In malingering, the patient will not accept hearing better in the occluded ear.

■ Audiometric Tests

Pure tone audiometry (PTA) is a commonly used test to measure the auditory sensitivity of a patient. An audiometer is an electronic device that produces pure tones, the intensity of which can be increased or decreased in 5-db steps. Frequency is the number of vibrations per second documented in cycles per second or hertz (Hz). The range of hearing for the human ear in frequencies is from 16 Hz to 20 kHz. The speech frequency ranges from 125 to 3,000 Hz. In audiometry, the test can be done from 125 Hz to 8 kHz in octaves. Mid-octaves are checked only if the hearing between two octaves is more than 20 dB. High frequencies, those above 2 kHz, are useful for speech discrimination.

Principle

An object that vibrates in a fixed single frequency creates sound waves that will form a sinusoidal wave pattern known as sine wave. This sound sensation formed by a sine wave is called a pure tone. Pure tones are delivered to the ear by AC and BC at various frequencies. PTA uses both AC and BC; therefore, the type of loss is identified by reduction in BC (sensorineural loss), an air–bone (A-B) gap (conductive loss), or both (mixed loss).

> **Pearl**
>
> Auditory threshold is defined as the lowest signal intensity at which the signal is identified 50% of the time. Decibel is the unit to measure the intensity of sound.

Role of Audiometry

When compared to tuning fork tests, audiometry is a qualitative and quantitative test.

Advantages of PTA:
- To assess the type of hearing loss: Conductive, sensory, and neural.
- To assess the degree of hearing loss: Mild, moderate, severe, or profound.
- It is a recorded document of hearing (audiogram) that can be used for handicap certificates.
- It is a medicolegal document.
- PTA can be used to check for postoperative improvement or deterioration of hearing.
- It is used for prescribing a hearing aid.
- It will help document the speech reception threshold. There is no ambient sound as it is done in a sound-treated room. The masking when used is controlled.

> **Pearl**
>
> In the equal loudness contour (Fletcher–Munson curve), it is noted that the ear is more sensitive at mid-frequencies and least at the extremes. This concept is used in manufacturing an audiometer where the 0-dB dial setting will vary depending on frequency. Regular calibration of the audiometer has to be done.

Procedure: Modified Hughson–Westlake Method

The patient is seated comfortably in a soundproof room. This is to avoid ambient sound (**Fig. 4.7**).

The parts of the audiometer include the following:
- A pure tone generator.
- Amplifier.
- Frequency selector switch (hertz).
- Intensity dial (in decibels).
- Interrupter.

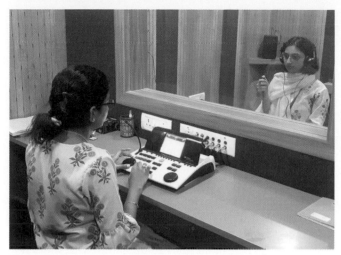

Fig. 4.7 Pure tone audiometry being performed.

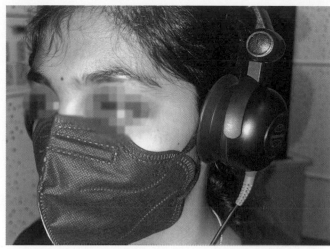

Fig. 4.8 Pure tone audiometry: Air conduction being tested.

- Masking dial.
- Headphones.
- BC vibrator.
- Provisions for speech audiometry and suprathreshold audiometry.

Earphones are color coded (red for the right ear and blue for the left ear). Masking sound is delivered to the nontest ear. This is a constant noise to prevent crossover from the test ear, when required, to prevent the nontest ear from detecting the signal (**Fig. 4.8**).

A pure tone is presented well above the hearing threshold, at 30 to 40 dB. After the first response, the intensity is decreased in 10-dB steps until the patient stops responding. If the patient stops responding, the intensity is increased by 5 dB until a positive response is obtained. If the initial level still yields a negative response, then the intensity is increased in 5-dB steps until a positive response is obtained. The duration of pure tone stimulus is 1 to 2 seconds and the stimuli separated by toneless intervals. The threshold of hearing, from 250 to 8,000 Hz, is marked on the audiogram paper. The points are then joined to make an AC audiogram.

Next, the bone vibrator is placed over the mastoid process (**Fig. 4.9**). Sound is delivered through the vibrator and the threshold of hearing for different frequencies of sound is recorded. Similar procedure is repeated on the other ear. This is for the BC audiogram.

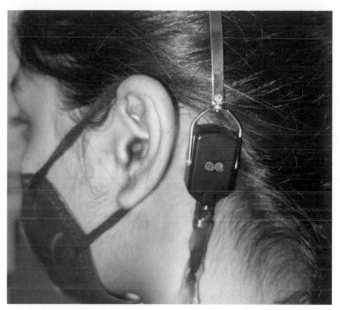

Fig. 4.9 Pure tone audiometry: Bone conduction being tested.

Interpretation of Audiogram

Air Conduction (AC) Threshold

It is the lowest level of decibel hearing loss (dB HL) at which 50% of pure tones introduced via earphones or speakers is heard. It represents conduction from the auricle to the cochlea. It is measured between 125 and 8,000 Hz. Frequencies less than 125 Hz are difficult to distinguish from the vibratory sensations and with frequencies greater than 8,000 Hz, sound pressures cannot be accurately calibrated for ordinary headphones.

Bone Conduction (BC) Threshold

It is the lowest level, in dB HL, at which 50% of pure tones introduced via a bone oscillator apparatus are heard. It

---

Pearl

Audiogram is a graphical recording of hearing sensitivity. AC is done first as it tests the AC pathway of hearing through the external, middle, and inner ear. BC is an indirect test of the cochlear reserve. The A-B gap shows the magnitude of the middle ear pathology, that is, conduction loss. An A-B gap of more than 50 dB may signify ossicular pathology.

represents conduction from the bones of the skull to the inner ear, bypassing the tympanic membrane and ossicles, and is measured from 250 to 4,000 Hz.

Pure Tone Average

It is the average thresholds for speech frequencies (500, 1,000, 2,000 Hz). It should be within 10 db of the speech reception threshold.

Air–Bone Gap

It is the decibel difference between BC and AC thresholds. AC thresholds can only be equal to or greater than BC thresholds.
    The commonly used symbols in audiometry are depicted in **Fig. 4.10**.

Masking

It is the presentation of a constant noise to the nontest ear. It is done to prevent crossover of a pure tone from the poorer ear to the better ear. It is used in unilateral deafness and in bilateral asymmetrical hearing loss. It is usually done when the A-B gap is greater than 10 dB, and the difference between the AC thresholds of right and left ears is greater than 40 dB.

Pure Tone Audiogram Interpretation

In a pure tone audiogram, the frequency in kilohertz is plotted along the X axis and the intensity of sound in decibels, along the Y axis. A *normal audiogram* is shown in **Fig. 4.11**, where all the hearing thresholds are less than 25 dB.
    In *conductive hearing loss*, there is an A-B gap between the AC and BC thresholds. For this to be significant, the gap should be more than 10 dB (**Fig. 4.12**).
    Normal: AC threshold not >25 dB and BC threshold not >25 dB.
    Therefore, in conductive hearing loss:
- AC threshold >25 dB.
- BC threshold <25 dB.
- A-B gap >10 dB.

The BC threshold is normal with the presence of an A-B gap. The maximum conductive hearing loss is 60 dB as seen in ossicular chain discontinuity with an intact tympanic membrane.
    In sensorineural hearing loss (**Fig. 4.13**):
- AC threshold >25 dB.
- BC threshold >25 dB.
- A-B gap <10 db.

AC and BC thresholds are below normal and are similar with no A-B gap. In mixed hearing loss (**Fig. 4.14**):
- AC threshold >25 dB.
- BC threshold > 25 dB.
- A-B gap >10 dB.

In addition to the patterns of conductive, sensorineural, and mixed hearing loss, audiograms can be used to diagnose special conditions. Various etiologies show characteristic patterns.
- Low-frequency sensorineural hearing loss is seen in the early stages of endolymphatic hydrops or Meniere's disease (**Fig. 4.15**).
- Bilateral high-frequency sensorineural hearing loss can be seen in presbycusis, ototoxicity, and acoustic neuroma (**Fig. 4.16**).
- Carhart's notch is a dip in BC at 2,000 Hz. This is seen in otosclerosis (**Fig. 4.17**).
- Boiler's notch is a high-frequency dip at 4,000 Hz. This is from noise-induced trauma. The dip is for AC and BC (**Fig. 4.18**).
- Cookie bite audiograms (*U*-shaped) are seen in congenital hearing loss. In this condition, there is a dip in the mid-frequencies centered around 1 kHz (**Fig. 4.19**).

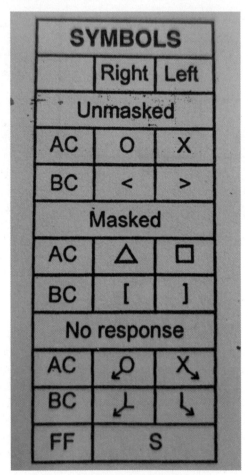

Fig. 4.10   Symbols used in audiometry.

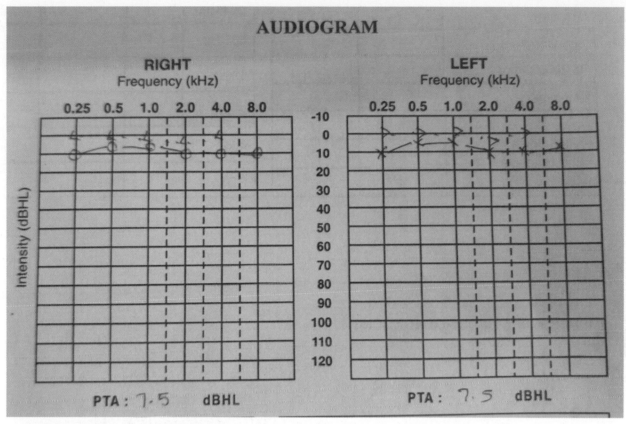

Fig. 4.11   Normal pure tone audiogram.

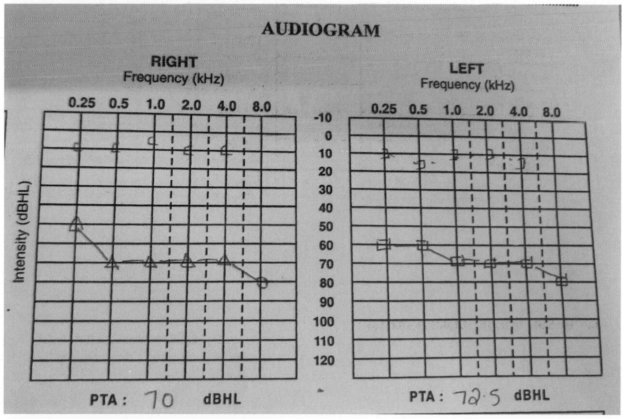

Fig. 4.12   Conductive hearing loss seen in both ears.

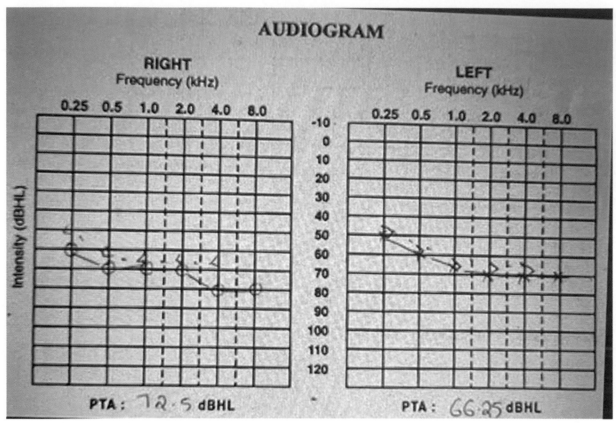

Fig. 4.13 Pure tone audiogram of sensorineural hearing loss.

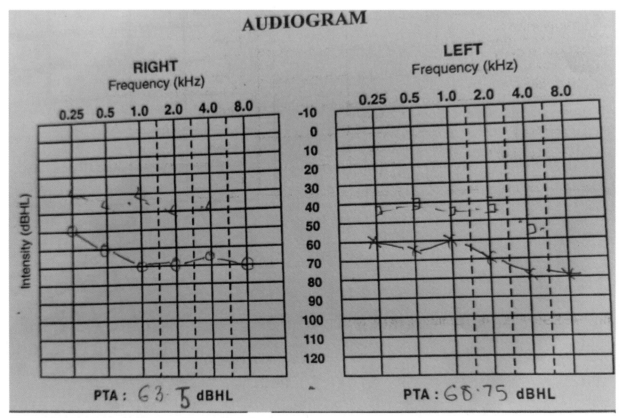

Fig. 4.14 Pure tone audiogram of mixed hearing loss.

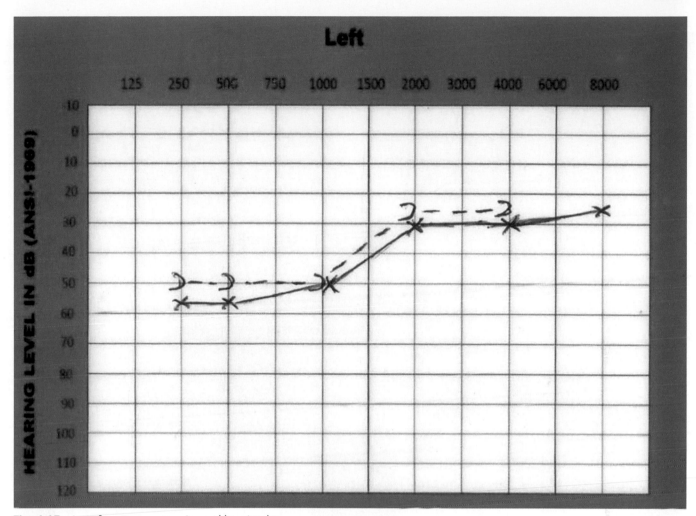

Fig. 4.15 Low-frequency sensorineural hearing loss.

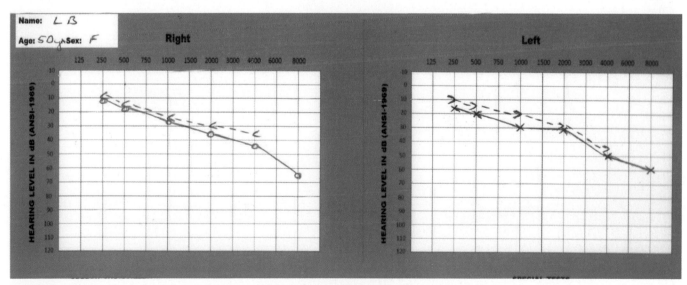

Fig. 4.16 Bilateral high-frequency sensorineural hearing loss.

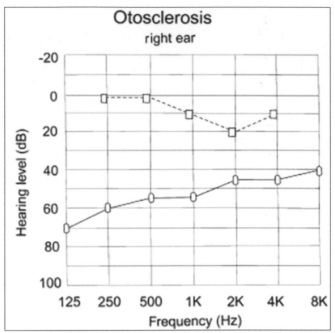

Fig. 4.17 Carhart's notch. Dip at 2 kHz.

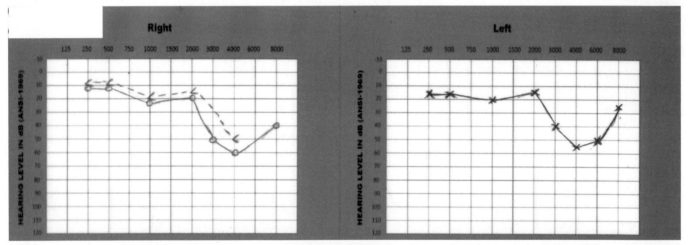

Fig. 4.18 Boiler's notch. Dip at 4 kHz.

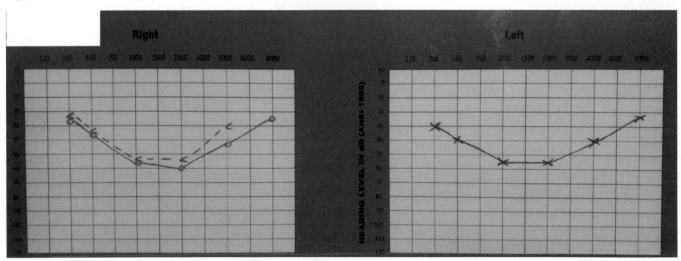

Fig. 4.19 Cookie bite audiogram. There is a dip in the midfrequencies.

Speech Audiometry

The stimulus used is speech, instead of pure tones, as it is more familiar and natural.

Speech Reception Threshold (SRT)

This is similar to pure tone threshold, but the patient should be able to discriminate speech. Spondee words, which are two-syllable words with equal stress, like ice-cream and airplane, are used. The lowest intensity, in decibels, at which a subject can repeat 50% of the stimulus is documented. The difference between speech reception threshold and PTA should not exceed ±12 dB, which, if present, may signify a faulty audiometer or malingering.

Speech Discrimination Score (PB max)

It uses phonetically balanced words in such a way that sounds occur in proportion to their language. Monosyllables like man and tan are used when English is the language. The right responses for 20 syllables are recorded as a percentage. The suprathreshold test is done 40 dB above the speech reception threshold. To make it comfortable for the patient, use a carrier phrase like "say the word." It is calculated by the number of correct responses divided by the total number of words multiplied by 100.

- In normal and conductive hearing loss, the score is 100%.
- In cochlear (sensory) loss, the score is 60 to 70%.
- In retrocochlear hearing loss where there is a neural pathology, poor scores are documented due to adaptation or tone decay.
- The other clinical application of speech discrimination is that it will enable one to determine the benefit of a hearing aid and amplification. In bilateral hearing loss, the ear with the better speech discrimination is selected for the hearing aid as the speech will be better understood with amplification.

Suprathreshold Audiometry

Tests for Recruitment

Recruitment is the abnormal growth of loudness seen in cochlear lesions. Gradual increase in loudness will be perceived as very loud sounds by a patient who has recruitment.

Short Increment Sensitivity Index

This is a common audiometric test done for recruitment. Initially, the pure tone threshold is noted. The test is done at 20 dB above the hearing threshold. A tone is presented to the patient 20 dB above hearing threshold and is kept there for 2 minutes. Every 5 seconds, the tone is increased by 1 dB. The patient has to indicate when he perceives the change in 1-dB sound. Twenty such sounds are given and the total number indicated by the patient is calculated as a percentage.

- In cochlear pathology, high scores of 70 to 100% are obtained.
- Forty to 60% scores are questionable for cochlear pathology.
- Less than 40% rules out recruitment.

Modified Short Increment Sensitivity Index is based on the principle that normal ears can detect 1-dB increment at higher levels. The presentation level is increased to 70 to 80 dB. At this intensity, the ears with normal hearing and cochlear deafness will behave similarly giving higher scores. In retrocochlear pathology, there will be low scores. It is an indirect way of detecting retrocochlear pathology.

Tests for Tone Decay

Tone decay or adaptation is reduction in the sensitivity or responsiveness of the auditory system to a prolonged stimulus and is seen in *retrocochlear* (neural) *pathology*. These tests measure the ability of the ear to sustain a tone continuously for 1 minute. In normal hearing, and in conductive and cochlear deafness, it is possible to sustain. In retrocochlear pathology, it is not possible.

Carhart's Tone Decay Test

It is done 5 dB above threshold. The patient is instructed to keep the finger raised as long as he hears the tone and to keep the finger down when he stops hearing the tone. The stop clock is started simultaneously and the test is terminated at 1 minute. The intensity is increased by 5 dB if the patient puts the finger down before 1 minute and the stop clock is restarted. The final level when the patient can hear for 1 minute continuously gives the tone decay. If the difference between hearing threshold and tone decay is more than 30 dB, the tone decay is positive. Between 15 and 20 dB is considered mild, and it may be cochlear or retrocochlear. Less than 15 dB is considered as normal. It is a time-consuming test.

Modified Carhart's Test

It is a screening test in which the stop clock keeps running, but the intensity is changed immediately when the patient puts the finger down, that is, when the tone fades. It is done for 1 minute. Less than 15 dB is normal. If above 15 dB, do the Carhart's test.

Impedance Audiogram or Tympanometry

It is an objective audiometric test used to assess the middle ear function. It can also be used to assess eustachian tube dysfunction. Acoustic impedance refers to resistance to flow of acoustic energy. The three factors that impede the flow of sound are the following:

- Stiffness (tympanic membrane and ossicles).
- Mass (ossicles).
- Friction or resistance (ligaments in the middle ear).

Impedance can be expressed by the term compliance or admittance, expressed in cubic centimeters of air.

Principle

Impedance is mainly determined by the stiffness of the middle ear system and friction has a negligible effect. Since a stiff system offers more impedance, less sound is conducted through it offering less admittance. In a flaccid system, impedance is less and admittance is more. Maximum admittance occurs when the pressures in the external ear and middle ear are equal.

Procedure

Apparatus 1: It consists of an ear probe and probe tip containing three tubes that can be placed into the ear canal. The tube is used to deliver the probe tone generated by a 220-Hz oscillator driving a miniature receiver. A microphone is used to pick up the energy in the canal, which is reflected back depending on the impedance. Manometer is devised to increase or decrease the pressure in the external canal using an air pump.

Apparatus 2: It is placed in the opposite ear, which consists of a conventional earphone connected to a suitable sound source that delivers signals (pure tone or noise) used to measure the acoustic reflex threshold.

Wax or debris in the external ear is cleared. An otoscopy is done to assess the tympanic membrane. Choose a proper ear tip that will give an airtight seal. The patient is instructed not to move, to avoid deep respiration, and to avoid talking and swallowing. The probe is put in the ear. The pressure is increased to +200 mm of water. The tympanic membrane is pushed inward and becomes fixed leading to more reflection and less compliance. Reduce the pressure serially to 100, 50, and 0 till maximum compliance. –100 and –200 make the tympanic membrane more rigid, that is, reduced compliance. Draw a graph with pressure on the X-axis and compliance on the Y-axis. This is the pressure versus compliance function curve. The graphical representation is called a tympanogram. The normal middle ear pressure is ±25 mm of water, but for practical purposes ±100 mm of water is taken as normal.

Inference

Static compliance is the difference between maximum compliance and the compliance at +200 mm of water, that is, pressure at 0 (ear canal + middle ear) minus pressure at +200 (value of ear canal admittance). The normal range is 0.3 to 1.7 mL. If it is more than 1.7 mL, it suggests a highly loose ossicular system (laxity); less than 0.3 mL means a stiff ossicular system. Positive middle ear pressure is rarely

encountered in conditions like early stage of acute otitis media, after blowing the nose and while crying.

Types of Tympanogram Curves

Jerger described five types of tympanograms (**Fig. 4.20**):
- *Type A*: Peak is near 0 pressure; it is seen in normal ears.
- *Type As*: Peak is at 0, but the amplitude of the peak is low (stiff); it seen in otosclerosis, tympanosclerosis, and thick graft (postmyringoplasty).
- *Type Ad*: Peak is around 0, but the peak amplitude is abnormally high, which means the system is more compliant than normal; it is seen in ossicular discontinuity and flaccid or monomeric membrane.
- *Type B*: Flat curve denoting that the pressure changes do not have much effect on the compliance; it is seen in impacted wax, foreign body, secretory otitis media, adhesive otitis media, perforated tympanic membrane, and a patent grommet.
- *Type C*: The peak is shifted to the negative side; it is seen in eustachian tube dysfunction and early secretory otitis media.

Acoustic Reflex or (Stapedial Reflex) Threshold

It is based on involuntary contraction of the stapedius muscle on both sides following a stimulus of a loud sound given to one ear. The unilateral, ipsilateral, contralateral, and bilateral reflexes can be measured. The stimulus is given at 70 to 90 dB sensation level (SL). The threshold is the lowest intensity at which the reflex is obtained.

It is a useful test in the following:
- Conductive hearing loss (ossicular fixation).
- Retrocochlear pathology.
- In children to decide on further assessment of hearing.
- As a topodiagnostic test in facial palsy (**Video 4.1**).

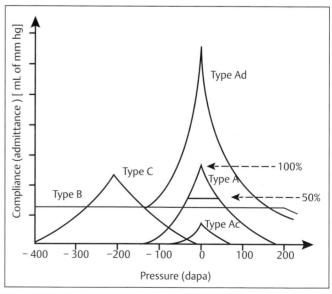

Fig. 4.20 Tympanogram showing various curves.

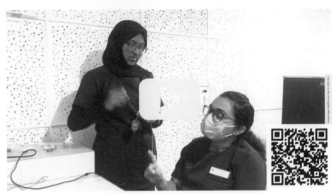

Video 4.1 Pure tone audiometry and tympanometry.

■ Otoacoustic Emission

An otoacoustic emission (OAE) is a sound that is produced in the basilar membrane of the cochlea through a cellular and mechanical process. It can be spontaneous or induced by an external stimulus. A small ear probe is placed in the ear canal, which delivers a low sound stimulus.

The low-intensity acoustic signals generated by active mechanical contraction of the outer hair cells (OHCs) of the cochlea are propagated through the middle ear into the ear canal where the signals are recorded. These signals may not be essential for hearing, but these indicate the functioning of OHCs. These have been predicted by Thomas Gold in 1948. These were first demonstrated by David Kemp, hence these are also referred to as "Kemp's echoes or cochlear echoes." These are the by-products of active processing by OHCs.

> ### Pearl
> OAEs are extensively used in neonatal hearing assessment. An individual's OAE is as unique as fingerprints!

Mechanism

Following an auditory stimulus, the movement of the basilar membrane causes movement or deflection of the OHCs. When the OHCs move, the stereocilia deflect to one or the other direction. This results in movement of the ions in and out of the cells, changing the membrane potential, which in turn changes the voltage across the plasma membrane. This results in changes in length of the OHCs referred to as electromotility. Vibration of the basilar membrane occurs, which forms the principle of OAE signal generation. Further, the motility of the OHCs causes amplification of signals, which stimulates the inner hair cells (IHCs). Following this, the IHCs send signals to the brain and we hear. Thus, the OHC motility helps pick up softer sounds by the IHCs, which is referred to as active processing. Louder sounds result in direct stimulation of the IHCs, which is referred to as passive processing.

Types of Otoacoustic Emissions

- *Spontaneous otoacoustic emissions (SOAEs)* are signals that occur spontaneously without introducing any signal into the ear canal. This is seen in 50% of normal-hearing individuals. It is found to be absent in all ears with hearing loss of more than 30 dB.
  - *Procedure*: A microphone attached to a probe is used to record SOAEs. The probe is placed in the external auditory canal with a flexible cuff. The signals detected are routed to a spectrum analyzer, which provides frequency analysis of the signal. SOAEs occur as peaks of energy along the frequency spectrum. Multiple recordings are obtained to ensure replicability.
  - *Interpretation*: SOAEs occur in 40 to 50% individuals with normal hearing. It is usually considered a sign of cochlear health, but its absence is not a sign of abnormality.

    SOAEs usually occur in the range of 1,000 to 2,000 Hz, and the amplitudes are between 5 and 15 db sound pressure level (SPL). It is bilateral in occurrence, more commonly found in females.
- *Evoked otoacoustic emissions (EOAEs)* consist of two types, namely, transient evoked OAE (TEOAE) and distortion product OAE (DPOAE).

  TEOAEs are elicited with transient signals or clicks. A series of click stimuli are presented, at intensity levels of 80 to 85dB SPL. In newborns, TEOAEs are elicited when clicks are more than 20 dB SPL, whereas in children and adults, responses range between 10 and 15 dB SPL.
  - *Interpretation*: TEOAEs are recorded in the range of 250 to 4,000 Hz for children and 500 to 6,000 Hz for adults at a stimulus level of around 80 dB. TEOAEs evaluate the OHC status in the resting state. It is reliable and fast, but it is poor at higher frequencies and the results can be affected by background noise.
- *DPOAEs* are responses elicited when two pure tones are presented to the cochlea simultaneously. These are rapidly elicited in newborns and are used in the newborn screening process. These reflect OHC integrity and cochlear function.

The pathological causes resulting in absence of OAEs are the following:
- *Outer ear*: Stenosis, otitis externa, and polyp.
- *Tympanic membrane*: Perforation.
- *Middle ear*: Otosclerosis, middle ear disarticulation, and cholesteatoma.
- *Cochlea*: Any cochlear diseases and ototoxic medications.

Uses

- Screening test for hearing in neonates, infants, or individual with developmental disabilities
- Differentiates between sensory and neural components (cochlear vs. retrocochlear loss).
- Test for functional hearing loss (malingering).

■ Brainstem Evoked Response Audiometry

Introduction

It is an objective and noninvasive method of hearing assessment that is based on the generation of electrical activity from the inner ear to the inferior colliculus due to external sounds. It was first described by Jewett and Williston in 1971. The administration and evaluation of the test is usually performed by an audiologist.

Principle

A sound in the form of a brief click or tone pip is introduced into the ear through an earphone or headphone. The electrical activity generated by the sound is recorded by the electrodes placed on the vertex of the scalp and the earlobes (**Fig. 4.21**). The amplitude of the waves (in microvolts), and the time (in milliseconds), is charted on a graph, like an electrocardiographic (ECG) wave.

The waveforms that develop, as the sound passes through the auditory pathway, are labeled from I to VII. All

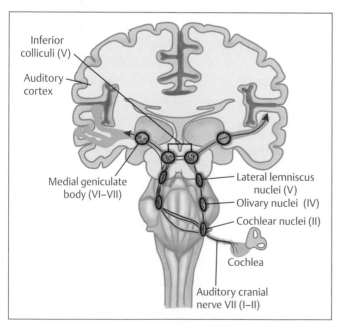

Fig. 4.21 Brainstem evoked response audiometry (BERA) being performed. Electrodes are placed over the earlobes and the forehead. A click is introduced through the headphone.

the waveforms develop within 10 milliseconds of a click stimulus, which are presented at high sound intensities of 70 to 90 dB.

Waveform Components

The waveform components are presented in **Figs. 4.22** and **4.23**:

- *Wave I*: This is due to action potential generated by the distal portion of the vestibulocochlear nerve as it leaves the cochlea and enters the internal auditory canal.
- *Wave II*: It is generated by the proximal vestibulocochlear nerve as it enters the brainstem.
- *Wave III*: This arises from the cochlear nucleus of the pons.
- *Wave IV*: This arises from the superior olivary complex.
- *Wave V*: This arises from the inferior colliculus. This wave is the one most often analyzed for clinical applications.
- *Wave VI and VII*: These arise from the medial geniculate body.

The two events measured in the waves are the following:

- Peaks in millivolts.
- Peak latencies between the waves in order to determine the site of pathology in the auditory pathway.

The peak latencies between waves I and III, III and V, and I and V, and the interaural latency differences are clinically relevant.

Applications

- Screening tool for deafness in newborns.
- Screening tool for evaluating patients with retrocochlear pathology.
- Monitoring intensive care unit patients.

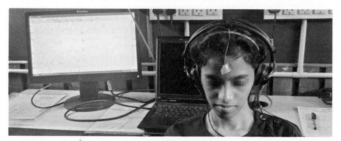

Fig. 4.22 Anatomical location of the various waves generated during brainstem evoked response audiometry (BERA).

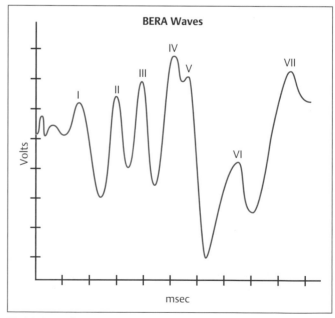

Fig. 4.23 The various waves represented in a graphical format.

Table 4.1 Classification of hearing loss

Average threshold level in dB	Degree of hearing loss
–10 to 15	Normal hearing
16–25	Minimal hearing loss
26–40	Mild hearing loss
41–55	Moderate hearing loss
56–70	Moderately severe hearing loss
71–90	Severe hearing loss
90 and above	Profound hearing loss

- Intraoperative monitoring of central and peripheral nervous system.
- Evaluation of suspected demyelination disorders.
- Evaluation of malingering.

Limitations

- Normal brainstem evoked response audiometry (BERA) does not rule out intrinsic brainstem lesions and nonacoustic tumors of the cerebellopontine angle.
- It is time consuming and requires training for interpretation.
- It is not frequency specific.

The classification of hearing loss given by the American Speech-Language-Hearing Association (ASHA) is given in **Table 4.1**.

Hearing Assessment in Children below 2 Years of Age

■ Acoustic Startle Reflex

It is a quick test for hearing wherein an abrupt, loud noise is used and the movement of the patient is noted in response to the sound.

■ Cribogram

This is an automatic system where the child is tested in the crib itself. It was used in high-risk babies. The crib has in-built speakers and motion sensors connected to a graph. The movement with sound is studied from the strip chart.

■ Otoacoustic Emissions

It is used as a screening test in newborns, especially in high-risk infants.

■ Brainstem Evoked Response Audiometry

It is a good objective test to assess hearing, especially in those who fail the initial screening.

Subjective Hearing Assessment in Children above 2 Years

■ Visual Reinforcement Audiometry

This is based on the principle of conditioning. The presentation of the stimulus is paired with visual stimulus of a moving doll. Initially, a tone is given to check the level at which the child has heard. The conditioned orientation reflex audiometry is when the child is conditioned with visual and sound stimulus.

■ Play Audiometry

This is done in the 3- to 4-year age group. The child responds to tones by doing something like putting blocks or throwing a ball. All frequencies are not tested to avoid the child getting fatigued or losing interest. Common BC is used for both ears. The degree of hearing impairment can be assessed but not the nature. The child does not understand the concept of masking, which is, therefore, not used.

■ Pure Tone Audiometry

It is used in children older than 4 to 5 years when the child is able to comprehend and give appropriate responses.

Objective Hearing Assessment in Children

- *Impedance audiometry* is used to measure the acoustic reflex threshold. Severe deafness is when there are no reflexes and no middle ear pathology. It is a guide for approximate thresholds.
- *BERA.*
- *OAEs.*

Points to Ponder

- There are three types of hearing loss: conductive, sensorineural, and mixed hearing loss.
- The frequencies of the three tuning forks used in ear, nose, and throat (ENT) are 256, 512, and 1,024 Hz.
- Rinne's, Weber's, and absolute BC tests are performed with tuning forks to assess the degree of hearing loss.
- PTA is the commonly used test for assessment of hearing in the ENT outpatient department (OPD).
- Carhart's notch is a dip in the BC curve at 2 kHz associated with otosclerosis.
- Impedance audiometry can be used to identify the pressures in the middle ear and also the presence of fluid.
- OAE is a newborn screening procedure.

Case-Based Questions

1. **A 43-year-old man was involved in a road traffic accident and had a head injury. He later presented with a left-sided hearing loss. The tuning fork tests showed a negative Rinne test on the left (with 265, 512, and 1,024 Hz), Weber was lateralized to the right, and the ABC was reduced when compared to the examiner.**

   a. What is the type of hearing loss he may have?

   b. How would you quantify it?

   c. How would you confirm the hearing loss?

   Answers

   a. Either a mixed hearing loss or a severe sensorineural hearing loss on the left. The Rinne test could be false negative.

   b. PTA.

   c. BERA is an objective test and will be a document of the hearing loss in medicolegal cases.

2. **A 3-year-old girl developed meningitis. Following the recovery, it was noted that the child was not responding to call.**

   a. What is the method for hearing assessment in this child?

   b. What is the radiological investigation to be done?

   c. How can the child be rehabilitated?

   Answers

   a. BERA. Meningitis can cause sensorineural hearing loss.

   b. High-resolution computed tomography (HRCT) scan of temporal bone as ossification of the labyrinth can occur.

   c. It depends on the degree of hearing loss: hearing aid for moderate to severe hearing loss and cochlear implant in severe to profound hearing loss. Early cochlear implantation is recommended when there is evidence of ossification of the labyrinth.

3. **A 26-year-old man was involved in a road traffic accident. He had a head injury and bleeding from the ear. There was a later claim regarding hearing loss with a summons to the doctor to testify in court.**

   a. What is the initial radiological investigation to be done and what should be looked for?

   b. What are the examination findings to be documented?

   c. What are the tests for hearing assessment to be done and why?

   Answers

   a. Other than a CT scan or magnetic resonance imaging (MRI) of the head, an HRCT of the temporal bone should be done. It will help detect the presence and type of fracture. Defects of cerebrospinal fluid (CSF) otorrhea, site of injury in case of facial palsy, and possibly ossicular chain status can be assessed.

   b. The ear should be examined by otoscopy (or later it can be confirmed under the microscope if the patient is stable). Look for external auditory canal laceration, anterior canal wall fracture, tympanic membrane perforation, and hemotympanum. One should assess for facial nerve palsy. If the patient is stable, tuning fork tests should be done. The presence or absence of nystagmus should be documented.

   c. PTA is done. If PTA shows a hearing loss, a BERA should be done to confirm, as it is an objective test that is required as documentation for claims in court, that is, for disability.

Frequently Asked Questions

1. How is Rinne's test performed and what are the inferences?

2. How is Weber's test done and what are the inferences?

3. How is modified Schwabach test (ABC test) done and what are the inferences?

4. What is recruitment?

5. What are the indications for doing a BERA?

6. What is the role of PTA in hearing assessment?

7. What are the various types of curves in a tympanogram and the interpretation?

Endnote

The tuning fork was invented in 1711 and it was mainly used by musicians. It came into the field of otology and physiology only after 100 years. It was Ernst Heinrich Weber, a physiologist from Germany, who in 1834 described the phenomenon of hearing better in the ear when it is occluded than when it is not occluded. Weber did the test by keeping the vibrating tuning fork on the incisor teeth. It is not followed nowadays as it causes discomfort to the patient and is unhygienic. In 1855, Adolf Rinne, a physician from Germany described the test named after him, but he never used it in clinical practice. The tuning fork tests were controversial till the beginning of the 20th century.

5 Hearing Loss and Rehabilitation

Ajoy Mathew Varghese

The competencies covered in this chapter are as follows:

PY10.16 Describe and discuss the pathophysiology of deafness.

EN4.12 Elicit, document, and present a correct history; demonstrate and describe the clinical features; choose the correct investigations; and describe the principles of management of hearing loss.

EN4.15 Describe the clinical features, investigations, and principles of management of noise-induced hearing loss.

IM24.17 Describe and discuss the etiopathogenesis, clinical presentation, identification, functional changes, acute care, stabilization, management, and rehabilitation of hearing loss in the elderly.

EN4.14 Describe the clinical features, investigations, and principles of management of sudden sensorineural hearing loss.

Hearing Loss Pathophysiology

Hearing loss is partial or complete inability to hear in one or both the ears. It can occur due to a defect in any part of the auditory system or its central connections. Based on the site, it may be conductive when either the outer or middle part of the ear is involved or sensorineural where the inner ear or neural connection (the auditory nerve) is involved.

Classification of Hearing Loss

Although functional hearing loss and malingering are well-established entities, traditionally hearing loss is classified into three types: conductive, sensorineural, and mixed hearing loss (**Flowchart 5.1**).

■ Conductive Hearing Loss

Conductive hearing loss occurs due to disruption of the mechanical transmission of sound anywhere from the external auditory canal to the stapediovestibular joint. It can be due to mechanical obstruction of the external canal due to impacted wax, perforation of the tympanic membrane, fluid in the middle ear, or fixation or disruption of the ossicular chain. Hearing loss can usually be corrected by treating the underlying pathology medically or surgically.

In conductive hearing loss, there is disruption of the mechanical transmission of sound. Based on the location, the severity of hearing loss varies (**Table 5.1**).

■ Sensorineural Hearing Loss

Sensorineural hearing loss (SNHL) is caused by lesions of either the inner ear (sensory) or the auditory (eighth) nerve (neural). This distinction is important because sensory hearing loss is sometimes reversible and is seldom life threatening. A neural hearing loss is rarely recoverable and may be due to a potentially life-threatening brain tumor—commonly a cerebellopontine angle tumor.

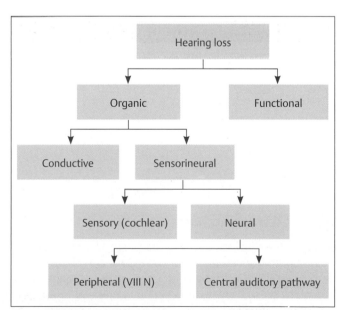

Flowchart 5.1 Diagram showing the various types of hearing loss.

Table 5.1 Site of hearing loss and severity of hearing loss in conductive deafness

Cause	History and examination	Audiometry
External canal		
Impacted wax	Sudden-onset painless hearing loss Cerumen in the canal	30 dB
Otitis externa	Sudden-onset painful hearing loss with discharge Narrow external auditory canal with debris	20–30 dB
Foreign body ear	History of foreign body ear Foreign body may be seen in the canal	20–30 dB
Tympanic membrane		
Acute otitis media	Typically, a child with earache and hearing loss following URTI Normal canal with red, immobile tympanic membrane	30–40 dB (hearing improves when eardrum perforates)
Chronic otitis media	Painless loss of hearing with discharge Perforation in the tympanic membrane	Negligible to 50 dB, based on the size and site of the perforation
Ossicles		
Otosclerosis (stapes fixation)	Bilateral progressive painless hearing loss Intact tympanic membrane	60 dB
Malleus fixation	Congenital hearing loss Intact tympanic membrane	15–25 dB
Ossicular disruption with perforation	As a part of chronic otitis media Perforation in the tympanic membrane	40–50 dB
Ossicular disruption with intact tympanic membrane	History of trauma Intact tympanic membrane	60 dB
Middle ear		
Middle ear effusion	Gradual painless loss of hearing Immobile tympanic membrane	30–35 dB

Abbreviation: URTI, upper respiratory tract infection.

Pearl

Retrocochlear hearing loss is used to describe a neural or central hearing loss that occurs beyond the cochlea, affecting the vestibulocochlear nerve or the central auditory system.

Auditory neuropathy spectrum disorder is a type of SNHL where the sound signal is not sent correctly to the brain, and is thought to be due to an abnormality of the inner hair cells or the neurons that innervate them within the cochlea.

■ Mixed Hearing Loss

In mixed hearing loss, as the name suggests, there are components of both conductive hearing loss and SNHL. It may be seen in head injury with fracture of the temporal bone or may be seen following inner ear involvement in a patient with conductive hearing loss (e.g., chronic otitis media and otosclerosis).

Sensorineural Hearing Loss

SNHL is the more common type of hearing loss that prompts evaluation by an otolaryngologist.

■ Etiology

The most common causes of SNHL are the following:
- Congenital: Syndromic and nonsyndromic.
- Presbycusis.
- Noise-induced hearing loss (NIHL).
- Head injury.
- Ménière's disease.
- Ototoxicity: Aminoglycosides and loop diuretics.
- Systemic conditions: Meningitis and diabetes.
- Vestibular schwannoma.
- Others: Autoimmune, barotrauma, and perilymphatic fistula.

■ Pathophysiology

SNHL results from damage to the hair cells within the inner ear, the vestibulocochlear nerve, or the brain's central processing centers.

There are several pathophysiological mechanisms by which damage to the inner ear results in SNHL (**Table 5.2**):

- *Structural* abnormality of the cochlea, for example, trauma or congenital conditions.
- Aberrant *metabolic* activity leading to changes in the endolymph, for example, genetic.
- Interference with *vascular supply* to the cochlea, for example, noise trauma, ototoxicity, and systemic vascular events.
- *Noise* trauma leading to damage to the stereocilia of the outer hair cells.

Hearing loss is a common problem affecting all ages. As discussed earlier, hearing loss can be conductive, sensorineural, or mixed, and can be due to varied causes. This section gives an overview of the evaluation of an adult with hearing loss.

■ Evaluation

A detailed history, thorough physical examination, followed by audiometric evaluation are essential to the diagnosis and treatment of hearing loss.

History

A comprehensive history can point toward diagnosis of patients with hearing loss. Patients may present with perceived hearing loss, inability to understand conversation, asking others to repeat things, or having difficulty hearing with background noise.

The clinician should ask about the duration of hearing loss, onset, and progression of the hearing loss. Hearing loss may be unilateral or bilateral, continuous or fluctuating, constant or progressive. The evaluation should also include other symptoms related to the ear, and related nose and throat symptoms. A systemic review of comorbidities and family history of ear disorders and hearing loss is also sought.

Some of the pertinent questions include the following:

Duration	When did your hearing loss begin?
Onset	Was your hearing loss sudden or gradual in onset?
Progression	Has your hearing slowly been getting worse?
Functional handicap	Do you have a problem understanding speech?
	Is your problem mainly with background noise (e.g., restaurants, parties) or is it just as bad in quiet settings?
	Does your hearing loss involve one or both ears?
	Have you had any previous ear surgery?
	Have you had any significant trauma, including noise and barotrauma?
	What medicines are you currently taking? Have you received any intravenous antibiotics, diuretics, salicylates, or chemotherapy?
Other ear symptoms	Is there pain or drainage out of the ear associated with the hearing loss?
	Is there associated tinnitus, vertigo, or disequilibrium?
	Do you have any nose or throat problems?
Past history	Do you have a history of stroke, diabetes, or heart disease?
Family history	Is there any one in your family who has hearing loss?

Physical Examination

Examination of the ear begins by visualization of the external ear. An otoscope is used to examine the external auditory canal and the tympanic membrane. The color, the surface anatomy, and the mobility of the tympanic membrane are evaluated. A tuning fork test (usually using a 512-Hz tuning fork) is used to determine the type of hearing loss. Commonly Rinne's, Weber's, and absolute bone conduction tuning fork tests are performed.

Table 5.2 Etiology of SNHL and correlation with examination findings and audiogram

Cause	History and examination	Audiogram
Presbycusis	Elderly, gradual hearing loss Normal tympanic membrane	Bilateral, symmetric high-frequency loss, above 2 kHz
Noise-induced traumatic loss	Noise exposure, gradual hearing loss, and tinnitus Normal tympanic membrane	Bilateral, symmetric loss centered at 4 kHz
Autoimmune hearing loss	Joint pain, rash, eye symptoms, rapidly progressive, possibly fluctuating, bilateral loss Normal tympanic membrane, possible disequilibrium	Any abnormal configuration with poor speech discrimination
Perilymph fistula	Head trauma, sudden pressure change (straining), sudden unilateral hearing loss, and vertigo Normal tympanic membrane; positive fistula sign	Any unilateral abnormal configuration
Ménière's disease	Episodes of sudden, fluctuating, unilateral hearing loss, tinnitus, and episodic vertigo Normal tympanic membrane	Unilateral low-frequency loss
Acoustic neuroma (vestibular schwannoma)	Gradual unilateral hearing loss, tinnitus Normal tympanic membrane, unsteadiness, and possible facial paresis	Any unilateral abnormal configuration

Table 5.3 Types of tympanograms and their etiology

Type	Finding	Etiology
Type A	Normal middle ear pressure	Normal
Type B	Little or no mobility of tympanic membrane	Otitis media with effusion or perforation of the tympanic membrane
Type C	Negative pressure in the middle ear	Eustachian tube dysfunction
Type As	Stiff middle ear system; minimal mobility of tympanic membrane	Otosclerosis and tympanosclerosis
Type Ad	Highly compliant tympanic membrane	Ossicular chain discontinuity Thin tympanic membrane

Investigations

- All patients will require an audiometric evaluation:
  - A *pure tone audiometry* (PTA) will identify the type and severity of hearing loss.
  - In a patient with conductive hearing loss and an intact tympanic membrane, *tympanometry* will help differentiate the cause of conductive hearing loss.
  - In cases of SNHL, *speech audiometry* can differentiate between cochlear and retrocochlear hearing loss.
- Based on the history and examination, other investigations may be needed. *Laboratory investigations* may include complete blood counts, blood sugar, thyroid function test, and serology as indicated.
- *Imaging studies* include contrast-enhanced computed tomography (CT) scan or magnetic resonance imaging (MRI) in case of SNHL, tumors, or cholesteatoma.

Audiological Evaluation

Formal audiologic evaluation is performed in a soundproof room by an audiologist. PTA with tympanogram and site of lesion testing provides accurate and definitive information about the patient's hearing ability.

Pure Tone Audiometry

Commonly known as audiogram, PTA evaluates both air and bone conduction to assess the type and severity of hearing loss. Specific audiometric patterns may suggest possible etiology (e.g., Carhart's notch for otosclerosis and dip at 4 kHz in bone conduction in NIHL).

Impedance Audiometry

Impedance audiometry has two parts: Tympanometry and stapedial reflex testing. Tympanometry is an objective measure of the change in impedance of the middle ear in response to changes in pressure. Tympanometry helps identify etiology in patients with conductive hearing loss (**Table 5.3**).

Stapedial reflex can be done as part of the evaluation of an otosclerosis or for site of lesion testing.

Speech Audiometry

Speech Reception Threshold

Speech reception threshold (SRT) is the lowest intensity at which a person is capable of repeating 50% of spondee words (bisyllabic, equally stressed, words). Poor SRT is suggestive of retrocochlear pathology. Examples of spondee words include "base-ball" and "bus-stop."

Speech Discrimination Score

Speech discrimination score (SDS) is the percentage of correctly repeatable, phonetically balanced, monosyllabic words, presented at the suprathreshold level (40 dB SL). SDS is reduced in sensorineural loss cases and a score <30% is suggestive of retrocochlear lesions.

Tone Decay Test

Tone decay test (TDT) is the most commonly used tests to diagnose neural lesions like acoustic neuroma. A sustained air conducted ear tone is presented and the changes in auditory threshold is noted. Marked tone decay is suggestive of *retrocochlear pathology*.

Results of TDT	Value
Normal	0.5 dB in 60 seconds
Mild	10–15 dB in 60 seconds
Moderate	20–25 dB in 60 seconds

Short Increment Sensitivity Index

Short Increment Sensitivity Index (SISI) test determines the ability of a patient to detect a 1-dB increment at the 20-dB suprathreshold tone. The patient is asked to count the increments, while 20 1-dB increments are presented. The correctly identified number is multiplied by 5 to give the percentage of SISI score.

Score	Site of lesion
Positive (>70%)	Cochlear pathology
Negative (<30%)	Retrocochlear pathology

Pearl

Recruitment is an abnormally rapid rise in loudness in response to increased stimulus intensity. It is seen in cochlear pathology.

Loudness Discomfort Level

Narrow dynamic range (normal discomfort threshold 90–105 dB) indicates recruitment.

Alternate Binaural Loudness Balance

Alternate binaural loudness balance (ABLB) is a test for recruitment in unilateral hearing loss. The test compares the growth of loudness in the ear with hearing loss compared that in the normal.

Brainstem Evoked Response Audiometry

Brainstem evoked response audiometry (BERA) is an objective electrophysiological test that evaluates the electrical potential generated at various levels of the auditory system from the cochlea to the brainstem (see Chapter 4 "Assessment of Hearing" for details of BERA).

Table 5.4 depicts the differences between conductive, cochlear, and retrocochlear hearing loss.

■ Management of Hearing Loss

The American Academy of Family Physicians has suggested the SCREAM mnemonic for the management of hearing loss: Sudden hearing loss, cerumen impaction, education, auditory rehabilitation, assistive devices, and medications.

Sudden Hearing Loss

This has been dealt with in another section.

Cerumen Impaction

Occlusion of the external auditory canal with cerumen can result in conductive hearing loss and removal can be curative. Cerumen can be removed by syringing (irrigation), manual removal using wax hooks, using wax dissolving medication, or a combination of the three.

Auditory Rehabilitation

Auditory rehabilitation refers to strategies for listening and speaking to make the environment optimal for the hearing-impaired person. Strategies include facing the person while talking, reducing background noise, improving lighting, and speaking at a reasonable speed and loudness. It also helps if, in groups, the hearing-impaired persons are included in conversation and are encouraged to be positive and relaxed.

Education

It is important that doctors provide information about the nature and cause of hearing loss and the rehabilitative process. Patient expectations and perceived benefit of the rehabilitative process are key to compliance.

Table 5.4 Characteristics of different types of hearing loss on evaluation

	Conductive	Cochlear	Retrocochlear
Understanding speech	Good	Poor	Poor
Intolerance to loud sound	Absent	Present	Absent
Other ear symptoms	Ear discharge may be present	Tinnitus	Tinnitus
Tuning fork test			
Rinne's test	Negative	Positive	Positive
Weber's test	Lateralized to "bad ear"	Lateralized to normal ear	Lateralized to normal ear
Absolute bone conduction	Normal	Reduced	Reduced
Pure tone thresholds			
Air conduction	Abnormal	Abnormal	Variable
Bone conduction	Normal	Abnormal	Variable
Speech reception threshold	Abnormal	Abnormal	Variable
Speech discrimination	Normal	Abnormal	Abnormal
Impedance battery			
Static compliance	Abnormal	Normal	Normal
Tympanometry	Abnormal	Normal	Normal
Reflex threshold	Absent	Absent/abnormal	Absent/decay
Reflex decay	N/A	Normal/absent	Absent/abnormal
Diagnostic battery			
ABLB	Normal	Abnormal	Normal
SISI	Normal	Abnormal	Normal
Tone decay	Normal	Normal	Abnormal
Bekesy	Type I	Type II	Type III or IV
PI-PB	No rollover	Plateau	Rollover
BERA	Variable	Normal/variable	Abnormal

Abbreviations: ABLB, alternate binaural loudness balance; BERA, brainstem evoked response audiometry; PI-PB, performance intensity using phonetically balanced words; SISI, Short Increment Sensitivity Index.

Assistive Devices

The key to hearing rehabilitation is assistive devices. The doctor should be able to suggest the appropriate device to the patients.

Hearing Aids

Although a hearing aid does not restore hearing to normal, the amplification of sound with a hearing aid helps people who have either conductive hearing loss or SNHL. Hearing aids improve hearing-related quality of life and overall health-related quality of life in mild to moderate hearing loss.

The hearing aid consists of the following:
- A microphone to pick up sound.
- An amplifier to increase the volume.
- A speaker to transmit sound to the ear.

Hearing aids can be the following types:
- Behind the ear.
- Receiver in the canal (RIC).
- Completely in the canal (CIC).

The RIC and CIC are more discrete but need more dexterity and are contraindicated in patients with a tympanic membrane perforation.

Cochlear Implantation

Many of the causes of conductive hearing loss can be corrected with surgery. Mild to moderate SNHL can be rehabilitated with hearing aids. For severe to profound hearing loss, not adequately rehabilitated with hearing aids, cochlear implantation may be an acceptable option. A cochlear implant (CI) is an electrode placed surgically in the cochlea to bypass the ear and directly stimulate the auditory nerves. An external microphone and processor pick up sound signals and convert the sound signals into electrical signals, which are transmitted to an internal coil electromagnetically. The electrodes connected to the internal coil stimulate the auditory nerve.

Brainstem Implants

In patients with absence of acoustic nerves, electrodes can be surgically implanted to the area of the brain responsible for hearing in the brainstem. It may be used in patients with:

- Fractures of the skull base with damage to the acoustic nerves.
- In children with congenital absence of acoustic nerves.
- Bilateral vestibular schwannoma.

Table 5.5 can be used as a guide to manage hearing loss in various conditions.

Other Assistive Devices

- Frequency modulated hearing device.
- Light alerting systems (e.g., doorbells).
- Closed captioning for TV programs.
- Vibrating alarm in phones.
- Teletext for telecommunication devices.

Medications

Physicians should ask about current and past medications and minimize the use of ototoxic drugs. In patients with chronic renal disease, dose adjustment and close monitoring are needed.

The management of conductive hearing loss and SNHL is shown in **Flowchart 5.2**.

Noise-Induced Hearing Loss

NIHL is a reduction in the hearing acuity as a consequence of excessive noise exposure (**Flowchart 5.3**).

> **Pearl**
>
> NIHL is the second most common form of SNHL after presbycusis, but the leading preventable cause of hearing loss.

■ Acoustic Trauma

Acoustic trauma has been used to describe the situation where a single exposure to an intense sound (like a gunfire) leads to an immediate hearing loss. Damage can be due to the following:

- Rupture of the tympanic membrane.
- Disruption of the ossicular chain.
- Damage to hair cell.
- Damage to Reissner's membrane.

■ Noise-Induced Hearing Loss

NIHL is SNHL caused due to overexposure to excessively loud sound. Hearing deteriorates gradually from chronic and repeated noise exposure (such as with loud music in rock concerts or power tools or machinery).

Temporary Threshold Shift

A temporary hearing loss due to transient hair cell dysfunction is called temporary threshold shift. It is normally caused by exposure to intense and/or loud sounds or noise

Table 5.5 Etiology and management of hearing loss

Cause of conductive hearing loss	Surgical option
Chronic otitis media (mucosal type)	Tympanoplasty
Chronic otitis media (squamous)	Mastoidectomy ± ossiculoplasty
Otitis media with effusion	Myringotomy with grommet insertion
Otosclerosis	Stapedotomy
Aural atresia with microtia	Atresia repair (canalplasty) with microtia reconstruction or bone-anchored hearing aid
Malformed ear and discharging ear	Bone-anchored hearing aid
Cause of sensorineural hearing loss	**Surgical options**
Profound hearing loss	Cochlear implantation
Ménière's disease	Endolymphatic sac decompression, vestibular nerve section, and labyrinthectomy
Unilateral profound hearing loss	Bone-anchored hearing aid
Mixed hearing loss	**Surgical option**
Moderate to severe SNHL with preserved word recognition score	Implantable middle ear hearing devices

Abbreviation: SNHL, sensorineural hearing loss.

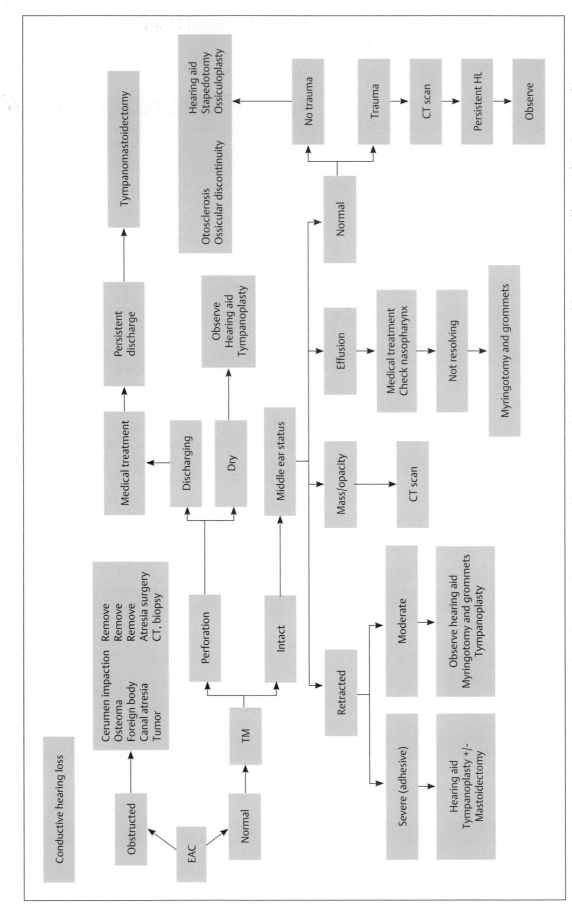

Flowchart 5.2 Algorithm for management of conductive and sensorineural hearing loss. Abbreviation: SSHL, sudden sensorineural hearing loss. (*Continued*)

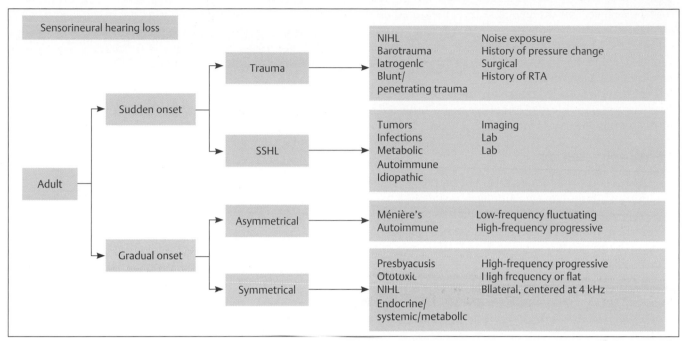

Flowchart 5.2 *(Continued)* Algorithm for management of conductive and sensorineural hearing loss. Abbreviation: SSHL, sudden sensorineural hearing loss.

levels for a short time. This could be an explosion or a concert. These shifts usually involve the 3- to 8-kHz range. They tend to resolve within minutes to hours, whereas complete recovery depends on the degree of shift and type of noise trauma.

Permanent Threshold Shift

A permanent threshold shift is when the ability to hear is reduced permanently, due to prolonged or repeated noise exposure irreversibly damaging the hair cells.

■ Acoustic Shock

Acoustic shock is an acute stress reaction to noise exposure causing psychological distress without objective hearing loss. It is thought to be due to myoclonic activity of the tensor tympani muscle.

■ Etiology

NIHL, by definition, is caused by noise exposure. It may be recreational like use of personal music device at high level or regular attendance at music concert, or occupational as in using power tools or machinery in industries (**Table 5.6**).

Table 5.6 Noise level in decibel for various appliances and equipment

Industry	Noise level (dBA)
Jackhammer	130
Textile loom	110
Tractor	100
Newspaper press	100
Power tools	90
Diesel generator	85

Pearl

Noise can cause permanent hearing loss at chronic exposures over 80 dB. Workplace noise level equal to an average sound pressure level (SPL) of 85 dB(A) or higher for an 8-hour period is at high risk of NIHL. If noise level increases to 88 dB (doubling of intensity), risk of NIHL can occur after 4 hours. The greater the noise level, the lesser the time before damage can occur. Noise intensity exceeding 140 dB causes severe deafness and tinnitus immediately after the noise exposure.

"High noise level" means any noise level measured on the A-weighted scale is ≥85 dB.

Table 5.7 shows the noise level in decibel and the number of hours that a human ear can be exposed to before noise-induced damage sets in.

Noise that carries a sudden, sharp sound for a brief period like clicks and pops is called impulsive noise. **Table 5.8** sets out the permissible levels for impulsive noise.

Pathophysiology

The cochlea is the predominant site for pathological manifestation of noise damage. Although metabolic changes play a role in temporary threshold shift, structural changes are considered to play a role in permanent threshold shift. Sound pressure exerts a shearing force on the stereocilia of the hair cells.

Pearl

Outer hair cells are first affected by noise-induced trauma.

Clinical Features

- History of exposure to excessive noise.
- Progressive bilateral symmetrical hearing loss. Patients usually have difficulty in hearing in noisy environments.
- Tinnitus often occurs early in the course.
- Psychological issues like social isolation and depression. In addition, there is an increased risk of accidents, increasing the stress to the person.

Screening questionnaires are available for early detection of hearing loss.

Investigations

- *PTA* is the cornerstone of investigation. The classical audiometric pattern is of a high-tone SNHL with a notched appearance centered on 4 kHz *(Boiler's notch)* or 6 kHz, with some recovery at 8 kHz (**Fig. 5.1**).
- *Tympanometry* helps exclude middle ear pathology.
- *Tests of malingering* like Stenger's test with tuning forks can be done.
- *Otoacoustic emissions and BERA* are objective tests of hearing.
- *MRI* is done in patients with asymmetrical loss to rule out acoustic neuroma.

Principles of Management

Flowchart 5.4 presents the principles of management of NIHL.

Primary Prevention

NIHL is a preventable form of hearing loss. Early diagnosis and management can reduce irreparable damage. Regular

Table 5.7 Permissible exposure in cases of continuous noise

Total time of exposure (continuous short-term exposure) in hours	Sound pressure level (dBA)
8	85
6	87
4	90
3	92
2	95
1.5	97
1	100
0.75	102
0.5	105
0.25	110

Note: No exposure in excess of 110 dBA is to be permitted.

Table 5.8 Permissible exposure levels of impulsive or impact noise

Peak sound pressure level in dB	Permitted number of impulses or impact per day
140	100
135	315
130	1,000
125	3,160
120	10,000

Source: Model rules part-II MR 120 and Schedules specifying Requirements in Respect of Dangerous Processes and Operations Notified under Section 87 of the Factories Act.
Note: No exposure in excess of 140-dB peak sound pressure level is permitted.

screening questionnaires and audiometry are the key to primary prevention.

Personal Protective Equipment

When hearing loss is detected or if there is likelihood of significant noise exposure, attenuation of the sound can be provided by the use of earplugs or earmuffs. Earplugs give about 10- to 15-dB attenuation in the real world, mainly in the lower and upper frequencies, whereas earmuffs give about 15-dB attenuation in the midrange. Active noise reduction uses electronics to mask the sound inside the earmuffs. This is very effective, especially for lower frequencies (around 1,000 Hz).

Occupational Hearing Conservation

An occupational hearing conservation program includes engineering (making quieter machines) and acoustic measures (sound isolation) to reduce noise exposures in

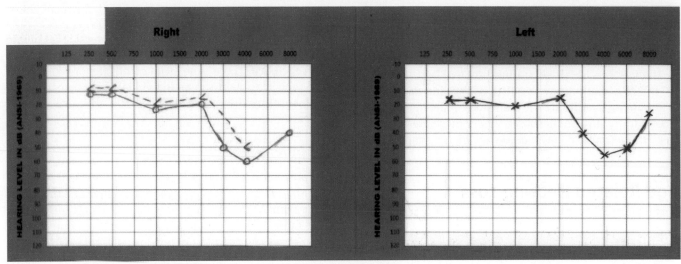

Fig. 5.1 Bilateral dip in hearing thresholds at 4 kHz (Boiler's notch).

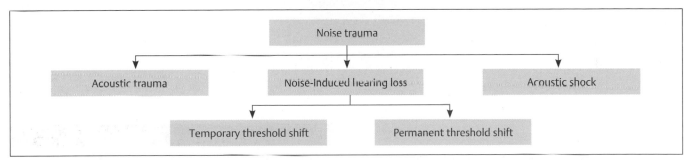

Flowchart 5.3 Algorithm outlining the classification of noise trauma.

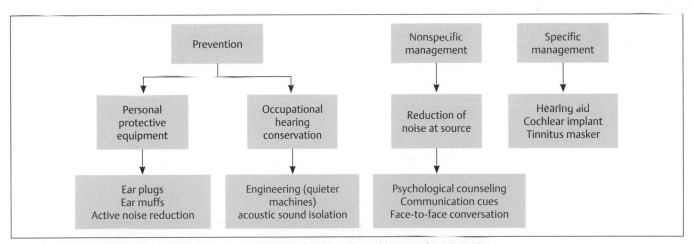

Flowchart 5.4 Algorithm outlining the management of noise-induced hearing loss (NIHL).

workplaces where noise levels exceed 85 dB for an 8-hour time-weighted average.

Nonspecific Management

- *Psychological counseling* regarding the hearing loss and management of anxiety can reduce depression and social isolation.

- *Communication cues* are used when reduction of noise is not possible. Nonverbal cues and face-to-face conversation can optimize communication.

Specific Management

Currently, definitive management of NIHL is limited to the use of hearing amplification:

- *Hearing aids* provide significant benefit in severe hearing loss. However, despite technologic advances, aids often cannot fully correct problems of speech discrimination. In profound hearing loss, a CI may be helpful.
- *Tinnitus* can be a debilitating problem and is seen 60 to 70% of patients with NIHL. Counseling and *tinnitus retraining therapy* are the mainstays in the management of tinnitus. In a small subset, where these measures fail, a *tinnitus masker* can be used to mask the sound.

Age-Related Hearing Loss

Pearl

Age-related hearing loss is the most common cause of hearing loss.

Although there are many causes for reduced hearing in the elderly, age-related hearing loss (ARHL) or presbycusis refers to a complex degenerative process characterized by a decline in auditory function. ARHL is multifactorial, involving both intrinsic (e.g., genetic predisposition) and extrinsic (e.g., noise exposure) factors.

Table 5.9 Prevalence of hearing impairment with age

Age group (y)	Prevalence (%)
18–30	2
31–40	5
41–50	10
51–60	17
61–71	30
71–80	53

Source: Reproduced with permission of Davis A. Hearing in adults. London: Whurr Publishers; 1995:14.
Note: Average threshold >30 dB HL; all causes; both ear average.

■ Definition

ARHL may be defined as a progressive bilateral SNHL of mid to late adult onset, where other underlying causes have been excluded. There is no strict cutoff age for ARHL, but a high tone hearing loss in an individual over 50 years in the absence of any alternative explanation is arbitrarily considered as ARHL.

■ Epidemiology

The prevalence of hearing loss increases with age. Over half the adults over the age of 75 years and almost all the adults older than 90 years have functionally significant hearing loss. **Table 5.9** depicts the percentage of the population in various age groups with hearing loss.

■ Etiopathogenesis

ARHL is the end-stage effect of the interplay of various pathways and interactions of multiple complex factors including ageing, genetic, epigenetic, environmental, and comorbidities. It is possible that all these processes affect the cochlea in a similar way, but with its own unique course (**Table 5.10**). Some of the risk factors for developing ARHL is outlined in **Table 5.11**.

Pearl

Stria vascularis atrophy, diminished Na$^+$ K$^+$ ATPase activity, and its effect on endolymphatic potential (EP) are the predominant factors in the aging cochlea.

■ Clinical Presentation

- *Hearing loss* begins in the sixth decade of life and is typically symmetrical, beginning in the high-frequency range with a variable but progressive decline with age. The initial description may be a lack of clarity, especially in the presence of background noise. Later, as the hearing loss progresses, the deafness becomes more

Table 5.10 Type of ARHL and the pathology in the ear

Type	Audiogram	Defining features
Sensory	Abrupt high-frequency hearing loss	Atrophy of the basal part of the organ of Corti
Neural	Diminished word discrimination	Degeneration and loss of spiral ganglion cells
Vascular or metabolic	Overall reduced pure tone thresholds	Atrophy of the cochlear stria vascularis
Mechanical or cochlear conductive	Down-sloping audiogram	Stiffened cochlear basilar membrane
Intermediate	Flat or high-frequency loss	No consistent change Possible changes in the intracellular organelles involved in cell metabolism
Mixed		A combination of the other five subtypes

Abbreviation: ARHL, age-related hearing loss.

Table 5.11   Risk factors for ARHL

Nonmodifiable factors	Modifiable factors	
	Environmental factors	**Health comorbidities**
Increasing age	Noise exposure	Hypertension
Male gender	Cigarette smoking and alcohol use	Diabetes mellitus
Possible genetic predisposition	Medication like NSAID and diuretics	Blood hyperviscosity
		Cardiovascular disease
		Cerebrovascular disease

Abbreviations: ARHL, age-related hearing loss; NSAID, nonsteroidal anti-inflammatory drug.

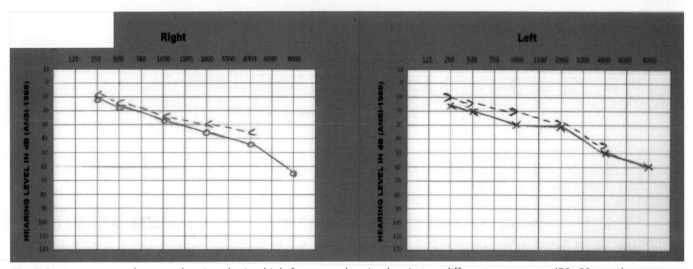

Fig. 5.2   Pure tone audiogram showing sloping high-frequency hearing loss in two different age groups (50–60 years).

apparent with TV often getting louder or asking others to repeat themselves. In the later stages, there may be a paradoxical hypersensitivity to loud sounds due to "recruitment."

- *Tinnitus* can be distressing and may be the presenting symptom. Tinnitus is most commonly a steady ringing, rushing, or "static" sound.
- *Dizziness*, although uncommon, ARHL may be associated with loss of vestibular end-organ function (presbyastasis). They often present with disequilibrium and falls. Dizziness is exacerbated by the presence of coexisting disorders, such as peripheral neuropathy, arthritis, peripheral vascular disease, and decreased visual acuity.
- *Functional changes*: ARHL is a part of a complex degenerative process involving cognition, hearing, neurological, and visual changes. The degenerative process in the central nervous system leads to relative loss of neural plasticity, and loss of cognitive abilities and sensory modalities, including hearing, sight, and loss of dexterity of fingers.
- Hearing loss has an adverse impact on the *psychological well-being* in addition to the *physical ability*. Associated with an increased incidence of falls, hearing loss can

lead to social isolation and anxiety. This can lead to further reduction of higher cognitive function, depression, and dementia.

■ Investigations

- *Screening questionnaire*: The Hearing Handicap Inventory for the Elderly-Screening (HHIE-S) is a simple questionnaire that can help identify older adult patients with significant hearing impairment.
- *PTA* is the first and often the only investigation required for ARHL. Initially, the audiogram will show a downward-sloping pure tone thresholds with relative preservation of word recognition scores. Hearing loss is seen above 2 kHz, with the mid and low frequencies affected late (**Figs. 5.2** and **5.3**).

■ Management

There is no definite treatment that can prevent or reverse the effects of ARHL. Treatment is directed at compensating for hearing loss and to improve daily function and well-being. The strategies can be directed to three broad areas: Psychological, nonspecific, and specific.

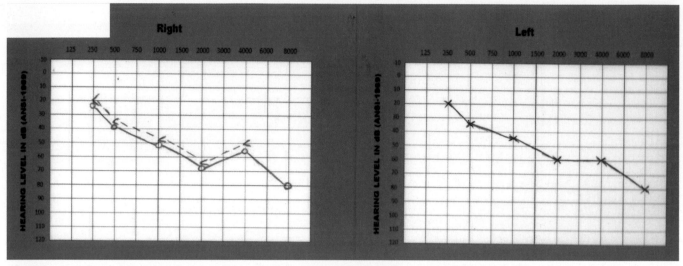

Fig. 5.3 Pure tone audiogram showing sloping high-frequency hearing loss in two different age groups (70–80 years).

Psychological Counseling and Support

This is essential in cases of severe hearing loss, especially in the presence of other comorbidities. A holistic approach including cognition and other sensory inputs like sight and dexterity of fingers need to be considered while planning rehabilitation.

Nonspecific Management

This includes the reduction of background noise, face-to-face conversation, and nonverbal cues, which can optimize the individual's acoustic environment.

Specific Management

Hearing Aids

Even in mild or moderate hearing loss, hearing aids have been found to be beneficial. Binaural hearing aids provide an additional 10-dB signal to noise gain. They also can be used to mask tinnitus if other nonspecific measures fail. Cognition and dexterity of fingers are the main considerations while selecting hearing aids.

Assistive Listening Devices

These can be linked to hearing aids like telecoil for telephone or frequency-modulated systems or independent of hearing aid like wireless headphones for use with their television and flashing light with doorbell.

Cochlear Implantation

This can be considered an option in bilateral severe to profound hearing loss with no significant benefit from hearing aids.

■ Future Interventions

Research to induce regeneration of hair cells to address the fundamental defect in ARHL is ongoing. These include genetic, cellular, and pharmacotherapeutic strategies.

Sudden Sensorineural Hearing Loss

Introduction

Sudden sensorineural hearing loss (SSHL) or sudden deafness is an unexplained rapid loss of hearing occurring at once or within a few days. It is defined as SNHL of 30 dB or greater occurring over three contiguous audiometric frequencies occurring over 72 hours.

■ Epidemiology

Although the estimated incidence of SSHL is 5-20 per 100,000, the true incidence may be much higher. The peak incidence is in the fifth and sixth decades, with no gender difference. Almost all cases are unilateral with less than 2% cases being bilateral.

■ Clinical Features

Sudden deafness is a medical emergency. SSHL is an alarming rapid-onset hearing loss, typically unilateral, occurring within a few days. SSHL may be associated with tinnitus (41–90%) and dizziness (29–56%).

Pearl

Red flags associated with SSHL are as follows:

- Concurrent head trauma.
- Neurological signs and symptoms.
- Unilateral middle ear effusion (suggestive of naso-pharyngeal malignancy).

Etiology

The majority of unilateral SSHL are *idiopathic*, that is *idiopathic* SNHL (ISSHL), with only 10% of patients having an identifiable cause (**Table 5.12**).

Pearl

Theories for etiology of ISSHL are the following:

- Labyrinthine viral infection.
- Labyrinthine vascular compromise.
- Intracochlear membrane ruptures.
- Immune-mediated inner ear disease.

Evaluation

The main aim of evaluation of SSHL is to establish the diagnosis and to rule out an identifiable underlying cause for the hearing loss. In addition, it will help in planning appropriate treatment and predict prognosis. A thorough history including onset, associated symptoms, and course may be helpful. Past medical and treatment history can reveal risk factors for hearing loss. Clinical examination can rule out local pathology. The investigations required in a patient with SSHL is outlined in **Flowchart 5.5**.

Audiogram

Serial PTA has value not only in diagnosis but also in prognosis and documenting the recovery of the patient. If malingering is suspected, tests for malingering like Stenger's test or BERA can be performed. Speech audiometry helps in documenting the functional handicap.

Ruling out Retrocochlear Pathology

MRI with gadolinium is the gold standard for ruling out a vestibular schwannoma or other retrocochlear pathology with a sensitivity of 99%. A stacked auditory brainstem response (ABR) has a sensitivity of 95% as compared to a traditional ABR (79–88%) for tumors less than 1 cm in size.

Pearl

A total of 1 to 6% of patients with SSNHL on average will have positive findings on MRI (approximately 1–2% of patients with ISSHL have internal auditory canal [IAC] or cerebellopontine angle [CPA]) tumors. Conversely, 3–12% of patients with vestibular schwannomas present with sudden hearing loss).

Pearl

Stacked ABR is an investigation tool to pick up small, unilateral, acoustic neuromas that are less than 1 cm in size. These are sometimes missed by the standard BERA. It is formed by aligning all the V wave peaks and adding the waveforms together.

Table 5.12 Identifiable causes of sudden sensorineural hearing loss

Autoimmune	Autoimmune inner ear disease	*Infectious*	Bacterial meningitis
	Behcet's disease		Mumps
	Cogan's syndrome		Mycoplasma
	Systemic lupus erythematosus		Syphilis
			Herpes zoster oticus
Metabolic	Diabetes mellitus	*Neurologic*	Migraine
	Hypothyroidism		Pontine ischemia
			Multiple sclerosis
Neoplastic	Vestibular schwannoma	*Otologic*	Ménière's disease
	cerebellopontine angle (CPA) or petrous tumors		Enlarged vestibular aqueduct
Traumatic	Head trauma causing inner ear concussion	*Toxic*	Aminoglycosides
	Perilymph fistula		Chemotherapeutic agents
	Acoustic trauma	*Central hearing disorder*	Psychogenic hearing loss
	Temporal bone fracture		

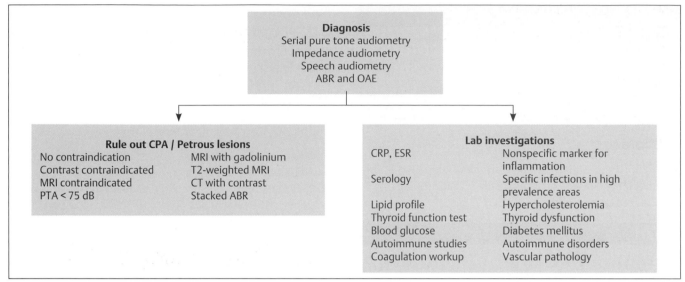

Flowchart 5.5 Algorithm to outline the investigations required for a patient with sudden sensorineural hearing loss (SSHL). Abbreviations: ABR, auditory brainstem response; CPA, cerebellopontine angle; CRP, C-reactive protein; CT, computed tomography; ESR, erythrocyte sedimentation rate; MRI, magnetic resonance imaging; OAE, otoacoustic emission.

■ Principles of Management

Placebo-controlled studies have shown about 45% spontaneous recovery to 10 dB of contralateral ear, within 2 weeks of onset of hearing loss. However, longer duration of hearing loss is associated with reduced chance of recovery of hearing loss.

Factors impacting hearing recovery include the following:
- Age at onset of hearing loss.
- Hearing loss severity.
- Frequencies affected.
- Presence of vertigo.
- Time between onset of hearing loss and visit with the treating physician.

Many of the etiological agents cause irreversible hearing loss. However, identifying these conditions and treating them can prevent further damage. Also, some of the underlying conditions like vestibular schwannoma have a broader implication on health.

Steroids

Corticosteroids may be offered as initial treatment to patients with SSHL within 2 weeks of onset of hearing loss. Oral prednisolone (1 mg/kg for 2 weeks followed by tapering over 6 weeks) and dexamethasone are the commonly used steroids.

Steroids reduce the inflammation and edema in the inner ear. *Intratympanic steroids* (dexamethasone 10 mg/ml, twice a week for 2 successive weeks) may be used in patients with an incomplete recovery from SSHL. Intratympanic injection increases the steroid concentration in the perilymph.

Hyperbaric Oxygen Therapy

If facilities are available, hyperbaric oxygen therapy (HBOT), in combination with steroid therapy, may be offered either as initial treatment within 2 weeks of onset or as salvage therapy to patients with SSHL within 1 month of onset.

Antiviral Agents

Acyclovir or newer agents like famciclovir and valacyclovir have been used in combination with steroids for treatment of SSHL presuming a viral etiology. However, there is lack of evidence of efficacy in treating SSHL.

Vasodilators and Rheologic Agents

Vasodilators, like papaverine and nicotinic acid, reverse hypoxia of the cochlea by improving the blood supply. Carbogen (5% carbon dioxide) has been shown to increase oxygen concentration in the perilymph. Rheological agents like dextran and pentoxifylline improve blood flow by reducing viscosity.

Prognosis

Factors influencing prognosis are presented in **Table 5.13**.

Ototoxicity

The harmful effect of certain therapeutic agents and chemical substances on the structures of the inner ear, that is, the end organs and neurons of the cochlear and vestibular divisions of the eighth nerve, that can cause functional

Table 5.13 Factors influencing prognosis

Factors	Positive impact	Negative impact
Age	<60 y	>60 y
Duration of hearing loss	<2 wk	>3 mo
Hearing loss in the opposite ear	Absent	Present
Vertigo	Absent	Present
Audiologic characteristics	Low or mid frequency (**Fig. 5.4**)	Down-sloping
Hearing loss	Mild-moderate	Severe or profound (**Fig. 5.5**)
Erythrocyte sedimentation rate	<25	>25 mm/h

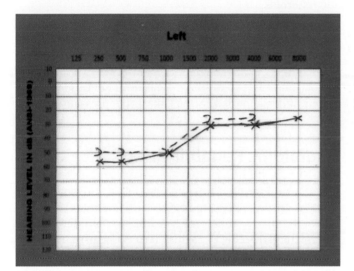

Fig. 5.4 Pure tone audiogram shows sensorineural hearing loss in the low to mid-frequencies.

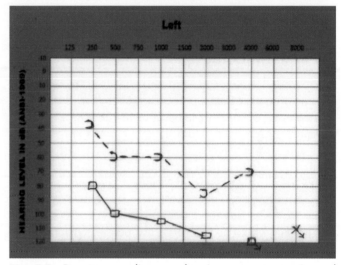

Fig. 5.5 Pure tone audiogram showing severe sensorineural hearing loss.

impairment is called ototoxicity. The effect of the substance can be cochleotoxic or vestibulotoxic or both, unilateral or bilateral, or temporary or permanent. The ototoxicity occurs at therapeutic doses.

Note: Neurotoxicity is when the effect of a drug is on the brainstem or the central connections of the cochlear or vestibular nuclei, which can affect the hearing and/or balance.

■ List of Ototoxic Drugs/Substances

- Antibiotics:
  - Aminoglycosides like gentamicin, amikacin, tobramycin, and streptomycin.
  - Macrolides like erythromycin and azithromycin.
  - Vancomycin.
- Antineoplastic agents:
  - Cisplatin and carboplatin.
  - Nitrogen mustard.
  - Bleomycin.
- Loop diuretics:
  - Furosemide

- Ethacrynic acid
- Analgesics:
  - Salicylates.
  - Hydrocodone.
  - Methadone.
- Antimalarial drugs:
  - Quinine.
  - Chloroquine.
- Chelating agents:
  - Deferoxamine.
- Chemicals:
  - Alcohol.
  - Nicotine.
  - Arsenic.
  - Carbon monoxide.
- Heavy metals:
  - Lead.
  - Gold.
- Solvents:
  - Polyethylene glycol.
  - Propylene glycol.

■ Risk Factors for Ototoxicity

The risk factors for ototoxicity are the following:
- Type of drug.
- Simultaneous use of other ototoxic drugs, for example, aminoglycoside with loop diuretic.
- Deranged renal or liver function.
- Duration of treatment and total dose.
- Age and sex.
- Familial tendency.
- Prior treatment with ototoxic drugs.
- Dehydration.

Note: Topical agents like neomycin and polymyxin B have been shown to cause ototoxicity in animal studies. In humans, it has not been substantiated.

■ Pathophysiology

The pathophysiology depends on the drug. In the cochlea, most of the effects are on the inner row of the outer hair cells, especially at the basal turn. The stria vascularis, Reissner's membrane, spiral ligament, and spiral ganglion cells can also be involved. In the vestibular system, type I hair cells of the crista ampullaris are more commonly involved along with vacuolization of the remaining hair cells. Aminoglycosides have a strong tissue binding capacity and tends to remain in the inner ear even after the drug is stopped, which accounts for the possible deterioration in hearing later. The effect of the drug may sometimes be unilateral.

■ Clinical Features

Tinnitus is an early symptom of ototoxicity. In erythromycin-related ototoxicity, the tinnitus is typically the "blowing" type. The hearing loss (sensorineural) may not be noticed initially as it involves the higher frequencies (above 4 kHz). The vestibular symptoms may be of gait abnormalities, oscillopsia, and imbalance. Vertigo with change in posture can occur. The symptoms may be unilateral. Often the symptoms are reversible on stopping the drug. With aminoglycosides, the effect on the inner ear may start later, that is, even after stopping the drug.

■ Management

- Pre- and posttreatment biweekly testing of hearing by PTA should be done, especially when known ototoxic drugs are used. Preferably an ultra-high-frequency audiometer, which tests the higher frequencies, is used to detect the early SNHL. Hearing loss of more than 15 dB at two or more frequencies in one or both ears is considered significant.
- Distortion product otoacoustic emissions (DPOAEs) are useful in detecting early hearing loss.
- BERA.
- Vestibular tests like caloric tests may show a decrease of the peak slow phase by 50%.
- Bedside evaluation for vestibular dysfunction: nystagmus (spontaneous, headshake).
- Reduction of the ototoxicity can be done by the following:
  - Use of an alternative drug.
  - Reduce/adjust dose as per the creatinine clearance.
  - Avoid simultaneous use of other ototoxic drugs.
  - Use of otoprotective compounds like N-acetylcysteine, D-methionine, caspase inhibitors, and intratympanic steroids.
- For hearing loss, hearing rehabilitation by hearing aids and CI.
- For vestibular dysfunction: vestibular rehabilitation therapy.
- For tinnitus, counseling, masking devices, tinnitus retraining, and medications like antidepressants.

Audiologic Rehabilitation

Patients who have residual hearing loss or tinnitus should be explained about the potential benefits of hearing rehabilitation. In unilateral hearing loss, options include contralateral routing of signal (CROS) hearing aids and bone-anchored hearing aid (BAHA). In bilateral hearing loss, hearing aids, assistive listening devices, or CIs may be considered.

Pearl

In the elderlies with comorbidities, and more prone for transient ischemic attacks and stroke, vascular compromise can cause SSHL.

Hearing Rehabilitation with Aids

■ Hearing Aids

Hearing aids amplify the sound vibration to improve hearing and speech comprehension in patients with hearing loss. The electronic hearing aid, or more correctly the electroacoustic hearing aid, detects sound in the environment, amplifies it, and then delivers it into the ear canal. By making sound louder, the hearing aid increases the sound transmission to stimulate the remaining hair cells within the inner ear.

All hearing aids have a microphone, processor, receiver, and battery compartment. Sound enters the microphone, is amplified, and shaped by the processor, converted back into sound by the receiver, and directed out to the ear canal (**Fig. 5.6**).

Hearing aid selection is a complex part of hearing rehabilitation. The process involves the clinician's assessment of a patient's candidacy for amplification, followed by the fitting and verification processes. The clinical considerations include the type and severity of hearing loss, sensitivity to sound and dynamic range, the psychological attitude of the patient, physical conditions like size and shape of the external auditory canal, dexterity of the patient, and the cosmetic appearance.

Hearing aids may be fitted in one or both ears. In patients with unilateral hearing loss, a CROS hearing aid can be used.

Hearing aids may be analog or digital. They can further be classified into programmable or nonprogrammable. They are available in four styles: Body-worn, eyeglass, behind the ear (BTE), and in the ear (ITE). The ITE includes in-the-canal (ITC) and CIC hearing aids (**Fig. 5.7**).

■ Implantable Hearing Systems

Implantable hearing systems are recommended for patients who cannot use or are not getting significant benefit from a conventional hearing aid, either due to medical or audiological reasons:

- Sensory hearing disorder not benefiting from a conventional hearing aid.
- Malformations of the ear where conventional aid cannot be fitted.
- Chronic otitis externa or eczema of the auditory canal or chronic diseases of the outer ear.

In single-sided deafness (SSD), bone conduction systems bypass the deaf ear entirely and deliver sound directly to the hearing ear's cochlea. SSD candidates with a large transcranial attenuation or an SNHL developing in the hearing ear may benefit from the additional amplification provided by the Baha Connect System or the Osia System.

The functional principle of implantable hearing systems consists of transforming the registered sound into electric signals and then into micromechanical vibrations that are transmitted to the ossicular chain or directly into the inner ear. Due to the better amplification, implantable hearing systems provide not only a better sound quality but also a more differentiated speech recognition based on less distortion.

Implantable hearing systems are classified into partially and fully implantable hearing systems (**Flowchart 5.6**).

■ Bone Conduction Implants

Bone conduction implants (BCIs) are used in patients with conductive hearing loss whose inner ear function is mostly intact or in SSD for contralateral routing of hearing. Since the sound energy is transmitted via bone conduction, the amplification of the inner ear is limited.

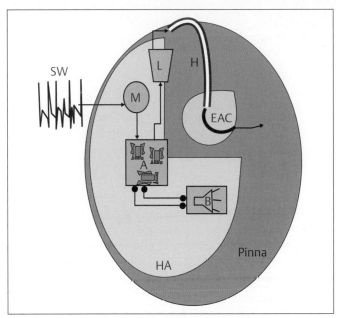

Fig. 5.6   Working of a hearing aid. A, amplifier (increases the strength of the signal); B, battery (powers the hearing aid); EAC, external auditory canal; H, hook (a tube that passes through the earmold to play sound into the EAC); HA, hearing aid; L, loudspeaker (plays sound into the ear hook); M, microphone (picks sound and converts it to an electrical signal); SW, sound waves (travel toward the ear).

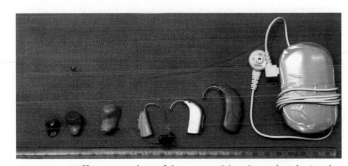

Fig. 5.7   Different styles of hearing aids. Completely in the canal (CIC), in the canal (ITC), in the ear (ITE), receiver in the canal (RIC), Mini BTE, behind the ear (BTE), body worn from left to right.

The idea of sound transmissions was known as early as 1757. Jorrissen published his doctoral thesis "hearing by means of the teeth and part of the hard palate." Itard developed the first bone conduction hearing system by connecting a megaphone fixed to the patient's teeth. Dentiphone was used in the 1930s and bone conduction glasses in the 1950s. BAHAs were first developed as a dental implant in the 1970s and then with a fixing screw onto the temporal bone.

Passive Bone Conduction Implants

In 1977, a partially implantable hearing system was developed, the BAHA, by coupling a hearing aid to a fixing screw/

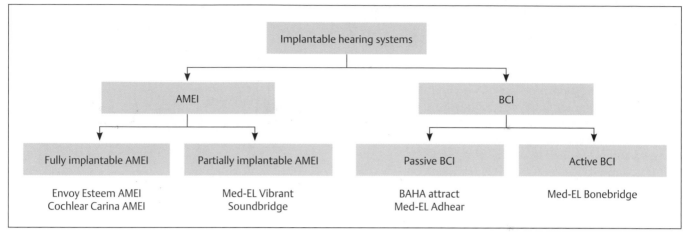

Flowchart 5.6 Classification of implantable hearing systems. Abbreviations: AMEI, active middle ear implants; BAHA, bone-anchored hearing aid; BCI, bone conduction implants.

implant anchored in the cranial bone. The sound vibrations were transmitted through bone conduction to the inner ear bypassing the eardrum. The transcutaneous devices have now been modified into percutaneous systems, by using magnets to keep the sound processor over the implant. Examples of passive BCI include BAHA and Sophono alpha.

Active Bone Conduction Implants

An abutment anchored in the bone transmits sound in the form of vibrations from the sound processor to the implant and then further through the bone to the inner ear. The sound processor can be adjusted independently from the system. Examples include BAHA connect and Oticon Ponto. Med-EL Bonebridge is an active partially implantable bone conduction system in which an electromagnetic transducer (bone conduction floating mass transducer, BC-FMT) is fixed at the skull bone and transmits actively sound waves via the bone to the inner ear.

■ Active Middle Ear Implants

In active middle ear implant (AMEIs), the amplified electric signals are transformed into mechanical vibrations and transmitted either to the sound conduction apparatus of the *middle ear* (tympanic membrane and ossicles) or to the cochlea.

The AMEI may work on an electromagnetic or piezoelectric basis. The vibrations in the electromagnetic transducers are generated between a current-supplied coil and a magnet, whereas in piezoelectric transducers, the vibrations are generated by the current-induced relative change in the length of a piezoelectric crystal (**Table 5.14**).

Electromagnetic transducers have a higher maximal output amplitude but consume more energy for the same acoustic performance. Furthermore, these are not MRI compatible. The piezoelectric transducers are less distorting, but the stiffness of these transducers leads to higher

Table 5.14 Overview of AMEI

	Fully implantable	**Partially implantable**
Piezoelectric	Envoy Esteem	Rion Device
	Implex TICA	
Electromagnetic	Cochlear Carina	Cochlear MET
		Cochlear Codacs
		Ototronix Maxum

Abbreviations: AMEI, active middle ear implants; MET, middle ear transducer; TICA, total implantable cochlear amplifier.

resistance of the sound conduction apparatus when these are coupled to the ossicles.

■ Cochlear Implant

A CI is a surgically implanted device for the treatment of severe to profound SNHL in both children and adults. Acoustic energy is converted into an electrical signal, to stimulate surviving spiral ganglion cells of the auditory nerve.

These implants usually consist of two main components:
- *External system*: Microphone, sound processor, and transmitter system.
- *Implanted system*: Receiver-stimulator and electrode array.

Indications for Cochlear Implants in Adults

- Bilateral moderate to profound levels of hearing loss with limited benefit from conventional amplification (**Fig. 5.8**).
- Less than and equal to 50% speech recognition ability in the ear to be implanted or ≤60% in the binaural best-aided condition.

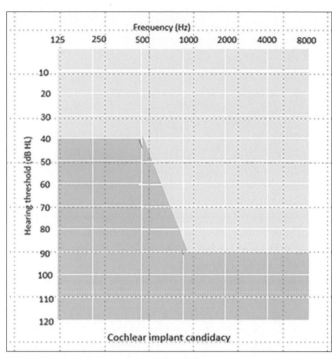

Fig. 5.8 Cochlear implant (CI) candidacy.

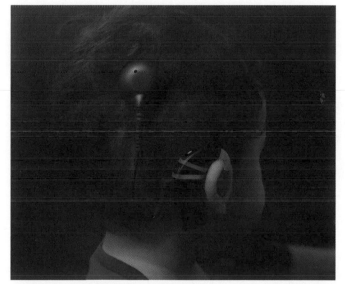

Fig. 5.9 A child with cochlear implant.

- Patients with residual low-frequency hearing, electric-acoustic stimulation with a shortened electrode array for unilateral consonant-nucleus-consonant (CNC) word scores ≤60%.
- Patients with SSD.

Indications for Cochlear Implants in Children

- Children aged 9 months to 2 years with profound (>90 dB HL) bilateral SNHL (**Fig. 5.9**).
- Children aged 2 to 17 years with severe to profound bilateral SNHL (>70 dB HL).
- Little to no benefit with appropriately fitted hearing aids.
- Children aged 5 years and older who have an SSD or asymmetric hearing loss with extremely poor word recognition (<5%).

A summary of the CI summary guidelines is given in **Table 5.15**.

Contraindication

Patients with cochlear nerve aplasia are not suitable for cochlear implantation.

Principle of Cochlear Implant

Sound detected by the microphone is converted into an electrical signal. The external sound processor transforms the signal into an electronic code. This digital signal is transmitted transcutaneously by a transmitting coil via radiofrequency to the receiver-stimulator. The receiver-stimulator translates the signal into electrical impulses distributed to multiple electrodes on an array implanted within the cochlea. This electrically stimulates spiral ganglion cells and auditory nerve axons. By different processing strategies in the sound processor, it is possible to convey the timing, frequency, and intensity of sound.

The electrodes are placed into the cochlea via the round window or a cochleostomy. The approach is by a posterior tympanotomy or the transcanal (Veria technique).

Table 5.15 Cochlear implant candidacy guidelines

	Adult	Children (2–17 y)	Children (12–24 mo)
Hearing threshold	Moderate to profound SNHL in both ears (>40 dB)	Severe to profound SNHL (>70 dB)	Profound SNHL (>90 dB)
Word recognition	Limited benefit from binaural amplification defined by ≤50% sentence recognition in the ear to be implanted (or ≤40% by CMS criteria) and ≤60% in the contralateral ear or binaurally	Limited benefit from binaural amplification defined by ≤20–30% word recognition scores	Limited benefit from binaural amplification trial based on the MAIS

Abbreviations: CMS, Centers for Medicare & Medicaid Services; MAIS, meaningful auditory integration scale; SNHL, sensorineural hearing loss.

■ Auditory Brainstem Implants

For patients with profound SNHL, who cannot benefit from a CI, the only remaining option of hearing rehabilitation of the ipsilateral ear is an auditory brainstem implant (ABI). The ABI is implanted near the surface of the cochlear nucleus on the brainstem and directly stimulates the auditory pathway.

Indications

Indications for ABI include patients with a disrupted or absent cochlear nerve or those with a cochlea that is not suitable for implantation. The most commonly implanted patients are those with neurofibromatosis type 2 (NF2). Nontumor indications for ABI include the following:

- Deafness secondary to bilateral temporal bone fractures with cochlear nerve avulsion.
- Labyrinthine ossifications.
- Severe congenital inner ear malformation with no receiving cavity to house a CI electrode array and/or a nerve to propagate the signal to the brainstem (e.g., bilateral cochlear nerve deficiency/aplasia, cochlear aplasia, or complete labyrinthine aplasia).

Points to Ponder

- NIHL is the leading preventable cause of hearing loss.
- NIHL can cause a temporary threshold shift initially, which is reversible but later leads to a permanent threshold shift.
- Workplace noise level equal to an average SPL of 85 dBA or higher for an 8-hour period is at high risk of NIHL.
- The classical early audiometric pattern of NIHL is of a high-tone SNHL with a notched appearance centered on 4 or 6 kHz, with some recovery at 8 kHz.
- ARHL is the most common cause of hearing loss.
- ARHL may be defined as a progressive bilateral SNHL of mid to late adult onset, where underlying causes have been excluded.
- PTA shows symmetrical down-sloping loss over 2 kHz.
- SSHL is defined as SNHL ≥30 dB occurring over three contiguous audiometric frequencies occurring over 72 hours.
- PTA should be performed as soon as possible to confirm a diagnosis.
- Patients with SSNHL should undergo MRI or ABR to evaluate for retrocochlear pathology.
- Corticosteroids, systemic or intratympanic, may be offered to patients with SSNHL.
- Antiviral therapy, thrombolytic therapy, vasodilator therapy, and vasoactive substances should not be routinely prescribed to patients with SSNHL.

Case-Based Questions

1. A 42-year-old man working in the engine room of a ship presented with bilateral tinnitus. Examination of the ear did not reveal any significant abnormality. A PTA done showed a dip in the audiogram at 4 kHz on both sides. He wants to continue in his profession.

   a. What is the diagnosis?
   b. How would you counsel this patient?
   c. What is the treatment if the hearing loss progresses to bilateral moderate/severe SNHL?
   d. What is the treatment available if the hearing loss progresses to bilateral profound hearing loss?

   Answers
   a. NIHL.
   b. Counseling would revolve around protection of the ear from loud sounds as long as he is working in that environment. Otherwise, his hearing and tinnitus will continue to deteriorate.
   c. Hearing aid.
   d. CI.

2. A 56-year-old male patient with pneumonia was responsive or sensitive to only drugs like amikacin and he was started on the same. After 6 days of treatment, the patient developed tinnitus on both sides and the renal function tests showed an increase in the creatinine levels.

   a. What is the possible cause for tinnitus?
   b. What test would aid in the diagnosis?
   c. What would be the further management options?

   Answers
   a. Ototoxicity due to the use of aminoglycosides like amikacin.
   b. PTA.
   c. Since the tinnitus is drug induced, the drug has to be stopped and an alternative drug that is not ototoxic has to be administered. Serial PTAs have to be done over a period of time to note any deterioration. If there is hearing loss, hearing aid must be considered. If tinnitus persists, tinnitus retraining therapy or TRT can be started.

Frequently Asked Questions

1. Enumerate the ototoxic drugs.
2. What is acoustic trauma and NIHL?
3. What are the indications for cochlear implantation in an adult?
4. Enumerate the various types of hearing aids.
5. What is the principle behind a hearing aid? What are the parts of a hearing aid?
6. What is presbycusis? Discuss the management of presbycusis.
7. What is SSHL?
8. How will you differentiate a cochlear deafness from a retrocochlear deafness?

Endnote

The first hearing aid created in the 17th century was the ear trumpet. Some of the first hearing aids were external hearing aids. The first electronic hearing aid was invented in 1898 by Harvey Fletcher while working at Bell Laboratories. By the late 20th century, digital hearing aids were commercially available.

In 1790, Alessandro Volta observed that electrical stimulation of the auditory pathway can create the perception of sound. William House with Jack Urban in the 1960s created the first implantable device that could stimulate the auditory nerve, making CIs a clinical reality. In the late 1970s, Graeme Clark in Australia developed the first multichannel CI with improved speech recognition abilities.

6 Otalgia

Vinay V. Rao

The competency covered in this chapter is as follows:

EN4.1 Elicit, document, and present a correct history; demonstrate and describe the clinical features; choose the correct investigations; and describe the principles of management of otalgia.

Introduction

Ear pain is called otalgia. Thees are of two types:
- Primary otalgia.
- Secondary or referred otalgia.

Pathophysiology

In primary otalgia, the pain is due to inflammatory, traumatic, and neoplastic causes affecting the ear.

In secondary/referred otalgia, the pain is referred to the ear from other head and neck sites that are supplied by the same nerve (**Fig. 6.1**). The following nerves are implicated:
- Trigeminal nerve (fifth cranial nerve): The nerve responsible is the auriculotemporal nerve, which is a branch of the mandibular division of the trigeminal nerve. It supplies the pinna, external auditory canal, and middle ear, and carries pain sensations from the oral cavity, nose and paranasal sinuses, face, nasopharynx, and temporomandibular joint.
- Facial nerve (seventh cranial nerve): It innervates the conchal skin and has a minor supply to adjacent area around the pinna.
- Glossopharyngeal nerve (ninth cranial nerve): The preganglionic secretomotor fibers to the parotid gland forms a part of tympanic plexus (Jacobson's nerve). It also supplies oropharynx (tonsil, soft palate, base of the tongue, and posterior pharyngeal wall).
- Vagus nerve (10th cranial nerve): It supplies the posterior canal wall and concha and is called Arnold's nerve. It also supplies sensation to the pharynx.
- C2 and C3 nerves: These include greater auricular and lesser occipital nerves.

Causes of Otalgia

■ Primary Otalgia

- *Pinna*: Perichondritis, trauma.
- *External auditory canal*: Furuncle, impacted wax, otitis externa (otomycosis, viral, and bacterial), foreign bodies, trauma, and herpes zoster oticus.

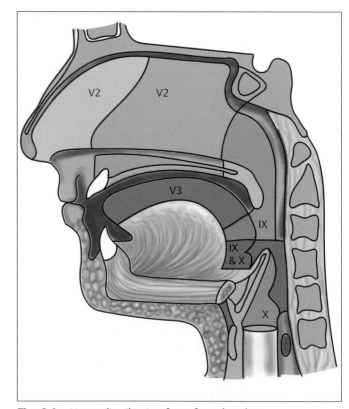

Fig. 6.1 Nerve distribution for referred otalgia.

- *Middle ear*: Acute otitis media, eustachian tube dysfunction, mastoiditis, trauma (barotrauma, direct trauma), malignancy, and granulomatous infection.

■ Secondary/Referred Otalgia

- Fifth cranial nerve (**Fig. 6.2**):
  - Dental: Caries, impacted molar, and apical infection.
  - Oral cavity: Stomatitis, aphthous ulcer, and malignant ulcers.
  - Salivary glands: Infection and malignancy.
  - Temporomandibular joint: Costen's syndrome, osteoarthritis, recurrent dislocation, and trauma.
  - Nose and paranasal sinuses: Trauma and sinusitis.
  - Nasopharynx: Space-occupying lesions like tumors.
  - Headache and atypical facial pain.
- Ninth cranial nerve:
  - Oropharynx: Tonsillitis, peritonsillar abscess, and palatal ulcers.
  - Elongated styloid process.
  - Glossopharyngeal neuralgia.
- Tenth cranial nerve:
  - Larynx, laryngopharynx, oropharynx, and esophagus: Inflammation, trauma, and malignancy.
- Seventh cranial nerve:
  - Herpes zoster oticus and Bell's palsy.
- C2 and C3:
  - Cervical spine disease through the trigeminal nerve can lead to referred pain.
- Psychogenic.

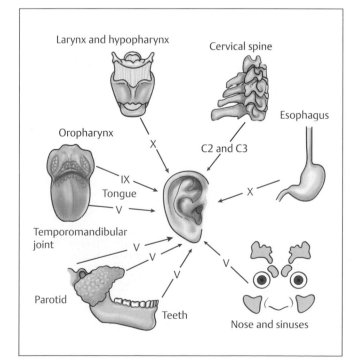

Fig. 6.2   Causes of referred otalgia.

Pearl

Neuralgias like trigeminal neuralgia can cause otalgia also. Tension headache and atypical facial pain can involve the ear. Cardiac otalgia refers to an atypical presentation of ear pain, unilateral or bilateral, due to myocardial infarction. The pain is referred through the auricular branch of the vagus.

Clinical Features of a Patient with Otalgia

■ History

The following points are to be noted:
- Onset.
- Duration.
- Type or quality:
  - Sharp and throbbing: Acute otitis media.
  - Dull and continuous throbbing: Furuncle.
- Localization:
  - Positive tragal sign: Furuncle in the anterior wall of the external auditory canal.
  - Postaural pain: Mastoiditis.
  - Deep-seated pain with blocking sensation: Acute otitis media.
  - Pain on chewing: Temporomandibular joint arthralgia and furuncle in the ear canal.
  - Associated symptoms with pain could be otorrhea, hearing loss, and swelling.
- History of prior surgery.

Pearl

Chronic suppurative otitis media, mucosal type, usually does not cause pain. The squamosal type can be associated with ear pain due to impending complications like mastoiditis.

Clinical Examination

- Ear, nose, and throat examination.
- Dental examination (remove dentures if present and reexamine).
- Temporomandibular joint examination.
- Neck examination.
- Neurological examination including cranial nerves.

Pearl

If the severity of the pain is more than the finding in the ear, consider the possibility of a referred otalgia and evaluate for the same.

Investigations

- Endoscopic examination of the nose and nasopharynx.
- Endoscopic evaluation of pharynx and larynx.
- Cervical spine, styloid process, and temporomandibular joint: X-ray or computed tomography (CT) scan.
- Orthopantomogram.

Management

- Appropriate investigations to confirm the diagnosis.
- When diagnosis is in doubt and there is a suspicious lesion, a biopsy for tissue diagnosis would be helpful, especially when considering malignancy or granulomatous conditions.
- In case of referred otalgia, treat the primary cause.

Points to Ponder

- Usual causes of primary otalgia include inflammation of the pinna, otitis externa, otitis media, and mastoiditis.
- Difficulty in diagnosis arises when the ear is normal; therefore, a search beyond the ear has to be carried out to identify referred otalgia.
- The common causes of referred otalgia include temporomandibular joint dysfunction, dental caries, throat infections like tonsillitis, malignancies of oropharynx, and elongated styloid process.
- Treatment is directed at the cause.

Case-Based Question

1. **A 45-year-old woman was seen in the ear, nose, and throat (ENT) clinic with complaints of pain over the right ear for the last 2 years. She had been examined by various ENT surgeons who have reassured her that the right ear is normal. On further enquiry, she says the pain starts sometimes in the upper neck on the right side and spreads to the ear. Examination of the throat is normal. Tonsils are not enlarged or congested. Palpation of the right tonsillar region elicited tenderness.**

   a. What is the provisional diagnosis?
   b. What investigation would you do to confirm your diagnosis?
   c. What is the treatment?

Answers

a. Pain radiating from the neck to the ear with a tender tonsillar region is suggestive of stylalgia or Eagle's syndrome.
b. Radiological investigations like an orthopantomogram or CT scan will reveal the presence of a medialized elongated styloid process.
c. Excision of the styloid process through a transoral route, after tonsillectomy.

Frequently Asked Questions

1. What is the difference between primary otalgia and secondary or referred otalgia?
2. Enumerate the causes of referred otalgia.
3. What are the causes of primary otalgia due to middle ear diseases?
4. Describe the nerves implicated in referred otalgia?
5. What is Eagle syndrome?

Endnote

Earache or otalgia and its remedies have been around for thousands of years, ever since the time of Hippocrates. It was the Roman physician Celsus who first wrote that "severe ear pain unsettles the mind" and suggested remedies that would not be accepted in today's medical world. Ancient remedies include the placement of boiled earthworms into the ear or inducing vomiting or as Galen wrote, "pouring a mixture of opium, musk and the white of an egg into the ear."

7 Diseases of the External Ear

K.S. Gangadhara Somayaji and A. Rajeshwary

The competencies covered in this chapter are as follows:

EN4.2 Elicit document and present a correct history; demonstrate and describe the clinical features; choose the correct investigations; and describe the principles of management of diseases of the external ear.

EN4.9 Demonstrate the correct technique for syringing wax from the ear in a simulated environment.

EN3.4 Observe and describe the indications for and steps involved in the removal of foreign bodies from the ear, nose, and throat.

Introduction

Diseases of the external ear can involve the auricle or the external auditory canal (EAC). Classification of the diseases of the external ear is described in the following sections (**Table 7.1**).

Diseases of the Auricle

■ Congenital Disorders

The congenital disorders of the external ear can involve the auricle or the EAC or both. As the development of external and middle ear is different from that of the inner ear, the inner ear is often normal in these anomalies.

Bat Ear or Protruding Ear

It is the most common congenital deformity of the ear and is caused by underdeveloped antihelical fold, which may be associated with hypertrophy or excessive curvature of the conchal cartilage. The auricle will be more than 2 cm from the side of the head and at an angle of more than 30 degrees. Although there are no functional impairments, psychological and emotional trauma, especially in childhood, necessitates surgical correction. Surgery can be performed any time after 4 to 6 years of age. Ear splinting may be tried in the neonatal period before the age of 3 months (**Fig. 7.1**).

Lop/Cup Ear

The lower part of the auricle appears normal with deformed upper portion, resembling hanging down ears of a rabbit.

Table 7.1 Classification of the diseases of the external ear

Type of disorder	Etiology	Disease
Congenital		Bat ear, lop ear, preauricular pits and sinuses, accessory auricles, anotia, microtia, macrotia, Mozart's ear, Wildermuth's ear, atresia of the auditory canal, and collaural fistula
Acquired	Traumatic	Lacerations, hematoma, seroma, and keloid
	Infective	Chondritis, perichondritis, acute and chronic otitis externa (bacterial, fungal, viral), and malignant otitis externa
	Tumors	
	Benign	Cysts, horns, osteoma, exostosis, ceruminoma, and adenoma
	Malignant	Squamous cell carcinoma, basal cell carcinoma, and melanoma
	Miscellaneous	Wax, keratosis obturans, canal wall cholesteatoma, and foreign body

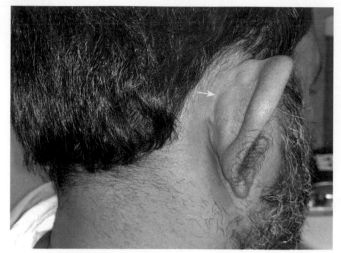

Fig. 7.1 Protruding ear or bat ear where the mastoid–helix angle is more than 35 degrees.

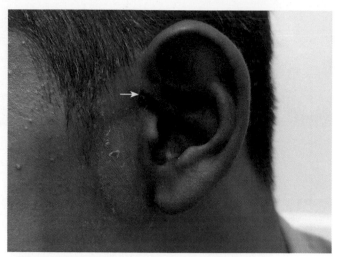

Fig. 7.2 Preauricular sinus (*arrow*), with abscess.

There are no functional problems. Surgical correction may be necessary for cosmetic purposes.

Minor Variations

Darwin's tubercle: Small elevation on the posterosuperior part of the helix, representing the apex of the pinna in some of the animals.

Mozart's ear: Bulging anterosuperior portion of the auricle due to fusion of the crura of the antihelix with protruding conchal cave.

Wildermuth's ear: The antihelix is more prominent than the helix.

Stahl's ear: It is characterized by flat helix and duplication of the upper crus of the antihelix.

Barbula hirci: This is excessive hair seen over the tragus. Similar growth of hair may be seen over the rim of helix, which is linked to Y-linked genetic inheritance and is seen only in males.

Pearls

- The surgical correction of malformed ears is called otoplasty. The ear grows during childhood. It reaches the adult size at 5 years of age; therefore, the ideal age for surgery for bat ears is 5 years.
- Minor variations like Darwin's tubercle are not that uncommon and do not need correction.

■ Preauricular Sinus and Cysts

Preauricular pit or sinus is a common congenital condition caused by faulty union of hillocks of His of the first and the second branchial arches during the development of the pinna. It is often seen at the root of the helix just above the tragus. The tract is lined by squamous epithelium. A sinus ends as a blind tract opening to the exterior, whereas a fistula is a tract that connects two epithelial surfaces. Three groups can be distinguished on the basis of the embryologic association and site:

- Preauricular sinus between the angle of the mouth and the tragus.
- Fistulas that begin in front of the ascending helix and lead toward the meatus, or open externally inferior to the angle of the mandible.
- A small fistula or pitted depression affecting any part of the auricle.

Clinical Features

The sinus can remain asymptomatic throughout life or get infected and form a painful swelling and abscess, which may discharge pus repeatedly (**Fig. 7.2**).

Treatment

Preauricular pits do not require treatment unless they become repeatedly infected. Abscess requires an incision and drainage followed by antibiotics. Complete excision of the sinus or fistula is the treatment of choice, which should be performed after controlling the infection. The tract can be delineated using methylene blue or cannulation. Incomplete removal results in recurrence. Asymptomatic patients need not be treated.

■ Skin Tags

They are mostly seen in the preauricular area, single or multiple, and in some cases may contain cartilage. They are due to incomplete closure of the first branchial cleft or incomplete fusion of the auricular hillocks. They require removal only for cosmetic purpose (**Fig. 7.3**).

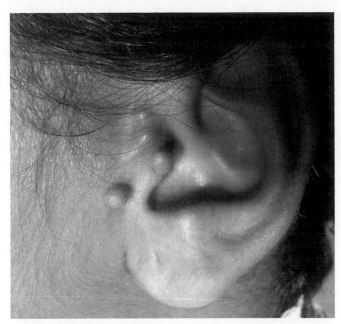

Fig. 7.3 Accessory skin tags in front of the auricle.

■ Microtia

Microtia is hypoplasia of the auricle, while anotia is the total absence of the auricle. Similarly, there can be polyotia and macrotia, which are rare. The incidence of microtia is around 1 to 3 per 10,000 live births. The condition is usually associated with canal atresia. It is found more commonly in males and more than 75% of cases are unilateral and seen on the right side. Microtia may be seen alone or in association with other malformations or syndromes such as Treacher Collins' syndrome, hemifacial microstomia, and Goldenhar's syndrome. Prenatal exposure to isotretinoin, thalidomide, and alcohol can increase the risk of microtia. The different grades of abnormalities are shown in **Table 7.2**.

Management

These cases require a complete audiological and radiological workup. Radiological evaluation includes a high-resolution computed tomography (HRCT) scans of the temporal bone and a magnetic resonance imaging (MRI) to rule out middle and inner ear abnormalities. Audiological tests like pure tone audiometry should be done to assess the type and degree of hearing loss. Surgical correction of the deformity using autologous costal cartilage is the treatment of choice. Ideal age for correction is 5 to 6 years and is usually done as the first surgery when there is an associated atresia of the canal. Staged surgery is necessary and atresia of the auditory canal is corrected at a second sitting. Multiple revisions may be required. Skin covering for the new auricle can be provided by rotating and advancing flaps from the neck and from the region of the hairline. Prostheses should

Table 7.2 Grades of auricular malformations

Grades	Characteristic features
I	Abnormal auricle with all identifiable subunits
II	Smaller than grade I auricle with severely under-developed or absent subunits, lower half of the ear is often more developed than the upper half
III	"Peanut ear" with a small piece of disorganized cartilage and malformed lobule
IV	Anotia (complete absence of the auricle and lobule)

be considered as an alternative in difficult cases and for those not willing for surgery.

■ Treacher Collins' Syndrome

Synonym: Mandibulofacial dysostosis.

It is an autosomal dominant condition involving the first and second branchial arches. The syndrome consists of microtia and atresia of the EAC, hypoplasia of the mandible and middle third of the face and malar prominence, and antimongoloid palpebral fissures along with conductive hearing loss. Reconstructive surgical procedures are needed for cosmetic purpose.

■ Keloids and Hypertrophic Scars

Keloids and hypertrophic scars occur as a result of an abnormal response to tissue injury causing an excessive growth of the tissues and scar formation. While hypertrophic scars are limited to the area of injury, keloids can grow beyond the area of the wound. Patients with darker skin, genetic predisposition, and wounds closed under tension have more tendency to form a keloid. In the pinna, it can occur at the site of ear piercings (**Fig. 7.4a, b**).

Treatment

Surgical excision is the treatment of choice with intralesional triamcinolone injection postoperatively. Laser and cryotherapy have also been used. Keloids have a high chance of recurrence, while hypertrophic scars tend to regress with time.

Traumatic Disorders

Lacerations and Avulsions of the Auricle

Many of these injuries are secondary to road traffic accidents, while a few can also be due to assaults. Lacerations can be superficial involving only the skin or deep, extending into the cartilage (**Fig. 7.5**). There is a risk of perichondritis and chondritis in both cases. Repair at the earliest possible time is the treatment of choice in order to prevent

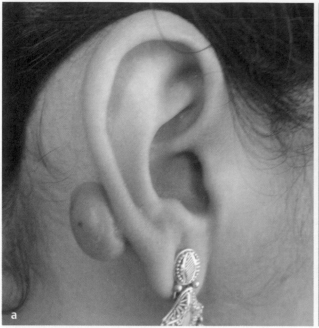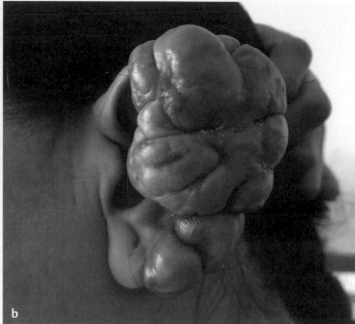

Fig. 7.4 (a, b) A small and an extensive keloid of the auricle.

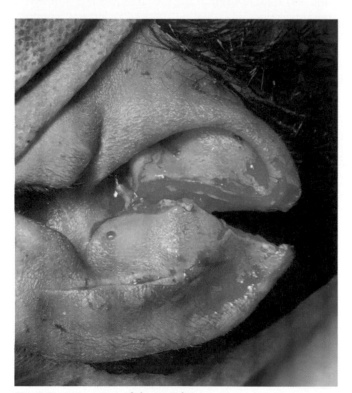

Fig. 7.5 Laceration of the auricle.

infection. Care should be taken to prevent stripping the perichondrium from the cartilage. Most of the lacerations without significant tissue loss can be closed primarily after irrigation with hydrogen peroxide and saline and wound debridement under cover of appropriate antibiotics. If the cartilage is exposed, it may be excised and covered

with local flaps or buried in a postauricular pocket for later reconstruction. Fine nonabsorbable monofilament suture materials (6–0 or 7–0) need to be used for suturing. Completely avulsed pinna can be reimplanted by microvascular surgery.

■ Hematoma/Seroma of the Auricle

It is the collection of blood or serous fluid between the perichondrium and the cartilage. The condition is most commonly seen in boxers, wrestlers, and rugby players. It is often due to repeated blunt trauma. However, it can also be induced by minor trauma like sleeping with the auricle folded. Seroma is also called pseudocyst of the auricle.

Clinical Features

Painless swelling of the auricle over the scaphoid and triangular fossa often obliterating the conchal bowl is the commonest presentation (**Fig. 7.6**). The condition is mostly seen on the lateral surface of the auricle where skin is tightly adherent to the perichondrium. The separation of the cartilage from its blood supply can lead to ischemia, necrosis, and a cauliflower deformity.

Treatment

A small hematoma may respond to aspiration and pressure dressing. However, larger ones and those that recur after aspiration require incision and drainage. When draining from the anterior aspect, the incision can be made in the fossa of the helix (scapha). Following curettage and readaptation of the skin with monofilament suture material,

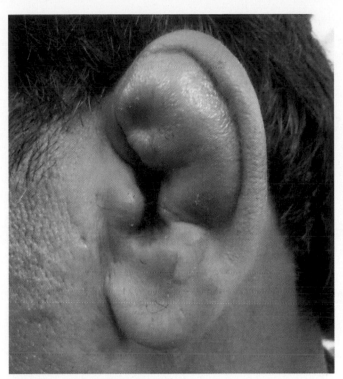

Fig. 7.6 Hematoma of the auricle.

pressure dressing for 3 to 5 days with a dental roll, secured with through-and-through sutures, is recommended. For drainage from the posterior surface of the auricle, incision has to be made in the cartilage to reach a seroma/hematoma on the anterior surface, and a cartilage window may be necessary (window operation). Pressure dressing will be required for a few days with dental rolls or buttons on either side tied with sutures. Broad-spectrum antibiotics are needed to prevent infection.

Complications

Infection can lead to perichondritis, organization, secondary calcification, and subsequently thickening, leading to a cauliflower deformity of the auricle.

> **Pearls**
>
> - Repeated aspiration of a seroma may lead to perichondritis.
> - Pressure dressing for 3 to 5 days is needed to prevent recurrence.

■ Frostbite

This condition occurs due to exposure to extreme cold temperature.

The disease can progress through three grades:
- Grade 1: Cyanosis of the skin due to vascular spasm.
- Grade 2: Ischemia with formation of vesicles.
- Grade 3: Necrosis of tissue.

Patients present with erythema, edema, bullae, or complete necrosis of the affected part. Treatment involves rewarming the pinna with moist cotton pledgets at a temperature of 38–42°C, and systemic and topical antibiotics and analgesics. Vasodilators and stellate ganglion blocks have also been tried. Surgical debridement may be required in selected cases.

■ Impetigo and Erysipelas

Impetigo is a superficial skin infection confined to epidermis, caused by *Staphylococcus aureus*. The typical appearance is formation of honey colored crusts. Itching and mild pain are the common symptoms. Treatment is with topical antibiotics.

Erysipelas (St Antony's fire) is the skin infection caused by beta hemolytic *streptococcus* extending to the dermis and presents with diffuse erythema and swelling of the auricle with a well demarcated border. Patient presents with pain, redness and may have systemic symptoms like fever. It is treated with a combination of topical and systemic antibiotics.

■ Perichondritis/Chondritis

This is an inflammatory condition involving the perichondrium (perichondritis) and/or the auricular cartilage (chondritis). It can be secondary to infections such as direct extension of otitis externa, and blunt, penetrating trauma and postsurgical trauma can be a manifestation of relapsing polychondritis. The most common associated pathogen is *Pseudomonas aeruginosa*. Uncontrolled diabetes mellitus leads to rapid progression of symptoms. In relapsing polychondritis, the cartilages of nose, trachea, ribs, and joints are also inflamed.

Clinical Features

It presents as painful erythematous swelling of the pinna, which is tender and indurated to touch (**Fig. 7.7**).

Treatment

Oral/parenteral antibiotics along with anti-inflammatory medications may be given in early cases. However, more severe cases will require incision and drainage and debridement with resection of the necrosed cartilage followed by regular dressing and postoperative antibiotics. Corticosteroids and immunosuppressant drugs are recommended in relapsing polychondritis.

> **Pearl**
>
> Perichondritis is a difficult entity to treat and requires thorough debridement and prolonged course of antibiotics.

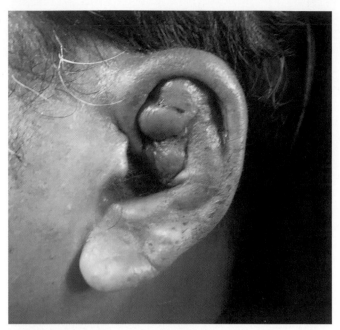

Fig. 7.7 Perichondritis of the auricle.

■ Miscellaneous

The auricle may be affected by many other disorders such as seborrheic dermatitis, allergic contact dermatitis, gout (tophi), psoriasis, ochronosis, chondrodermatitis nodularis chronica helicis, and many more conditions, the description of which can be read from the standard reference books.

Diseases of External Auditory Canal

■ Congenital Disorders

Atresia of the Canal

This condition can be partial or total, sporadic, or associated with deformities of the auricle. It can be a part of syndromes like Treacher Collins, Crouzon, Nager, or Goldenhar. The incidence is around 0.8 to 1.6 per 10,000 live births. It can be bilateral in one-third of the cases. It may occur alone or in association with microtia. Isolated atresia is due to failure of canalization of the first branchial cleft and it is usually associated with a normal middle and inner ear. When presenting with microtia, there can be associated middle ear and inner ear anomalies. Fusion of malleus and incus is the most common middle ear anomaly with a normal stapes footplate. The facial nerve is typically displaced either superiorly or laterally.

Investigations

Audiological assessment and imaging of the temporal bone are essential for planning the treatment.

Treatment

Unilateral atresia does not require immediate intervention if the hearing on the opposite side is normal. Bilateral atresia with significant hearing loss on both the sides requires hearing amplification. The preferred options are bone-anchored hearing aid (BAHA) or any other middle ear implantable device such as vibrant soundbridge or Bonebridge.

The surgical repair can be performed at the age of 6 to 7 years after microtia repair, if present. Patients with poor mastoid pneumatization, abnormal or absent oval window/footplate, abnormal facial nerve course, and abnormalities of the inner ear are poor candidates for surgical repair. Canal restenosis and residual hearing loss are the most common complications of the surgery.

Acquired atresia are secondary to chronic otitis externa, trauma, or burns. Such cases need meatoplasty and split skin grafting for the canal.

> **Pearls**
> - Prenatal exposure to isotretinoin, thalidomide, and alcohol can increase the risk of microtia.
> - The surgical repair of aural atresia can be performed at the age of 6 to 7 years as a second step after microtia repair, if present.

Collaural Fistula

It is an abnormality of the first branchial cleft associated with a skin-lined tract extending from the floor or the anterior wall of the EAC till the neck just below and behind the angle of the mandible. The track goes through the parotid gland in proximity to the branches of the facial nerve. If symptomatic with recurrent infection and discharge, it may be excised through a transcervical approach.

■ Trauma to the External Auditory Canal

Minor injuries are often secondary to attempts at cleaning, either self-cleaning or through the use of unskilled instrumentation for removal of wax and foreign bodies. Generally, the wound will heal rapidly without any complications. However, repeated stimulation of the bony auditory canal may predispose to osteitis.

Major lacerations of the ear canal are due to road traffic accidents, gunshot wounds, or assaults. The bleeding and clots may obscure the view of the deeper structures. All such cases need appropriate surgical management to establish proper skin lining of the ear canal to prevent subsequent stenosis.

■ Otitis Externa

Otitis externa is the inflammation of the EAC, which can be acute or chronic. Based on the causative organism, it can be bacterial, fungal, or viral. It can be localized or generalized.

Classification

- Infective:
  - Bacterial: Localized, diffuse, and malignant.
  - Fungal: Otomycosis.
  - Viral: Herpes zoster oticus and myringitis bullosa.
- Reactive:
  - Eczematoid otitis externa.
  - Seborrheic otitis externa.
  - Neurodermatitis.

■ Acute Otitis Externa and Furuncle

Furuncle or boil is the localized form, while acute otitis externa is mostly generalized or diffuse.

Predisposing Factors

Otitis externa is an inflammatory condition of the EAC usually caused by a breach in the skin through direct injury (while cleaning the EAC) or obstruction (hearing aid, foreign body, cerumen impaction) or change to alkaline environment (swimming). It is more commonly seen in hot and humid climate (Singapore ear). Furuncle (or boil) is the localized type of infection of the root of hair follicle, confined to the outer one-third of the cartilaginous canal. People with diabetes mellitus are more prone for recurrent furunculosis.

Causative Organisms

Most commonly isolated pathogens include *P. aeruginosa* for diffuse type and *S. aureus* for localized infection. Root of the hair follicle is often involved when *staphylococcus* is the causative organism causing a furuncle. Nasal vestibule, rarely the perineum, may be the carrier site for recurrent furunculosis.

Clinical Features

Severe ear pain aggravating with touch, chewing, and opening the mouth, itching, and purulent otorrhea in case of diffuse skin involvement are the common symptoms. Examination reveals tragal tenderness, canal edema, purulent discharge with epithelial debris, and erythema (**Fig. 7.8**). Pre- and postauricular lymph nodes can be enlarged in severe cases. Furuncle is often single; however, it may be multiple (**Fig. 7.9**). Posterior wall furuncle often obliterates the retroauricular grove, and there is pain on moving the pinna during examination. In such cases, differentiation from acute mastoiditis may be necessary (**Table 7.3**).

Investigations

Investigation is generally not required in acute cases. Ear swab may be taken for culture and sensitivity if the patient does not respond to conventional medications and in recurrent cases.

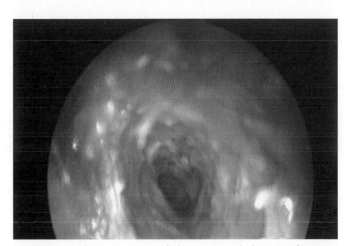

Fig. 7.8 Endoscopic view of the ear canal showing features of diffuse otitis externa along with central perforation of the tympanic membrane.

Table 7.3 Differences between furuncle and acute mastoiditis of the external auditory canal

Features	Furuncle of the ear canal	Acute mastoiditis
History of ear discharge	No	Mucopurulent discharge may be there
Pain	Severe; aggravates with chewing and yawning	Continuous dull acne
Hearing loss	Absent or minimal because of canal edema	Present
Tenderness	Over the tragus	Over the mastoid
Movements of the auricle	Painful	Painless
Displacement of the auricle	Anterior and lateral	Anterior, lateral, and inferior
Retroauricular groove	Obliterated in the posterior wall furuncle	Not obliterated
External auditory canal	Swelling in the cartilaginous part or edema	Sagging of the posterior and superior bony canal wall
Tympanic membrane	Normal	May have a perforation
X-ray of the mastoid	Normal	Clouding of the mastoid air cells

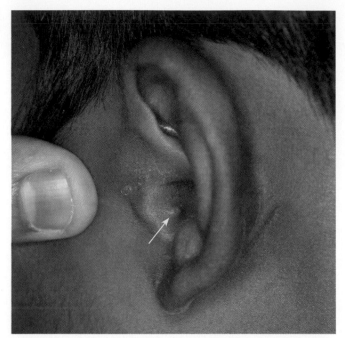

Fig. 7.9 Furuncle seen on the anterior canal wall of the left ear.

Treatment

Proper ear toileting with removal of infected material and debris is required to deliver the topical medications effectively. Suction clearance using a dilute solution of hydrogen peroxide will be helpful in thorough cleaning. Topical antibiotics with steroids can be applied through a cotton wick or merocele or gauze pack, which is changed on a daily basis. Acetic acid applied locally will be beneficial. Cases with furuncle require anti-staphylococcal oral antibiotics like clindamycin, lincomycin, linezolid, penicillinase-resistant penicillins like dicloxacillin, or a quinolone. Topical mupirocin can also be used. Ten percent ichthammol glycerin pack will reduce pain and canal edema by providing splintage and acting as an antiseptic agent. If an abscess has formed, incision and drainage may be needed. Systemic antibiotics are usually not required in diffuse infections unless there is concurrent otitis media, persistent or severe symptoms, cellulitis, chondritis, or perichondritis. Analgesic/anti-inflammatory drugs may be added for symptomatic relief.

■ Chronic Otitis Externa

Normally, low pH values of the canal skin, fatty acids in the secretions from the glands, lysosomes in the secretions of the ceruminous glands, and the normal self-cleaning mechanism caused by the external migration of the epithelium protect the ear canal from infection.

Chronic infections of the auditory canal are often associated with skin conditions like dermatitis and psoriasis, or irritation by a foreign body or earmold. It could also be secondary to allergy to topical medications or hair dyes and shampoo. The resulting maceration and reduction in the elasticity of the skin with associated atrophy of the glands lead to dryness, and disturbance in the pH and chemical balance resulting in increased susceptibility to infection.

Clinical Features

The condition is often painless, but will be associated with intense itching and irritation. Repeated itching may cause self-inflicted injuries while cleaning bleeding and discharge due to secondary infection. Canal will be edematous with epithelial debris. Skin may appear thickened.

Treatment

A thorough debridement of the ear canal is necessary (if required, under the microscope) to facilitate effective delivery of topical medications. An antibiotic with steroid cream may be applied over a cotton wick or merocele or gauze pack and replaced daily till the healing is complete. Certain antibiotics like neomycin can themselves cause allergic reaction, which needs to be kept in mind. If the canal is not edematous, antibiotic with steroid drops or spirit-boric acid drops may be used. Topical acetic acid in alcohol may also be helpful. The offending cause should also be simultaneously treated. Thick meatal skin in chronic cases may need to be excised and a split skin grafting done, that is, canalplasty. This procedure may be done with meatoplasty for better results.

■ Eczema of the Ear

This is often due to contact allergen like jewelry, cosmetics, or secondary to seborrheic dermatitis. The entry of sweat or water, and the presence of a moist exudate promotes colonization by pathogenic bacteria or fungi in the canal. There may be intense irritation with swelling and scaling of the affected part.

Treatment

It can be treated by elimination of the allergen, use of oral antihistamines, and topical treatment with steroid cream.

■ Seborrheic Otitis Externa

It is scaly dermatitis of the EAC, which is associated with seborrheic dermatitis in the scalp. Itching is the primary complaint. Yellow greasy crusts are seen in the canal. The underlying cause needs treatment along with topical antibiotic–steroid drops to the ear.

■ Neurodermatitis

It is a condition associated with compulsive itching due to psychological factors. It may lead to secondary otitis externa

- *Middle ear*: Acute otitis media, eustachian tube dysfunction, mastoiditis, trauma (barotrauma, direct trauma), malignancy, and granulomatous infection.

Secondary/Referred Otalgia

- Fifth cranial nerve (**Fig. 6.2**):
  - Dental: Caries, impacted molar, and apical infection.
  - Oral cavity: Stomatitis, aphthous ulcer, and malignant ulcers.
  - Salivary glands: Infection and malignancy.
  - Temporomandibular joint: Costen's syndrome, osteoarthritis, recurrent dislocation, and trauma.
  - Nose and paranasal sinuses: Trauma and sinusitis.
  - Nasopharynx: Space-occupying lesions like tumors.
  - Headache and atypical facial pain.
- Ninth cranial nerve:
  - Oropharynx: Tonsillitis, peritonsillar abscess, and palatal ulcers.
  - Elongated styloid process.
  - Glossopharyngeal neuralgia.
- Tenth cranial nerve:
  - Larynx, laryngopharynx, oropharynx, and esophagus: Inflammation, trauma, and malignancy.
- Seventh cranial nerve:
  - Herpes zoster oticus and Bell's palsy.
- C2 and C3:
  - Cervical spine disease through the trigeminal nerve can lead to referred pain.
- Psychogenic.

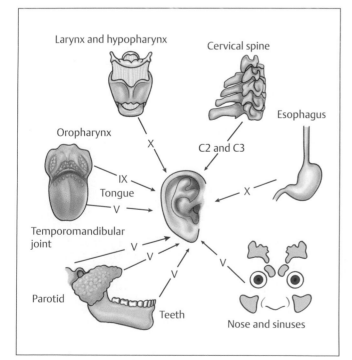

Fig. 6.2 Causes of referred otalgia.

Pearl

Neuralgias like trigeminal neuralgia can cause otalgia also. Tension headache and atypical facial pain can involve the ear. Cardiac otalgia refers to an atypical presentation of ear pain, unilateral or bilateral, due to myocardial infarction. The pain is referred through the auricular branch of the vagus.

Clinical Features of a Patient with Otalgia

History

The following points are to be noted:
- Onset.
- Duration.
- Type or quality:
  - Sharp and throbbing: Acute otitis media.
  - Dull and continuous throbbing: Furuncle.
- Localization:
  - Positive tragal sign: Furuncle in the anterior wall of the external auditory canal.
  - Postaural pain: Mastoiditis.
  - Deep-seated pain with blocking sensation: Acute otitis media.
  - Pain on chewing: Temporomandibular joint arthralgia and furuncle in the ear canal.
  - Associated symptoms with pain could be otorrhea, hearing loss, and swelling.
- History of prior surgery.

Pearl

Chronic suppurative otitis media, mucosal type, usually does not cause pain. The squamosal type can be associated with ear pain due to impending complications like mastoiditis.

Clinical Examination

- Ear, nose, and throat examination.
- Dental examination (remove dentures if present and reexamine).
- Temporomandibular joint examination.
- Neck examination.
- Neurological examination including cranial nerves.

Pearl

If the severity of the pain is more than the finding in the ear, consider the possibility of a referred otalgia and evaluate for the same.

Investigations

- Endoscopic examination of the nose and nasopharynx.
- Endoscopic evaluation of pharynx and larynx.
- Cervical spine, styloid process, and temporomandibular joint: X-ray or computed tomography (CT) scan.
- Orthopantomogram.

Management

- Appropriate investigations to confirm the diagnosis.
- When diagnosis is in doubt and there is a suspicious lesion, a biopsy for tissue diagnosis would be helpful, especially when considering malignancy or granulomatous conditions.
- In case of referred otalgia, treat the primary cause.

Points to Ponder

- Usual causes of primary otalgia include inflammation of the pinna, otitis externa, otitis media, and mastoiditis.
- Difficulty in diagnosis arises when the ear is normal; therefore, a search beyond the ear has to be carried out to identify referred otalgia.
- The common causes of referred otalgia include temporomandibular joint dysfunction, dental caries, throat infections like tonsillitis, malignancies of oropharynx, and elongated styloid process.
- Treatment is directed at the cause.

Case-Based Question

1. **A 45-year-old woman was seen in the ear, nose, and throat (ENT) clinic with complaints of pain over the right ear for the last 2 years. She had been examined by various ENT surgeons who have reassured her that the right ear is normal. On further enquiry, she says the pain starts sometimes in the upper neck on the right side and spreads to the ear. Examination of the throat is normal. Tonsils are not enlarged or congested. Palpation of the right tonsillar region elicited tenderness.**

   a. What is the provisional diagnosis?
   b. What investigation would you do to confirm your diagnosis?
   c. What is the treatment?

Answers

a. Pain radiating from the neck to the ear with a tender tonsillar region is suggestive of stylalgia or Eagle's syndrome.
b. Radiological investigations like an orthopantomogram or CT scan will reveal the presence of a medialized elongated styloid process.
c. Excision of the styloid process through a transoral route, after tonsillectomy.

Frequently Asked Questions

1. What is the difference between primary otalgia and secondary or referred otalgia?
2. Enumerate the causes of referred otalgia.
3. What are the causes of primary otalgia due to middle ear diseases?
4. Describe the nerves implicated in referred otalgia?
5. What is Eagle syndrome?

Endnote

Earache or otalgia and its remedies have been around for thousands of years, ever since the time of Hippocrates. It was the Roman physician Celsus who first wrote that "severe ear pain unsettles the mind" and suggested remedies that would not be accepted in today's medical world. Ancient remedies include the placement of boiled earthworms into the ear or inducing vomiting or as Galen wrote, "pouring a mixture of opium, musk and the white of an egg into the ear."

because of trauma while attempting to scratch. Treatment is psychotherapy and covering the ear with a bandage to avoid scratching the ear and subsequent trauma.

■ Malignant Otitis Externa

Synonyms: Skull base osteomyelitis and necrotizing otitis externa.

This is an aggressive and relatively fatal infection of the EAC and adjacent soft tissues, which is known to spread rapidly along the skull base. It is more commonly seen in the immunocompromised diabetic patients and those on anticancer drugs and organ transplant recipients. *P. aeruginosa* is the most common causative pathogen. *S. aureus* and fungi have also been reported to be associated in some of the cases. The infection may present as cellulitis, chondritis, osteitis, and osteomyelitis. Initial spread from the canal is through fissures of Santorini in the floor and involving the haversian system of compact bone. Involvement of the pneumatized portion is seen only at a later stage. The infection spreads through the tissue clefts of the cartilaginous meatus and extends into the retromandibular fossa and along the base of the skull as far as the jugular foramen. It leads to an insidious osteomyelitis of the temporal bone. If left untreated, the infection can spread along the skull base and involve the cranial nerves, more commonly the facial nerve (60% of cases). Locally, the infection can spread into the mastoid, middle ear, and petrous apex. Otic capsule is usually spared. Anteriorly, it can spread to the temporomandibular joint. Mortality is reported to be around 10%.

Clinical Features

Patients present with severe ear pain, often continuous, dull, and refractory to initial treatment. The pain is more at night. There is purulent ear discharge, which is occasionally blood stained. Examination reveals granulation tissue at the bony cartilaginous junction commonly on the floor of the EAC (**Fig. 7.10**). There may be lower motor neuron facial nerve palsy. Other cranial nerves especially the lower cranial nerves (IX–XI) are involved in advanced disease.

Based on the nature of spread, there can be four stages:
- Stage 1: The disease is limited to soft tissue and cartilage with negative technetium-99.
- Stage 2: There is bone involvement and erosion with positive technetium-99.
- Stage 3: This is associated with cranial nerve palsies.
- Stage 4: This is associated with intracranial spread. Other complications include sinus thrombosis, sepsis, intracranial infections, and death.

Investigations

Diagnosis is based on the patient's history, clinical examination, culture and sensitivity, and radiological findings. Erythrocyte sedimentation rate (ESR) is elevated. CT scan of the temporal bone helps in detecting bony erosion and MRI is helpful in detecting bone marrow edema, soft-tissue abnormalities, and intracranial complications. Technetium-99m bone scan can pick up areas of osteoblastic activity and can be useful in detecting the early changes. Biopsy of the granulation or the sequestrum may be done to exclude malignancy. Follow-up is monitored with gallium-67 citrate scan for soft-tissue disease. Blood sugar levels have to be monitored as a majority will have uncontrolled diabetes.

Treatment

Along with control of diabetes, the medical management involves the prolonged use of systemic and topical antibiotics, mostly quinolones like ciprofloxacin for 6 to 8 weeks. It can be administered both orally as tablets and by topical ear drops.

Many cases require parenteral third-generation cephalosporins like ceftazidime and penems like imipenem when they are resistant to ciprofloxacin. Aminoglycosides may be added if the renal function is normal. Local treatment of the external auditory meatus helps in the drainage of infective secretions.

A gallium scan will help determine for how long antibiotics should be continued. A scan should ideally be repeated every 6 weeks till the osteomyletic lesions disappear. Antibiotics should be continued for 2 weeks to 1 month after the scan comes back to normal.

The role of surgery in malignant otitis externa is confined to drainage of abscess, removal of bony sequestrum, or wound debridement to remove necrotic tissues.

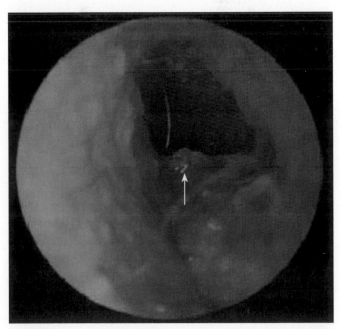

Fig. 7.10 Endoscopic view of the ear canal showing granulation tissue at the bony cartilaginous junction (*yellow arrow*).

Hyperbaric oxygen has been used in some cases as an adjuvant treatment. Blood sugar levels need to be kept under control. Prognosis is generally poor. Reduction in pain and ESR level is a good indicator of recovery.

Pearls

- *P. aeruginosa* is the most common pathogen associated with perichondritis and malignant otitis externa.
- Blood glucose levels should be checked in patients with recurrent furunculosis of the external auditory meatus.
- Malignant otitis externa requires long-term antibiotic therapy.

■ Otomycosis

It is the superficial fungal infection of the EAC. Many of the cases are associated with superadded bacterial infection. The most common pathogens include *Aspergillus niger* and *Candida albicans*.

Predisposing Factors

The predisposing factors are immunocompromised patients, hearing aid users, and the overuse of topical antibiotics (especially quinolones) with steroids.

Clinical Features

The clinical features are intense itching and ear fullness with occasional watery discharge with a musty odor. There may be associated pain. Examination reveals blackish brown or dotted gray membrane with an appearance of "tissue paper" or wet newspaper appearance in cases of *Aspergillus* infection. The debris may appear whitish in case of candida infection. Fungal hyphae can occasionally be seen through otoscopy (**Fig. 7.11**).

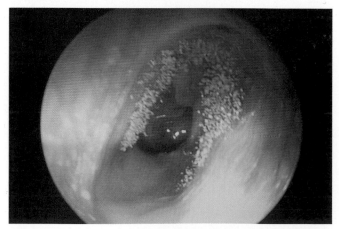

Fig. 7.11 Endoscopic picture of the canal showing debris with fungal hyphae, *Aspergillus flavus*.

Treatment

Treatment is removal of the fungus with suction followed by the use of topical antifungal agents like clotrimazole, salicylic acid in alcohol, or topical nystatin for a minimum period of 3 weeks to prevent recurrence. Oral antihistamines may be added for symptomatic relief. Topical antibiotic drops may be added if there is an associated edema and inflammation of the canal.

■ Herpes Zoster Oticus

Synonym: Ramsay Hunt syndrome; geniculate neuralgia.
This condition is caused by reactivated varicella zoster virus that remains dormant in geniculate ganglion of the facial nerve and in the spiral and vestibular ganglion of the vestibulocochlear nerve, after an attack of chicken pox. It is often predisposed by an immunocompromised state and stress.

Clinical Features

It presents with severe ear pain. There are vesicles in the concha and posterior ear canal skin in the outer one-third, spreading along the dermatomes. This is followed by lower motor neuron type of facial palsy on the same side 2 to 3 days later. Nearly 25% of the patients may complain of vertigo and tinnitus. Sensorineural hearing loss has been reported in 6% of the cases.

Management

Diagnosis is by history and clinical examination. However, a gadolinium-enhanced MRI may demonstrate enhancement in the area of geniculate ganglion. Polymerase chain reaction (PCR) assay of the vesicle fluid may demonstrate varicella zoster viral DNA. Antiviral drugs are the mainstay of treatment. Oral acyclovir 800 mg five times a day, famciclovir 500 mg three times a day, or valacyclovir 1 g three times a day for 7 days may be used. Oral prednisolone 1 mg/kg body weight over a period of a week will reduce the inflammation. Local application of antibacterial steroid cream has been found to be useful. Proper eye care is required till the facial paresis recovers. Overall, 50% of adults and 80% of children will achieve full recovery from facial palsy, if the treatment is initiated early. Labyrinthine sedatives may be required if there is vertigo.

■ Myringitis Bullosa

Synonym: Hemorrhagic or bullous otitis externa.
It is an inflammatory condition of the tympanic membrane that can be primary or secondary to an EAC infection. Although it is said to be viral in origin, *Mycoplasma pneumoniae*, *Haemophilus influenzae*, and *S. pneumoniae* are also frequently associated with this condition.

because of trauma while attempting to scratch. Treatment is psychotherapy and covering the ear with a bandage to avoid scratching the ear and subsequent trauma.

■ Malignant Otitis Externa

Synonyms: Skull base osteomyelitis and necrotizing otitis externa.

This is an aggressive and relatively fatal infection of the EAC and adjacent soft tissues, which is known to spread rapidly along the skull base. It is more commonly seen in the immunocompromised diabetic patients and those on anticancer drugs and organ transplant recipients. *P. aeruginosa* is the most common causative pathogen. *S. aureus* and fungi have also been reported to be associated in some of the cases. The infection may present as cellulitis, chondritis, osteitis, and osteomyelitis. Initial spread from the canal is through fissures of Santorini in the floor and involving the haversian system of compact bone. Involvement of the pneumatized portion is seen only at a later stage. The infection spreads through the tissue clefts of the cartilaginous meatus and extends into the retromandibular fossa and along the base of the skull as far as the jugular foramen. It leads to an insidious osteomyelitis of the temporal bone. If left untreated, the infection can spread along the skull base and involve the cranial nerves, more commonly the facial nerve (60% of cases). Locally, the infection can spread into the mastoid, middle ear, and petrous apex. Otic capsule is usually spared. Anteriorly, it can spread to the temporomandibular joint. Mortality is reported to be around 10%.

Clinical Features

Patients present with severe ear pain, often continuous, dull, and refractory to initial treatment. The pain is more at night. There is purulent ear discharge, which is occasionally blood stained. Examination reveals granulation tissue at the bony cartilaginous junction commonly on the floor of the EAC (**Fig. 7.10**). There may be lower motor neuron facial nerve palsy. Other cranial nerves especially the lower cranial nerves (IX–XI) are involved in advanced disease.

Based on the nature of spread, there can be four stages:
* Stage1: The disease is limited to soft tissue and cartilage with negative technetium-99.
* Stage 2: There is bone involvement and erosion with positive technetium-99.
* Stage 3: This is associated with cranial nerve palsies.
* Stage 4: This is associated with intracranial spread. Other complications include sinus thrombosis, sepsis, intracranial infections, and death.

Investigations

Diagnosis is based on the patient's history, clinical examination, culture and sensitivity, and radiological findings. Erythrocyte sedimentation rate (ESR) is elevated. CT scan of the temporal bone helps in detecting bony erosion and MRI is helpful in detecting bone marrow edema, soft-tissue abnormalities, and intracranial complications. Technetium-99m bone scan can pick up areas of osteoblastic activity and can be useful in detecting the early changes. Biopsy of the granulation or the sequestrum may be done to exclude malignancy. Follow-up is monitored with gallium-67 citrate scan for soft-tissue disease. Blood sugar levels have to be monitored as a majority will have uncontrolled diabetes.

Treatment

Along with control of diabetes, the medical management involves the prolonged use of systemic and topical antibiotics, mostly quinolones like ciprofloxacin for 6 to 8 weeks. It can be administered both orally as tablets and by topical ear drops.

Many cases require parenteral third-generation cephalosporins like ceftazidime and penems like imipenem when they are resistant to ciprofloxacin. Aminoglycosides may be added if the renal function is normal. Local treatment of the external auditory meatus helps in the drainage of infective secretions.

A gallium scan will help determine for how long antibiotics should be continued. A scan should ideally be repeated every 6 weeks till the osteomyletic lesions disappear. Antibiotics should be continued for 2 weeks to 1 month after the scan comes back to normal.

The role of surgery in malignant otitis externa is confined to drainage of abscess, removal of bony sequestrum, or wound debridement to remove necrotic tissues.

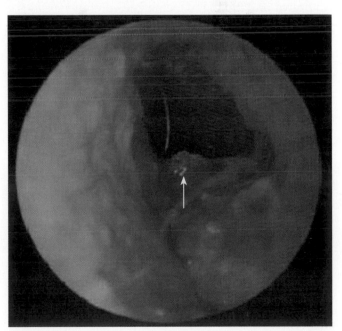

Fig. 7.10 Endoscopic view of the ear canal showing granulation tissue at the bony cartilaginous junction (*yellow arrow*).

Hyperbaric oxygen has been used in some cases as an adjuvant treatment. Blood sugar levels need to be kept under control. Prognosis is generally poor. Reduction in pain and ESR level is a good indicator of recovery.

Pearls

- *P. aeruginosa* is the most common pathogen associated with perichondritis and malignant otitis externa.
- Blood glucose levels should be checked in patients with recurrent furunculosis of the external auditory meatus.
- Malignant otitis externa requires long-term antibiotic therapy.

■ Otomycosis

It is the superficial fungal infection of the EAC. Many of the cases are associated with superadded bacterial infection. The most common pathogens include *Aspergillus niger* and *Candida albicans*.

Predisposing Factors

The predisposing factors are immunocompromised patients, hearing aid users, and the overuse of topical antibiotics (especially quinolones) with steroids.

Clinical Features

The clinical features are intense itching and ear fullness with occasional watery discharge with a musty odor. There may be associated pain. Examination reveals blackish brown or dotted gray membrane with an appearance of "tissue paper" or wet newspaper appearance in cases of *Aspergillus* infection. The debris may appear whitish in case of candida infection. Fungal hyphae can occasionally be seen through otoscopy (**Fig. 7.11**).

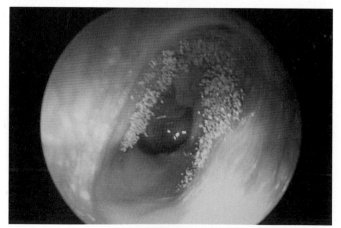

Fig. 7.11 Endoscopic picture of the canal showing debris with fungal hyphae, *Aspergillus flavus*.

Treatment

Treatment is removal of the fungus with suction followed by the use of topical antifungal agents like clotrimazole, salicylic acid in alcohol, or topical nystatin for a minimum period of 3 weeks to prevent recurrence. Oral antihistamines may be added for symptomatic relief. Topical antibiotic drops may be added if there is an associated edema and inflammation of the canal.

■ Herpes Zoster Oticus

Synonym: Ramsay Hunt syndrome; geniculate neuralgia. This condition is caused by reactivated varicella zoster virus that remains dormant in geniculate ganglion of the facial nerve and in the spiral and vestibular ganglion of the vestibulocochlear nerve, after an attack of chicken pox. It is often predisposed by an immunocompromised state and stress.

Clinical Features

It presents with severe ear pain. There are vesicles in the concha and posterior ear canal skin in the outer one-third, spreading along the dermatomes. This is followed by lower motor neuron type of facial palsy on the same side 2 to 3 days later. Nearly 25% of the patients may complain of vertigo and tinnitus. Sensorineural hearing loss has been reported in 6% of the cases.

Management

Diagnosis is by history and clinical examination. However, a gadolinium-enhanced MRI may demonstrate enhancement in the area of geniculate ganglion. Polymerase chain reaction (PCR) assay of the vesicle fluid may demonstrate varicella zoster viral DNA. Antiviral drugs are the mainstay of treatment. Oral acyclovir 800 mg five times a day, famciclovir 500 mg three times a day, or valacyclovir 1 g three times a day for 7 days may be used. Oral prednisolone 1 mg/kg body weight over a period of a week will reduce the inflammation. Local application of antibacterial steroid cream has been found to be useful. Proper eye care is required till the facial paresis recovers. Overall, 50% of adults and 80% of children will achieve full recovery from facial palsy, if the treatment is initiated early. Labyrinthine sedatives may be required if there is vertigo.

■ Myringitis Bullosa

Synonym: Hemorrhagic or bullous otitis externa. It is an inflammatory condition of the tympanic membrane that can be primary or secondary to an EAC infection. Although it is said to be viral in origin, *Mycoplasma pneumoniae*, *Haemophilus influenzae*, and *S. pneumoniae* are also frequently associated with this condition.

Clinical Features

Patients present with severe ear pain and blood-stained, serous discharge. Hemorrhagic bullae or vesicles may be seen on the surface of the tympanic membrane and deeper portion of the EAC. There can be conductive (20%) or sensorineural (30%) or mixed hearing loss (50%). Some of these cases may progress onto granular myringitis wherein patches of granulation tissue with mucosalization appear on the tympanic membrane causing persistent ear discharge. The granular appearance may also follow long-standing foreign body or impacted wax.

Treatment

Oral macrolides or fluoroquinolones may be given along with analgesic/anti-inflammatory drugs. Topical antibacterial steroid ear drops can also be added. Hearing loss recovers in majority of the cases within 3 to 6 months.

■ Keratosis Obturans

It represents an abnormal accumulation of a dense plug of keratin in the deeper portion of the EAC without bony erosion. It is secondary to a faulty pattern of epithelial migration.

Clinical Features

It is usually a bilateral disorder and affects young adults in the age group of 20 to 40 years. It presents with severe ear pain and otorrhea secondary to otitis externa. There is widening of the EAC. Pearly white keratin mass may be seen filling the ear canal. There will be conductive hearing loss. Rare cases of associated facial nerve palsy have been reported. Some of the cases are associated with bronchiectasis and chronic sinusitis.

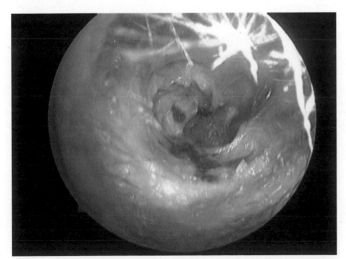

Fig. 7.12 Endoscopic picture of the canal showing widening with granulation tissue and collection of debris.

Management

HRCT scan of the temporal bone shows significantly diffuse widening of the EAC without bone erosion. Treatment involves careful and complete removal of keratin plugs under the microscope, which needs to be repeated at regular intervals (sometimes may have to be done under sedation or general anesthesia). Antibiotic with steroid drops is used if there is associated infection. Two percent salicylic acid in alcohol may be used prophylactically to prevent future accumulation of keratin.

■ External Auditory Canal Cholesteatoma

This condition is associated with collection of squamous epithelium in the EAC causing ulceration and erosion of the underlying bone of the inferior and posterior part of the canal. The reported incidence is 60 times less than middle ear cholesteatoma. Periostitis of the bony canal is the commonest associated feature (**Fig. 7.12**).

Clinical Features

It is usually unilateral and affects elderly patients. The differentiating features of EAC cholesteatoma and keratosis obturans are listed in **Table 7.4**. Patients present with severe ear pain, discharge, and conductive hearing loss. Examination may reveal destruction of the posterior meatal or outer attic wall. This condition needs to be differentiated from squamosal otitis media, malignant otitis externa, and malignancy.

Management

HRCT scan of the temporal bone shows a soft-tissue filling EAC and bony erosion. Treatment is complete debridement and removal of the epithelium under the microscope. Topical antibiotic and steroid drops may be given if there is

Table 7.4 Differences between keratosis obturans and external auditory canal cholesteatoma

Features	Keratosis obturans	External auditory canal cholesteatoma
Age	Young adults	Elderly
Side	Bilateral	Unilateral
Pathology	Disorder of epithelial migration	Periostitis
Ear pain	Severe pain	Dull pain
Ear discharge	Absent	Present
Bone erosion	Absent	present
Treatment	Medical	Medical and surgical

an associated infection. Exploration and canalplasty may be required in extensive and refractory cases to remove chole-steatoma matrix and necrotic bone.

■ Earwax or Cerumen

Wax is a yellowish-brown mass consisting of lipid and peptide secretions of the sebaceous and ceruminous glands, respectively, along with desquamated epithelial cells, hair, keratin, and particles of dirt. Wax serves to lubricate the ear canal and may trap small foreign objects and dust from damaging the deeper canal and tympanic membrane. It maintains an acidic pH in the canal. It has bacteriostatic and fungistatic properties due to the presence of lysosomes, hyaluronic acid, and immunoglobulins.

Predisposing Factors

The factors increasing the chances of wax accumulation or impaction are a narrow and tortuous canal, repeated use of cotton buds, earplugs, earphones, dry skin, stiff hairs, and obstruction in the form of exostosis. In some cases, there may be a genetic predisposition. Normally, the wax gets extruded through the movements of the jaw. Disorders of the temporomandibular joint may also contribute to impaction of wax.

There are two types of earwax, the wet type and the dry type. The wet type is autosomal dominant and the dry type is recessive.

Clinical Features

Patients present with ear fullness, tinnitus, mild pain, sudden reduction in hearing with entry of water, occasionally giddiness, and itching. Reflex cough because of the stimulation of the auricular branch of the vagus can occur. Long-standing wax may lead to thinning and unhealthy meatal skin. It is visualized in the canal as brownish black, soft to semi-hard mass, and partially or completely occluding the canal.

Treatment

Wax needs to be removed when the patient is symptomatic or to visualize the deeper canal or the tympanic membrane. Hard and impacted wax requires softening with 2% paradichlorobenzene, 5% sodium bicarbonate, 3% hydrogen peroxide, or olive oil. Dilute hydrogen peroxide instillation in the canal may facilitate removal of the wax.

Semi-hard wax can be removed without prior softening with a wax hook or probe. The auricle needs to be pulled gently superiorly and posteriorly so as to create a space in the posterosuperior canal wall through which the instrument can be passed beyond the wax plug and it can be pulled out. General anesthesia might be required to remove hard wax in children.

Soft wax can be removed either with suction or by syringing.

Ear Syringing

Ear syringing is a common procedure that is usually performed in the primary care setting for a variety of conditions from removal of wax to nonhygroscopic foreign bodies. Hygroscopic foreign bodies tend to absorb water and swell up. The primary aim is to remove matter from the EAC by injecting fluid (either boiled water cooled to body temperature of 37°C or normal saline) into the canal with a syringing. In a tertiary care center, foreign bodies and wax are removed under vision using a microscope and suction apparatus.

Indications are earwax impaction and nonorganic foreign body in the ear.

Contraindication:
- Perforation of the tympanic membrane as otitis media may get reactivated with entry of water into the middle ear.
- Hygroscopic or living foreign bodies and otitis externa are other contraindications.

Technique: Water or saline at body temperature can be used for syringing so that the semicircular canals are not stimulated. With the patient sitting on a chair, the pinna is pulled upward, laterally, and backward to straighten the cartilaginous canal. A kidney tray is placed below the pinna in contact with the skin to collect the syringed fluid with debris and wax. The nozzle of the syringe should be directed posteriorly and superiorly in the canal. The jet of water goes behind the wax plug and pushes the wax out. After the procedure, the canal has to be mopped dry (**Fig. 7.13**).

Complications:
- Wax can be pushed deeper.
- The tympanic membrane can be perforated by using too much of force, in which case, the patient will complain of pain and there may be blood-tinged discharge.
- Extremes of temperature can induce giddiness.

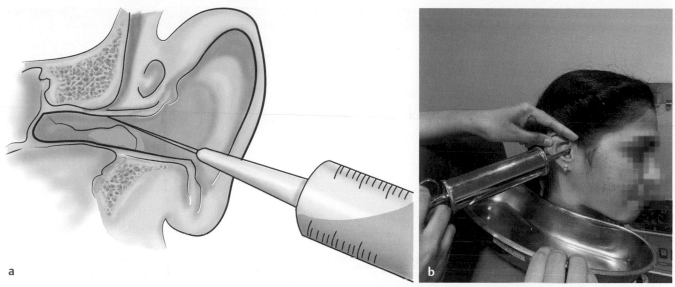

a

b

Fig. 7.13 **(a, b)** Technique of ear syringing to explain how foreign bodies and earwax are expelled by a jet of water.

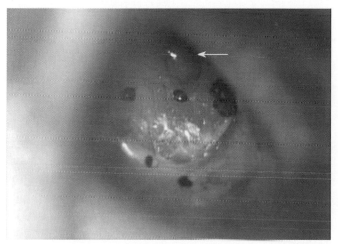

Fig. 7.14 Otoendoscopic picture of the ear canal showing a tick on the tympanic membrane.

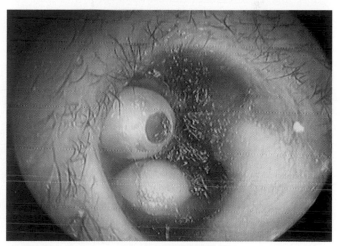

Fig. 7.15 Otoendoscopic picture of the ear showing beads in the ear canal.

■ Foreign Bodies in the Ear

Foreign bodies are more common in children, although they can also be seen in adults, especially in mentally challenged individuals.

Classification

Foreign bodies can be divided into the following:
- Living (animate) like cockroaches, ticks, or maggots (**Fig. 7.14**).
- Nonliving foreign bodies: These can be organic, like seeds, peas, or beans, or inorganic like paper, button, rubber, batteries, beads, etc. (**Fig. 7.15**).

Nonliving foreign bodies are found to be more common on the right side because right handedness is more common.

These are mostly introduced by children while playing. Patients may be asymptomatic. These objects can be removed in the clinic using crocodile forceps, hook, or syringing. Syringing is not recommended for hygroscopic objects like seeds as they may get impacted after swelling up. General anesthesia may be needed in uncooperative patients and children. Living objects must be killed before removal using water, saline, or lignocaine. Maggots may be killed using chloroform or ether. Animate objects are usually removed with forceps. Button batteries must be removed at the earliest to avoid corrosive injury to the canal skin. The postaural approach may sometimes be needed to remove foreign bodies impacted beyond the isthmus of the EAC. Unskilled attempts at removal may cause injury to the ear canal, the tympanic membrane, and the ossicles.

■ Aural Polyps

Aural polyps are essentially granulation tissue masses arising as a response to an underlying inflammatory process. Commonly associated conditions include foreign bodies, keratosis, wax, chronic ear infections, granulomatous conditions like tuberculosis, otitis media (both mucosal and squamosal), and rarely malignancy. Granulation polyps may be differentiated from the mucosal polyps associated with chronic otitis media by the lack of epithelial lining. Nearly 60% of aural polyps in children are associated with cholesteatoma (**Figs. 7.16** and **7.17**).

Symptoms are related to the underlying disease.

Treatment

Treatment of the underlying cause is cauterization with silver nitrate followed by the use of topical steroid with antibiotic drops. Excisional biopsy is indicated in case of an unresolved polyp. The polyp may be attached to deeper structures like ossicles and the facial nerve and therefore should not be avulsed. Occasionally, they may arise through an intracranial defect like meningoencephalocele and encephalocele. Hence, imaging studies are mandatory before considering excision.

Benign Neoplasms

Tumors involving the external ear are rare (refer to Chapter 19 for tumors of the ear). The common ones are adenoma, osteoma, and exostosis.

■ Ivory Exostosis

This condition is seen as multiple outgrowths at the bony portion of the EAC near the tympanic annulus along tympanomastoid and tympanosquamous suture lines, usually in patients having repeated exposure to cold water such as swimmers. There is usually periostitis and new bone formation. Exostosis needs to be differentiated from hyperostosis, caused by periosteal stimulation with progressive narrowing of the lumen of the meatus.

Clinical Features

It is usually asymptomatic but it may cause narrowing of the canal. There can be frequent wax impaction. Rarely, there can be mild conductive hearing loss or symptoms of recurrent otitis externa. Examination reveals multiple, bilateral, smooth broad-based sessile hard masses.

Treatment

It is required only in symptomatic cases or to allow a proper hearing aid fitting. Audiological tests like pure

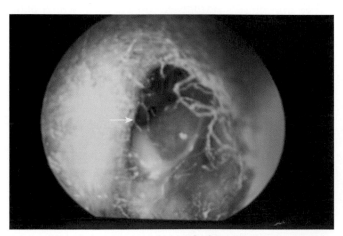

Fig. 7.16 Endoscopic picture of the ear canal showing granulation polyp.

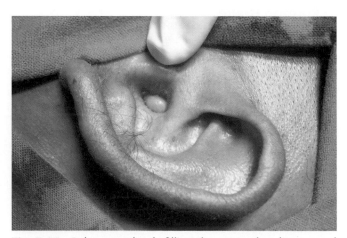

Fig. 7.17 Polyp completely filling the external auditory canal of the left ear.

Table 7.5 Differences between osteoma and exostosis

Features	Exostosis	Osteoma
Number	Multiple	Single
Predisposing factors	Frequent exposure to cold water	Nil
Site	More medial to the suture lines involving the tympanic bone	More lateral: along the suture lines at the bony cartilaginous junction
Side	Often bilateral	Mostly unilateral
Base	Sessile	Pedunculated
Histology	Layers of dense compact bone	Irregularly oriented bony lamella
Fibrovascular channels	Absent	Present

tone audiometry and radiological investigations including HRCT scan of the temporal bone may be done preoperatively. Surgery can be challenging because of the limited space. Drilling may be done either through the transcanal or postaural route. Facial nerve course and the location of temporomandibular joint has to be kept in mind during the procedure. Maximum care should be taken to preserve the meatal skin.

■ Osteoma

It is a solitary bony growth seen at the bony cartilaginous junction.

Clinical Features

It is often asymptomatic and appears as narrowing of the canal. Occasional cases may have hearing loss, recurrent infection, or wax impaction.

Treatment

It is not required unless symptomatic. Drilling is done either through transcanal or postaural route. The pedicle can be fractured and drilled in line with the bony canal.

Table 7.5 depicts the contrast between *osteoma* and *exostosis*.

Senile keratosis, Bowen's disease, and cutaneous horns are often recognized as premalignant lesions and need to be followed up.

Malignant Neoplasms

Primary cancers of the auricle and the EAC are rare and include basal cell carcinoma, squamous cell carcinoma, melanoma, and rarely ceruminous gland tumors (refer to Chapter 19 for tumors of the ear). Tumors from the surrounding areas like parotid malignancy may invade the EAC.

Basal cell carcinoma (rodent ulcer) is the most common malignancy seen in the auricle and preauricular area, while *squamous cell carcinoma* is more common in the canal. Adenoid cystic carcinoma can also occur in the ear canal. While basal cell carcinoma rarely spreads to the regional nodes, squamous cell carcinoma may spread to the lymph nodes in 20% of the cases. In *malignant melanoma*, both local and distant metastasis can occur. Squamous cell carcinoma can occur secondary to chronic ear discharge. Blood-stained discharge along with a friable proliferative mass in the canal should raise the suspicion of malignancy. There may be associated facial nerve palsy.

Surgery is the mainstay of treatment in all the cases ranging from wide excision to radical surgery with neck dissection and postoperative radiotherapy. Surgery for the EAC malignancy varies from lateral temporal bone resection to subtotal/total temporal bone resection depending on the extent of the tumor. Chemotherapy and immunotherapy may be required depending on the type of tumor.

Points to Ponder

- Among the congenital conditions of the pinna, preauricular sinus is frequently encountered above the tragus at the root of the helix. If infected, it can become an abscess.
- Keloids develop on the pinna due to trauma. They grow beyond the boundaries of the injury and are difficult to treat. Surgical excision can be attempted along with injection of steroids to reduce recurrence.
- Perichondritis of the pinna is a low-grade inflammation caused by trauma leading to a thickened and deformed pinna. If not treated adequately, it can lead to a cauliflower ear.
- Malignant otitis externa is an aggressive infection of the EAC and skull base mostly seen in immunocompromised individuals and diabetics. They present with granulation tissue on the floor of the EAC with or without cranial nerve palsies. The facial nerve is the commonest cranial nerve to be affected.

- Otomycosis or fungal infection is usually caused by either *Aspergillus* or *Candida*. Patients present with itching and blocked sensation of the ear. Antifungal ear drops will be required for 3 weeks along with regular aural toilet.

- Wax is formed by the secretions of the ceruminous and sebaceous glands of the cartilaginous part of the external ear. It has a protective function. It can be removed by suctioning, syringing, or instrumentation.

Case-Based Questions

1. **A 37-year-old man presented to the ENT OPD with a 2-week history of intense itching and blocked sensation of the left ear. He had a history of diabetes. On otoscopic examination of the left ear, there was thick whitish debris (wet newspaper appearance) studded with black fungal hyphae. How will you manage this condition?**

Answer

The history and clinical appearance are suggestive of a fungal infection of the ear or otomycosis. The organism is *A. niger* due to the color. Examination of the ear is performed under the microscope to confirm the diagnosis and to suction out the debris and fungus. Topical antifungal ear drops must be given for 3 weeks.

2. **A 65-year-old woman presented to the OPD with a 1-month history of severe pain of the right ear with purulent blood-stained discharge. The pain was so severe** that she had difficulty sleeping at night. Along with this, there was deviation of the angle of the mouth to the left side. She is a known diabetic on irregular medication. Examination of the ear revealed granulation tissue on the floor of the EAC and lack of movement of one-half of the face including the forehead on the right side. What is the likely diagnosis and management of this condition?

Answer

The diagnosis is malignant otitis externa of the right ear with lower motor neuron facial palsy on the right side. Investigations include biopsy from the mass in the EAC, CT scan to look for bony erosion of the temporal bone including the fallopian canal, and gallium or technetium scan to know the extent of osteomyelitis of the skull base. Treatment should be in the form of aural toilet, topical antibiotic ear drops, and parenteral antibiotics, either ciprofloxacin or a third-generation cephalosporin like ceftazidime, long term.

Frequently Asked Questions

1. What is a preauricular sinus?
2. What is the etiology of perichondritis of the pinna? How will you manage this condition?
3. Describe the technique of ear syringing. What are the contraindications to this procedure?
4. How do you classify foreign bodies in the ear?
5. Name the common organisms associated with fungal infections of the ear. Describe the clinical features and treatment of otomycosis.

Endnote

The famous composer Wolfgang Amadeus Mozart had a deformed left pinna, which was famously called "Mozart's ear." In this condition, the antihelix is prominent and fuses with the helix of the upper part of the pinna to form a flat surface, and the earlobe is absent. This peculiar shape was thought to confer musical talent, although there is no scientific proof for this. Mozart's portraits usually show his left ear covered by a wig.

8 Diseases of the Middle Ear

Vijayalakshmi Subramaniam and Harsh Ajay Suri

> **The competencies covered in this chapter are as follows:**
>
> EN4.6 Elicit, document, and present a correct history; demonstrate, describe clinical features, choose the correct investigations, and describe the principles of management of the discharging ear.
>
> EN4.5 Elicit, document, and present a correct history; demonstrate and describe the clinical features, choose the correct investigations, and describe the principles of management of otitis media with effusion.
>
> EN4.3 Elicit, document, and present a correct history; demonstrate and describe the clinical features, choose the correct investigations, and describe the principles of management of acute suppurative otitis media (ASOM).
>
> PE28.4 Discuss the etiopathogenesis, clinical features, and management of acute otitis media.
>
> EN4.7 Elicit, document, and present a correct history; demonstrate and describe the clinical features, choose the correct investigations, and describe the principles of management of chronic suppurative otitis media.
>
> EN4.8 Elicit, document, and present a correct history; demonstrate and describe the clinical features, choose the correct investigations, and describe the principles of management of squamous chronic otitis media.

The Discharging Ear

■ Introduction

Ear discharge, also known as otorrhea, is a common complaint that patients present to the otorhinolaryngologist. A properly elicited history most often points toward the cause for the ear discharge.

Ear discharge could be wax, which is the normal secretion of the ceruminous glands in the external auditory canal, or it could be arising out of other diseases of the external or middle ear when it could be purulent or mucoid/mucopurulent, respectively. Clear discharge could be due to cerebrospinal fluid (CSF) otorrhea.

■ Causes of Ear Discharge

- Otitis externa.
- Granular myringitis.
- Acute otitis media (AOM).
- Chronic otitis media (COM): Mucosal or squamous type.
- Tuberculous otitis media.
- Postmastoidectomy cavity.
- External or middle ear neoplasms.
- Foreign body in the ear canal.
- CSF otorrhea.

■ Evaluation of a Patient Presenting with Ear Discharge

A detailed history pertaining to the type of ear discharge, the mode of onset, duration, and associated complaints is elicited. Infections of the external ear are associated with purulent ear discharge and often accompanied by ear pain. Middle ear infections are characterized by mucoid or mucopurulent ear discharge. In AOM, there is usually history of a preceding upper respiratory tract infection followed by ear block and ear pain, which begins to reduce with the onset of discharge.

Mucoid or mucopurulent discharge that is profuse, intermittent, and aggravated by the upper respiratory infections is a feature of mucosal COM (tubotympanic).

In the squamous (atticoantral) COM, the discharge is typically foul smelling, scanty, purulent, and continuous. It could be blood stained when the disease is associated with the formation of granulation tissue.

Blood-stained ear discharge is also seen in tumors of the external and middle ear, and trauma.

One should also enquire into the details of hearing loss, tinnitus, and vertigo when a patient presents with ear discharge. Ear discharge may be associated with vertigo in patients having complications like labyrinthitis or labyrinthine fistula. Associated hearing loss could be due to a blocked external canal, tympanic membrane perforation, cholesteatoma, or tumors.

Facial palsy is seen with otorrhea in patients who develop it as a complication of AOM, cholesteatoma, malignant otitis externa, temporal bone trauma, tuberculous otitis media, and herpes zoster oticus (Ramsay Hunt syndrome). In patients with petrositis, discharge is associated with a deep-seated retro-orbital pain, due to involvement of the trigeminal ganglion, and diplopia, due to inflammation of the abducens nerve (*Gradenigo's syndrome*).

If there is history of head injury or mastoid surgery, the possibility of CSF leak should be ruled out, especially when the discharge is watery.

■ Examination of the Ear

This will establish the diagnosis:
- Tragal tenderness is seen in otitis externa, whereas mastoid tenderness is seen in acute mastoiditis.
- Otoscopic examination will identify the cause of ear discharge based on the clinical features in the external auditory canal and the tympanic membrane.
- Skin of the external auditory canal will be inflamed and swollen in otitis externa. Otomycotic debris may be present.
- Granulation tissue in the floor of the external auditory canal at the bony–cartilaginous junction is typically seen in malignant otitis externa.
- Perforation in the anteroinferior quadrant with pulsatile ear discharge is seen in AOM. The rest of the pars tensa is usually congested.
- Sagging of the posterosuperior canal wall is seen in acute mastoiditis.
- Mucosal COM is characterized by the presence of a central perforation. A central perforation is a perforation of the pars tensa whose margins are formed by the remnants of the pars tensa.
- Squamous COM is characterized by marginal, total, or attic perforation, or presence of a retraction pocket usually in the posterosuperior quadrant or attic with cholesteatoma.
- Recurrent or persistent discharge can occur in a *postmastoidectomy cavity* (modified radical mastoidectomy [post-MRM]). This may be due to the following:
  - Recurrent or residual disease.
  - Large cavity.
  - Deep recess at the mastoid tip.
  - High facial ridge.
  - Inadequate saucerization of the cavity.
  - Inadequate meatoplasty.
  - Exposed eustachian tube area.
  - Ulceration and granulation, or mucosalization of the lining of the cavity.

- Tuberculous otitis media is characterized by the presence of multiple perforations of the tympanic membrane initially, which coalesce later to form a large perforation and the presence of pale granulations in the middle ear.

■ Investigations

- Otomicroscopy/otoendoscopy should be performed to confirm the diagnosis. If discharge is present, a swab should be taken and sent for culture and antibiotic sensitivity test. During the otomicroscopic examination, the ear discharge can be cleaned using suction or dry mopping (for profuse discharge) or wet mopping (for dried discharge in the canal or on the membrane).
- Audiometry is done to document the type and degree of hearing loss.
- Radiological investigations like high-resolution computed tomography (HRCT) scan are required only in cases with temporal bone trauma and malignant otitis externa. Contrast-enhanced CT scan or magnetic resonance imaging (MRI) is done for those with complications of otitis media or neoplastic lesions.
- If there is a lesion in the external auditory canal or middle ear that is not responding to medication, a biopsy should be taken after imaging.

■ Treatment of Ear Discharge

It is directed toward treating the underlying cause and preventing further complications.

Otitis Media

■ Introduction

Otitis media refers to the inflammation or infection of the middle ear space. It comprises a spectrum of diseases that include AOM, COM, and otitis media with effusion (OME). Most inflammatory diseases of the middle ear cleft are related to eustachian tube dysfunction.

Otitis media can be further classified as suppurative or nonsuppurative depending on whether there is formation of pus.

The term "nonsuppurative otitis media" encompasses a group of conditions affecting the middle ear, which are of inflammatory origin but without any evidence of suppuration. These include the following:
- Eustachian tube dysfunction.
- OME.
- Atelectasis.
- Adhesive otitis media.
- Tympanosclerosis.
- Otitic barotrauma (aerotitis).

■ Otitis Media with Effusion

The synonyms of OME are secretory otitis media, serous otitis media, seromucinous otitis media, and glue ear. OME is defined as the presence of an effusion in the middle ear space without signs and symptoms of acute ear infection. OME is characterized by the presence of nonpurulent fluid in the middle ear which is usually thick and viscid (like glue), more commonly in children (2–5 years of age). It could also be thin and watery (serous), which is usually seen in adults.

Etiology

Eustachian Tube Dysfunction

This affects ventilation and drainage of the middle ear. The conditions that cause eustachian tube dysfunction include the following:
- Congenital palatal abnormalities like cleft palate where the eustachian tube fails to open on swallowing due to limitation of action of the tensor veli palatini muscle.
- Syndromic children with craniofacial anomalies and trisomy 21.
- Infections of the nose and paranasal sinuses, nasopharynx, and adenoids.
- Ciliary dysfunction seen in Kartagener's syndrome and due to smoking.
- Surfactant deficiency.
- Benign and malignant tumors of the nose, paranasal sinuses, and nasopharynx.
- Trauma.
- Allergy, which also increases susceptibility to upper respiratory infections.
- Hormonal factors like high estrogen levels and hypothyroidism.
- Palatal paralysis.
- Postradiotherapy.

Unresolved Acute Otitis Media (in Children)

Impaired drainage of the middle ear and presence of low-grade infection stimulate the middle ear mucosa to secrete more fluid.

Bacterial Biofilms

These have been shown as a possible cause for middle ear effusion with eustachian tube dysfunction as a secondary factor.

Other predisposing factors are parental smoking and stay in the day care.

Pearl

A nasopharyngeal tumor should be suspected in adult patients presenting with features of unilateral OME. The tumor can block the eustachian tube opening at the nasopharyngeal end leading to OME.

■ Clinical Features

Symptoms

- Patients with OME may report no symptoms. Some may present with hearing loss with seasonal fluctuation.
- Conductive hearing loss in children with OME goes unnoticed as it usually does not exceed 40 dB. However, these children are often labeled as inattentive in the class and the hearing loss affects their scholastic performance.
- Speech and language development get delayed in younger children. They may not respond to call or environmental sounds.
- Some children may present with problems with balance or unexplained clumsiness. There may be a gross motor development delay.
- Children with craniofacial anomalies, syndromes, autism, or blindness are more likely to be adversely affected by the OME.
- There is a prior history of repeated episodes of upper respiratory infection with otalgia, which is followed by reduced hearing.
- Adult patients often complain of ear block, tinnitus, decreased hearing, and autophony; occasionally, vertigo may be present.

Signs

- Otoscopic (otoendoscopic/microscopic) examination may show one or more of the following features:
  - Opaque with amber or gray colored tympanic membrane.
  - Distorted or absent cone of light.
  - Foreshortened handle of the malleus.
  - Mild to severe retraction of tympanic membrane with prominent (sickle-shaped) anterior and posterior malleolar folds (**Table 8.1**).
  - Reduced or absent mobility of the tympanic membrane on air insufflation (Valsalva's maneuver or Siegelization).
  - Air–fluid level or bubbles of air may be visible through the tympanic membrane.
- Pneumatic otoscopy should be routinely done to aid diagnosis. Movement of the tympanic membrane during release of the already compressed bulb should be noted.

Table 8.1 Grades of retractions of the tympanic membrane

Grade	Pars tensa (Sade)	Pars flaccida (Tos and Paulsen)
1	Slight retraction of tympanic membrane over its annular fold	Small attic dimple
2	Severe retraction of the tympanic membrane. It is draped over the long process of incus and incudostapedial joint	Pars flaccida is retracted and in contact with the neck of the malleus
3	Atelectasis: the tympanic membrane is in contact with the promontory but is mobile with Valsalva's maneuver	Here in addition to grade 2 features, there is minimal erosion of the outer attic wall
4	Adhesive otitis: the tympanic membrane is adherent or stuck to the promontory. It does not move with Valsalva's maneuver	Deep retraction with severe erosion of the outer attic wall

- Tuning fork tests reveal mild to moderate conductive hearing loss. This may be difficult to elicit in younger children.

Investigations

- *Pure tone audiometry (PTA)*: Mild-to-moderate conductive hearing loss may be noted.
- *Tympanometry*: Flat tympanogram ("B" type) is obtained due to reduced compliance of the tympanic membrane. The test is reliable in infants older than 4 months. It is important for documentation.
- Tests for speech delays.
- In children, the nasopharynx should be evaluated for adenoid hypertrophy by taking an X-ray of the nasopharynx (lateral view).
- In adults, a diagnostic nasal endoscopy should be done to rule out a lesion in the nasopharynx.

Treatment

If the OME has been present for less than 3 months and the hearing loss is mild with no significant speech and language delay or the child is doing well in school, the child should be kept on follow-up and reassessed after 3 months. Improvement is evidenced by pneumatic otoscopy, which allows you to note the movement of the tympanic membrane or a change in the tympanogram from "B" type to "non-B" type.

- Antibiotics such as erythromycin, co-trimoxazole, and co-amoxiclav are controversial. Recent studies have demonstrated the presence of metabolically active bacteria in culture-negative middle ear effusions using polymerase chain reaction. Therefore, antibiotics may only have short-term benefits.
- Nasal decongestants and antihistamines have been used with limited success. A short course of corticosteroids in adults for resistant cases is recommended by some, but its effectiveness is uncertain.
- Exercises such as Valsalva's maneuver, Toynbee's manoeuvre, or politzerization to ventilate middle ear are recommended by some. Otovent autoinflation device, which increases the pressure in the nose thereby

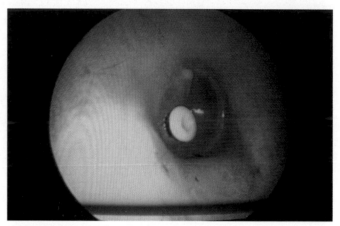

Fig. 8.1 Post myringotomy with a grommet in situ.

opening the eustachian tube to equalize the pressure in the middle ear, is useful in the children older than 3 years. These maneuvers should not be done in the presence of an upper respiratory tract infection.

Surgery is performed to restore ventilation of the middle ear by eliminating the primary source of infection or cause for eustachian tube obstruction and to drain the middle ear effusion.

- *Myringotomy and grommet insertion* is the procedure commonly done. Aspiration of the middle ear fluid is done by making a radial incision in the anteroinferior quadrant of the tympanic membrane. A grommet (ventilation tube) is inserted to allow ventilation of the middle ear (**Fig. 8.1**).
- *Adenoidectomy* is used to remove obstruction to the eustachian tube at the nasopharyngeal end and also to remove any focus of infection in the adenoids.
- *Eustachian tuboplasty* using laser, microdebrider, and balloon dilatation has been tried for persistent or recurrent OME to improve the dilatory function of the eustachian tube with fairly good results. The long-term results need to be assessed.
- *Steroids* have been tried for the treatment of OME, but it is controversial. Topical steroid nasal sprays like mometasone have been prescribed, but there is no clear evidence to show that it is effective in the treatment of OME.

If there is a *cause* for OME like nasopharyngeal carcinoma, it should be treated. Some patients may have persistent OME after treatment for this condition, which will warrant a myringotomy and grommet insertion.

Sequelae of OME

- Atelectasis of the middle ear.
- Adhesive otitis media.
- Atrophy of the tympanic membrane or thinning of the tympanic membrane. This is due to the absence of the middle fibrous layer due to persistent negative middle ear pressure (**Figs. 8.2** and **8.3**).
- Formation of a retraction pocket.
- Ossicular necrosis commonly involves the lenticular and long process of the incus (**Fig. 8.3**).
- Tympanosclerosis is the hyaline degeneration of the middle fibrous layer followed by subsequent calcification. The overlying mucosa is thin and lacks vascularity (**Fig. 8.2**).
- Cholesterol granuloma consists of cholesterol crystals surrounded by foreign body giant cells embedded in fibrous connective tissue along with inflammatory cell infiltration and blood vessels.

Atelectasis

- Retraction of the tympanic membrane onto the promontory due to inadequate ventilation of the middle ear consequent to eustachian tube dysfunction is called middle ear atelectasis.
- The tympanic membrane becomes thin, transparent, and atrophic. Necrosis of the ossicles may occur with formation of granulations.

Adhesive Otitis Media

- This condition is also called chronic middle ear catarrh where fibrous adhesions are formed in the middle ear, and the tympanic membrane becomes adherent to the promontory and ossicles.

Pearl

The conditions causing conductive hearing loss with intact tympanic membrane are the following:
- Otitis media with effusion.
- Tympanosclerosis.
- Ossicular discontinuity.
- Otosclerosis.
- Congenital cholesteatoma.
- Congenital fixation of the malleus head or stapes.
- Persistent stapedial artery.
- Glomus tympanicum.

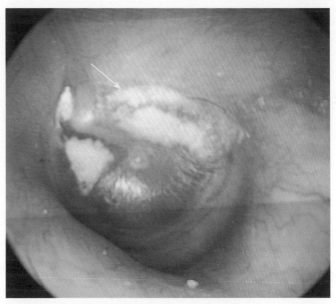

Fig. 8.2 Atrophic tympanic membrane with white patches of tympanosclerosis (*yellow arrow*).

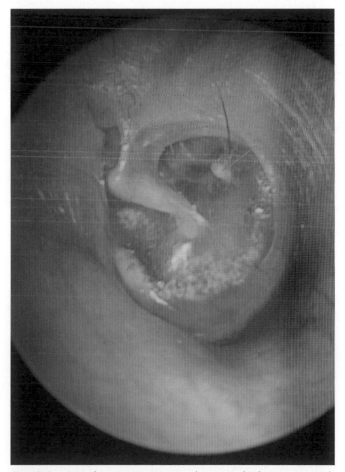

Fig. 8.3 Atrophic tympanic membrane, which is retracted. The head of the stapes can be seen with absent incus (*green arrow*). Retraction of the pars flaccida with mild erosion of the lateral attic wall is also noted (*orange arrow*).

Otitic Barotrauma

The synonyms of otitic barotrauma are aerotitis media and barotitis media.

It is a condition resulting from failure of the eustachian tube to maintain middle ear pressure at ambient atmospheric level. The symptoms manifest during deep sea or scuba diving or on descent from an altitude during air travel. The changes can occur under conditions of less marked ambient pressure fluctuation. The incidence would be more in nonpressurized aircrafts.

▪ Predisposing Factors

- Poor eustachian tube function.
- Recent upper respiratory tract infection.
- Sleeping during the flight or alcohol consumption prior to or during the flight.
- Nasal conditions like a deviated nasal septum may also predispose to otitic barotrauma as the patient may not be able to equalize the pressure effectively.

▪ Clinical Features

The patient complaints of aural fullness, popping sensation, discomfort, and/or pain. Patients are typically asymptomatic once they return to ground level. In some cases, significant barotrauma may cause temporary middle ear effusion or hemotympanum (**Fig. 8.4**). This occurs when the atmospheric pressure is more than the middle ear pressure by 90 mm Hg and the eustachian tube gets locked. This causes negative pressure in the middle ear, which leads to tympanic membrane retraction and transudation or hemorrhage. In these cases, middle ear effusion or hemotympanum may be evident on otoscopy. At times, when there is rapid change in pressure, rupture of the tympanic membrane can occur.

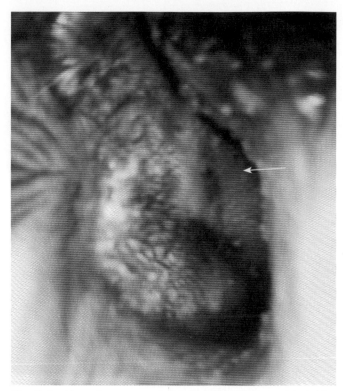

Fig. 8.4 Hemotympanum behind an intact drum (*dark blue areas*).

The change in pressure can also affect the inner ear. Due to a bleed in the inner ear or rupture of the intralabyrinthine membranes, there can be sensorineural hearing loss and vertigo.

The diagnosis is by history. PTA may show a conductive hearing loss; rarely, the hearing loss may be sensorineural or mixed.

▪ Treatment

The treatment is mainly symptomatic with decongestants and analgesics when required.

Topical nasal decongestants like xylometazoline or oxymetazoline help open the eustachian tube. Oral decongestants like phenylephrine are helpful.

Eustachian tuboplasty may be helpful in frequent flyers. A long-standing ventilation tube is also useful in professional and frequent flyers.

▪ Prevention

Otitic barotraumas can be prevented in some cases by avoiding traveling during an upper respiratory tract infection. Correction of a deviated nasal septum may allow for proper equalization of the pressure. Use of oral or topical nasal decongestants prior to travel may be helpful.

Acute Otitis Media

■ Introduction

AOM is the acute infection of the mucoperiosteum of the middle ear cleft caused by pyogenic organisms. It is one of the commonest infections seen in preschool children. The prevalence of AOM in India is reported to be around 17 to 20%. It is commonly seen during winter months and children who are not breastfed. *Recurrent AOM* is when there are more than three episodes in 6 months or four to six episodes in 1 year. The infection is considered *resistant* when it persists despite 3 to 5 days of antibiotics.

■ Predisposing Factors

- Age: Six months to 3 years.
- Allergies and genetic factors.
- Bottle feeding at an early age (especially in the supine position) and use of pacifiers.
- Craniofacial anomalies: Cleft palate and Down's syndrome.
- Crowded living conditions and low socioeconomic status.
- Cystic fibrosis and primary ciliary dyskinesia.
- Anemia.
- Immunoglobulin deficiency (immunoglobulin G [IgG] and immunoglobulin M [IgM]).
- Exposure to smoke.
- Exposure to viral infections in day-care centers.
- Gastroesophageal reflux.
- Immunodeficiency.

■ Etiopathogenesis

- A viral upper respiratory tract infection can involve the middle ear through the eustachian tube. There is release of inflammatory mediators, reduction in ciliated cells, and increased mucous production. This increased fluid in the middle ear along with impaired drainage may later lead to a secondary bacterial infection.
- In children, the immature immune system may be a contributing factor.

- In infants, the eustachian tube is wider, shorter, and more horizontal, which makes them prone to AOM. If infants are bottle-fed in the supine position, milk may enter the middle ear through the eustachian tube.
- Infections such as adenoiditis, tonsillitis, pharyngitis, and rhinosinusitis can spread to the middle ear through the eustachian tube. Forceful blowing of the nose or performing Valsalva's maneuver in the presence of rhinitis may force the infection into the middle ear through the eustachian tube.
- Deep sea diving, barotrauma, and swimming can cause AOM. Flying in an unpressurized aircraft, especially in the presence of rhinitis, can cause AOM.
- Traumatic perforations can facilitate spread of infection into the middle ear via the external ear.
- Infection of the middle ear is rarely blood borne.

■ Causative Organisms

Streptococcus pneumoniae, *Moraxella catarrhalis*, and *Haemophilus influenza* are the common causative organisms. The other organisms responsible are *Staphylococcus aureus* and *S. haemolyticus*. Rarely, gram-negative bacilli like *Proteus* and *Escherichia coli* can cause AOM.

■ Clinical Features

AOM is usually preceded by a viral upper respiratory tract infection. There will be rapid onset of ear pain, which is more severe at night. Infants usually present with irritability and intense crying. They may not feed well. Toddlers clutch or rub the ear due to pain and cry. Their sleep is affected. The clinical features of the disease may be described under five stages based on the course of the disease starting from the stage of tubal occlusion to the stage of resolution or complications (**Table 8.2**).

■ Stage of Complications

Continuing inflammation when untreated or inadequately treated can lead to complications particularly if the immunity of the host is reduced or the virulence of organism is high. Infection can spread to the mastoid air cell system leading to acute mastoiditis and abscess. Other complications that can occur include labyrinthitis, petrositis, facial paralysis, lateral sinus thrombophlebitis, meningitis, extradural abscess, and brain abscess.

Table 8.2 Five stages based on the course of the disease

Stage	Symptoms	Signs
Stage of tubal occlusion (catarrhal stage): Eustachian tube obstruction resulting from inflammatory edema in the nasopharynx causes absorption of oxygen and increase in carbon dioxide in the middle ear	• Blocking sensation/fullness in the ear • Mild ear pain • Mild deafness • Fever and malaise	• Retracted tympanic membrane with loss of light reflex • Tuning fork tests show conductive hearing loss
Stage of presuppuration: Persistent occlusion of the eustachian tube causes exudation from capillaries in the middle ear due to mucosal congestion	• Severe throbbing type of ear pain, which worsens during sleep because of venous congestion in the recumbent position • Tinnitus, i.e., bubbling sounds are heard • Deafness, which goes unnoticed due to the severity of pain • Fever and malaise. The patient looks toxic	• Congested tympanic membrane with prominent blood vessels in the pars tensa giving it a *cartwheel* appearance • Congestion of the pars flaccid due to epitympanitis (**Fig. 8.5a**) • Tuning fork tests show a conductive hearing loss
Stage of suppuration: There is accumulation of pus in the middle ear. Tympanic membrane bulges laterally due to pus under tension	• Excruciating ear pain • Deafness • Fever and other constitutional symptoms	• Congested and bulged tympanic membrane with loss of landmarks (**Fig. 8.5b**) • A yellow nipple is seen on one spot of the tympanic membrane suggesting impending rupture • Tenderness over the suprameatal triangle due to mastoiditis
Stage of resolution: The tympanic membrane ruptures at its weakest part causing otorrhea while other symptoms begin to abate	• Blood-stained mucopurulent ear discharge • Fever, ear pain, and constitutional symptoms subside	• Perforation in the anteroinferior quadrant of the pars tensa with blood-stained mucopurulent ear discharge coming out under pressure, which may be pulsatile. This is also known as the light house sign (**Fig. 8.5c**) • Conductive hearing loss

■ Management

Diagnosis of AOM is essentially clinical. Ear discharge is sent for culture and sensitivity to determine the causative organism and the antibiotics to which they are sensitive. Investigations like CT scan or MRI of the temporal bone or head are considered only when complications are suspected and when there is failure to improve with medications. A complete blood picture, C-reactive protein, and blood culture are done in severe complications.

■ Treatment

The principles of treatment include the following:
- Relief from symptom.
- To control and eradicate middle ear infection.
- Ensuring eustachian tube patency for ventilation of the middle ear and drainage of the middle ear cleft.
- Return of auditory function.

■ Prevention

Vaccination for *H. influenza*, *Pneumococcus*, and *Influenza A virus* has reduced the incidence and severity of AOM. Breastfeeding of infants up to 6 months of age is known to be protective.

■ Medical Treatment

- In the catarrhal stage, antibiotics are usually not required and most cases resolve spontaneously. Topical (nasal) decongestants like oxymetazoline (0.025% in children and 0.05% in adults) or xylometazoline (0.05% in children and 0.1% in adults) or oral decongestants with or without antihistamines help relieve mucosal edema around the eustachian tube, thereby improving middle ear ventilation. It is important to point out that some studies have concluded that decongestants and antihistamines do not have a role to play, but they can reduce nasal symptoms in a preexisting rhinitis.

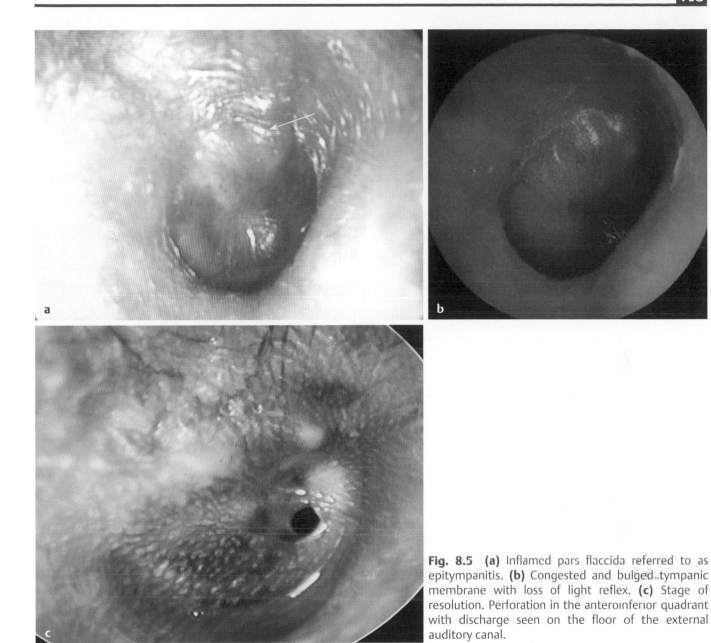

Fig. 8.5 **(a)** Inflamed pars flaccida referred to as epitympanitis. **(b)** Congested and bulged tympanic membrane with loss of light reflex. **(c)** Stage of resolution. Perforation in the anteroinferior quadrant with discharge seen on the floor of the external auditory canal.

- Antibiotics are started at the earliest suspicion of suppuration. Amoxicillin 40 mg/kg/d in three divided doses is recommended for 7 to 10 days. Amoxicillin with clavulanate, cefixime, or cefuroxime is recommended for beta-lactamase producing organisms. Oral cephalosporins (like cefdinir, cefuroxime, or cefpodoxime) or macrolides (like clarithromycin) are given when the patient has penicillin allergy. Parenteral antibiotics (amoxicillin with clavulanate or ceftriaxone) for 24 to 48 hours followed by oral antibiotics for 7 days are to be considered in severe infection.
- Topical antibiotic ear drops should *not* be given in the presence of ear discharge or when the perforation is pinhole or small as they may not enter the middle ear to

be effective. Aural toilet is carried out for removing the discharge, if present.
- Analgesics and antipyretics (ibuprofen and/or acetaminophen) should be given to relieve pain and fever.

■ Surgical Treatment

The surgical management of AOM is resorted to when the medical management fails or when there are impending complications. There are three types of surgical procedures that can be carried out and the indications for these are diagnostic, therapeutic, or prophylactic.

- *Tympanocentesis* is a diagnostic procedure that allows the fluid in the middle ear to be aspirated with a needle.

The aspirate is sent for culture and antibiotic sensitivity test. This also allows the middle ear pressure to be relieved and the pain to reduce.

- *Myringotomy* is a therapeutic procedure where an incision is made (a curvilinear incision) in the posteroinferior quadrant of the tympanic membrane, midway between the annulus and umbo, to enable drainage and ventilation of the middle ear cleft. Myringotomy is usually performed in the following:
  - In the exudative stage when the tympanic membrane is bulging due to pus under tension.
  - In the suppurative stage when there is a small perforation with inadequate drainage of the middle ear.
  - In AOM with impending complications.
- *Myringotomy and grommet* insertion may be carried out in recurrent AOM.

■ Sequelae of Acute Otitis Media

- Conductive hearing loss due to failure of resolution.
- Sensorineural hearing loss due to damage to the inner ear through absorption of toxins from the middle ear via the round window membrane.
- Persistent perforation due to eustachian tube pathology. This occurs more commonly in a large perforation that is kidney shaped or in a poorly pneumatized mastoid.
- Atelectasis of the tympanic membrane due to persistence of eustachian tube pathology.
- Healing of perforation with scarring of the tympanic membrane or tympanosclerosis.
- Healing with the formation of a dimeric membrane at the perforation site. The middle fibrous layer is absent.

Pearl

Most central perforations of the tympanic membrane (pars tensa) are kidney shaped because the parts of the membrane with abundant blood supply are in the peripheral annular region and along the handle of the malleus. The region in between is relatively avascular.

■ Acute Necrotizing Otitis Media

This is a severe, virulent form of AOM where there is necrosis of the tympanic cavity. It was common during the pre-antibiotic days, but it is less common now.

This infection is of rapid onset and progression and is usually seen in children suffering from influenza, typhoid, measles, or scarlet fever. Immunocompromised and malnourished children are at greater risk of developing acute necrotizing otitis media.

It occurs due to secondary infection by β-hemolytic streptococci, which causes necrosis of considerable areas of the tympanic membrane including the annulus, ossicular chain, middle ear mucosa, and mastoid air cells.

The condition is characterized by profuse otorrhea with a kidney-shaped or near-total perforation and a moderate to severe hearing loss that may be conductive or mixed.

Treatment comprised early institution of antibiotic therapy, which is continued for at least 10 to 14 days. Cortical mastoidectomy is considered when medical treatment fails or when complicated by acute mastoiditis. Healing leads to fibrosis of the tympanic membrane, or ingrowth of the squamous epithelium from the external auditory meatus may occur.

Chronic Otitis Media (Chronic Suppurative Otitis Media)

■ Types of Chronic Otitis Media

Traditionally, COM is classified into two:
- Mucosal type or tubotympanic disease (TTD).
- Squamous type or atticoantral disease (AAD).

■ Mucosal Type or Tubotympanic Disease

This type of COM mainly involves the anteroinferior part of the middle ear cleft. It is associated with perforation of the pars tensa and ear discharge. The perforation present is called a *central perforation* because it is in the pars tensa and surrounded by part of the pars tensa remnant on all sides. The ear discharge is usually mucoid in consistency because of the presence of goblet cells in the anteroinferior part of the middle ear cleft. It can also be mucopurulent.

Mucosal COM can be either active or inactive.

Active Disease

It is termed active where there is perforation of the pars tensa with the presence of ear discharge and/or middle ear inflammation, granulation tissue, or polyps. The discharge is present at the time of examination.

Inactive Disease

It is termed inactive when there is perforation of the pars tensa and absence of ear discharge and/or middle ear inflammation or polyps. There is no discharge at the time of examination.

- *Note*: In the previous nomenclature, namely, chronic suppurative otitis media (CSOM)–tubotympanic type, four stages are described: (1) The *active stage*: there is presence of discharge and/or congested middle ear mucosa, granulation, or polyp. (2) The *quiescent stage*: there is a perforation of the tympanic membrane but no discharge at the time of examination; the last discharge occurred within the last 6 months. (3) The *inactive stage*: There is a perforation and the last discharge was more than 6 months ago. (4) The *healed stage*: In dry (non-discharging) ears, sometimes the tympanic membrane perforation heals by itself in two layers with the absence of the middle fibrous layer (called dimeric membrane), which may be associated with tympanosclerosis and conductive hearing loss.

- *Permanent perforation*: In long-standing infections, when the squamous epithelium lines the edges of the perforation, it is called permanent perforation. The outer epithelial layer of the tympanic membrane and the inner mucosal layer come into contact and stop growing around the margins of the perforation. This is called contact inhibition. This can occur when there is insufficient blood supply, connective tissue hyperproliferation, and less growth factors at the margins of the perforation.

■ Squamous Type or Atticoantral Disease

It is a chronic inflammatory condition of the middle ear cleft usually involving the posterosuperior part of the mesotympanum, attic, and antrum, and associated with entrapment of the keratinizing squamous epithelium (cholesteatoma) in the middle ear space, which can erode and destroy adjacent tissues in the temporal bone.

It is also called the AAD or the unsafe type of CSOM because of its site of involvement in the middle ear cleft and its potential for causing intratemporal and intracranial complications.

The squamous CSOM has two stages, namely:
- **Active:** In this stage, cholesteatoma and granulation tissue are present.
- **Inactive:** In this stage, there is a retraction pocket but no cholesteatoma, or granulation tissue. When the nomenclature CSOM, atticoantral type, is used, based on the disease (retraction pocket or cholesteatoma), no stages are mentioned.

■ Types of Perforations of the Tympanic Membrane

The tympanic membrane comprises the pars tensa and the pars flaccida (**Fig. 8.6**). The pars tensa can be divided into four quadrants (anterosuperior, anteroinferior, posterosuperior, and posteroinferior) by a vertical line drawn along the handle of the malleus and a horizontal line drawn at the level of the umbo. Perforations of the tympanic membrane are characterized by the site, type, and the involvement of the annulus.

Perforation of Pars Tensa

Central Perforation

It is the perforation of the pars tensa where the margins of the perforation is formed by the remnants of the pars tensa. This is also known as a safe perforation. It can be the following:
- *Small perforation*: Perforation involving only one quadrant or <10% of the pars tensa.
- *Medium perforation*: Perforation involving two quadrants or 10 to 40% of the pars tensa.
- *Large perforation*: Perforation involving three or more quadrants or >40% of the pars tensa.
- *Subtotal perforation*: It is perforation of the pars tensa, which involves all four quadrants and reaches up to the fibrous annulus but not involving it. The handle of the malleus may be skeletonized.

Marginal Perforation

A perforation in the pars tensa, more commonly in the posterosuperior quadrant, which erodes the annulus and one margin, is formed by the sulcus tympanicus. This is an unsafe perforation.

Total Perforation

It is complete perforation of the pars tensa where the margins are formed by the bony annulus. Total perforation is an unsafe perforation.

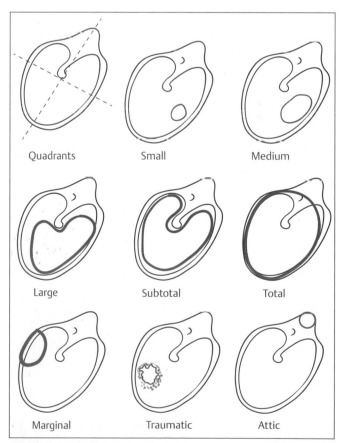

Quadrants   Small   Medium

Large   Subtotal   Total

Marginal   Traumatic   Attic

Fig. 8.6 Perforations of the tympanic membrane depending on the site and extent.

Traumatic Perforation

The perforation usually occurs in the posteroinferior quadrant, and the edges of the perforation will be ragged with blood clots. This is usually caused by trauma like a slap on the ear, insertion of a sharp foreign body into the ear, or an iatrogenic or blast injury.

Perforation of the Pars Flaccida

Attic Perforation

This type of perforation is seen in the pars flaccida. It is associated with cholesteatoma formation. It is an unsafe perforation and is seen in squamous COM or AAD.

■ Traumatic Tympanic Membrane Perforation

It can occur following a slap to the region of the ear, blast injury, attempted self-cleaning with buds or sticks, pressure changes, or as an iatrogenic injury during wax or foreign body removal, syringing, or any instrumentation.

Clinical Features

The patient will have pain, bleeding from the ear, and tinnitus, which usually subsides. Vertigo may be present. Depending on the type and intensity of trauma, the ossicular chain (conductive) and the inner ear (sensorineural) may be involved, which can affect the hearing.

On examination, commonly the perforation will be in the posteroinferior quadrant of the pars tensa, due to curvature of the external auditory canal. The perforation will have ragged edges with blood clots in the margins. A recent trauma may have blood in the canal and over the perforation (**Fig. 8.7**). Tuning fork tests will help in the initial assessment of hearing.

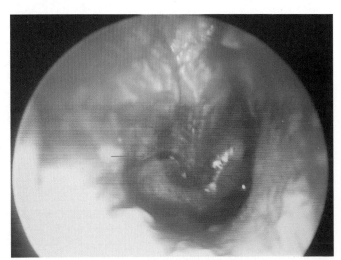

Fig. 8.7 Traumatic perforation covered with blood (*blue arrow*).

Treatment

Treatment is mainly reassurance, a wait-and-watch policy, and regular follow-up to assess the membrane. A PTA should be done to document hearing, especially in medicolegal cases. Aural hygiene to prevent ear infection is to be explained to the patient. This includes preventing water from entering the ear and avoiding use of earbuds. The margins may be brought together under vision, with the help of a microscope, for early healing. Topical ear drops should not be used. For contaminated injuries, cleaning should be done under the microscope and oral antibiotics should be started. Most traumatic perforations heal spontaneously. If the perforation persists, a myringoplasty is done.

Chronic Otitis Media–Mucosal Type or Chronic Suppurative Otitis Media–TTD

■ Definition

Mucosal COM is a chronic inflammatory condition of the middle ear cleft (eustachian tube, tympanic cavity, aditus, antrum, and mastoid air cells) characterized by a permanent perforation of the pars tensa with or without intermittent otorrhea and hearing loss.

The mucosal type is also known as the following:

- CSOM–tubotympanic type as the disease mainly involves the anteroinferior part of the middle ear cleft or tympanic cavity adjacent to the eustachian tube.
- Safe ear or the benign type of CSOM as inflammation in this area leads to profuse discharge from the mucous glands and goblet cells (based on the lining epithelium) and there are no important structures that can be involved by the disease, and there are less chances of complications.

> **Pearl**
>
> A central perforation of the pars tensa is the hallmark of mucosal COM disease.

■ Epidemiology

It is a common cause of conductive hearing loss, especially in the rural population due to lack of health education and less accessibility to specialists. Poor socioeconomic status and improper nutrition are contributing factors.

■ Etiology

It is commonly seen in the younger age group, that is, in school-going children. Both sexes and all age groups can be affected. Inadequately treated or untreated episodes of AOM, which results in perforation of the tympanic membrane, leads to mucosal COM disease.

Other causes include a traumatic perforation and following extrusion of a grommet in which the perforation of the tympanic membrane does not heal leading to a permanent perforation. The perforation becomes permanent when the outer epithelial layer and the inner mucosal layer come in contact and stop growing (contact inhibition).

Infections of the tonsils, adenoids, nasopharynx, nose, and paranasal sinuses reach the middle ear via the eustachian tube, which results in recurrent infection and ear discharge. Middle ear mucosa is known to act as a shock organ in response to allergic reactions to ingested food or dust or hay causing persistent otorrhea.

■ Causative Organisms

Pseudomonas aeruginosa is the most common organism implicated. Other organisms that have been isolated are *Proteus, E. coli, S. pneumoniae,* and *S. aureus.* Several studies have shown the presence of bacterial biofilms on the middle ear mucosa of children with COM supporting the concept that biofilms play a major role in chronic ear infections.

> ### Pearl
>
> Biofilms represent a form of survival mechanism for bacteria. The organisms in contact with a surface are enveloped in an extracellular matrix made of polysaccharide. This makes it difficult for antibiotics to penetrate and is often a cause for antibiotic resistance.

■ Clinical Features

Symptoms

- Patients present with mucoid, non-foul-smelling, painless, non-blood-stained *ear discharge.* Ear discharge may be profuse and intermittent. It may aggravate in the presence of upper respiratory infections, in cold climate, and after water entering the ear while bathing or swimming. The discharge usually reduces with medication.
- Causes for intermittent/persistent discharge in mucosal disease:
  - *Anteriorly, through the eustachian tube*: Sinonasal infection, infection from the nasopharynx including adenoids, and upper respiratory allergy.
  - *Laterally, through the perforation*: Water entering the ear, foreign body (patient may use a thin stick/feather due to irritation, part of which may get retained), or use of cotton buds.
  - *Posteriorly*: Mastoid reservoir of infection.
  - *In the middle ear*: Resistant organisms (in persistent discharge not responsive to medication, one must rule out tuberculous otitis media).
    - *Bacterial biofilms* may play a role in persistent ear discharge due to their resistance to antibiotics.
    - *Poor patient compliance* for treatment.
    - *Systemic causes* like diabetes and immunocompromised states.
- *Hearing loss* is usually of conductive type. It may be mild to severe.

Round window shielding effect is when the patient hears better in the presence of discharge as it helps maintain the *phase differential.* In case of dry ear, the sound from external environment strikes the round window and oval window simultaneously, thus cancelling each other's effect.

A slowly progressive conductive hearing loss can be due to tympanosclerosis or fibrosis involving the ossicular chain. There may be a mixed hearing loss due to the absorption of bacterial toxins, cytokines, or ototoxic drugs into the cochlea from the oval window or the round window.

- Tinnitus may be present. It may be due to loss of the ambient sound, or due to the bacterial toxins or ototoxic drugs affecting the inner ear.
- Otalgia is not common. Pain is usually due to otitis externa, which can be caused secondary to the ear discharge from the middle ear.

Signs

- Perforation of the tympanic membrane. It is usually central and may lie anterior, inferior, or posterior to the handle of the malleus. It may be of varying size (**Figs. 8.8, 8.9, 8.10,** and **8.11**).
- Middle ear mucosa may be pale pink or moist (inactive) or congested and edematous (active; **Fig. 8.12**); occasionally, a polyp might also be seen. There may be otomycosis in the external auditory canal (**Fig. 8.13**), which may be secondary to the ear discharge or due to overuse of the quinolone and/or steroid ear drops.
- Polyp is a pale smooth glistening mass of edematous mucosa that protrudes through a preexisting perforation and enters the external auditory canal. It may be congested in appearance and covered in discharge in case of active infection.
- Ossicular chain is usually intact and normal, but in long-standing cases, there can be erosion of the ossicles, commonly the long process of the incus.
- Tympanosclerosis appears as white chalky deposits over the tympanic membrane and may be present over the ossicles, promontory, tendons, and joints in the middle ear leading to conductive hearing loss.
- The external auditory canal may be filled with discharge and may have dried discharge or debris of otomycosis debris (**Fig. 8.12**). The canal may be edematous due to secondary otitis externa.

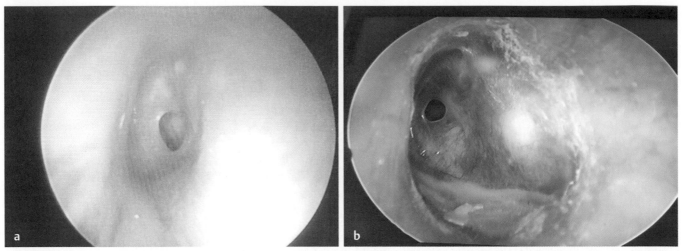

Fig. 8.8 **(a)** Small central perforation with congested membrane and middle ear mucosa. **(b)** Active discharge with mucopurulent discharge on the floor.

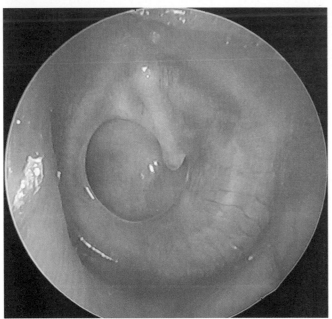

Fig. 8.9 Medium-sized central perforation in the pars tensa (left-side tympanic membrane). (This image is provided courtesy of Dr. H. Vijayendra, Director, Vijaya ENT Care Centre, Bangalore.)

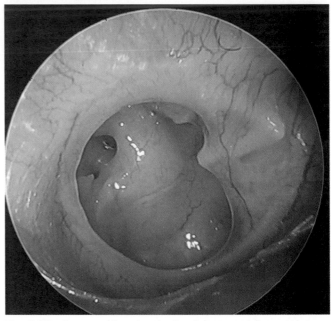

Fig. 8.10 Large perforation in the right tympanic membrane. (This image is provided courtesy of Dr. H. Vijayendra, Director, Vijaya ENT Care Centre, Bangalore.)

■ Investigations

Pure Tone Audiometry

This is done to assess the degree and type of hearing loss. It is a documentation of the hearing loss and will help in comparing the postoperative hearing status with the preoperative hearing. When the conductive hearing loss (air–bone gap) is more than 40 dB, ossicular chain involvement (discontinuity or fixity) should be suspected.

Patch Test

It is carried out when the air–bone gap (conductive hearing loss) on audiometry is more than 40 dB. After the initial PTA, a cigarette paper or thin filter paper is cut and shaped so as to just cover the perforation and rest on the remnant of the tympanic membrane. The paper should not be resting on the ear canal. A little liquid paraffin on the margins will help the placement. The PTA is repeated. If there is improvement in hearing, the ossicular chain is not

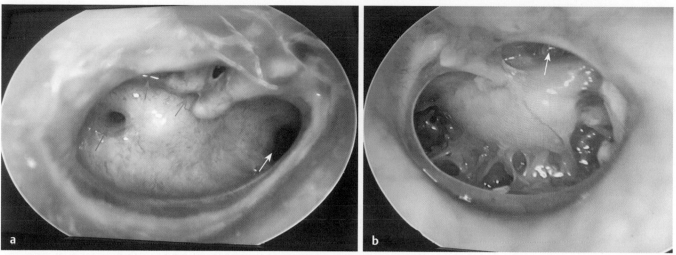

Fig. 8.11 Subtotal perforation. **(a)** Eustachian tube opening (*white arrow*), round window niche (*orange arrow*), incudostapedial joint (*blue arrow*), and stapedius tendon (*green arrow*) are visualized. **(b)** The footplate of the stapes (*white arrow*) is visualized due to the absence of the incus and the stapes suprastructure.

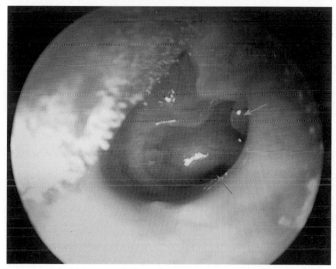

Fig. 8.12 Central perforation with active discharge from the middle ear (*green arrow*). The incudostapedial joint (*blue arrow*) and round window niche (*orange arrow*) are seen.

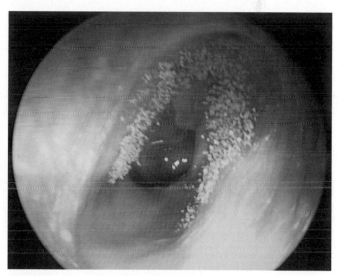

Fig. 8.13 Central perforation with otomycosis.

involved, and a myringoplasty is sufficient. If there is worsening of the air–bone gap, there is likely to be ossicular discontinuity, which would require a tympanoplasty. If there is no change, either the test has not been done properly or there is an ossicular fixity (tympanosclerosis or fibrosis involving the ossicular chain).

Culture and Sensitivity of Ear Discharge

The organisms causing ear discharge usually are *P. aeruginosa* (commonest), *Proteus*, *E. coli*, *S. aureus*, *Bacteroides*, and anaerobic streptococci. The swab should preferably be taken from the discharge in the middle ear after cleaning the discharge from the external auditory canal.

X-Ray of the Mastoid

This is done prior to a planned opening of the mastoid antrum or for cortical mastoidectomy. It gives information regarding the type of mastoid, and the level of the dural plate superiorly and the sinus plate posteriorly. Most often in chronic middle ear disease, X-ray of the mastoid will show a secondary sclerotic mastoid.

High-Resolution CT Scan of the Temporal Bone

It may be required when a mastoid reservoir of infection is suspected. Complications of the otitis media are rare in mucosal disease, but when present, a contrast-enhanced MRI should be done to look for intracranial pathology.

Diagnostic Nasal Endoscopy

It should be done when there are symptoms of nasal and paranasal sinus disease, which can be a source of infection.

■ Treatment

Aim

The aim of the treatment is to eliminate infection, recreate the barrier between the tympanic cavity and the external auditory canal, and restore hearing.

Medical Management

Aural Toilet

It is the removal of discharge and debris from the external auditory canal, which is done by dry mopping with cotton on a probe such as the Jobson-Horne probe or suction clearance under a microscope. For dried discharge or ear drops in the ear canal, wet mopping (saline-soaked cotton on a probe) is used.

Topical Ear Drops

Topical ear drops are used in an actively discharging ear. Antibiotic ear drops should be instilled for about three to four times a day for a period of up to 2 weeks. Topical antibiotics usually have a high drug concentration with a low minimum inhibitory concentration (MIC), which may be helpful in some resistant organisms. It can be combined with steroids, which act as an anti-inflammatory agent. Commonly used drops include the quinolones (a combination of ciprofloxacin and ofloxacin) with dexamethasone. Instillation of 1.5% acetic acid drops is useful to create an acidic medium in the ear canal. The acidic pH of ear drops helps eliminate *Pseudomonas* infection.

Instillation of Ear Drops

- To use ear drops, the patient is made to lie supine with the affected ear upward. After instilling the drops, the tragus is pressed inward intermittently (tragal pumping), which helps the drops to reach the middle ear.
- It is to be stopped if the ear becomes dry. Care should be taken as sometimes ear drops may cause local allergy, skin maceration, growth of fungus, and resistance of

organisms. Long-term use of quinolone and/or steroid drops can predispose to otomycosis.

- Ototoxic drugs should be avoided.

Systemic Antibiotics

Systemic antibiotics are useful when topical antibiotic drops have failed or cannot reach the infected areas, such as the mastoid air cells. Systemic therapy is also started when there is a source of infection outside the middle ear cleftlike tonsillitis, adenoiditis, or rhinosinusitis. Culture and sensitivity tests are required before starting systemic antibiotic therapy.

Precautions

Patients should be instructed to avoid water entry into the ear while having a head bath (by using cotton with Vaseline or sterile ear plugs) and to avoid swimming. Forceful blowing of the nose should be avoided to prevent infections from the nasopharynx reaching the middle ear. Use of ears buds should be discouraged.

Surgical Treatment

Removal of Aural Polyps or Granulation Tissue

Aural polyps should be removed before starting the local medical therapy to facilitate the topical antibiotics reaching the middle ear. The polyps should be removed carefully and should not be avulsed as it may be attached to the stapes, facial nerve, or horizontal semicircular canal. This can result in giddiness with sensorineural hearing loss, facial nerve palsy, or labyrinthitis.

Cortical Mastoidectomy

This is carried out when there is a mastoid reservoir of infection. Some authors advocate it in the presence of a eustachian tube dysfunction as the air in the mastoid acts as a buffer.

Reconstructive Surgery

- There are various surgical procedures that can be performed to close the defect in the tympanic membrane and to improve the hearing loss. This includes myringoplasty and tympanoplasty. The details of these surgical procedures are given in Chapter 15.
- *Myringoplasty*: Myringoplasty is surgical repair of the tympanic membrane.
- *Tympanoplasty*: It is a surgical procedure to eradicate the disease from the middle ear and to reconstruct the hearing mechanism.

■ Chronic Otitis Media–Squamous Type or Chronic Suppurative Otitis Media–AAD

Introduction

The squamous COM is a chronic inflammatory condition of the middle ear cleft usually involving the posterosuperior part of the mesotympanum, attic, and antrum, and is associated with entrapment of the keratinizing squamous epithelium in the middle ear space, known as a cholesteatoma, that can erode bone and destroy adjacent tissues in the temporal bone.

The squamous COM is also known as the following:
- CSOM–AAD.
- Unsafe ear.
- Dangerous type of CSOM.

The hallmark of this type of COM is the presence of cholesteatoma or granulations. It is associated with a greater risk of complications.

Cholesteatoma

Synonyms: Epidermosis or keratoma

The term "cholesteatoma" was coined by Johannes Mueller in 1838. The term cholesteatoma is a misnomer. It is not a tumor and does not contain cholesterol. It was also known as *skin in the wrong place.*

It is a sac lined by stratified squamous epithelium with a central mass of keratin debris that has bone-eroding properties.

Cholesteatoma consists of two parts (**Figs. 8.14** and **8.15**):
- A matrix made up of squamous epithelium (consisting of the stratum basale, stratum superficiale, and stratum corneum) and resting on a thin fibrous stroma (perimatrix).
- A central white mass consisting of keratin debris produced by the matrix.

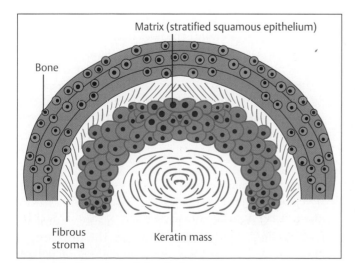

Fig. 8.14 Structure of the cholesteatoma.

Causes of bone destruction by cholesteatoma include the following:
- Hyperemic decalcification.
- *Osteoclastic bone resorption by cholesteatoma:* This may be due to enzymes like acid phosphatase, collagenase, acid proteases, proteolytic enzymes, leukotrienes, and cytokines, which may cause resorption of bone.
- Pressure necrosis.

Types of Cholesteatoma

Flowchart 8.1 shows the different types of cholesteatoma.

Congenital Cholesteatoma

It originates from the embryonal inclusion of the squamous epithelium (cell rests) in the middle ear cleft or the temporal bone. The usual sites of persistence of epithelial cell rests are the tympanic cavity, petrous apex, and the cerebellopontine angle. It presents as a white mass behind an intact tympanic membrane with conductive hearing loss.

The diagnostic criteria are the following:
- An intact tympanic membrane.
- No previous history of otitis media.

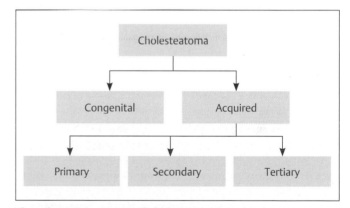

Flowchart 8.1 Types of cholesteatoma.

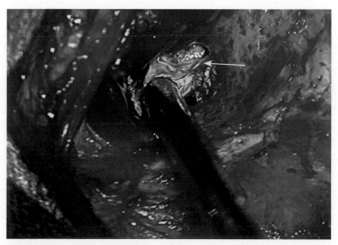

Fig. 8.15 Cholesteatoma seen in the middle ear during surgery.

Acquired Cholesteatoma

- *Primary acquired cholesteatoma* is formed in an attic (pars flaccida) or a posterosuperior quadrant (pars tensa), retraction pocket. There is little or no history of ear discharge (**Fig. 8.16**).
- *Secondary acquired cholesteatoma* occurs in a marginal perforation, usually in the posterosuperior quadrant of the pars tensa or in a long-standing pars tensa perforation with growth of the epithelium from the margins onto the medial wall of the middle ear. It is characterized by foul-smelling ear discharge. Granulation tissue and polyps may be seen.
- *Tertiary acquired cholesteatoma* can occur following trauma or after tympanoplasty (graft cholesteatoma can occur after an onlay technique of myringoplasty).

Pathogenesis of Acquired Cholesteatoma

Impaired functioning of the eustachian tube causes fluctuations in the middle ear pressure. When the eustachian tube is blocked, air in the middle ear is absorbed leading to negative middle ear pressure. This causes retraction of both the pars flaccida and the pars tensa.

Theories of Cholesteatoma Formation

Invagination or Retraction Pocket Theory (Wittmack)

This is one of the primary mechanisms of cholesteatoma formation where a retraction pocket develops in the attic or posterosuperior quadrant of the pars tensa with erosion of the adjacent canal wall. The eustachian tube dysfunction and/or epitympanic dysventilation (failure of ventilation) leads to retraction. The retraction pocket deepens because of negative middle ear pressure and repeated inflammation. The sac loses its self-cleansing mechanism and there is secondary infection of the keratin matrix by bacteria. The sac expands further resulting in an attic perforation or it can progress medially.

Epithelial Invasion/Migration Theory (Habermann)

Keratinizing squamous epithelium from the surface of the tympanic membrane or the external auditory canal migrates into the middle ear through a preexisting perforation in the tympanic membrane. The epithelial cells have been shown to migrate along a surface by a process called contact guidance. When these cells encounter another epithelial surface, they stop migrating (contact inhibition).

Basal Cell Hyperplasia (Ruedi and Lange)

It is postulated that in response to an inflammatory stimulus, epithelial cells (basal cells of stratum corneum) from the keratinizing epithelium of the pars flaccida could invade into the sub epithelial space and form an attic cholesteatoma.

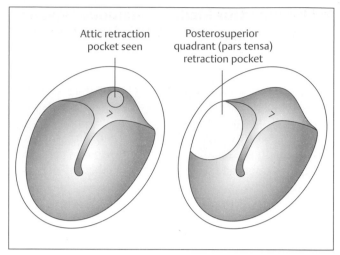

Fig. 8.16 The tympanic membrane showing the attic retraction pocket and the posterosuperior retraction pocket.

Metaplasia (Wendt)

It has been pointed out that the pluripotent middle ear epithelium could be stimulated by inflammation to transform into a metaplastic stratified squamous epithelium with keratinization.

Implantation Theory

Iatrogenic implantation of skin into the middle ear can occur following surgery like tympanoplasty. It can also occur as a rare complication of myringotomy and grommet insertion. Entrapment of the epithelium can also occur through a fracture line following trauma.

Expansion of Cholesteatoma

Cholesteatoma enters the middle ear cleft and invades the surrounding structures by first following the path of least resistance, and then by enzymatic bone destruction. Pars flaccida cholesteatoma originates in *Prussak's space*, the area just below the scutum, which is limited by the tympanic membrane (laterally), the neck of the malleus (medially); and the lateral ligament of the malleus (inferiorly), and then extends laterally toward the ossicular chain and into the epitympanum. Pars tensa cholesteatoma begins posterosuperiorly and extends posteriorly toward the facial recess and tympanic sinus, and medially toward the ossicular chain.

Clinical Features

Symptoms

- There is a history of persistent, scanty, purulent, foul-smelling, painless ear discharge. The discharge is blood stained when there are granulations or polyps.

There is no relation (increase) of the discharge to upper respiratory tract infection, and usually does not completely subside with medication.

- The hearing loss is usually conductive. In limited disease of the pars flaccida, the hearing may be normal. *Cholesteatoma hearer* is the term applied when there is erosion of the ossicular chain, but the gap is bridged by the cholesteatoma mass, so the hearing is normal.
- The progressive hearing loss can be conductive due to the ossicular involvement, or mixed (conductive and sensory), where, in addition to the tympanic cavity, there is involvement of the inner ear by the bacterial toxins, ototoxic drugs, or erosion of the cochlea or lateral semicircular canal (labyrinthitis).
- Ear pain is due to otitis externa secondary to the irritation of the ear discharge. A dull pain due to cholesteatoma filling the mastoid antrum may be present.
- There may be tinnitus and giddiness.

The symptoms associated with complications are the following:

- Sudden onset of severe vertigo may be due to the disease eroding into the lateral semicircular canal of the inner ear.
- Sudden onset of severe deafness can be due to the disease eroding into the cochlea.
- A paralyzed face could be due to the disease affecting the facial nerve.
- Swelling around the ear associated with pain due to mastoiditis.
- Fever, neck stiffness, and severe headache due to meningitis.
- Headache, retro-orbital pain, and diplopia due to petrositis.
- Headache, blurred vision, and projectile vomiting due to intracranial complications.

Signs

- Retraction pocket or an invagination of the tympanic membrane is seen in the attic (**Fig. 8.17**) or posterosuperior area of the pars tensa (squamous—inactive).
- Perforation is seen either in the attic (pars flaccida; **Fig. 8.18**) or the posterosuperior quadrant of the pars tensa with involvement of the margin (**Fig. 8.19**). An attic perforation may be hidden behind dried-up discharge or crusts. The attic disease can erode the lateral attic wall resulting in an *auto-atticotomy cavity*. With posterior extension of the erosion by the disease from the attic into the antrum, an *auto-mastoidectomy cavity* can form.
- Crusts over the pars flaccida should be removed as it can hide an attic disease.
- Even when there is a pars tensa (central) perforation, the pars flaccida should be examined to rule out a double pathology in which case the squamous disease takes precedence.
- A total perforation is one that involves the fibrous annulus (**Figs. 8.20** and **8.21**).
- Cholesteatoma debris or flakes can be seen in the retraction pocket and also in other parts of the middle ear cleft.
- Granulation tissue may be seen in the pars flaccida (**Fig. 8.22**), posterosuperior quadrant of pars tensa (**Fig. 8.23**), or posterosuperior deep meatus adjacent to the tympanic membrane. During mastoidectomy, granulation may be seen in the middle ear and mastoid.
- There may be a perforation in the pars tensa with ingrowing epithelium (commonly the posterior margin), spreading onto the medial wall of the tympanic cavity, which has a velvety appearance (**Fig. 8.24**).
- The aural polyp may be seen filling the external auditory meatus (**Fig. 8.25**).

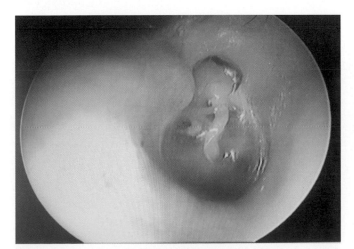

Fig. 8.17 Grade IV retraction of the pars flaccida.

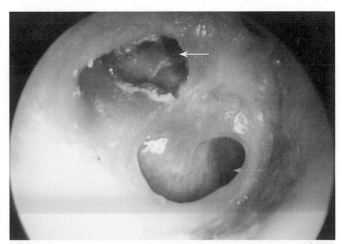

Fig. 8.18 Attic perforation (*yellow arrow*) with pars tensa perforation (*blue arrow*).

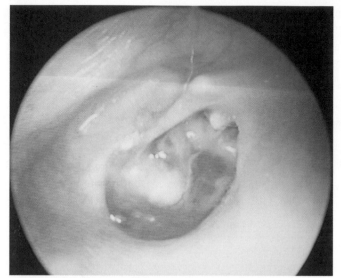

Fig. 8.19 Posterior marginal perforation with cholesteatoma.

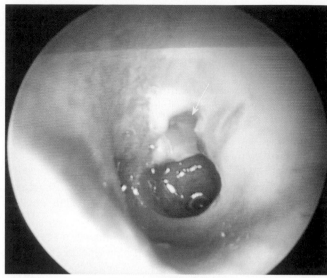

Fig. 8.20 Total perforation with cholesteatoma.

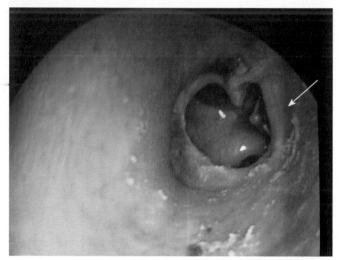

Fig. 8.21 Perforation involving the posterior margin. The head of the stapes (*yellow arrow*) and the stapedius tendon are seen.

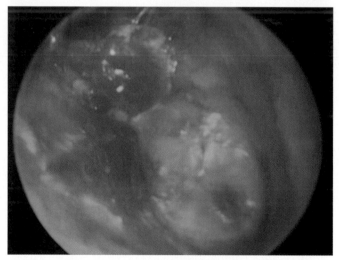

Fig. 8.22 Attic granulation.

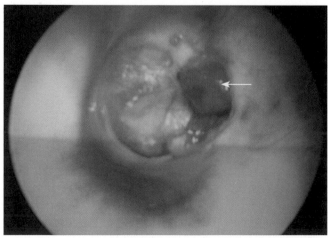

Fig. 8.23 Posterosuperior quadrant granulation tissue (*yellow arrow*).

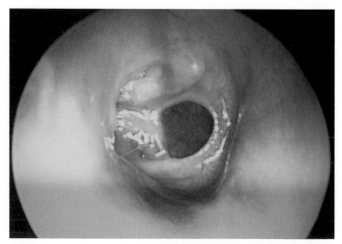

Fig. 8.24 Perforation with ingrowing epithelium (*blue arrow*).

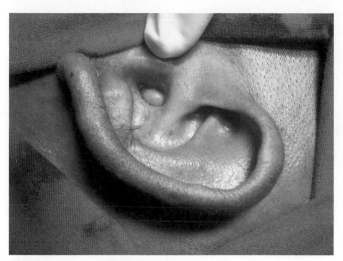

Fig. 8.25 Aural polyp.

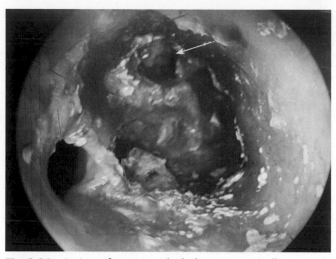

Fig. 8.26 Attic perforation with cholesteatoma (*yellow arrow*), posterosuperior retraction pocket (*green arrow*), and erosion of the posterior canal wall (*blue arrow*).

- There may be erosion of the posterior canal wall by the disease (**Fig. 8.26**).
- Tuning fork tests will be suggestive of the type of hearing loss (conductive or mixed).
- The fistula sign will be positive in the presence of a labyrinthine fistula. It more commonly affects the lateral semicircular canal.
- Signs of facial weakness will be seen if there is facial paralysis.

The various clinical signs seen in the squamous type of COM have been simplified into line diagrams (**Figs. 8.27** and **8.28**).

Pearl

When there is presence of crusts over the pars flaccida, it should be cleaned to look for underlying squamous disease. When there is a pars tensa perforation, one should examine the pars flaccida also to look for any pathology as there may be signs of squamous COM.

Investigations

- Examination under microscope to confirm the findings of clinical examination.
- Pure tone audiogram (PTA) to document the presence, type, and degree of hearing loss.
- X-ray of the mastoid if done will show a secondary sclerotic mastoid in the long-standing disease. A cholesteatoma cavity may be seen in the mastoid as an outer zone of sclerosis and a cotton wool appearance within the cavity and a translucent zone in between. This is referred to as the cotton wool appearance on X-ray of the mastoid.
- HRCT scan of the temporal bone is done to know the extent of disease, status of the ossicular chain, and type

of mastoid, and to identify any erosion of the sinus plate, dural plate, facial canal, or lateral semicircular canal.
- Culture and sensitivity of ear discharge is usually of not much significance as it reduces after the surgical procedure. The organisms commonly isolated are *P. aeruginosa* (commonest), *Proteus*, *E. coli*, *S. aureus*, *Bacteroides*, and anaerobic streptococci.

Treatment

Treatment of cholesteatoma is essentially surgical. The aim of surgery is to make the ear safe by eliminating the cholesteatoma and chronic infection, to conserve residual hearing, to improve hearing where possible, and to achieve a dry ear.

Disease clearance is usually accomplished by a canal wall up or canal wall down procedure. Canal wall up procedures include *atticotomy and atticoantrostomy* in which the posterior canal wall is largely preserved. These are done for limited disease involving the epitympanum. The canal wall down procedure includes *modified radical mastoidectomy*. This is done for extensive disease.

A *tympanoplasty* is performed for reconstruction of the hearing mechanism. A *conchomeatoplasty* is also carried out if there is a canal wall down procedure to widen the external auditory canal. This allows easy inspection and cleaning when required.

- *Modified radical mastoidectomy* is a canal wall down procedure performed to eradicate disease in the middle ear cleft involving exenteration of all accessible air cells of the mastoid air cell system and converting the tympanic cavity, mastoid antrum, and external auditory canal into a common cavity by removing the posterior canal wall. The disease is exteriorized through the external auditory meatus by widening it through a conchomeatoplasty.

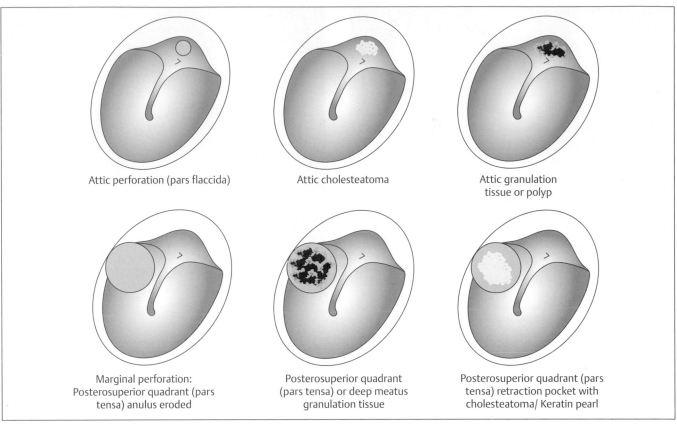

Attic perforation (pars flaccida)

Attic cholesteatoma

Attic granulation tissue or polyp

Marginal perforation: Posterosuperior quadrant (pars tensa) anulus eroded

Posterosuperior quadrant (pars tensa) or deep meatus granulation tissue

Posterosuperior quadrant (pars tensa) retraction pocket with cholesteatoma/ Keratin pearl

Fig. 8.27 Clinical findings seen in squamous chronic otitis media.

Fig. 8.28 Additional clinical findings suggestive of squamous chronic otitis media.

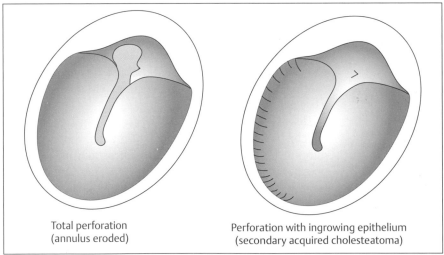

Total perforation (annulus eroded)

Perforation with ingrowing epithelium (secondary acquired cholesteatoma)

The parts of the tympanic membrane and ossicular chain not involved by disease are retained.

Cavity problems: The post–canal wall down mastoidectomy cavity problems include dizziness, deafness, discharge, debris collection, and dependence on regular follow-up. Conservative management comprising topical antibiotic ear drops and suction clearance has a very limited role and is used only in the following situations:

- Early disease with shallow retraction pocket.
- Only hearing ear with cholesteatoma.

- Elderly patients and those who are not fit for surgery under general anesthesia.
- Patients with inactive squamous disease who can come for regular follow-up.

Complications of Otitis Media

Complications of otitis media occur when the normal barriers of the middle ear are overcome, permitting infection to spread to the adjacent structures. These should be distinguished from the sequelae of otitis media, namely, tympanosclerosis, atelectasis, adhesive otitis media, ossicular erosion, perforation of tympanic membrane, cholesteatoma formation, or hearing loss (conductive or sensorineural) which occur as a direct result of the disease process but do not present as an acute medical or surgical emergency.

These complications can occur due to AOM or squamous COM (atticoantral type of CSOM). Complications in the mucosal COM is not common.

The factors favoring the development of complications include the following:

- Bacteria with high virulence and antibiotic resistance.
- Patient factors such as age, immunosuppression, malnutrition, systemic diseases like tuberculosis and diabetes mellitus, or malignancy.
- *Inadequate treatment* include inadequate course or dose of antibiotic, wrong choice of antibiotic, and lack of patient compliance to treatment.
- Poorly pneumatized mastoid.

■ Pathophysiology and Routes of Spread

- Extension through the bone that has been demineralized during the acute infection or has undergone resorption by cholesteatoma or osteitis in chronic disease.
- Retrograde thrombophlebitis or periphlebitis of small veins through bone and dura to venous sinuses.
- Through normal anatomical pathways such as the following:
  – Oval and round window to the inner ear.
  – Cochlear or vestibular aqueducts.
  – Dehiscence of the thin bony covering of the jugular bulb.
  – Dehiscence of the tegmen tympani.
  – Dehiscence of suture lines of the temporal bone.
- Through nonanatomical defects caused by accidental or surgical trauma or neoplastic erosion.
- Through other surgical defects such as vestibular opening created during stapedectomy or lateral semicircular canal fenestration.

- Extension into brain tissue along the periarteriolar spaces of Virchow–Robin.

Squamous COM can cause complications due to the bone-eroding properties of cholesteatoma. The complications produced by this disease are shown in **Table 8.3**.

■ Intratemporal Complications

Acute Mastoiditis

Most suppurative infections of the middle ear are associated with inflammation of the mastoid air cells to some extent owing to the proximity of the mastoid air cell system to the middle ear and the continuity of the lining mucosa. The term mastoiditis with osteitis is used when infection spreads from the mucosa to involve the bony walls of the mastoid air cell system. The breakdown of the cells leads to *acute coalescent mastoiditis*, also known as acute surgical mastoiditis.

Predisposing Factors

It is more common in children. It is associated with reduced host resistance like malnutrition, immunosuppression, exanthematous fever, and diabetes mellitus. It usually occurs in a cellular mastoid.

Causative organisms are *S. pneumoniae*, β-hemolytic streptococci, and *H. influenza*. Occasionally, it may be gram-negative organisms like *Pseudomonas*, *Proteus*, and *E. coli*.

Pathogenesis

Flowchart 8.2 depicts the pathogenesis of acute mastoiditis.

Clinical Features

Acute coalescent mastoiditis classically occurs 2 weeks after the onset of otorrhea. The symptoms are similar to AOM (**Table 8.4**).

On examination, there may be a perforation of the tympanic membrane and conductive hearing loss. Constitutional symptoms like fever, malaise, and toxic look may be present.

Table 8.3 Complications produced by squamous chronic otitis media

Intratemporal	Extratemporal	Intracranial
• Acute coalescent mastoiditis • Masked mastoiditis • Acute petrositis • Facial paralysis • Labyrinthitis	• Postauricular abscess • Bezold's abscess (sternomastoid) • Zygomatic abscess • Luc's abscess (meatal) • Citelli's abscess (digastric) • Parapharyngeal abscess • Retropharyngeal abscess	• Meningitis • Lateral sinus thrombophlebitis • Extradural abscess • Subdural abscess • Brain abscess: temporal lobe/cerebellum • Otitic hydrocephalus

Table 8.4 Suggestive and definitive symptoms and signs

Otorrhea persisting beyond 2 wk	Presence of postauricular abscess
Persistent or recurrent pain behind the ear	Mastoid tenderness and swelling over the mastoid region—*ironed out mastoid*
Erythema and edema over the mastoid tip	Sagging of the posterosuperior meatal wall resulting from thickening of the periosteum of the bony external auditory meatus

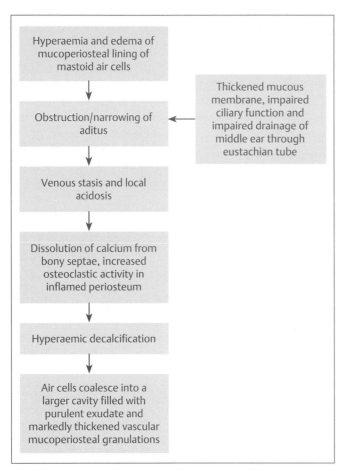

Flowchart 8.2 Pathogenesis of acute mastoiditis.

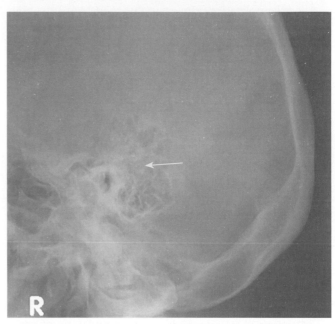

Fig. 8.29 X-ray of the left mastoid showing haziness of the air cells.

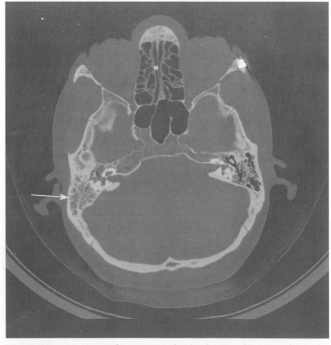

Fig. 8.30 Computed tomography (CT) scan showing the right mastoiditis.

Investigations

- *Complete blood count* will show polymorphonuclear leukocytosis, and raised erythrocyte sedimentation rate (ESR).
- *Swab of the discharge for culture and sensitivity*: The ear canal should be cleaned and the swab should be taken from the discharge coming through the perforation.
- *X-ray of the mastoids* (lateral oblique Schuller's view) will show diffuse clouding of the air cells (**Fig. 8.29**) due to replacement of air by fluid followed by destruction of the bony septal walls of the air cells.
- *HRCT of the temporal bone* will show haziness of the air cells (**Fig. 8.30**), followed by loss of bony trabeculae within the mastoid process.

Differential Diagnosis

- Postauricular suppurative lymphadenitis.
- *Otitis externa:* Furunculosis of the external auditory canal involving the posterior canal wall.

Treatment

- High-dose intravenous antibiotics based on culture and sensitivity report.
- Myringotomy to facilitate drainage of pus under tension if there is no perforation.
- Cortical mastoidectomy to exenterate all the accessible mastoid air cells is carried out when there is:
  - Subperiosteal abscess.
  - Sagging of the posterosuperior meatal wall.
  - Positive reservoir sign (persistent discharge in the canal, which fills up after cleaning).
  - No change or worsening of patient's condition even after 48 hours of antibiotics.
  - Mastoiditis with complications like facial nerve palsy, labyrinthitis, or intracranial complications.

Complications

- Subperiosteal abscess.
- Petrositis.
- Facial nerve paralysis.
- Labyrinthitis.
- Lateral sinus thrombophlebitis.
- Extradural abscess.
- Brain abscess.
- Otitic hydrocephalus.

Subperiosteal Abscess

Postauricular Abscess or Wilde's Abscess

It forms as a result of the hematogenous spread of infection through minute vascular channels in the suprameatal triangle. The abscess displaces the pinna forward, outward, and downward. The abscess can present in the subperiosteal plane, subcutaneous tissue, or open up with discharge from the mastoid cutaneous fistula (**Figs. 8.31, 8.32,** and **8.33**).

Zygomatic Abscess

It is formed when infection in the zygomatic air cells erodes through the cortical bone at the zygoma. There is a swelling above and in front of the ear.

Meatal or Luc's Abscess

When pus breaks through the bony wall of the antrum and the external auditory meatus, swelling is visible in the deep part of the bony meatus.

Citelli's Abscess

Pus may travel along the mastoid emissary vein or the occipitotemporal suture and hence there is a swelling posterior to the mastoid. The pus can also track along the

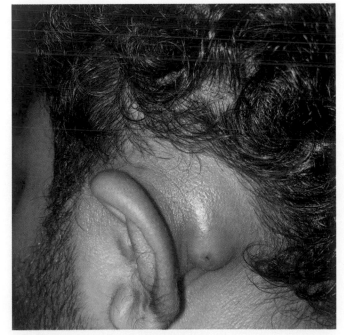

Fig. 8.31 Left postauricular abscess.

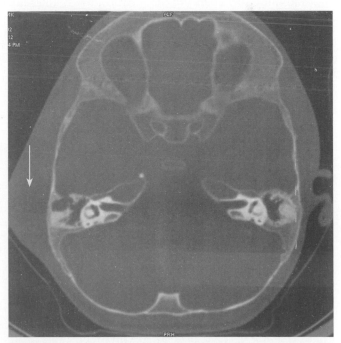

Fig. 8.32 Computed tomography (CT) scan showing the right subperiosteal abscess.

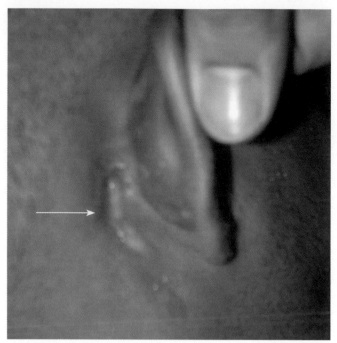

Fig. 8.33 Spontaneous rupture of postauricular abscess can lead to a mastoid cutaneous fistula.

posterior belly of the digastric muscle from the mastoid tip, anteriorly.

Bezold's Abscess

Pus can break through the medial side of the tip of the mastoid and track down beneath the sheath of the sternocleidomastoid muscle into the neck.

Treatment

It can be treated with intravenous antibiotics followed by incision and drainage of the abscess and cortical mastoidectomy.

Masked Mastoiditis

Synonyms of masked mastoiditis are latent mastoiditis and subacute mastoiditis.

This term is used in cases of mastoiditis without a draining ear or other usual signs and symptoms of mastoiditis. There is slow destruction of mastoid air cells without acute signs and symptoms. It is often seen in acute mastoiditis modified by treatment with antibiotics. The clinical features include mild pain over the mastoid region, persistent conductive hearing loss, and a thick tympanic membrane. A radiograph of the mastoid will show extensive decalcification and coalescence of mastoid air cells. The condition is treated with cortical mastoidectomy. Antibiotics based on culture and sensitivity are administered. Granulation tissue and dark gelatinous material are seen in the mastoid during the mastoidectomy.

Petrositis

Petrositis occurs when the infection spreads from the middle ear and mastoid to the petrous part of the temporal bone involving the anterior or posterior petrous apex.

Etiology

Petrositis is usually associated with acute coalescent mastoiditis, latent mastoiditis, and cholesteatoma. The common causative organisms are *Pneumococcus*, *H. influenza*, and β-hemolytic streptococci.

Pathology

The petrous apex is closely related to the abducens nerve and trigeminal ganglion. It is pneumatized in 30% of individuals. Two groups of air cells lead to the petrous apex from the mastoid and the middle ear:

- The posterosuperior tract that starts in the attic and antrum and runs around semicircular canals to the petrous apex.
- The anteroinferior tract that starts in the hypotympanum and passes around the eustachian tube and cochlea to the petrous apex.

Infection spreads along these tracts to the petrous apex and can involve the abducens nerve (in Dorello's canal) and trigeminal ganglion (in Meckel's cave).

Clinical Features

Gradenigo's Syndrome

- Lateral rectus palsy, due to paralysis of the sixth cranial nerve (abducens nerve), causing diplopia.
- Deep seated retro-orbital pain due to involvement of the trigeminal ganglion.
- Persistent otorrhea.

Other clinical features include transient facial paresis, mild recurrent vertigo, low-grade intermittent fever, vomiting, and headache.

Investigations

HRCT scan of the temporal bone will show the haziness in the cells in the petrous apex. MRI will better define the involvement of the cells along with involvement of the abducens nerve and the trigeminal ganglion. Spread to the cavernous sinus will also be better delineated on MRI. Swab should be sent for culture and sensitivity.

Treatment

Treatment is with high-dose antibiotics for 5 to 7 days followed by complete mastoidectomy. For persistence of disease, the petrous apex should be approached surgically to clear the disease. This can be done by a transcochlear or translabyrinthine approach, which will affect the hearing and balance, or by an infracochlear, retrolabyrinthine, or subarcuate approach, which may preserve the hearing and balance.

Labyrinthitis

Infection can spread to the inner ear causing labyrinthitis. In AOM, bacterial toxins can enter the inner ear through oval and round windows. Other predisposing factors for spread of infection are a Mondini malformation and a labyrinthine fistula, which can be detected with a CT scan.

Erosion of bone, usually of the lateral semicircular canal, by cholesteatoma can lead to the formation of a labyrinthine fistula. The patient will present with recurrent and transient episodes of vertigo and fluctuant sensorineural hearing loss. Nystagmus will be observed on examination with a positive fistula sign if there is a labyrinthine fistula. Bony erosion of the lateral semicircular canal will be seen on HRCT of the temporal bone in patients with labyrinthine fistula.

Spread of infection from the labyrinth to the subarachnoid space via the cochlear aqueduct can cause meningitis. Infection can also spread from meningitis into the labyrinth via the same route.

The treatment comprises antibiotics and labyrinthine sedatives. Steroids are also given. A canal wall down mastoidectomy for disease clearance should be done in patients with cholesteatoma. Only after complete removal of the cholesteatoma can the fistula be covered by a graft; otherwise, the cholesteatoma sac should be everted to epithelialize without an overlying graft.

Facial Nerve Paralysis

Facial nerve paralysis can occur in AOM or with cholesteatoma.

When it occurs within 2 weeks of onset of AOM, it is usually due to inflammatory edema, either by compression within the fallopian canal or by irritation of the nerve due to osteitis. Exposure of the dehiscent segment of the facial nerve, commonly in the tympanic segment above the oval window, to active infection causes direct irritation of the nerve.

Erosion of the bony fallopian canal by cholesteatoma causes exposure of the nerve to active infection, compression, or invasion by the disease leading to facial nerve paralysis.

Management

Management of facial palsy following AOM includes myringotomy to release the pus under tension and antibiotics. Mastoidectomy is indicated:
- If paralysis has occurred 2 weeks after onset of otitis media.
- In patients with COM.

- If paralysis fails to resolve after adequate management of otitis media.
- If electroneuronography (ENoG) indicates degeneration of more than 90% of motor nerve fibers within 6 days of onset of paralysis.

Exploration of the facial canal and removal of granulations should be done. In patients with cholesteatoma, modified radical mastoidectomy with complete removal of cholesteatoma is carried out with or without facial nerve decompression, depending on the nerve involvement noted on MRI or intraoperatively.

■ Intracranial Complications

Extradural Abscess

The *synonym* of extradural abscess is epidural abscess (**Fig. 8.34**).

It is the collection of pus between the bone and the dura. It can occur due to AOM or cholesteatoma. It may precede a brain abscess and may coexist with sinus thrombophlebitis.

Pathology

The overlying dural bone is destroyed by hyperemic decalcification in AOM and due to enzymatic activity in cholesteatoma resulting in pus collection in the epidural space. The affected dura gets covered with granulation and appears unhealthy and discolored.

An extradural abscess may lie in the middle cranial fossa, posterior cranial fossa, or as a perisinus abscess, outside the dura of the lateral venous sinus.

Clinical Features

Some cases remain asymptomatic and may be discovered accidentally during mastoidectomy:
- Persistent headache, which disappears with free flow of pus from the ear (spontaneous drainage of abscess), occurs on the affected side.

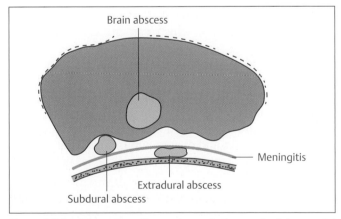

Fig. 8.34 Diagrammatic representation of intracranial complications.

- Severe ear pain.
- Generalized malaise and low-grade fever.
- Pulsatile discharge, which is purulent.

Diagnosis

Contrast-enhanced CT or MRI will show dural elevation, which is indicative of extradural abscess.

Treatment

- Antibiotic therapy is mandatory before and after surgery.
- *Mastoidectomy*: The overlying bone is removed until the healthy dura appears. In case of strong suspicion, the overlying intact tegmen tympani bone may be removed deliberately to check and evacuate any collection of pus. Such patients should be closely observed to look for other intracranial complications.
- The primary disease should be treated.

Subdural Abscess

It is the collection of pus in the subdural space between the dura and the arachnoid mater. It is a rare complication and used to be fatal in the preantibiotic era.

Pathology

The spread of infection usually occurs due to erosion of the bone and dura or by a thrombophlebitic process. Pus in the subdural space lies against the cerebral hemisphere and results in pressure symptoms. Later, it gets loculated in various places in the subdural space, which may result in a fatal mass that can rupture.

Clinical Features

The symptoms are sudden and severe and may progress rapidly. Severe and throbbing headache associated with fever, vomiting, and rapid deterioration of the patient point toward subdural abscess. The clinical features are due to meningeal irritation, thrombophlebitis of the cortical veins of the cerebrum, and raised CSF pressure.

Meningeal irritation, which can present with headache, high-grade fever, malaise, progressive drowsiness, neck rigidity, and Kernig's sign, may be seen. Some of these features may be masked due to prior antibiotic use. Thrombophlebitis of the cortical veins and cerebrum leads to aphasia, contralateral hemiplegia and hemianopia, and seizures. The raised CSF pressure presents with papilledema, ptosis, and dilated pupils due to the involvement of the third cranial nerve. Other cranial nerves may also be involved.

Diagnosis

An MRI is superior to a CT scan. It can distinguish between an epidural and a subdural abscess. A CT scan will show a loculated subdural abscess. Lumbar puncture is contraindicated as it can result in herniation of the cerebellar tonsil.

Treatment

It is a surgical emergency. Burr holes have to be drilled to drain the subdural abscess. High-dose broad-spectrum intravenous antibiotics are started. Mastoidectomy is done once the abscess resolves and the general condition of the patient improves.

Otogenic Brain Abscess

It is the focal suppurative infection of the brain parenchyma. Approximately 50% of brain abscesses in adults and 25% in children are otogenic in origin.

In adults, abscess usually follows CSOM with cholesteatoma, whereas in children, it is usually the result of an AOM. Cerebral abscesses (temporal lobe) occur more frequently than cerebellar abscesses.

It has a bimodal age distribution as seen in the pediatric population and in the fourth decade of life.

Route of Infection

- Otogenic brain abscesses are usually a result of direct extension of middle ear infection or through retrograde thrombophlebitis of the dural vessels.
- A cerebral abscess is often associated with an extradural abscess.
- A cerebellar abscess also develops as a direct extension through retrograde thrombophlebitis from the sigmoid sinus, which is related to the posterior wall of the mastoid.

Bacteriology

Both aerobic and anaerobic organisms are seen. Polymicrobial cultures are influenced by the immune status of the host.

- Aerobic organisms include gram-positive bacteria like pyogenic staphylococci, *S. pneumoniae*, and *S. haemolyticus*, and gram-negative bacteria like *P. mirabilis*, *E. coli*, and *P. aeruginosa*.
- Anaerobic organisms include *Peptostreptococcus* and *B. fragilis*.
- *H. influenza* is found rarely.

Pathogenesis

A brain abscess develops through four stages.

- *Invasion (initial encephalitis)*: It often includes mild symptoms like headache, low-grade fever, malaise, and drowsiness. These may often go unnoticed. It lasts for 1 to 3 days.
- *Localization (latent abscess)*: The pus starts getting localized with the formation of a capsule. Patients may

remain asymptomatic for several days or weeks. It lasts for 4 to 10 days.

- *Enlargement (manifest abscess)*: The abscess begins to enlarge. A zone of edema appears around the abscess and is responsible for aggravation of symptoms. Clinical features at this stage are due to the following:
  - Raised intracranial tension.
  - Disturbance of function in the cerebrum or cerebellum, causing focal symptoms and signs.

  This stage lasts for 10 to 13 days.
- *Termination (rupture of abscess)*: An expanding abscess in the white matter of the brain ruptures into the ventricle or the subarachnoid space resulting in fatal meningitis.

Clinical Features

A brain abscess is often associated with other complications such as extradural abscess, perisinus abscess, meningitis, sigmoid sinus thrombosis, and labyrinthitis. The clinical picture can overlap.

- The patient will appear to be toxic and drowsy.
- Dizziness, nystagmus, vomiting, and ataxia may indicate a cerebellar abscess. Temporal abscess may cause seizures.

Clinical features can be due to raised intracranial tension or due to the area of the brain affected, that is, the localizing features.

Symptoms and Signs of Raised Intracranial Tension

- Headache, which is often severe and generalized, is worse in the morning.
- Nausea and projectile vomiting are seen more often in cerebellar lesions.
- The level of consciousness alters with lethargy, which progresses to drowsiness, confusion, stupor, and finally, coma.
- Papilledema is absent in the early cases. It appears late when raised intracranial tension has persisted for 2 to 3 weeks. It appears early in a cerebellar abscess.
- Slow pulse and subnormal temperature cab be observed.

Localizing Features of a Temporal Lobe Abscess

- *Nominal aphasia* occurs if the lesion is of the dominant cerebral hemisphere, which is the left side in right-handed individuals. The patient may not be able to name common objects such as pen, key, and phone; however, the patient explains the use of the objects.
- *Contralateral homonymous hemianopia* indicates pressure on the optic radiations. The visual field defect is usually of the upper quadrant and can be recorded by perimetry. A confrontation test, that is, comparison of the visual field of the patient with that of the examiner

by standing in front of the patient, may be done depending on the patient's condition.

- *Contralateral motor paralysis, that is, upward spread* causes facial palsy followed by paralysis of the arms and legs or inward spread toward the internal capsule leads to paralysis of the leg followed by paralysis of the arm and face.
- *Epileptic fits, that is, small involuntary smacking movement of the lips and tongue* can be noted. Generalized fits may also occur.

Localizing Features of a Cerebellar Abscess

- Suboccipital headache with neck rigidity.
- Spontaneous nystagmus.
- Ipsilateral ataxia, that is, staggering to the side of the lesion.
- Finger–nose test, that is, past pointing, and intention tremor.
- Dysdiadochokinesia, that is, rapid pronation and supination movements become slower and irregular on the affected side.

Investigation

- Contrast-enhanced CT scan is done to confirm the site and size of the abscess. Other associated complications like extradural abscess or sigmoid sinus thrombosis can be detected. *Ring sign*: The brain abscess appears as a hypodense area surrounded by the area of edema (**Fig. 8.35**). The temporal bone is also better visualized on CT scan than on MRI.
- MRI helps detect subtle changes in the brain parenchyma and note the spread of the abscess.
- Lumbar puncture will show a rise in pressure, increase in protein with normal sugar content, and raised white blood cells (polymorphs or lymphocytes, depending on the severity of the infection).

Treatment

Medical Treatment

- Intravenous antibiotics like chloramphenicol, penicillin, or its derivatives. Metronidazole may be added to cover against anaerobic organisms. Aminoglycosides such as gentamicin covers *pseudomonas* and *proteus*. Antibiotics are later changed as per the culture and sensitivity report.
- Dexamethasone 4 mg given intravenously every 6 hours or 20% mannitol at a dose of 0.5 g/kg body weight helps reduce the associated edema and intracranial tension.

Surgical Treatment

- Life-saving neurosurgical intervention is more important than the otological management in such conditions.

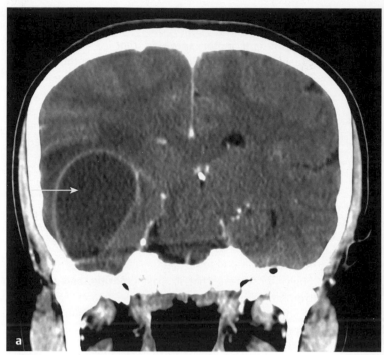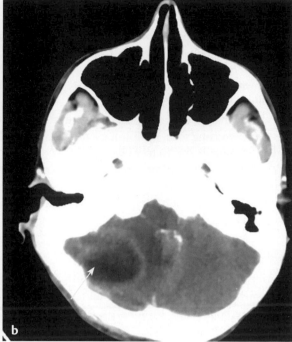

Fig. 8.35 Contrast-enhanced computed tomography (CT) scan. **(a)** Right temporal lobe abscess. **(b)** Right cerebellar abscess.

- Aspiration of pus for culture and sensitivity is followed by a repeat CT or MRI to see the resolution of the size of the abscess. Repeated aspirations may be done. If it does not decrease in size or is rapidly enlarging, then excision is required.
- After aspiration, penicillin can be instilled into the abscess.

Otological Intervention

Once neurologically stable, patients can be taken up for a tympanomastoid surgery. The presence of cholesteatoma requires a modified radical mastoidectomy, which removes the disease.

Meningitis

It is the inflammation of the leptomeninges (pia and arachnoid) along with CSF of the subarachnoid space. It is the most common intracranial complication and can occur in children and adults.

Causes

- After an episode of AOM in children.
- Squamous COM disease.
- Temporal bone fracture causing CSF leak.
- Following middle ear or mastoid surgeries (rare).

Route of Spread

The infection from the middle ear or mastoid can reach the meninges via the following pathway:

- Preformed pathways via the patent petrosquamous suture.
- Retrograde venous thrombophlebitis.
- Direct erosion of bone and dura.
- From labyrinthitis via the cochlear aqueduct.

The commonest organisms include *Haemophilus influenzae* and *S. pneumoniae*.

Clinical Features

The severity varies with the extent of the infection.
The earliest symptoms include the following:
- High-grade fever with chills and rigors.
- Throbbing headache and photophobia.
- Nausea and sometimes projectile vomiting.
- Irritability and restlessness.
- Infants may even develop seizures.

Signs (may be masked due to the use of antibiotics):
- Neck rigidity is the earliest sign.
- *Kernig's sign*: Extension of the leg with flexion of the thigh on the abdomen is painful.
- *Brudzinski's sign*: Flexion of the neck results in flexion of the hip and knee.
- Cranial nerve palsies and hemiplegia.
- Exaggerated deep tendon reflexes initially, which later becomes sluggish or absent.

Investigations

- HRCT of the temporal bone is the imaging modality of choice. It helps in providing details regarding the bony erosion, congenital malformations, or any fistula.

- MRI is done to rule out inflammatory changes in the brain and other related complications.
- Lumbar puncture and CSF analysis usually help in establishing a diagnosis.
  - Cloudy (turbid) or yellow (xanthochromic).
  - Raised cell count with predominance of polymorphs.
  - Raised protein level.
  - Low sugar and chlorides.
- Gram staining and culture: Sensitivity of the CSF to identify the organism and antibiotic sensitivity.
- Fundoscopy may show indistinct disc margins and choking of vessels.
- Ear swab is taken for culture and sensitivity.

Treatment

Medical treatment always takes precedence over surgery. Surgery is usually indicated in failed medical therapy. The antibiotics of choice are crystalline penicillin, ampicillin, chloramphenicol, or third-generation cephalosporins given intravenously for 7 to 10 days. Surgery is performed when the general condition of the patient improves. In AOM, myringotomy with or without cortical mastoidectomy is done. For cholesteatoma, a modified radical mastoidectomy is done for disease clearance.

Lateral Sinus Thrombophlebitis

Lateral sinus thrombophlebitis is also known as sigmoid sinus thrombosis.
This condition is characterized by inflammation of the inner wall of the lateral sinus with formation of a thrombosis, which later gets infected. The incidence has lately decreased due to newer antibiotics, yet the mortality remains high.

Etiology

- Acute coalescent mastoiditis.
- Masked mastoiditis.
- Cholesteatoma.

The common bacteriology includes β-hemolytic *Streptococcus*, *Pneumococcus*, *Bacillus*, *proteus*, and *pseudomonas*.

Clinical Features

- *Fever*: *Hectic picket fence type* of fever with chills and rigors. Fever has one or more peaks a day but does not touch the baseline as this coincides with the release of septic emboli into the bloodstream. Later, there is fall in the temperature with profuse sweating and a sense of well-being.
- *Headache*: Mild headache occurs due to the formation of a perisinus abscess. It may get severe with an increase in intracranial pressure.

- Deep-seated ear pain and ear discharge may be noticed in some patients.
- *Griesinger's sign*: Thrombosis of the mastoid emissary vein leads to tenderness and edema over the posterior part of the mastoid. It is a pathognomonic symptom of sigmoid sinus thrombosis.
- Tenderness along the internal jugular vein (in the neck) due to thrombosis of the jugular vein.
- Enlarged and tender jugular lymph nodes.
- Anemia.
- *Papilledema*: The fundus shows blurring of the disc margins, retinal hemorrhages, or dilated veins. It occurs when the clots extend to the superior sagittal sinus.
- *Crowe–Beck test (Lily–Crowe sign)*: When pressure is applied on the opposite side internal jugular vein, it causes engorgement of the retinal and supraorbital veins and subsides on release of pressure.
- Cavernous sinus thrombosis will cause proptosis, ptosis, chemosis, and ophthalmoplegia.

Investigations

- *Blood culture*: The antibiotic may be changed as per the sensitivity report.
- *Peripheral smear*: This is done to rule out malarial parasites in the blood.
- Culture sensitivity of the ear discharge, if present, is done.
- *Lumbar puncture*: Normal CSF findings with rise in pressure; it is done to rule out meningitis.
- *Tobey–Ayer test*: This test is done by recording the CSF pressure by a manometer while compressing one or both jugular veins. Compression of the affected side produces no effect, whereas compressing the opposite side vein causes rapid rise in the CSF pressure.
- *Contrast-enhanced CT scan*: Typical feature of sinus thrombosis is the "delta sign" seen on axial cuts. It is an empty triangular area with rim enhancement and central low density seen at the level of the sigmoid sinus.
- *MRI*: In Gadolinium-enhanced MRI, thrombus appears as a soft-tissue signal associated with vascular and bright appearance of the dural walls. MRI is more sensitive than a CT scan.
- MR angiography and venography will help demonstrate the thrombus by radiology.

Complications

If left untreated, it may lead to septicemia, meningitis, and brain abscess. The septic thrombi can cause pyogenic abscess in the lungs, bones, joints, and subcutaneous tissues. Thrombosis of the jugular bulb and jugular vein can involve the cranial nerves IX–XI. Cavernous sinus thrombosis and otitic hydrocephalus can occur.

Treatment

- Antibiotic therapy is started initially with 1 million units of intramuscular (IM) injection of crystalline penicillin every 6 hours to cover pyogenic organisms. Antibiotics should be given according to culture sensitivity report for a period of 10 to 14 days.
- *Mastoidectomy*: Cortical or modified radical mastoidectomy is done in cases of AOM or cholesteatoma, respectively. The bony sinus plate is removed to expose the dura and to drain the perisinus abscess.
- Ligation of the internal jugular vein is done when medical and surgical options fail. It is done to restrict the spread of thromboemboli.
- Blood transfusion is given to treat anemia.
- Improve general well-being of the patient with supportive and nutritional therapy.
- Anticoagulants may help reduce clot propagation, promote sinus recanalization, and reduce the risk of neurological deficits.

Otitic Hydrocephalus

It is also known as benign raised intracranial hypertension because there is no associated ventricular dilation. It is a rare complication that is characterized by raised intracranial pressure and normal CSF. It is seen in children and adolescents.

Mechanism

It occurs because of the following factors:
- Lateral sinus thrombosis due to middle ear infection causes obstruction to the venous return.
- The thrombosis extends into the superior sagittal sinus and also impedes the functioning of the arachnoid villi to absorb CSF.

Clinical Features

- Severe headache is the usual presenting complaint, associated with nausea and vomiting.
- Traction on the sixth cranial nerve causes diplopia.
- Increased intracranial pressure causes papilledema and optic atrophy causing blurring of vision.
- Papilledema may be accompanied with patches of exudates and hemorrhages.
- Nystagmus may be present.

Diagnosis

- MRI to evaluate the venous sinuses.

- *Lumbar puncture:* CSF is sterile and normal in cell count, sugar, and protein levels. Pressure is raised to about 300 mm of water (normal is 70–120 mm of water).

Treatment

The aim of medical treatment is to reduce the CSF pressure, which includes administration of corticosteroids, mannitol, and acetazolamide.

Surgical treatment is done to reduce CSF pressure and prevent optic atrophy and blindness. This can be achieved by a lumbar drain or repeated lumbar puncture or a lumboperitoneal shunt (to drain the CSF into the peritoneal cavity). Mastoidectomy and decompression of the sigmoid sinus is recommended. Optic sheath decompression may prevent optic atrophy.

Points to Ponder

- OME is a common condition seen in children where they present with hearing loss due to accumulation of fluid in the middle ear.
- Ear discharge is a common complaint and the nature of the discharge can lead to the diagnosis. Mucoid or mucopurulent discharge in the external auditory canal means there is a perforation of the tympanic membrane because mucoid discharge is secreted by the mucous glands and goblet cells of the middle ear mucosa.
- AOM is a common condition during infancy and early childhood because of the anatomy of the eustachian tube. The tube is shorter, wider, and more horizontal in children.
- COM can be mucosal or squamous. Both mucosal and squamous COM can be active or inactive. The old terminology was chronic suppurative otitis media or CSOM, and it was divided into TTD and AAD. TTD is now referred to as mucosal disease and AAD is referred to as squamous disease.
- CSOM-TTD is the safe type of CSOM because it is not usually associated with complications. CSOM-AAD is the dangerous type because it can cause complications due to the presence of cholesteatoma.
- Cholesteatoma is a sac lined by the squamous epithelium with a central mass of keratin. It has bone-eroding properties and is the cause of complications.
- The complications of CSOM can be classified into intratemporal, extratemporal, and intracranial.

Case-Based Questions

1. **A 5-year-old girl was brought to the ear, nose, and throat (ENT) clinic because she was inattentive in the class and her mother felt she had difficulty in hearing. There was no history of ear discharge or ear pain. Examination revealed a dull grayish tympanic membrane and the cone of light was distorted. Air bubbles could be seen through an intact eardrum.**

   a. What is the probable diagnosis?

   b. What investigations would you recommend?

   c. What is the treatment?

   Answer

   a. OME, which is very common in this age group where fluid accumulates behind an intact drum. Sometimes air bubbles can be seen behind the drum.

   b. PTA, which will show whether there is conductive hearing loss, and tympanometry, which will reveal a B type curve signifying fluid in the middle ear.

   c. Myringotomy and grommet insertion.

2. **A 35-year-old man presented with hearing loss and discharge from the left ear for the past 5 years. He had been seen by various doctors who had prescribed ear drops to stop the discharge. He had not had discharge from that ear for the past 7 months. On examination, there was a large central perforation in the pars tensa. What is the management of this patient?**

Answer

A central perforation reveals that he has mucosal COM disease or CSOM–TTD. It is in the inactive stage as the last discharge was more than 7 months back. He requires an examination under the microscope (EUM) to confirm the findings of a central perforation and a dry ear. PTA will help document his hearing loss, and he should be counseled for tympanoplasty as a permanent solution.

3. **A 44-year-old man had been complaining of constant ear discharge and foul smell from the right ear for the last 7 years. He also had reduced hearing. There were no other symptoms. On examination, there was mucopurulent discharge in the external auditory canal with an attic perforation. White flakes were seen covering the perforation. There was a foul smell emanating from the ear. What is the management of this condition?**

Answer

White flakes seen in the attic region of the tympanic membrane together with foul smell, discharge, and deafness signify CSOM–AAD or squamous COM. The white flakes are due to cholesteatoma. He needs to undergo modified radical mastoidectomy or MRM to remove the cholesteatoma and make the ear safe and dry. It should be done as early as possible to prevent any intratemporal or intracranial complications.

Frequently Asked Questions

1. What is the tympanometry finding in OME?

2. Where do you make an incision for myringotomy?

3. What is the function of a grommet?

4. What is the management of AOM?

5. What are the stages of AOM?

6. What is a central perforation?

7. How do you divide a tympanic membrane into various quadrants?

8. What is a cholesteatoma?

9. How does a cholesteatoma produce complications?

10. What are the complications of the atticoantral disease?

Endnote

Mastoidectomy or the surgical technique of opening up the diseased mastoid air cells became part of the ENT practice only after 1850. Before that time, the only surgery performed behind the ear was to drain a "red, warm, painful abscess" by incision and drainage, to let out the pus of a subcutaneous mastoid abscess. Although mastoidectomy was primarily carried out for clearing infections, many unscrupulous ENT surgeons performed this procedure for deafness and tinnitus. This led to the surgery becoming unpopular for some time. Then in 1873, Hermann Schwartze published an article clearly outlining the indications and steps of mastoidectomy and this procedure is now named after him as Schwartze's mastoidectomy.

9 Otosclerosis

Vijendra Shenoy S. and Sreenivas Kamath K.

The competency covered in this chapter is as follows:

EN4.13 Describe the clinical features, investigations, and principles of management of otosclerosis.

Introduction

Otosclerosis is a term that refers to "oto" meaning ear and "sclerosis" meaning hardening of body tissue. It is a disease caused by abnormal bone remodeling in the middle ear (stapes footplate), and occasionally involves the inner ear. It is a common cause of conductive deafness with an intact tympanic membrane.

The disease often progresses through two phases: (1) active phase where there is bone resorption and (2) inactive or remission phase, which is characterized by bone deposition. In this process, the normal enchondral layer of the bony otic capsule or the labyrinth of the inner ear is replaced by an irregularly laid immature bone. Incidence of the disease is difficult to assess, although the prevalence has been reported to be up to 5 to 18% of the general population.

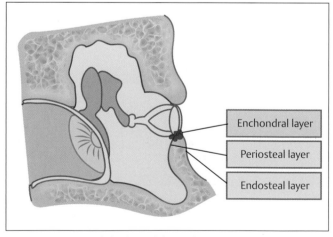

Fig. 9.1 Layers of the bony labyrinth.

Relevant Anatomy

The inner ear consists of (1) a bony labyrinth and (2) a membranous labyrinth. Otosclerosis is a disease of the bony labyrinth.

The bony labyrinth is basically a three-layered structure (**Fig. 9.1**):
- Periosteal layer.
- Enchondral layer.
- Endosteal layer.

Otosclerosis begins in the *enchondral layer.*

Etiology

Exact etiology is unknown. Following are the proposed theories regarding the causation of this disease.
- **Anatomical location:** "*Fissula ante fenestram,*" which is located anterior to the oval window, is the commonest site of occurrence as it may harbor a remnant of embryologic cartilage.
- **Genetic association:** Aberrations in genes involved with bone formation and remodeling have been found to have association with otosclerosis (e.g., *COL1A1* gene, transforming growth factor beta 1 [TGF-beta 1], angiotensin II, human leukocyte antigens [HLAs]).
- **Hereditary:** More than 50% individuals with otosclerosis have a positive family history. It has an autosomal dominant mode of transmission with reduced penetrance and variable expressivity.
- **Gender:** It is more common in females, with a male-to-female ratio of 1:2.
- **Ethnicity:** It is more common in Caucasians.
- **Age:** it is more prevalent in the age group of 20 to 30 years.

- **Pregnancy:** It may worsen the deafness (controversial).
- **Viral infection:** The role of the measles virus has been postulated. After measles infection, viral ribonucleic acid (RNA) was found in fixed stapes foot plate. The incidence of otosclerosis has dropped following successful vaccination against measles.

Clinical Classification

■ Clinical Classification Based on Location

Types of otosclerosis	Characteristics
Clinical otosclerosis	Involves the stapes, stapediovestibular ligament, or round window. The patient presents with conductive hearing loss
Cochlear otosclerosis	Involves the cochlear endosteum; hence, the patient presents with sensorineural hearing loss
Histological otosclerosis	Microscopic lesions found in regions other than the stapes or the round window or cochlea. The patient has no symptoms
Additional types	
Malignant otosclerosis (obliterative otosclerosis)	Severely active disease with progressive involvement of both the windows (oval and round) and the cochlea. The patient presents with progressive mixed hearing loss
FAO	Air conduction is no better than 95 dB and bone conduction is at 55–60 dB at one frequency only or air or bone conduction is not measurable

Abbreviation: FAO, far advanced otosclerosis.

■ Based on Site of Involvement of Stapedial Footplate (Clinical Otosclerosis) (Fig. 9.2)

Pathology of Otosclerosis

Otic capsule is made up of mature bone and has very less bone remodeling. The otic capsule has been noted to have small regions of immature cartilaginous tissue called the "globuli interossei," and these cells could be the cause of otosclerosis (**Flowchart 9.1**).

Clinical Presentation

■ Symptoms

- **Hearing loss:** Commonly, it is insidious in onset and slowly progressive, with bilateral conductive hearing loss in 70% of cases. It can be unilateral hearing loss initially or in sporadic cases only unilateral. The hearing loss

is mixed when the inner ear is also involved. The hearing loss will be sensorineural in cochlear otosclerosis.
- **Tinnitus:** This is more often seen in active disease due to high vascularity of the otosclerotic foci and in cochlear otosclerosis.
- **Vertigo:** This may be seen in a few individuals. Other coexistent causes must be ruled out especially prior to a planned surgery for otosclerosis.
- **Speech:** Due to conductive deafness, patients may develop a monotonous, soft speech.
- **Paracusis Willisii:** It is the ability to hear better in a noisy environment because people tend to talk loudly. The patient hears the words but not the ambient sound. This is seen in conditions with conductive hearing loss and is not an actual improvement in hearing (paradoxical improvement).

■ Signs

- Otoscopic examination: The tympanic membrane is intact and normal in 90% of patients. Rarely, a reddish hue (flamingo red in 10%) is noticed behind an intact tympanic membrane over the area of promontory due to the increased vascularity in an active otosclerotic foci. This is called *Schwartze's sign*.
- Pneumatic otoscopic examination reveals normal tympanic membrane movement.
- Types of tuning fork tests are depicted in **Table 9.1**.
- The Schwabach test will be lengthened as compared to the examiner. Gelle's test will be negative.

Differential Diagnosis of Conductive Hearing Loss

The differential diagnosis of conductive hearing loss is as follows:
- **External ear causes:** Wax, foreign body, osteoma, exostosis, otitis externa, otomycosis, congenital atresia,

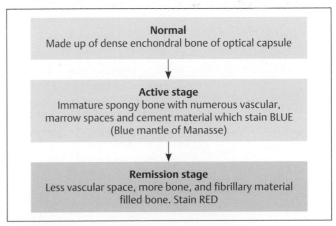

Flowchart 9.1 Pathophysiology of otosclerosis.

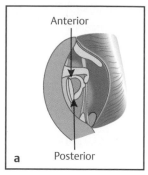

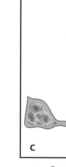

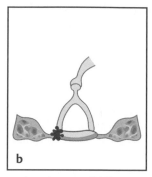

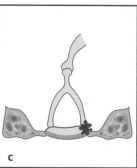

Normal · Anterior crura (MC) · Posterior crura

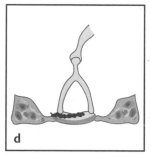

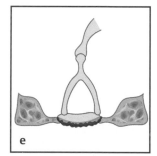

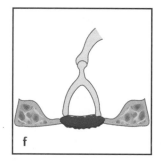

Biscuit type · Circumferential type · Obliterative type

Fig. 9.2 (a–f) Classification of otosclerosis based on the site of involvement of the stapedial footplate.

Table 9.1 Types of tuning fork test

Type	Rinne's test	Weber's test	Absolute bone conduction test
Clinical otosclerosis	Negative	Lateralized to worse ear	Same as examiner
Cochlear otosclerosis	Negative	Lateralized to normal ear	Reduced as compared to examiner

stenosis, myringitis, tympanic membrane perforation, myringosclerosis, and tumors.

- **Middle ear causes:** Congenital ossicle defects and fixation, acute otitis media, chronic otitis media, adhesive otitis media, barotrauma, hemotympanum, tympanosclerosis, *otosclerosis*, and tumors of middle ear.

Pearl

There are two other conditions that can lead to demineralization of the otic capsule and deafness.

- **Van der Hoeve's syndrome**: This is a genetic disorder that affects bones. This syndrome consists of the classic triad of hearing loss, spontaneous fracture, and blue sclera. Histologically, all three layers of the otic capsule are involved (endosteal, enchondral, and periosteal layers), whereas in otosclerosis, only the enchondral layer is affected.
- **Paget's disease**: This is a chronic disease of the skeletal bones affecting the spine, pelvis, and long bones of the limbs. If it affects the otic capsule, it can result in deafness due to stapedial fixation.

Investigation

- *Pure tone audiogram* will show a conductive deafness (air–bone gap will be present; **Fig. 9.3**).
  Carhart's notch: A dip at 2 kHz of bone conduction (sensorineural component) will be seen. This is a mechanical artifact that gets corrected after surgery.
  The audiogram may show a mixed hearing loss in far-advanced otosclerosis and a sensorineural hearing loss in cochlear otosclerosis.

Pearl

Carhart's notch is a characteristic finding in otosclerosis where there is a dip in the bone conduction thresholds at 2,000 Hz. The accurate testing of bone conduction depends on normal middle ear function. If there is a middle ear ossicular pathology, like stapes fixation, then there is an increase in bone conduction thresholds at 2,000 Hz because the natural frequency of vibration of the ossicular chain is close to 2,000 Hz.

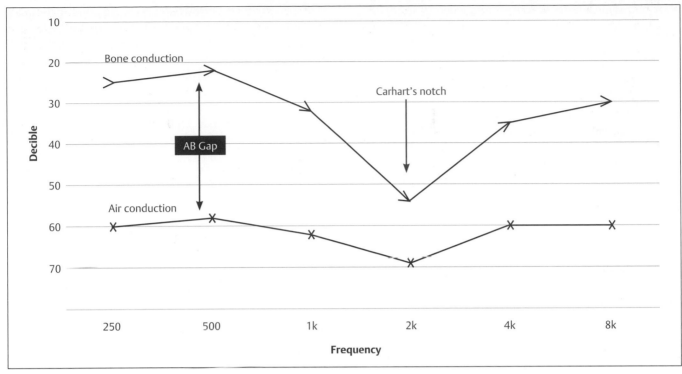

Fig. 9.3 Pure tone audiogram.

- **Impedance audiometry:** It is normal in the initial stages. With ossicular fixation, the tympanometric peak reduces, giving a type "*As*" curve on impedance audiometry (**Fig. 9.4**).
- **Acoustic reflex (stapedial reflex):** The first sign of otosclerosis is the "biphasic pattern" of acoustic reflex.
  The biphasic pattern is described as brief increase in compliance at the beginning and end of stimulus.
  In advanced disease when the footplate is fixed completely, the *stapedial reflex* will be *absent*.
- **Speech audiometry:** It is normal in otosclerosis, except in cases of cochlear otosclerosis.
- **Otoacoustic emission:** It is absent otoacoustic emissions (OAEs).
- **Imaging:** High-resolution computed tomography (HRCT) temporal bone with 1-mm slices will reveal the active otosclerotic lesions. In cochlear otosclerosis, a double-ring sign may be seen.

Treatment Principles of Otosclerosis

The treatment options for otosclerosis include the following:
- Nonsurgical management:
  - Hearing aids.
  - Medical management.
- Surgical management:
  - Stapedectomy.

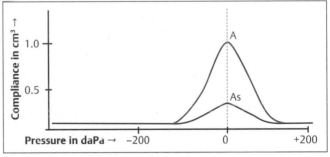

Fig. 9.4 Illustration of the normal tympanogram in *green color* and type As tympanogram in *red color*. Type As tympanogram suggests a less compliant middle ear system (<0.3 cm³) and normal peak pressure.

  - Stapedotomy.
  - Cochlear implantation.

■ Hearing Aid in Otosclerosis

Amplification via hearing aids is an alternative to surgical treatment for otosclerosis for those reluctant or unfit to undergo surgery.

■ Medical Management

- Management is directed toward arresting the progress of the disease.
- It is useful especially in the active phase of otosclerosis and in cochlear otosclerosis.

- Sodium fluoride is prescribed in divided doses of 20 to 40 mg daily.

How Does Sodium Fluoride Act?

- It reduces the bone resorption.
- It increases the osteoblastic activity.
- It prevents release of cytotoxic enzymes.
- Hydroxyapatite is replaced by fluorapatite, which is a harder and better-quality composition for bone formation.
- It promotes maturation of bone and reduces vascularity.

The indications and contraindications of sodium fluoride implementation are listed in **Table 9.2**.

■ Surgical Management

- Stapedectomy: The whole of the stapes is removed. A connective tissue graft is placed on the oval window. A prosthesis is placed from the long process of the incus to the graft (**Table 9.3**).

Table 9.2 Indications and contraindications of fluoride therapy

Indication for fluoride therapy	Contraindication for fluoride therapy
• Patient with sensorineural hearing loss • Rapidly progressing hearing loss • Schwartze's sign positive, and CT imaging showing spongiotic bone • Patient refusing surgery	• Renal insufficiency • Pregnancy • Young children • Skeletal fluorosis • Allergic to fluoride

- Stapedotomy: A fenestration is created on the footplate of the stapes, after the removal of stapes suprastructure. A prosthesis is placed from the long process of the incus into this fenestra with or without an intervening connective tissue graft (**Table 9.3**).
- Cochlear implant: It has good outcome in far-advanced otosclerosis.

Note: Stapedotomy has replaced stapedectomy as it has lesser complications and better surgical outcomes.

Stapedotomy

Principle

The goal of stapedotomy is creating a fenestra on the footplate of the stapes and placement of prosthesis. Commonly employed prostheses are made of Teflon, stainless steel, or titanium.

Steps of stapedotomy are illustrated in **Fig. 9.5**.

Indications

- Diagnosed case of clinical otosclerosis with 30-dB hearing loss.
- An air–bone gap of more than 20 dB.
- The speech discrimination score should be good.

Contraindications

The contraindications of stapedotomy are listed in **Table 9.4**.

For a detail description of the steps of stapedotomy, see Chapter 17 "Stapedotomy."

Table 9.3 Comparison of advantages and disadvantages of stapedotomy and stapedectomy

Types of surgical management	Advantages	Disadvantages
Stapedotomy	• Lesser trauma to inner ear • Stable long-term hearing • Fewer complications	• More difficult to perform • Closure of air–bone gap is not as good as stapedectomy
Stapedectomy	• Relatively easier to perform • Good closure of air–bone gap	• Relatively more traumatic to inner ear • Hearing results decline over time • More intraoperative complications

Table 9.4 Contraindications of stapedotomy

Absolute contraindication	Relative contraindication
• Only hearing ear • Active middle ear infection or inflammation • Patient with uncontrolled Meniere's disease • Atelectatic tympanic membrane	• Unfit for surgery • Patient with active focus of otosclerosis (Schwartze's sign +) • Pregnant patient • Professionals at risk of prosthesis displacement: boxer, wrestlers, etc. • Professionals at risk of vertigo due to prosthesis: skydivers, construction workers, pilots, etc.

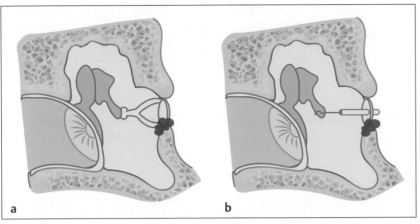

Fig. 9.5 **(a)** Fixed stapes footplate due to otosclerosis. **(b)** Footplate bypassed using a stapes prosthesis placed directly in contact with the inner ear by performing a stapedotomy.

Points to Ponder

- Otosclerosis is a metabolic bone disorder confined to the temporal bone resulting in hearing loss.
- In otosclerosis, enchondral bone of the otic capsule is resorbed by osteoclasts and new bone deposited by osteoblasts.
- The fissula ante fenestram is located anterior to the stapes footplate and is the commonest site for otosclerosis.
- Patients present with gradual onset of hearing loss, which is insidious in onset and usually bilateral.
- Pure tone audiogram will show a dip at 2,000 kHz in the bone conduction curve. This is called Carhart's notch. These patients are managed surgically by performing a stapedotomy.

Case-Based Question

1. **A 25-year-old woman came to the OPD with complaints of a 4-year history of hearing loss in the right ear. It was gradually progressive and she had no other complaints. On examination, the tympanic membrane had a reddish hue. The 512-Hz tuning fork Rinne test was negative for the right ear and positive for the left ear. Weber's test was lateralized to the right side and the absolute bone conduction (ABC) test was normal.**

   a. What is the condition the patient is suffering from?

   b. What is the reddish hue called?

   c. What type of hearing loss does the patient have?

   Answer

   a. Otosclerosis.

   b. Schwartz sign.

   c. Conductive hearing loss.

Frequently Asked Questions

1. Describe the etiopathogenesis of otosclerosis.
2. How do you classify otosclerosis?
3. What is Schwartze's sign?
4. What is the finding on tympanometry in a case of otosclerosis?
5. What is cochlear otosclerosis?
6. What is the difference between stapedotomy and stapedectomy?
7. What is the role of sodium fluoride in otosclerosis?

Endnote

Otosclerosis or fixation of the stapes was first described by Valsalva in 1704. The first attempt at improving the hearing in otosclerosis was by Kessel in 1875, who tried to mobilize the stapes without ossicular reconstruction. It fell into disrepute till Rosen again popularized it in 1952. The first stapedectomy was performed by John Shea in 1956 on a lady with hearing loss that did not improve with the use of a hearing aid.

10 Disorders of the Facial Nerve

Mahesh Santhraya G.

The competency covered in this chapter is as follows:

EN4.18 Describe the clinical features, investigations, and principles of management of facial nerve palsy.

Introduction

The facial nerve is the seventh cranial nerve. It is the longest cranial nerve within a bony canal. It is a mixed nerve containing motor fibers that control muscles of facial expression, special sense of taste sensation from the anterior two-third of the tongue and parasympathetic autonomic fibers for lacrimation. It also has small branches to muscles involved in moderating our sensitivity to external noise (stapedius muscle) and along with the vagus nerve supplies sensation to a part of the external auditory canal.

An individual nerve fiber of facial nerve is surrounded by the endoneurium. Groups of individual nerve fibers are bundled together into a fascicle with a sheath called a perineurium. Different fascicles are grouped together, surrounded by the epineurium to form the facial nerve.

Facial nerve palsy is a disorder in which there is partial or complete loss of function of the *facial nerve*. It is a debilitating disorder that poses a physical and psychological impact on the well-being of a patient. Identification of the etiology is of paramount importance since the management varies for different conditions. The site of involvement of the facial nerve can be systematically identified by clinical examination and relevant investigations which help with further management. This chapter gives a broad overview of facial nerve anatomy and physiology, differentiating features of the upper and lower motor neuron facial palsy, symptoms and grading system of facial palsy, investigations (topodiagnostic and electrodiagnostic), and treatment. It also gives a brief overview of the etiological classification of conditions causing facial palsy and etiology-directed treatment.

Anatomy

The facial nerve nucleus is located in the brainstem, that is, in the pons. The sensory and motor roots exit the pons separately to enter the internal acoustic meatus. It traverses the temporal bone in three parts: labyrinthine segment, horizontal (tympanic) segment, and the vertical (mastoid) segment before exiting the temporal bone through the stylomastoid foramen. The first genu, between the labyrinthine and horizontal segment, gives out the greater superficial petrosal nerve. The second genu, between the horizontal and vertical segment, gives out the nerve to the stapedius. The chorda tympani nerve arises in the vertical segment and traverses the middle ear adjacent to the malleus to enter the glaserian (petrotympanic) fissure on the anterior wall to supply the anterior two-third of the tongue (**Fig. 10.1**).

On its exit through the stylomastoid foramen, the posterior auricular nerve, the nerve to the stylohyoid, and the nerve to the digastric muscle are given out.

The nerve finally enters the parotid to divide into terminal branches (from cranial to caudal: temporal, zygomatic, buccal, marginal mandibular, and cervical) that supply the facial muscles involved in various human expressions (**Table 10.1**).

Upper Motor Neuron versus Lower Motor Neuron Facial Paralysis

Facial nerve palsy is a state of partial or complete loss of functionality of the seventh cranial nerve.

It can be categorized into two types, based on the location of the causal pathology:

- *Central or upper motor neuron facial palsy* due to involvement of the cranial nerve to the facial nucleus (between the cortex and the brainstem).
- *Peripheral or lower motor neuron facial palsy* due to involvement at or caudal to the facial nucleus (between the brainstem and the peripheral organs).

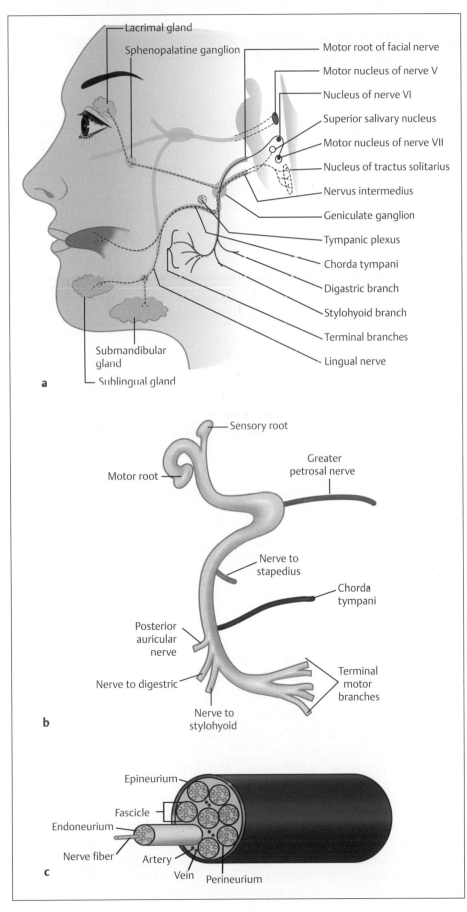

Fig. 10.1 **(a)** Branches of the facial nerve. **(b)** Diagramatic representation of the branches of the facial nerve. **(c)** Structure of nerve showing endoneurium, perineurium, and epineurium.

Table 10.1 Peripheral branches of facial nerve

Facial nerve branches	Functionality
Greater superficial petrosal nerve	Secretory function of the lacrimal and nasal glands (secretomotor)
Nerve to stapedius	Contraction of stapedius muscle (motor)
Chorda tympani	Taste sensation: anterior two-thirds of the tongue (special sensory)
Temporal	Contraction of forehead muscles (motor)
Zygomatic	Contraction of the orbicularis oculi (motor)
Buccal	Contraction of muscles involved in moving the nostril, upper lip, spontaneous eye blinking, and raising the corner of the mouth to smile (motor)
Marginal mandibular	Contraction of muscles involved in depression of the lower lip (motor)
Cervical	Contraction of the platysma (motor)

Table 10.2 Symptoms of lower motor neuron facial palsy

Appearance	Functional symptoms	Somatic symptoms
Drooping of the face	Salivary dribbling	Dry eye, i.e., reduced tear production (greater superficial petrosal nerve affected)
Difficulty in eye closure	Difficulty in food and fluid intake	Hyperacusis (nerve to stapedius affected)
Deviation of the angle of the mouth	Pronunciation of labial consonants (b, p, m, v, f) affected	Altered taste sensation (chorda tympani affected)

The upper half of the face receives innervation from motor fibers from both sides of the cerebral cortex. The lower half of the face receives innervation from the contralateral motor fibers only. Hence, in upper motor neuron facial palsy, there is involvement of the contralateral lower half of the face only, whereas in lower motor neuron facial paralysis, there is involvement of the ipsilateral upper and lower half of the face on the affected side, sparing of the opposite half of the face (**Fig. 10.2**).

Henceforth, we limit our discussion to lower motor neuron type of facial paralysis. The clinical features, investigations, and treatment of various conditions causing lower motor neuron facial paralysis are described.

■ Clinical Features of Lower Motor Neuron Facial Paralysis

Symptoms

Symptoms of lower motor neuron facial palsy are listed in detail in **Table 10.2**.

Signs

The *grading of facial paralysis* was proposed by House and Brackmann to describe and note the progression or improvement in facial nerve function (**Table 10.3**). They described six grades of lower motor neuron facial paralysis. (Remember: The angle of the mouth is affected first, then the eye and the forehead as the grading progresses.)

> **Pearl**
>
> *Bell's phenomenon* (palpebral oculogyric reflex) occurs when in facial palsy an attempt is made to close the eye, an upward and outward movement of the eyeball is observed.

Investigations

The site of injury of the facial nerve and extent of injury and recovery can be ascertained by topodiagnostic tests and electrodiagnostic tests, respectively. The specific tests related to etiology have been discussed under the specific etiology later in the chapter.

■ Topodiagnostic Tests

These tests are performed to localize the site of lesion.

- *Schirmer's test* (for greater superficial petrosal nerve): A long strip of filter paper is hooked on to the lower fornix of each eye and kept there for 5 minutes. The length of the moisture on the strip is then measured. If the moisture on the paper is less than 15 mm over a duration of 5 minutes, it is considered significant. This indicates that the lesion affecting the facial nerve is proximal to the geniculate ganglion because the greater superficial petrosal nerve arises from that ganglion (**Fig. 10.3**).
- *Stapedial reflex*: Contraction of the stapedius is a normal response on acoustic reflex testing during impedance

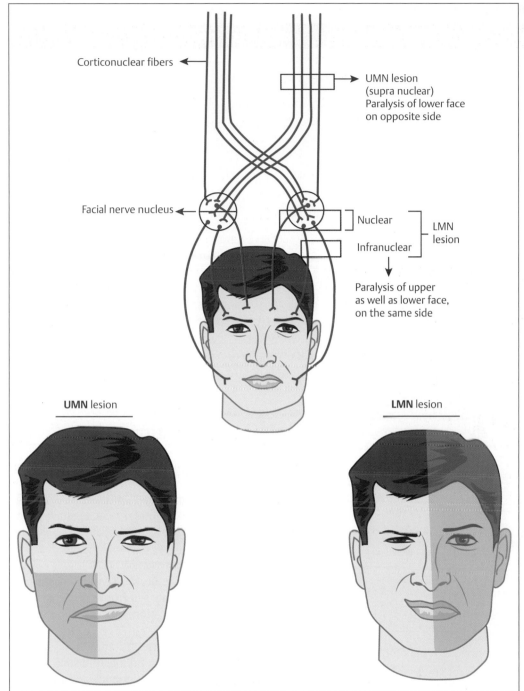

Fig. 10.2 Nerve pathway to explain the upper motor neuron (UMN) and lower motor neuron (LMN) features.

Corticonuclear fibers

UMN lesion (supra nuclear) Paralysis of lower face on opposite side

Facial nerve nucleus

Nuclear

Infranuclear

LMN lesion

Paralysis of upper as well as lower face, on the same side

UMN lesion

LMN lesion

audiometry. Absence of reflex suggests nerve injury proximal to the second genu of the facial nerve.

- *Salivary flow test*: A gustatory stimulus is given following cannulation of Wharton's duct. Salivary flow is measured subsequently. Reduction of ≥25% on the side of the facial palsy compared to the uninvolved side is suggestive of a nerve injury proximal to the first genu of the facial nerve.
- *Taste test*: Sugar or salt solution is applied to one side of the tongue to measure the integrity of the chorda tympani

nerve. Lack of taste sensation implies a lesion proximal to the chorda tympani nerve. Electrogustometry can also be done.

■ Electrodiagnostic Testing

- *Electroneuronography*: This test involves a quantitative analysis of the extent of degeneration by recording the summation potential. It checks the integrity of the nerve.
- *Nerve excitability test*: Stimulation of facial muscles with an excitable current stimulus is carried out.

Table 10.3 House–Brackmann grading of facial paralysis

Grades	Gross appearance	Facial muscles at rest	Muscle function during facial movement
Grade I	Normal		
Grade II	Minimal weakness	Normal tone and symmetry	*Forehead*: Good *Eye closure*: Complete without effort *Mouth*: Asymmetry present
Grade III	Obvious weakness but no facial disfigurement/asymmetry	Normal tone and symmetry	*Forehead*: Moderate movement *Eye closure*: Complete with effort *Mouth*: Movement only with maximum effort
Grade IV	Obvious weakness with facial disfigurement/asymmetry	Normal tone and symmetry	*Forehead*: None *Eye closure*: Incomplete *Mouth*: Asymmetry with maximum effort
Grade V	Barely perceptible motion	Abnormal tone and asymmetry	*Forehead*: None *Eye closure*: Incomplete *Mouth*: Minimal movement
Grade VI	Total paralysis		

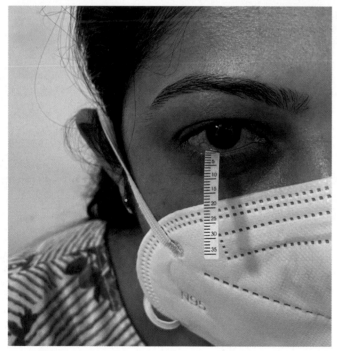

Fig. 10.3 Schirmer's test being performed. (This photograph is provided courtesy Dr. Aishwarya Kulkarni, resident, Department of Ophthalmology, KMC, Manipal.)

The minimum current required for stimulation is noted. A difference of 3.5 µA between the involved and uninvolved side is considered significant.

- *Maximal stimulation test*: This test uses maximal electrical stimulation to determine the neuromuscular unit status. If nerve conduction is neurapraxic, response is positive; if nerve conduction shows degeneration, response is absent. Injured nerve shows nerve activity up to 3 days following injury. Hence, the test is ideally done 3 days following nerve injury. The test is graded subjectively and compared with the normal side.

- *Electromyography*: This test notes the muscular activity of facial muscles. Polyphasic potentials are observed between 6 and 12 weeks prior to clinical improvement. The following section deals with etiological classification of lower motor neuron facial palsy and a brief overview of the disorders.

Etiological Classification

- The etiological classification of the lower motor neuron facial palsy is as follows:
  - *Bell's palsy or idiopathic facial paralysis*: It is a diagnosis of exclusion. All secondary causes have to be ruled out before a diagnosis of idiopathic facial palsy is made.
  - *Secondary causes (pneumonic: MITTENS)*:
    - Congenital: **M**oebius syndrome, **M**yotonic dystrophy.
    - **I**nfection: Ramsay Hunt syndrome, Lyme disease, herpes simplex reactivation, human immunodeficiency virus.
    - **T**rauma: Temporal bone fracture and surgical trauma (parotid surgery and mastoid surgery).
    - **T**umors: Parotid gland malignancy and tumors of the external auditory canal, middle ear, and internal acoustic meatus.
    - **E**ndocrine: diabetes mellitus, hyperthyroidism, and pregnancy.
    - **N**eurologic: Guillain–Barré syndrome, multiple sclerosis, and cerebrovascular accident.
    - **S**ystemic: Sarcoidosis and amyloidosis.

■ Herpes Zoster Oticus (Geniculate Neuralgia or Ramsay Hunt Syndrome)

Viral involvement of the sensory afferent neurons of the facial nerve by herpes zoster virus is characterized by severe earache and vesicles on the concha and external auditory canal (**Fig. 10.4**). It occurs due to the reactivation of the varicella zoster virus, which was latent in the cranial nerve neuron and dorsal ganglia. When the efferent motor axons of the facial nerve are involved, resulting in facial palsy, it is termed Ramsay Hunt syndrome. It is characterized by facial nerve palsy, vesicular eruptions, sensorineural hearing loss, and vertigo. It can also involve the anterior two-third of the tongue and soft palate. Occasionally, the vesicles may not be present (zoster sine herpete).

■ Trauma

Fractures of the temporal bone can cause acute or delayed-onset facial nerve paralysis. Fracture lines perpendicular to the petrous bone long axis, that is, transverse fractures, have a higher predisposition (40–50%) to cause facial nerve paralysis. It may present with hemotympanum, sensorineural deafness, and vertigo due to inner ear involvement.

Fracture lines parallel to the long axis of the temporal bone, that is, longitudinal fractures, have a lesser likelihood

(20%) of paralysis. It may present with ear bleeding, trauma and tear of the tympanic membrane, external auditory canal fracture, and conductive hearing loss.

The facial nerve can also be involved in trauma to the region of the parotid gland, which can be in the form of a penetrating injury or an iatrogenic injury.

In acute facial nerve injury, surgery is the mainstay of treatment, whereas in cases of delayed-onset facial paralysis, which occurs due to edema and inflammation surrounding the facial nerve, oral steroids form the mainstay of treatment. Parotid injuries require exploration and repair of the nerve.

■ Bell's Palsy

It is a type of acute-onset (occurs rapidly within 72 hours) lower motor neuron paralysis of idiopathic origin. It accounts for 70% of facial nerve palsies. Conversely, the remaining 30% need to be examined and investigated to determine a cause of lower motor neuron facial nerve paralysis. The etiology is not known. Swelling and inflammation of the nerve may be due to a subclinical viral infection. Rarely, it is bilateral. Recurrences are not common.

History suggestive of symptoms of Bell's palsy includes pain in the ear and postauricular region; weakness of facial muscles, including the inability to chew food without difficulty; incomplete eye closure; alteration of taste, occasional numbness or tingling of the cheek or mouth; and eye pain and tearing. There may be a family history of Bell's palsy. Other risk factors include pregnancy, uncontrolled diabetes, immunocompromised states, and people with upper respiratory illness (**Figs. 10.5** and **10.6**).

Although the most common cause of facial nerve palsy is Bell's palsy, this is a diagnosis of exclusion. In the presence of other neurological symptoms, sudden worsening of neurological symptoms, ocular symptoms, or persistence

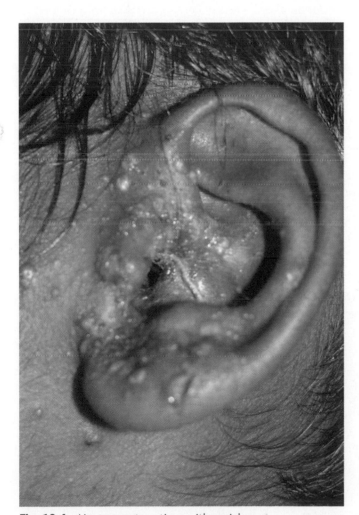

Fig. 10.4 Herpes zoster oticus with vesicles.

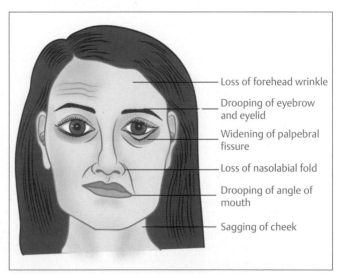

Fig. 10.5 Signs of Bell's palsy on clinical examination.

- Loss of forehead wrinkle
- Drooping of eyebrow and eyelid
- Widening of palpebral fissure
- Loss of nasolabial fold
- Drooping of angle of mouth
- Sagging of cheek

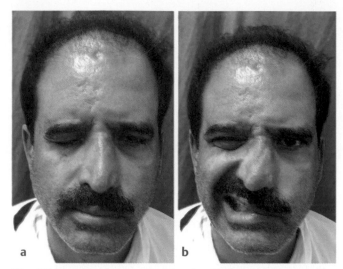

Fig. 10.6 **(a)** Left-sided facial palsy. The left eye cannot be closed completely even with effort. **(b)** Left-sided facial palsy. Eyes open, smiling with deviation to the right.

of palsy beyond 3 months, one should reassess for the possibility of another diagnosis.

Investigations

These are done to rule out secondary causes:

- Imaging studies: Computed tomography (CT) or magnetic resonance imaging (MRI) helps rule out inflammatory causes, tumors, and fractures.
- Serologic studies are done to rule out infectious causes.
- Audiological evaluation to determine cochlear or retro-cochlear pathology.
- Tests of vestibular function.

Treatment of Bell's Palsy

Most cases of Bell's palsy have spontaneous recovery. Hence, Bell's palsy has an excellent prognosis and is usually treated conservatively. Recovery begins approximately 2 to 3 weeks after symptom onset and completed within 3 months. Seventy percent of the patients with complete paralysis have complete recovery within 6 months compared to 94% with incomplete paralysis.

The goals of treatment are to minimize facial nerve damage and maximize nerve function.

Although usually self-limiting, the facial paralysis in Bell's palsy can cause significant temporary difficulties with speech and swallowing. In addition, the inability to completely close the eyelid can lead to dry eye and corneal injury, which may cause permanent vision problems. These problems along with facial asymmetry can lead to functional as well social problems that can precipitate depression. If the long-term outcome is poor, it can affect the quality of life. Treatment is generally designed to improve facial function and facilitate recovery.

Treatment options for Bell's palsy include general measures, medical therapy, surgical options, and complementary therapies such as physiotherapy.

General measures consist of reassuring the patient about the excellent prognosis in Bell's palsy, offering symptomatic relief of associated earache if present, and advising strict eye protection. Use of lubricating eye drops during the day, and gel at night, along with covering of the affected eye during sleep to prevent exposure keratitis due to drying of the eye avoids injury to the cornea.

Medical therapy consists of steroids alone or with antiviral agents. Steroids should ideally be started within 3 days of symptom onset. The recommended dose of prednisone is 1 mg/kg for a week followed by tapering dose of the steroid for another 2 weeks. Steroids are used with caution in patients with hypertension, tuberculosis, diabetes mellitus, sepsis, peptic ulcer disease, and renal dysfunction. Antiviral agents are given in Bell's palsy due to the possible viral etiology. The use of antiviral agents such as acyclovir may be considered in certain situations. The dosage of acyclovir is 800 mg five times a day for 10 days. Antivirals, if used, should be given along with corticosteroids. The modified Stennert's protocol has been tried with some success. It consists of hydrocortisone, low-molecular-weight dextran, pentoxifylline, and acyclovir given for 10 to 14 days. The treatment regimen is said to reduce inflammation and edema, improve microcirculation, and the additional antiviral action, which facilitates recovery with reduced sequelae.

Surgical treatment for Bell's palsy is controversial. Facial nerve decompression may be done in persistent palsy. The transmastoid or the middle cranial fossa approach is used.

Surgical Treatment for Other Causes of Facial Palsy

Restoring facial symmetry and movement is a challenging task for a surgeon. There are two types of surgical procedures that can be carried out in these patients, *dynamic procedures* and *static procedures*. Dynamic procedures help animate or restore some movement to the face after surgery, while static procedures help passively assist in moving the tissues of the face.

Following are some of the surgical procedures that can be carried out for restoring symmetry and function.

Acute facial palsy: Surgeries that can be attempted include facial nerve decompression, facial nerve repair, and nerve grafting. Facial nerve repair is reserved for those due to trauma where the nerve has been cut. Primary approximation and repair is done. When the primary approximation cannot be done due to distance between the cut margins, a nerve graft like greater auricular nerve or sural nerve (depending on the length required) is used.

Chronic facial paralysis: These procedures are aimed at protecting the cornea from exposure keratitis and for achieving facial symmetry. It is done for persistent facial palsy including some cases of Bell's palsy.

Gold weight implant can be placed into the eyelid where the added weight will allow the eyelids to close preventing exposure keratitis. The other procedure to be considered is lateral tarsorrhaphy where the lateral part of the upper and lower eyelids is sutured together to narrow the palpebral fissure.

Other surgical procedures that can be attempted include temporalis muscle transposition, hypoglossal to facial nerve anastomosis, masseter nerve to facial nerve transfer, and neuromuscular transplantation.

- In the temporalis muscle transposition, the muscle is transferred to the eyelid and the mouth in an attempt to dynamically reanimate the face for eye closure and lateral oral commissure movement, respectively. The muscle is made to contract by attempting to chew or clench the teeth.
- In the hypoglossal to facial nerve anastomosis, part of the intact hypoglossal nerve is mobilized and sutured to the distal part of the facial nerve trunk. By moving the tongue, the facial muscles can be reanimated.
- The masseteric nerve redirection to the facial nerve is a good option due to its proximity to the facial nerve, good motor impulse, less dissection, and short innervation time.
- In free neuromuscular transfer, the gracilis muscle is used.

Physical therapy may help prevent atrophy and contractures of the muscles. It includes galvanic current stimulation of the facial muscles and facial muscle movement exercises.

■ Role of COVID-19 and the Vaccine

Viruses have been identified as one of the possible etiological factors of Bell's palsy. Cases of idiopathic facial paralysis have been reported with COVID-19 disease and in those who were vaccinated. Further studies are required to find out the exact link.

Pearl

In trauma or during tumor removal, if the nerve is cut or if there is loss of a segment of the nerve, treatment can be carried out by re-approximating the cut ends with sutures or cable grafting using either the greater auricular nerve or the sural nerve.

Points to Ponder

- The facial nerve is a mixed nerve containing motor, special sensory, and parasympathetic autonomic fibers.
- The upper half of the face receives bilateral motor innervation, whereas the lower half of the face receives contralateral innervation enabling the differentiation between an upper and a lower motor neuron facial paralysis.
- Topognosis tests enable the detection of the specific site of the lower motor neuron facial paralysis.
- Electrodiagnostic tests enable the detection of neural regeneration of the paralyzed nerve.
- Bell's palsy is the most common idiopathic cause of facial paralysis of acute onset.

Case-Based Question

1. **A 47-year-old man woke up one morning with pain behind the left ear, deviation of angle of the mouth to the right side, and inability to close the left eye completely even with maximal effort. The symptoms were sudden in onset with no previous history.**

   a. What is the diagnosis? Using the House–Brackmann grading system, what is the grade of the facial paralysis?

   b. What are the problems associated with the eye and how would you manage it?

   c. On performing the topodiagnostic tests, the Schirmer's test was normal, taste was affected, but the stapedial reflex was present. Where is the site of lesion in the facial nerve?

   Answers

   a. Sudden onset of facial paralysis with no obvious cause is diagnosed as Bell's palsy. This is a grade IV palsy because of the incomplete closure of the eyes even on maximal effort.

b. Because of the inability to close the eye completely, the cornea is exposed leading to exposure keratitis. In addition, there may be lower lid ectropion and decreased tear production.

Eye care is an important component of the treatment of Bell's palsy. Artificial tears can be applied during the day and an eye ointment at night. The eyelids can be occluded by tape at night when the patient is asleep. Surgical procedures can be carried out to increase the weight of the upper eyelid through gold implants. Tarsorrhaphy can be performed to narrow the eye opening, and, where indicated, animation procedure like the hypoglossal to facial nerve anastomosis can be attempted.

c. The lesion is in the vertical or mastoid segment of the facial nerve between the nerve to stapedius and the chorda tympani nerve. Since Schirmer's test is normal, the geniculate ganglion is normal.

Frequently Asked Questions

1. What is the commonest cause of facial palsy?

2. Which type of fracture of the temporal bone is more commonly associated with facial nerve palsy, transverse or longitudinal fracture?

3. How can exposure to keratitis be prevented after facial nerve palsy?

4. What is the management of herpes zoster oticus?

5. If Schirmer's test is less than 5 mm on the paralyzed side, what is the inference?

Endnote

Italian anatomist, Fallopius in 1550, first described the stylomastoid foramen through which the facial nerve came out into the face from a bony canal. The facial canal is also called the fallopian canal.

Bell's palsy is named after Sir Charles Bell (1774–1842), a Scottish anatomist and surgeon, who was the first to note that the facial nerve supplied the muscles of the face. He also noted that the trigeminal nerve conducted sensation from the face. He was also an artist who combined his anatomical knowledge and artistic talent to produce detailed drawings of the human body and muscles of facial expression. His name is also associated with Bell's spasm and Bell's phenomenon.

11 Assessment and Disorders of the Vestibular System

Ajay Bhandarkar

Introduction

The balance system of our body is dependent on the reflex arc. The sensory component is composed of the labyrinth (vestibule and three semicircular canals), the visual system, and the proprioceptive system. These sensors collect the information on the static and dynamic body position with respect to the environment. The afferent neural pathway delivers the information to the vestibular nuclei located in the brainstem, which is responsible for integration of this information. The vestibular nuclei, with the support of the central nervous system (cerebellum, thalamus, reticular formation, and vestibular cortex), generate an output through the efferent pathway which is delivered to the muscles, that is, the eyes, limbs, and trunk, also known as the vestibuloocular reflex, vestibulospinal reflex, and vestibulocollic reflex. This reflex arc is responsible for maintenance of balance. It is also well supported by the vestibular cortex, which stores prior vestibular memory to generate quick responses for maintenance of balance. The gross mismatch or conflict in the sensory information delivered by any of the three sensors will produce vertigo.

History Taking

Vertigo is a symptom and not a disease. Hence, it is essential to evaluate the patient systematically. Neuro-otological history and examination forms a very important aspect of vertigo evaluation as it determines the site or organ of origin responsible for the symptom.

- Presenting complaint: The patient should always be asked to describe his or her complaint, which can be subjectively classified into four broad groups:
  - Vertigo: Feeling of spinning or rotation (self or surrounding), rocking, and rolling.
  - Instability: Feeling unsteady, swaying, or stumbling.
  - Light-headedness: Blackouts or fainting spells on postural change from supine to sitting position.
  - Visual disorientation: Inability to localize, depth of field perception defect, and oscillopsia.

Pearl

The patients should describe the first episode the way they perceived it for proper categorization of the symptom:

- Vertigo may be related to central or peripheral balance disorders.
- Instability is more commonly due to central disorders.
- Light-headedness is commonly due to cardiovascular or neurocardiogenic cause.
- Visual disorientation is commonly seen due to ocular causes.

The detailed characteristics of vertigo required to be mentioned in history are presented in **Tables 11.1, 11.2, 11.3, 11.4,** and **11.5**.

Past medical histories with respect to cardiovascular system (hypertension), endocrine system (thyroid and

Table 11.1 Duration of symptoms of vertigo

Duration	Types of vertigo
Seconds	Benign paroxysmal positional vertigo Small recurrent perilymph fistula
Minutes	Transient ischemic attacks (usually <20 min) Meniere's disease (>20 min) Perilymph fistula
Hours	Meniere's disease Migraine-related vertigo
Days	Vestibular neuronitis Labyrinthitis Central causes of vertigo

Table 11.2 Precipitating factors for vertigo

Precipitating factors	Types of vertigo
Head turning	Benign paroxysmal positional vertigo
Trauma	Benign paroxysmal positional vertigo Perilymph fistula
Viral upper respiratory infection	Vestibular neuronitis
Valsalva/sneezing/coughing/lifting weights	Perilymph fistula Superior semicircular canal dehiscence
Postural change	Orthostatic hypotension
Exposure to noise	Third window phenomenon Advanced Meniere's disease
Emotion	Psychogenic vertigo

Table11.3 Reproducibility of symptoms voluntarily

Symptoms	Conditions producing symptoms
Head turning	Benign paroxysmal position vertigo
Extreme lateral rotation of neck	Vertebral artery stenosis (bow hunter's syndrome)
Hyperventilation	Third window phenomenon
	Vestibular paroxysmia

Table 11.4 Associated features of vertigo

Associated features		Etiological cause
Otological symptoms like deafness, tinnitus, otalgia, and discharge		Likely to be an otological cause
Visual symptoms like diplopia and squint		Likely to be an ocular cause
Motor or sensory disturbance		Likely to be a central cause
Loss of consciousness		Likely to be a central cause
History of fall	Immediate recovery and mobilized without help	Otolithic cause
	Immediate recovery but mobilized with help	Transient ischemic attack
	With loss of consciousness	Syncope Epilepsy

diabetes mellitus), neurological system (migraine, stroke, and epilepsy), and hematological system (anemia, blood dyscrasias) are important as they may predispose to conditions that may produce vertigo.

Detailed history of current and past medications is important. Antibiotics like aminoglycosides, antimalarials

Table 11.5 Factors worsening vertigo

Factors	Vertiginous conditions
Stress	Meniere's disease
Sleep deprivation and hunger	Vestibular migraine
Crowded places	Chronic subjective dizziness
Stairs	Vestibular paroxysmia
Dark surroundings	Bilateral vestibulopathy
Unstable ground	Peripheral neuropathy

(quinine), antiepileptic drugs, antidiabetic drugs, sedatives, tranquilizers, and chemotherapeutic agents have a predisposition to cause vertigo.

Clinical Examination in Neuro-Otology

The clinical examination in a patient with vertigo should include a detailed otological examination, neurological examination, and examination of all the elements of the balance system.

■ Examination of Ears

Emphasis should be on examination of the tympanic membrane, preferably with a microscope or pneumatic otoscope and tuning fork tests. The detailed otological examination has been described in Chapter 3 "History Taking and Examination of the Ear."

■ Neurological Examination

- Cranial nerve examination: Testing of nerves of ocular motility (third, fourth, and sixth cranial nerves) and nerves for corneal reflex (afferent fifth and efferent seventh cranial nerves) plays a significant role. Ocular motility disorders or central nervous system disorders can affect the movement of the ocular muscles. Tumors at the pontomedullary junction may affect the integrity of the corneal reflex.
- Deep tendon reflexes and Babinski's reflex.
- Motor and sensory system.
Examination of the latter two may ascertain whether there are no neurodegenerative disorders or space-occupying lesions causing vertigo.

Tests for Equilibriometric System

Three important elements in testing the balance system are the cerebellum, vestibuloocular system, and the vestibulospinal system. For easy understanding, it has been divided into two parts: (1) vestibuloocular tests and

(2) vestibulospinal tests including cerebellar tests because of the overlap in examination of the vestibulospinal system and the cerebellum.

■ Vestibuloocular Tests

Nystagmus (Rapid, Repetitive Involuntary Movements of the Eyes)

How to check for nystagmus: The patient is seated comfortably in front of the examiner and at a distance of approximately 30 cm. The examiner observes for spontaneous nystagmus. The examiner then moves a finger or a pen 30 degrees from the center on either side to check for nystagmus. Care should be taken not to extend beyond 30 degrees from the center as it may elicit gaze evoked nystagmus.

The jerk nystagmus has an initial slow phase wherein the eye moves in one direction and a fast/recovery phase wherein the eye moves rapidly in the opposite direction. The direction of nystagmus is always noted as the direction of the fast phase.

Pearls

- Nystagmus is from the Greek words *nustagmos*, meaning drowsy or nodding, and *nystazein*, meaning sleepy.
- Horizontal semicircular canal produces a horizontal nystagmus.
- Superior semicircular canal produces a downbeating, torsional nystagmus.
- Posterior semicircular canal produces an upbeating, torsional nystagmus.
- Central disorders produce a pure vertical nystagmus, a pendular nystagmus, or a disconjugate nystagmus.

Paretic lesions produce nystagmus to the opposite side (vestibular neuronitis).

Labyrinthine irritative lesions produce nystagmus to the same side or canal (e.g., benign paroxysmal positional vertigo [BPPV], suppurative labyrinthitis, and irritative phase of Meniere's disease).

Degree of Nystagmus

This is based on Alexander's law for peripheral nystagmus. intensity based on the degree of asymmetry signifies the severity of nystagmus:

- First degree: It is present only in the direction of the fast component.
- Second degree: It is present in the direction of the fast component and in the neutral position.
- Third degree: It is present in the direction of the fast component, neutral position, and in the direction of the slow component.

■ Supranuclear Oculomotor System Testing

This is tested by the saccade test, smooth pursuit test, vergence test, and optokinetic test. Abnormalities in these tests may indicate a lesion in the central pathway.

■ Head Impulse Test

Sudden accelerating movements are performed horizontally to each side from the neutral position of the head with the patient keeping their vision fixed on an object in the neutral position. On sudden head movements, the vestibuloocular reflex is activated and the patient is able to stabilize vision on the central object. In case of a paretic labyrinthine lesion on one side, head impulse on the affected side shows a corrective saccade (quick movement of eyes between points of fixation) or a catch-up saccade to maintain fixation on the object after moving the head to the affected side.

■ Head Shaking Test

This test unmasks an underlying semicircular canal pathology (unilateral vestibular hypofunction) by producing nystagmus on rapid head shaking. The nystagmus is usually in the direction of the affected semicircular canal.

■ Dix–Hallpike Test

This test is designed to test BPPV involving the posterior semicircular canal. The head is turned to 45 degrees and the patient is rapidly positioned supine with the head hanging by 30 degrees for a period of at least 30 seconds (**Figs. 11.1** and **11.2**). In cases of BPPV, a fatigable nystagmus is produced to the side of the lesion. A vertical, upbeating, torsional nystagmus indicates a posterior semicircular

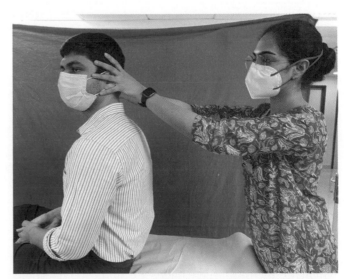

Fig. 11.1 Dix–Hallpike maneuver: The patient sitting with the head to one side.

Table 11.6 Contrast between central and peripheral nystagmus

Characteristics	Central nystagmus	Peripheral nystagmus
Latency period	Absent	Present
Fatigability	Not fatigable	Fatigable
Direction/plane of nystagmus	Any direction	Horizontal or torsional vertical
Direction: Changing or fixed	Direction changing	Direction fixed
Visual fixation	No change in nystagmus	Nystagmus suppressed

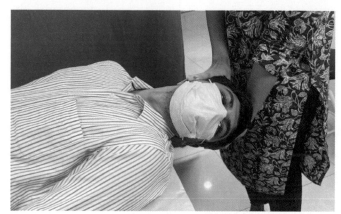

Fig. 11.2 Dix–Hallpike maneuver: The patient with head below the table at an angle of 30 degrees.

canal BPPV. A vertical, downbeating torsional nystagmus indicates a superior semicircular canal BPPV. Horizontal nystagmus indicates a horizontal semicircular canal BPPV. Vertical nystagmus indicates a central disorder.

Differences between Central and Peripheral Nystagmus

Differences between the central and peripheral nystagmus are highlighted in **Table 11.6**.

■ Fistula Test

The patient lies supine with a 30-degree head flexion. Siegel's speculum or a pneumatic otoscope is used to induce pressure changes in the external auditory canal. Alternately, intermittent pressure over the tragus can also be done to elicit the response. The patient's eyes should be observed for nystagmus.

A *positive fistula test* (nystagmus present) indicates a horizontal semicircular canal fistula, a perilymph fistula (at oval window or round window), or a surgical fistula (fenestration operation).

A *false-positive fistula test* (fistula absent but nystagmus present) indicates a hypermobile stapes as seen in congenital syphilis, also known as Hennebert's sign, or in endolymphatic hydrops where there are fibrous connections between the utricle and the footplate of the stapes.

A *negative fistula test* (no nystagmus) indicates a normal ear.

A *false-negative fistula test* (fistula present but nystagmus absent) is seen when cholesteatoma or granulation tissue covers the fistula and, therefore, there is no response to pressure changes induced in the external auditory canal. It is also seen in a dead labyrinth (end stage of labyrinthitis).

Vestibulospinal Tests and Cerebellar Tests

- *Standing test*: The patient stands in front of the examiner with eyes closed and arms by the side. The patient should be observed for swaying to one side. In patients with unilateral vestibular dysfunction, the head and trunk will be deviated to the side of the lesion, with the hand on the side of dysfunction lowered and the hand on the healthy side raised to balance the patient.
- *Walking test*: The patient is asked to perform tandem walking. Deviation or repeated fall to one side suggests a unilateral peripheral vestibular dysfunction on that side. Inability to do tandem walking and tendency to walk with a broad-based gait suggests a cerebellar pathology.
- *Unterberger's test (stepping test)*: The patient is asked to put the feet together, extend the arms, and close the eyes. The patient is then asked to march at the same spot quickly at around 90 times per minute. In unilateral peripheral vestibular dysfunction, the patient deviates to the side of vestibular dysfunction. In cerebellar or central lesions, there is swaying or side-to-side movement, that is, to both sides.
- *Past-pointing test*: The patient sits in front of the examiner with the arms and, in particular, the index finger extended. The patient is asked to touch the extended index finger of the examiner with open eyes. If the patient is unable to do so, then it is considered an abnormal past-pointing test. On multiple testing, if the patient past-points to the same side, it may suggest a peripheral vestibular dysfunction on the same side.
- *Fukuda writing test*: The patient is asked to write 10 capital letters vertically on a paper with their eyes closed. Care should be taken that the patient does not touch the table to avoid additional proprioceptive input from the upper limbs. Deviation of legible writing to one side is

suggestive of unilateral vestibular dysfunction. Illegible writing may be suggestive of a cerebellar lesion.

- *Romberg's test*: The patient stands with both feet together, arms extended, and eyes closed. Fall or sway to one side suggests a positive Romberg test. Since the eyes are closed, the visual input for balance is removed, and the fall or sway may suggest an abnormality with the proprioceptive or the vestibular system. Other tests should be corroborated with Romberg's test to ascertain the site of lesion, since Romberg's test is less sensitive.
- *Tests for incoordination*: Knee–heel test, finger–nose–finger test, and alternating tests (pronation and supination of palms) are done as an examination of cerebellar function.

Test for Orthostatic Hypotension

The blood pressure of the patient is measured in the supine and standing positions. A drop in systolic blood pressure of 20 mm Hg is diagnostic of orthostatic hypotension.

Test for Psychogenic Dizziness (Hyperventilation Test)

The patient is asked to take deep breaths for 3 minutes. Vertigo/dizziness/light-headedness during the test may indicate an underlying psychogenic cause for dizziness.

Investigations

They complement the clinical diagnosis and should cater to testing various aspects of the balance system when suspicion of a particular disorder arises.

Tests for the integrity of *vestibuloocular reflex*:
- Electronystagmography.
- Videonystagmography.

Tests for the integrity of *vestibulospinal reflex*:
- Craniocorpography.
- Computerized dynamic posturography.

Audiological investigations:
- Pure tone audiometry, brainstem evoked response audiometry, glycerol dehydration test (Meniere's disease), and electrocochleography.

Test to monitor *cerebral activity during vestibular input processing*:
- Vestibular evoked myogenic potential (VEMP).

Radiological imaging:
- Computed tomography (CT) scan, magnetic resonance imaging (MRI), functional MRI (f-MRI), positron emission tomography (PET), and single-photon emission computed tomography (SPECT).

Hematological and biochemical investigations:
- Hemogram, lipid profile, thyroid profile, renal function, and liver function.

Electronystagmography: It tests the integrity of vestibuloocular reflex, the supranuclear ocular reflex systems, and otolith function by measuring the electrical changes brought about by the eye movements as a graphical recording.

This comprises spontaneous nystagmus testing, gaze nystagmus testing, supranuclear ocular reflex tests (saccades, smooth pursuit, and optokinetic system), positional tests, rotational test, fistula test, and caloric test.

Videonystagmography (**Fig. 11.3**): This test is an advanced version of electronystagmography. This uses a high-resolution camera with sensor and scans the eye movements electronically and records the movements graphically. It consists of the similar testing battery as mentioned in electronystagmography.

Craniocorpography: This test records the Romberg and Unterberger tests in a dark room. The patient has LED lights attached to a crown, which is placed on the head, and

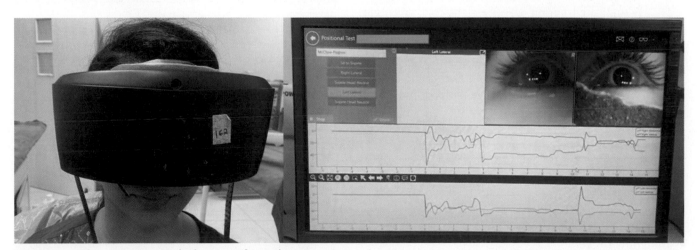

Fig. 11.3 Videonystagmography being performed.

a convex mirror is attached to the roof. The camera on the wall is directed to face the convex mirror. When the patient performs the tests, the camera records the movements of the LED lights. The displacement and angular changes are recorded.

Computerized dynamic posturography: This test detects the changes in gravity position of the patient.

VEMP: It records the myogenic potentials on stimulation of the ear with a sound. It has two components: ocular VEMP (oVEMP), which tests the integrity of the utricle by testing the ocular muscles, and cervical VEMP (cVEMP), which tests the integrity of the saccule and vestibular nerve by testing the cervical muscles (sternocleidomastoid).

Fitzgerald–Hallpike bithermal caloric test: It is a part of electronystagmography or videonystagmography in the current era. It tests the integrity of the horizontal semi-circular canals. It is based on the principle that cold (30°C) and warm (44°C) water irrigation in the semicircular canals changes the density of the endolymph in the semicircular canals causing nystagmus to the opposite side and the same side, respectively (mnemonic COWS = Cold – opposite side, Warm – same side).

- Procedure: The patient is placed in a 30-degree head flexed position to make the horizontal canal vertical. Each ear is irrigated, after a certain interval between the ears, with calibrated temperature water (30 and 44°C), alternately. Each irrigation should be done for a minimum of 40 seconds and there should be a gap of 10 minutes between each irrigation (cold and warm water).
    - Interpretations:
        o *Canal paresis*: It produces a reduced response on caloric testing.
        o *Dead labyrinth:* There is no response on caloric testing.
        o *Directional preponderance:* If there is 25% more nystagmus on one side (left beating nystagmus is indicated by left warm + right cold, and right beating nystagmus is indicated by right warm + left cold), it denotes a directional preponderance to one side. This may indicate a central lesion but does not localize it. It also states that the central lesion is away from the side of peripheral lesion.

Treatment of Vertigo

Drug therapy and surgical therapy will depend upon the specific etiology of vertigo.
Drugs used to control vertigo:
- Prochlorperazine.
- Dimenhydrinate.
- Cinnarizine.
- Betahistine.
- Meclizine.
- Diazepam.

Antioxidants, thrombolytics, and vasodilators are used for vascular events causing vertigo.
Drugs to reduce nausea and vomiting:
- Domperidone.
- Promethazine.
- Metoclopramide.
- Ondansetron.

■ Classification of Peripheral and Central Vestibular Disorders

Classification of the peripheral and central vestibular disorders is presented in detail in **Table 11.7**.

> **Pearl**
>
> Motion sickness, visual vertigo, and height-induced vertigo are physiological forms of vertigo.

Peripheral Vestibular Disorders

■ Benign Paroxysmal Positional Vertigo

It is the commonest cause of vertigo in clinical practice. It is characterized by paroxysmal events of spinning sensation triggered by changes in the head position. The lifetime prevalence of BPPV is 2.4% and the mean age at presentation is 50 years, but it can affect a person of any age.

Table 11.7 Classification of peripheral and central vestibular disorders

Peripheral vestibular disorders	Central vestibular disorders
Involvement of labyrinth: 1. Benign paroxysmal peripheral vertigo 2. Labyrinthitis 3. Meniere's disease 4. Vestibulotoxic drugs 5. Superior semicircular canal dehiscence	*Vascular origin*: 1. Vertebrobasilar insufficiency 2. Posterior inferior cerebellar artery syndrome 3. Basilar migraine
Involvement of vestibular nerve: 1. Vestibular neuronitis 2. Acoustic neuroma	*Degenerative disorders*: 1. Multiple sclerosis
Trauma: 1. Labyrinthine concussion 2. Perilymph fistula 3. Delayed endolymphatic hydrops	*Neuronal disorders*: 1. Epilepsy 2. Post head injury
	Brainstem tumors
	Cerebellar disorders

Etiology

- Idiopathic (39%).
- Posttraumatic: head trauma (61%).
- Elderly: Due to degeneration of the macula.

Pathogenesis

Otoconia get dislodged from the otolithic organ (utricle) to enter the semicircular canal, most commonly the posterior semicircular canal. Rarely, the lateral semicircular canal and the superior semicircular canal can be affected. Free-floating otolith in the semicircular canal produces momentary vertigo and nystagmus on positional changes (**Flowchart 11.1**).

Clinical Features

Symptoms: Acute spell of vertigo lasting for few seconds. This spell is aggravated by change in head position. The spell maybe associated with light-headedness.

Signs: The Dix–Hallpike test, described previously, confirms the diagnosis.

Investigations are not required to diagnose BPPV.

Treatment: Principle

The displaced otolith needs to be repositioned back in the utricle from the semicircular canals. This can be achieved by performing positional head maneuvers in a systematic manner.

- **Epley's maneuver** (**Fig. 11.4**): It is a commonly performed maneuver for posterior semicircular canal BPPV. The first two positions are similar to the Dix–Hallpike test to the side of the affected canal. Following this, the head is turned 180 degrees and the shoulder is turned 90 degrees in two steps. Finally, the patient is kept in the sitting position with the neck flexed.
- **Semont's maneuver**: The patient lies in the semiprone position on the side causing BPPV for 4 minutes and after that rapidly turns to the opposite side with the normal ear down.

Precautions: The patient is advised not to perform sudden head movements, not to bend down, and not to lift heavy weights for 2 weeks. Driving a vehicle should be prohibited. The maneuvers are contraindicated in patients with cervical spine problems, unstable cardiac disease, and stroke/transient ischemic attack. In case of severe vertigo, betahistine 8 mg can be given twice daily for 5 days.

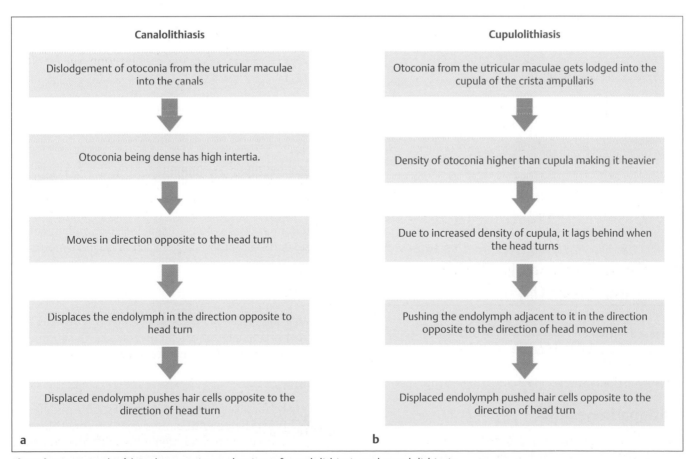

Flowchart 11.1   (**a, b**) Pathogenetic mechanism of canalolithiasis and cupulolithiasis.

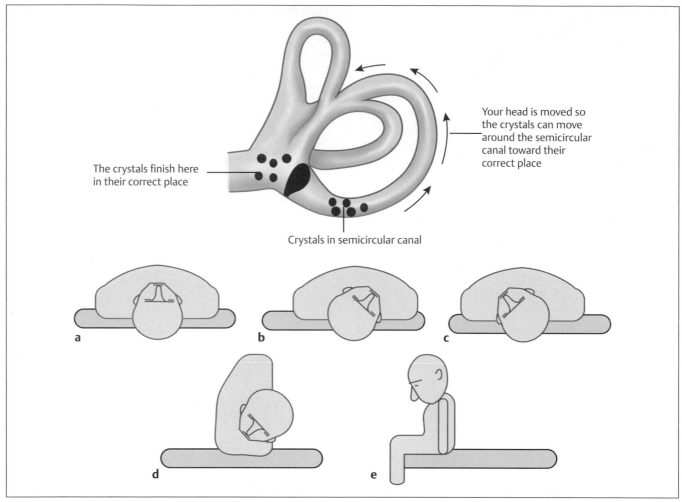

The crystals finish here in their correct place

Your head is moved so the crystals can move around the semicircular canal toward their correct place

Crystals in semicircular canal

a

b

c

d

e

Fig. 11.4 Epley's maneuver for right-sided benign paroxysmal positional vertigo (BPPV). **(a)** Neutral position of the head. **(b)** Head is turned 45 degrees to the right side (affected side). **(c)** Head is then turned 90 degrees to the opposite side (normal side) from the previous position. **(d)** Shoulder is rotated 90 degrees with head position unchanged with respect to the shoulder. **(e)** The patient is made to sit upright with the neck flexed.

For lateral semicircular canal BPPV, the corrective maneuver used is the barbecue roll maneuver.

Vestibular Neuronitis (Acute Vestibular Neuritis)

This is a disorder characterized by spontaneous, acute vertigo due to inflammation of the vestibular nerve. The superior vestibular nerve is more commonly involved than the inferior vestibular nerve.

■ Etiopathogenesis

Reactivation of latent herpes simplex virus (HSV-1) has been described as the most common cause of vestibular neuronitis. The superior vestibular nerve is longer when compared to the singular nerve and inferior vestibular nerve. The superior vestibular nerve also accompanies the arteriole in a narrow bony channel. Hence, inflammation and ischemia make the superior vestibular nerve more susceptible to involvement.

■ Clinical Features

The superior vestibular nerve innervates the utricle, and the superior and lateral semicircular canals. This forms the basis for the clinical signs and investigations.

Symptoms

• Acute spontaneous severe vertigo (lasts for minutes to days) is associated with nausea and vomiting. The vertigo increases with head mobility and reduces on lying down with eyes closed in a semiprone position.
• Hearing is usually normal.

Signs

- Nystagmus is horizontal or torsional with the fast component away from the side of lesion. It does not change directions. It is increased in the headshaking test.
- Patients will be unable to perform vestibulospinal tests. If they do, they tend to fall on the side of involvement.
- The head impulse test may show impaired responses on the side of involvement.

■ Investigations

The diagnosis is mostly clinical. Investigations only complement the diagnosis:

- Caloric test: Paresis may be noted on the affected side. This test may be difficult to perform in view of the acute/distressing symptoms.
- VEMP: It can be used to detect otolithic organ dysfunction in vestibular neuritis.

■ Treatment

Treatment is mainly symptomatic:

- Hospitalization and intravenous fluids: The patient may be dehydrated because of multiple episodes of nausea and vomiting.
- Vestibular suppressants (prochlorperazine, cinnarizine, or promethazine) may be used in acute phase to reduce vertigo, nausea, and vomiting.

- Oral steroids (prednisolone) are used to reduce the inflammation around the nerve.
- Taking diazepam (2–5 mg) thrice a day can reduce anxiety and provide a tranquilizing effect in patients, relieving them of the distressing symptoms during an acute attack.
- Vestibular rehabilitation therapy is done after the patient recovers from the acute phase to realign and improve the vestibuloocular reflex and vestibulospinal postural regulation.

Points to Ponder

- Vertigo is a symptom and not a disease.
- At the time of examination, there are very few clinical signs, unless the patient is suffering from an acute condition and diagnosis will have to rely on a detailed history.
- Balance depends on an intact vestibular system, proprioceptive impulses from the limbs, and inputs from the visual system. All these inputs are integrated in the central nervous system.
- In lesions of the peripheral vestibular system, Unterberger's test will be positive as the patient falls on the affected side.
- The Dix–Hallpike test is designed to identify BPPV involving the posterior semicircular canals.

Case-Based Questions

1. **A 45-year-old, hypertensive patient presented to the outpatient department with a single episode of severe vertigo that has been persistent for the last 2 days and increasing in intensity. On examination, there is a direction-changing, vertical nystagmus. Deep tendon reflexes are less brisk. The next line of investigation will be:**

   a. Video head impulse test.

   b. Videonystagmography.

   c. VEMP.

   d. MRI.

   Answers

   d.

   Clues to this question:

   - A 43-year-old hypertensive (predisposing factor) patient.
   - Single episode of severe vertigo increasing in intensity (peripheral or central causes).
   - Lasts 2 days (to rule out vestibular neuronitis and labyrinthitis in peripheral vs. central cause).
   - Vertical, direction-changing nystagmus (clinches central cause as first diagnosis: combine this with the

   predisposing factor of hypertension and increasing intensity of vertigo).

   Hence, the next line of management will be MRI as intracranial hemorrhage/stroke is the most likely pathology.

2. **A 35-year-old woman with history of trauma presents to the outpatient department with one episode of vertigo that lasted a few seconds when she woke up from the bed in the morning. The blood pressure was normal in the supine and standing positions. The next line of management would be:**

   a. Pure tone audiometry.

   b. VEMP.

   c. Dix–Hallpike test.

   d. Epley's Maneuver.

   Answers

   c.

   Clues to the question:

   - Postural change of vertigo.
   - Lasts a few seconds (possibly BPPV or postural hypotension).

- Previous history of trauma with normal blood pressure on postural change (possible points of diagnosis toward posttraumatic BPPV).

Hence, the next line of management would be a *Dix–Hallpike* maneuver to diagnose the canal involved in BPPV.

Frequently Asked Questions

1. What is nystagmus?
2. What is Alexander's law?
3. What are the differences between central and peripheral nystagmus?
4. What is the indication for Epley's maneuver?
5. What is the etiopathology of BPPV?
6. Name three drugs that act as labyrinthine sedatives.

Endnote

Robert Barany was a Hungarian otologist who described a condition of sudden vertigo caused by movements of the head which lasted for a few seconds or minutes. He attributed this to the movements of otoliths within the inner ear. For his work on the vestibular apparatus and BPPV, he was awarded the Nobel Prize in Physiology and Medicine in 1914. Dix and Hallpike took the research into BPPV further and developed a test to diagnose it in 1952. In his memory, a Barany Society was established in 1960 to facilitate vestibular research.

12 Ménière's Disease

Suja Sreedharan

The competency covered in this chapter is as follows:

EN4.20 Describe the clinical features, investigations, and principles of management of Ménière's disease.

Introduction

Ménière's disease is an inner ear disorder characterized by bouts of incapacitating vertigo, fluctuating hearing loss, and tinnitus preceded by aural fullness. If no specific cause can be found, the disorder is idiopathic and can be called Ménière's disease. However, in the presence of specific etiology (autoimmune, syphilis, or trauma), this tetrad of symptoms is called Ménière's syndrome.

Pathology

The primary pathology in Ménière's disease is endolymphatic hydrops, which is the abnormal accumulation and distension of the membranous compartment of the inner ear with endolymphatic fluid. This primarily occurs in the cochlear duct and saccule and to a lesser extent in the utricle and semicircular canals (**Fig. 12.1a,b**). As the membranous labyrinth dilates and distends with endolymph, it gives way (the membrane breaks), causing a sudden mixing of the inner ear fluids, resulting in debilitating vertigo and hearing loss. The membrane break heals, and both vertigo and hearing loss improve. However, in late stages of the disease, repeated membrane breaks damage the sensory cells of the inner ear (cochlea and vestibule), and the patient has permanent hearing loss with disequilibrium.

Etiology

Genetic variations: 5 to 15% of Ménière's disease is familial with the disease caused by the presence of genes linked to water and ion transport in the inner ear. The familial forms are more likely to be autoimmune in origin and usually affects both ears.

Autoimmune: Autoimmunity may cause Ménière's disease because of intolerance to inner ear antigens or autoimmunity-induced cytokine storm causing damage to the inner ear.

Vascular: Endolymphatic sac enlargement can cause venous obstruction, which may cause vertigo.

Allergy: An association with allergy has been observed, with studies showing deposition of circulating immune complexes in the blood vessels of the endolymphatic sac and stria vascularis.

Infective: Herpes simplex virus has been postulated as one of the etiologies of the disease.

Pearl

Ménière's disease and Ménière's syndrome are both caused by excess endolymph within the endolymphatic system. In *Ménière's disease*, the exact etiology is unknown, whereas *Ménière's syndrome* refers to a condition where a definite etiology has been identified.

Clinical Features

The disease occurs usually in the second to sixth decade of life with an equal prevalence in both men and women.

■ Early Stages

The disease is characterized by the symptom complex of vertigo, hearing loss, tinnitus, and aural fullness. The vertigo is sudden in onset, usually rotatory in character, lasts anywhere from 20 minutes to 24 hours, and debilitates the patient. It is associated with autonomic disturbances like vomiting, sweating, abdominal cramps, diarrhea, or bradycardia. The pressure symptoms in the ear (aural fullness)

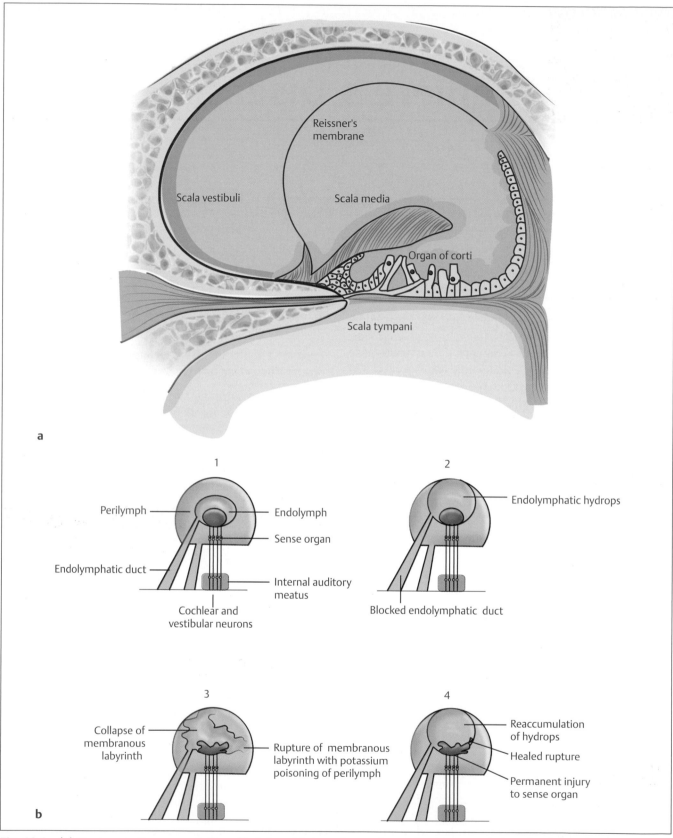

Fig. 12.1 **(a)** Diagrammatic representation of bulging of Reissner's membrane due to accumulation of endolymph in Scala media. **(b)** Pathogenesis of Ménière's disease showing (1) normal, (2) hydrops with distended membranous labyrinth, (3) rupture of membranous labyrinth with sudden mixing of endolymph and perilymph, and (4) healed labyrinth with recurring hydrops.

usually precede the vertigo, with onset of or change in characteristic of the tinnitus, if already present. The patient perceives a reduction in hearing during the episode. Examination of the patient at this point may reveal a nystagmus. The episodes occur in clusters and are punctuated by periods of remission when the patient is completely free of symptoms.

■ Late Stages

Hearing loss fails to recover between episodes and becomes persistent. Similarly, patients are free of episodic vertigo, but in a state of constant disequilibrium. Rarely, elderly patients in late stages develop abrupt attacks of fall, which are not associated with either vertigo or loss of consciousness. This is known as Tumarkin's otolithic crisis and is extremely distressing to the patient.

> ### Pearl
> Lermoyez's syndrome is a rare variant of Ménière's disease characterized by improvement of hearing and reduction of tinnitus during the acute episodes of vertigo.

Investigations

Pure tone audiogram: In the acute phase, the audiogram typically shows low-frequency hearing loss in the pure tones below 2 kHz, which may recover with time or after adequate medical management. In the late stages, the audiogram is a flat curve affecting all frequencies (**Figs. 12.2** and **12.3**).

Special tests done for hearing: These tests are performed to determine whether there is any sensorineural hearing loss in the patient.

Speech discrimination score is the number of words correctly repeated by the patient expressed as a percentage. In Ménière's disease, this is reduced because the number of words correctly repeated is less than 90%.

Short Increment Sensitivity Index (SISI) is the ability of the patient to recognize brief 1-dB increase in intensity of sound when a constant suprathreshold sound is presented to the ear. This is expressed as a percentage. When the patient is able to detect 1-dB increase 70% of the time or more, it is considered positive and is a sign of a cochlear lesion as you would expect in Ménière's disease.

Tone decay test: In this test, a sound above the hearing threshold is delivered to the ear for 60 seconds. If the patient can hear the tone for the full 60 seconds, the test is considered negative implying that it is a cochlear pathology due to Ménière's disease. If the patient does not hear for 60 seconds, the test is positive for a retrocochlear nerve lesion.

• *Speech discrimination*: The affected ears show reduced hearing.

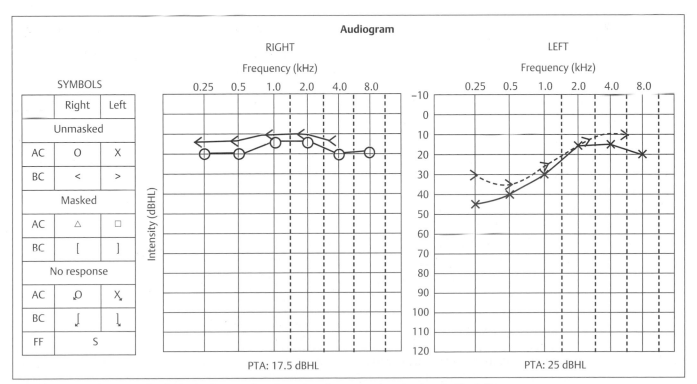

Fig. 12.2 Initial stages of Ménière's disease showing a low-frequency hearing loss in the left ear.

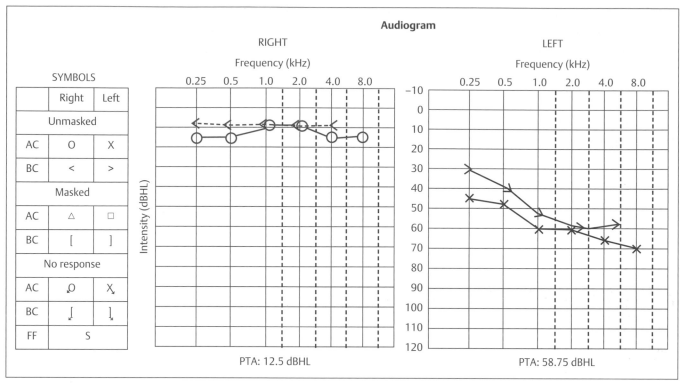

Fig. 12.3 Late stages of Ménière's disease showing a loss in both low and high frequencies in the left ear.

- *Tests for recruitment*: SISI is positive.
- *Tone decay test*: Negative.

Glycerol dehydration test: 1.5 mL/kg body weight of glycerol is mixed with equal quantities of water and given orally. Glycerol, on administration, reduces the volume of the endolymph and improves hearing. So an initial audiogram is performed and glycerol is administered. If a repeat audiogram after 1 hour shows an improvement in thresholds by 10 dB and improvement in speech discrimination by 10 dB, then it is suggestive of Ménière's disease.

Electrocochleogram: Electrocochleogram measures sound evoked electrical activity near the cochlea by transtympanic or extratympanic measurements. The two waveforms recorded after 10 milliseconds are the summating potential (SP) and the action potential (AP). The normal SP-to-AP ratio is 30%. An increase in the ratio (**Fig. 12.4**) due to a deep SP is seen in endolymphatic hydrops and aids in the diagnosis of Ménière's disease.

Gadolinium-enhanced magnetic resonance imaging (MRI): Gadolinium is a contrast agent that selectively enters the perilymphatic space when given intravenously 4 hours before the MRI. In normal ears, the endolymphatic space in the vestibule should not exceed 33% of the vestibule. In Ménière's disease, the endolymphatic compartment will be grossly enlarged. It will also help exclude a retrocochlear lesion–like vestibular schwannoma on the MRI.

Classification and Diagnostic Criteria for Ménière's Disease Revised by the American Academy of Otolaryngology

■ Definite Ménière's Disease

- Two or more spontaneous attacks of vertigo, each lasting 20 minutes to 12 hours.
- Audiometrically documented fluctuating low- to mid-frequency sensorineural hearing loss in the affected ear on at least one occasion before, during, or after one of the episodes of vertigo.
- Fluctuating aural symptoms (hearing loss, tinnitus, or fullness) in the affected ear.
- Other causes excluded by other tests.

■ Probable Ménière's Disease

- At least two episodes of vertigo or dizziness each lasting 20 minutes to 24 hours.

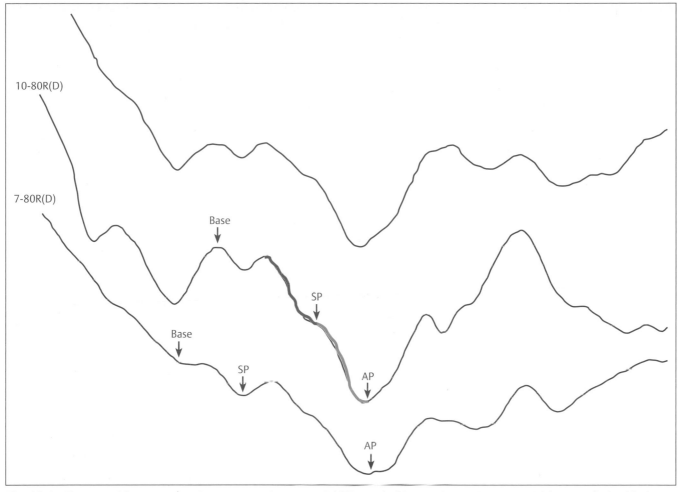

Fig. 12.4 Electrocochleogram showing a summating potential (SP; *marked in green*) to action potential (AP; *marked in blue*) ratio of more than one-third in Ménière's disease.

- Fluctuating aural symptoms (hearing loss, tinnitus, or fullness) in the affected ear.
- Other causes excluded by other tests.

Pearl

Differential diagnosis of Ménière's disease

Acute vestibular syndrome: This consists of sudden onset of vertigo, nausea, vomiting, and nystagmus lasting for more than 24 hours. The patients also have unsteadiness of gait. Vestibular neuronitis is often the cause, but in 20% of patients, posterior circulation stroke may induce this.

Vertiginous migraine: Recurrent episodes of vertigo in patients suffering from migraine, along with associated nausea and vomiting. The patients may or may not have headache at the time of presentation.

Treatment

■ Medical Management

Bed Rest during Acute Episodes and Reassurance

Labyrinthine sedatives include prochlorperazine oral tablet (5 mg), cinnarizine (25 mg or as 75 mg sustained release), Dramamine (50 mg), and prochlorperazine (25 mg), which is available as injection for parenteral use (deep IM). These are usually used in the treatment of acute attacks. However, long-term use is not recommended because of the extrapyramidal side effects, especially in the elderly.

Dietary modification: A low-sodium and caffeine-free diet improves outcome in Ménière's disease when followed for a period of 6 months.

Diuretics like hydrochlorothiazide, furosemide, and acetazolamide reduce the endolymphatic volume and pressure, which helps ameliorate the symptoms. The side effects related to diuretics include electrolyte imbalances. These drugs should be prescribed with caution in the elderly and those with metabolic disorders.

Betahistine hydrochloride: A weak H1 receptor agonist and potent H3 receptor antagonist available as an oral preparation is used in the prophylactic treatment of Ménière's disease. High doses for prolonged periods are required for good effects.

Intratympanic injection of steroids: Dexamethasone 4 mg/mL daily for 3 to 5 days or weekly injections for 4 weeks can be used in refractory cases of Ménière's disease with good hearing.

Intratympanic injection of gentamicin: The vestibulotoxic effect of gentamicin (0.3 mL of 40 mg/mL) instilled weekly into the middle ear directly or through a grommet is utilized for partial "chemical labyrinthectomy" in patients who are refractory to medical management. Both ataxia and sensorineural hearing loss can occur as side effects, so this treatment should be used with caution in the elderly. Chemical labyrinthectomy is a destructive procedure where ototoxic drugs are used to destroy the sensory inner ear hair cells.

Meniett's device produces repetitive pulses of low pressure (0–20 cm of H_2O) in the external ear, which is transmitted to the middle ear (and inner ear) via a grommet. A few reports have shown improvement of acute attacks as well as hearing loss with pressure therapy. However, there is no conclusive evidence of benefits.

■ Surgical Management

The majority of patients can be treated medically, but 10% of patients will suffer from debilitating recurrent vertigo despite medical management. For these patients, surgery can be considered. The primary aim in these procedures is to control the vertigo and preserve the hearing as far as possible unless the hearing is also affected by the disease. The following are some of the procedures that can be attempted:

Endolymphatic sac procedures: Surgical decompression of the endolymphatic sac with or without shunting of the fluid into the mastoid relieves endolymphatic pressure. It improves both the vertigo and hearing loss in Ménière's disease.

Labyrinthectomy: Surgical destruction of the membranous labyrinth may have to be done in refractory cases. Since this procedure results in complete hearing loss, it should be offered only to patients with poor hearing.

Vestibular nerve section: The vestibular nerve in the internal auditory meatus can be sectioned in refractory cases. The hearing is usually preserved.

■ Rehabilitation

Vestibular rehabilitation exercises (Cooksey–Cawthorne): This is useful for developing compensation due to the vestibular hypofunction. This is undertaken especially after an episode of vertigo or after surgical management.

Dizziness handicap inventory: This is a questionnaire with 25 items to assess the impact of dizziness on the daily life of the patient. The maximum score is 100 and the minimum score is 0. The higher the score, the greater the handicap due to the disease. It helps assess the quality of life and progress of the patient.

Summary of Treatment

- **Acute attacks**: Bed rest and labyrinthine sedatives.
- **Chronic disease**: Betahistine, diuretics, and dietary modification.
- **Refractory disease**: Intratympanic injection of steroids/gentamicin, sac procedures, and surgical labyrinthectomy/vestibular nerve section.

Points to Ponder

- Ménière's disease or endolymphatic hydrops is a disorder of the inner ear due to excessive production or decreased absorption of endolymph.
- The main symptoms include vertigo, hearing loss, tinnitus, and ear fullness.
- Clinical examination of the ear does not reveal any specific signs. A pure tone audiogram taken during the early stages of the disease will show hearing loss affecting the lower frequencies. As the disease progresses, the hearing loss affects all frequencies. Special tests of hearing will determine whether it is a cochlear (Ménière's disease) or retrocochlear pathology (affecting the cochlear nerve). Glycerol tests will show improvement in hearing.
- Medical management will give symptomatic relief. Intratympanic injection of steroids can help in patients' refractory to medical treatment and with good hearing. In persistent, intractable vertigo, surgery is an option. The prognosis of this disease is difficult to assess because of the pattern of exacerbation and remission.

Case-Based Questions

1. **A 43-year-old man presented with recurrent episodes of vertigo associated with fluctuating hearing loss and tinnitus. He suffers from nausea and vomiting during the attack, which lasts for a few hours.**

   a. Name two possible tests that will help pinpoint the diagnosis.

   b. What is the acute management of this condition?

   Answers

   This patient is suffering from Ménière's disease.

   a. Pure tone audiogram typically shows a low-frequency hearing loss in the early stage of the disease. This is due to the higher sensitivity of the apex of the cochlea to the pressure changes rather than the basal turn.

   The second test that can help confirm is the glycerol dehydration test where there is an improvement of 10 dB in hearing after administration of oral glycerol to the patient.

   b. Medical management during the acute phase will give symptomatic relief. Labyrinthine sedatives are used to control the nausea and vomiting; therefore, prochlorperazine injection (12.5 mg) is administered by deep IM route. The patient may not be able to take oral medications initially. Intravenous fluids will have to be given to overcome dehydration in these patients.

2. **A 50-year-old man presented with a 2-year history of persistent vertigo and hearing loss along with tinnitus. The vertigo was severe and disabling. Medical management did not help relieve the symptoms. What is the next step in the management?**

   Answer

   In patients with refractory, disabling vertigo, intratympanic injection with steroids can be attempted if they have good hearing. If there is already a hearing loss, intratympanic gentamicin can be administered because it is ototoxic. Surgery is the last option.

Frequently Asked Questions

1. What is the reason for episodic vertigo in Ménière's disease?

2. What are the main symptoms associated with Ménière's disease?

3. What is the characteristic finding in the pure tone audiogram, in the acute, early phase, and late stages of the disease?

4. What is the principle behind the glycerol dehydration test?

5. What drugs can be given during an acute attack of Ménière's disease?

6. Describe the surgical options available to the patient who has severe vertigo but hearing is preserved.

Endnote

Ménière's disease is named after Prosper Ménière, a French physician. In 1861, he presented a paper at the French Academy of Medicine that outlined his observations on vertigo and hearing loss. He concluded that semicircular canals of the inner ear were responsible for vertigo, which was controversial because the belief at that time was that the inner ear was responsible only for hearing. He was recognized for his work only after his death.

13 Tinnitus

Devaraja K.

The competency covered in this chapter is as follows:

EN4.21 Describe the clinical features, investigations, and principles of management of tinnitus.

Introduction

Tinnitus can be defined as a conscious auditory perception without an actual acoustic stimulus. It is a common clinical condition encountered in clinical practice. However, tinnitus is not a disease by itself; it is a symptom with varied etiopathological attributes. The prevalence of tinnitus is reported to range from 10 to 20% of the global population, although not all of them are troubled by it. In fact, only around 20% of the patients with tinnitus may seek medical attention, and in 1 to 2% of the affected patients, the tinnitus can be severely disabling, hampering their quality of life.

Classification

There are many ways in which tinnitus can be classified. The most common method is to classify tinnitus either as subjective, that is, when only the affected person perceives tinnitus, or as objective, that is, when the examiner can also hear the patient-perceived sound with the help of a stethoscope or a microphone placed in the ear canal.

Etiologically, the tinnitus could be idiopathic, without any identifiable cause, or could be due to *vascular*, *muscular*, or *neurological* causes. Idiopathic tinnitus can also be referred to as primary tinnitus as against the tinnitus that is secondary to a specific underlying condition, either local or systemic, as listed in **Table 13.1**.

Table 13.1 Common causes of secondary tinnitus

	Subjective tinnitus	Objective tinnitus
Local causes	• Cerumen • Otomycosis • Otitis media • Otosclerosis • Ménière's disease • Presbycusis • Noise-induced hearing loss • Ototoxicity • Sudden sensorineural hearing loss • Labyrinthitis • Acoustic neuroma	• Arteriovenous malformations • Temporal bone paragangliomas • High or dehiscent jugular bulb • Persistent stapedial artery • Intratympanic carotid artery • Neurovascular conflict at the cerebellopontine angle • Temporal bone fracture • Palatal myoclonus • Tensor tympani or stapedius myoclonus • Patulous eustachian tube • Temporomandibular joint disorders
Systemic causes	• Hypothyroidism • Meningitis • Encephalitis • Stroke • Multiple sclerosis • Vitamin deficiency • Drug-induced • Sleep deprivation • Psychogenic	• Carotid artery stenosis • Carotid artery dissection/aneurysm • Vertebral artery dissection/aneurysm • Thyrotoxicosis • Paget's disease • Increased cardiac output, anemia • Cardiac arrhythmias • Pregnancy • Pseudotumor cerebri

The most common type of tinnitus encountered in clinical practice is primary subjective tinnitus followed by secondary subjective tinnitus. Objective tinnitus is quite rare but is invariably secondary in nature.

Based on the duration, tinnitus that has been there for a short duration is referred to as *recent onset or acute tinnitus*, while the one that lasts for more than 6 months is referred to as *persistent* or *chronic tinnitus*. Tinnitus can be subcategorized, depending on the temporal characteristics of the sound perceived, as *continuous* or *intermittent*, *fluctuant* or *nonfluctuant*, or *pulsatile* or *nonpulsatile*. There are some specific variants of tinnitus, like *somatic tinnitus* and *typewriter tinnitus*, which require a different management strategy.

Etiopathology

Subjective tinnitus is the perception of sound in the absence of any auditory stimuli.

In most cases of subjective tinnitus, the actual mechanism and site of origin of tinnitus remain largely elusive. The postulated hypotheses include the following:

- Loss of outer hair cells.
- Spontaneous neural activity.

The commonly accepted theory suggests that the subjective tinnitus takes origin from abnormally activated neurons of the auditory pathway, secondary to auditory deprivation or altered somatosensory input. The functional imaging studies have also linked the origin of tinnitus to the interaction of auditory areas with other cortical networks related to emotion, memory, and attention centers. The co-activation of these nonauditory cortical centers seems to play a role in psychosomatic manifestations, prevalent in patients with disabling tinnitus.

Pearl

Although tinnitus can involve any age group, it is common in elderly males and particularly in individuals with a history of chronic noise exposure or ototoxicity.

Evaluation of a Patient with Tinnitus

■ History Taking

Tinnitus is a heterogeneous clinical symptom with a large spectrum of perceptual characteristics and accompanying symptoms. A detailed history is one of the crucial steps in managing a case of tinnitus. **Table 13.2** highlights the

Table 13.2 Clinical workup of tinnitus

History	1.	Onset: Sudden/insidious
	2.	Duration: Recent onset/chronic or persistent
	3.	Progression: Intermittent/continuous
	4.	Laterality: Unilateral/bilateral; if bilateral, symmetrical or not
	5.	Loudness: Scale of 1–10, or ordinal scale of gentle/loud/thumping
	6.	Severity: Grade I/II/III/IV
	7.	Pattern: Hissing/ringing/clicking/sizzling/whistling/swishing/roaring
	8.	Quality: Pure tone/polyphonic/noise
	9.	Pitch: Low/medium/high
	10.	Other characteristics: Pulsatile/synchronous with the heartbeat
	11.	Other complaints: Hearing loss/discharge/dizziness/neurological deficit
	12.	Comorbidities: Thyroid/diabetes/cardiovascular/medications
	13.	History of trauma: Head injury/neck injury
	14.	Family history: Head and neck tumors
	15.	Personal history: Occupation/smoking status/weight loss
Examination	1.	General physical examination
	2.	Local examination:
		a. Ear: Ear canal and tympanic membrane
		b. Functional test: Tuning fork tests and facial nerve
		c. Basic vestibular tests: Spontaneous nystagmus and fistula sign
	3.	Examination of the nose, oral cavity, throat, face, and neck
	4.	Neurological examination: Cranial nerves and motor functions
	5.	Cardiovascular system
Investigations	1.	Audiological evaluation:
		a. Pure tone audiogram (PTA)
		b. Impedance audiometry
		c. Otoacoustic emissions (OAE)
		d. Auditory brainstem response (ABR)
		e. Electrocochleography
	2.	Imaging techniques:
		a. Magnetic resonance imaging (MRI)
		b. Computed tomography (CT)
		c. Angiography (MR/CT)
	3.	Tools for assessing the impact of tinnitus:
		a. Tinnitus handicap inventory
		b. Tinnitus functional index
	4.	Blood tests: Complete blood count, blood sugar, thyroid function tests, lipid profile, antinuclear antibodies, and rheumatoid factor
	5.	Allergy workup in select cases

components of clinical evaluation in tinnitus, including critical elements of history taking. Along with the inquiry about the onset of tinnitus, its duration, and perceived intensity, one needs to pay attention to the detailed characteristics of the tinnitus:

- The perceptive nature of tinnitus can be described as hissing, ringing, clicking, sizzling, whistling, swishing, or roaring.
- Tinnitus can be continuous or intermittent, unilateral or bilateral, or pulsatile or nonpulsatile.
- It may be synchronous with breathing or heartbeat.

Typically, most patients report hearing the tinnitus in quiet surroundings in the absence of ambient noise, particularly at night or when the affected person pays more attention to it. Continuous tinnitus can be annoying to the patient.

Pearls

- Pulsatile tinnitus synchronous with the heartbeat is mostly vascular in origin. Pulsatile tinnitus that is asynchronous with the heartbeat suggests palatal or middle ear myoclonus. This is an objective tinnitus that can be appreciated by the examiner with the help of a stethoscope or a microphone placed in the ear canal.
- Continuous nonpulsatile subjective tinnitus can be seen in external ear problems like impacted cerumen or otomycosis and in middle ear conditions like serous otitis media, chronic otitis media, or otosclerosis. Subjective paroxysmal tinnitus could be a feature of cochlear pathology like Ménière's disease or a disorder of the auditory pathway.

The affected patients can also have a wide range of psychosomatic symptoms ranging from irritability, anxiety, stress, and insomnia to depression and suicidal tendencies. As shown in **Fig.13.1**, these psychosomatic symptoms are linked to the negative reinforcement associated with perceived tinnitus and subsequent activation of the limbic and autonomic nervous system (particularly a sympathetic response).

■ Grading of Tinnitus

Tinnitus severity can be classified into the following grades based on the discomfort and resultant consequences on day-to-day life:

- Grade I: Perceived tinnitus is rated by the patient as *not annoying.*
- Grade II: *Annoying in quiet environment* without impacting day-to-day life.
- Grade III: *Annoyance throughout the day; marginally disturbs personal and professional activities.*
- Grade IV: *Significantly hampers the daily routine* and severely impairs the quality of life.

■ Clinical Examination

- The general physical examination should identify any abnormalities in pulse rate, rhythm, and volume, blood pressure, respiratory rate, temperature, body mass index, pallor, icterus, or clubbing, as these signs reflect systemic causes of tinnitus.
- The otoscopic examination should look for a local source of tinnitus in the external auditory canal or middle ear. A detailed functional assessment of the ear can provide a clue about the status of the inner ear and auditory pathway.
- The oral cavity, pharynx, neck, and temporomandibular joint should be examined along with the functional status of lower cranial nerves.
- The systemic examination, particularly the examination of cardiovascular and neurological systems, needs to be done in detail to rule out the corresponding systemic causes that are listed in **Table 13.1**.

■ Differential Diagnosis of Similar Auditory Perception Disorders

Auditory hallucination: Contrary to the elementary sounds like hissing, clicking, or roaring perceived in tinnitus, the patients in auditory hallucination tend to hear spoken voice or music or any other organized sound that conveys a meaningful audiological perception.

Autophony: The patient hears his/her own voice that is unusually loud and disturbing. It is commonly seen in patulous eustachian tube or conductive hearing loss due to

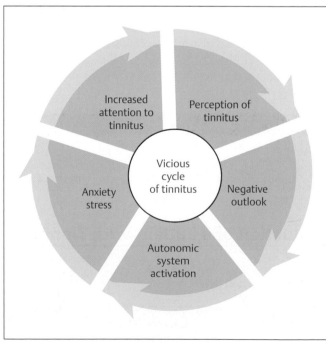

Fig. 13.1 The vicious cycle of tinnitus progression.

occlusion effect. The perceived sounds of autophony subside in a quiet environment.

Hyperacusis: It is an auditory perception disorder with an unknown cause. The affected patient exhibits unusual intolerance to day-to-day sounds of normal loudness or ambient noise of a particular frequency and volume. It may occur along with tinnitus.

Recruitment: In recruitment, there is rapid growth of loudness to uncomfortable levels with a slight increase in the level of external stimulus. The recruitment phenomenon is a feature of cochlear hearing loss and is not seen in neural causes of sensorineural hearing loss.

■ Investigations

A list of relevant investigations that could be useful for evaluating a case of tinnitus is provided in **Table 13.2**. The investigations required depends on the clinical context:

- Assessment of hearing threshold by *pure tone audiogram or auditory brainstem response* is done in most cases of idiopathic tinnitus (**Figs. 13.2** and **13.3**).
- *Examination under microscopy and impedance audiometry* is needed in cases of chronic otitis media and otitis media with effusion, respectively.
- Other adjuvant investigations like otoacoustic emission, vestibular function tests, and electrocochleography could be helpful in selected cases, where the middle ear and external ear are normal.
- Similarly, in subjects with suspected intracranial/skull base lesions or vascular abnormality, *magnetic resonance imaging or computed tomography with or without angiography* should be done. *Diffusion-weighted magnetic resonance imaging* or other functional imaging studies may help in identifying the area of abnormal neuronal activity in the central nervous system, which could be of prognostic and therapeutic relevance.

- As far as the psychosomatic consequences of tinnitus are concerned, the validated questionnaires like *tinnitus handicap inventory* or *tinnitus functional index* might be necessary for estimating the effects of tinnitus on the physical, mental, and overall health of the affected person.

> **Pearl**
>
> Recent-onset high-pitched pulsatile tinnitus, tinnitus with sudden sensorineural hearing loss, acute post-traumatic tinnitus, and loud tinnitus with serious psychological symptoms like depression or suicidal tendencies need to be investigated for early therapeutic intervention.

Treatment

■ General Measures

Treatment includes protection from noise, quitting caffeine/nicotine/smoking, reduction of physical/emotional stress, and stopping/altering existing ototoxic medications.

■ Treat Underlying Conditions (for Known Causes)

Medical management or surgical intervention for known ailments like cerumen, otomycosis, otitis media, otosclerosis, Ménière's disease, vascular causes, myoclonus, patulous eustachian tube, and cerebellopontine angle/skull base tumors can abolish tinnitus.

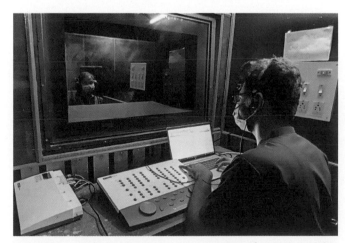

Fig. 13.2 Basic audiometric assessment of tinnitus. (This image is provided courtesy of Dr. Hari Prakash P.)

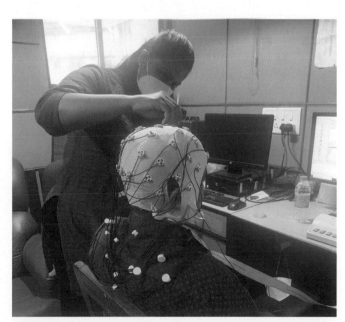

Fig. 13.3 Advance electroencephalogram and event-related potential (ERP) recording system for assessment of tinnitus. (This image is provided courtesy of Dr. Hari Prakash P.)

However, in the majority of the cases, there may not be a clear identifiable cause for tinnitus. In these cases, the therapeutic focus should be aimed at reducing the severity of tinnitus and its affective components.

◼ Behavioral and Psychological Treatment: Habituation of Tinnitus

This approach is very effective in patients with grade I/II tinnitus.

Education and Counseling

- It includes *the provision of basic information* to the affected individuals about the innocuous nature of tinnitus to aid the patients to achieve habituation, empower them to cope with the negative thoughts, and ensure compliance.
- *Cognitive-behavioral therapy (CBT)* helps *modify the maladaptive cognitive*, *emotional*, and *behavioral responses* to tinnitus by cognitive restructuring and behavioral modification, that is, to mainly reduce attention toward tinnitus.

◼ Auditory Stimulation

Auditory stimulation is an essential component of tinnitus treatment. There are numerous acoustic delivery strategies for tinnitus, each one with peculiar working principles, and the preference is guided by the patient characteristics.

- **Use of ambient sounds:** Divert attention toward some of the typical household sounds like the one produced by rotating fan or air conditioner, or toward ambient environmental sounds produced by a blowing wind, insect buzz, or rain.
- **Sound-generator therapy (sound therapy; masking devices):** The principle is to use an auditory device to generate and deliver acceptable environmental sounds like waterfalls, rain, sea waves, or simple white noise, so as to *mask the tinnitus or reduce its perception* (**Fig. 13.4**). A tinnitus-tailored sound whose frequency and loudness can be adjusted to mask the tinnitus can even be integrated with hearing aids.

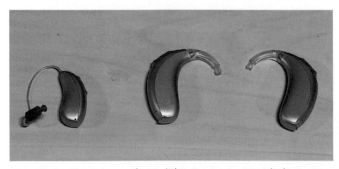

Fig. 13.4 Tinnitus maskers. (This image is provided courtesy of Dr. Hari Prakash P.)

- **Hearing aid and cochlear implant:** Improvement of hearing using a hearing aid or a cochlear implant (depending on the severity of hearing loss) can effectively mask tinnitus.

◼ Retraining Therapy

The primary objective of this approach is to reduce the symptoms of tinnitus by eliminating the central neuroplasticity in the auditory and nonauditory cortex.

Tinnitus retraining therapy (TRT): TRT involves a combination of counseling and sound-generator therapy for habituation to tinnitus and reducing the strength of the tinnitus signal.

Auditory perceptual training (acoustic neuromodulation; acoustic desensitization protocol): Using sound-based active training exercises helps tinnitus patients change their behavioral and passive responses to the tinnitus. The aim is to facilitate a coordinated reset of the abnormal neuronal activity responsible for tinnitus. The auditory training procedures like frequency discrimination training, intensity discrimination training, and auditory object identification and localization are some of the techniques used.

◼ Pharmacotherapy

No medication has demonstrated a direct therapeutic benefit in relieving tinnitus. Some of the commonly used drugs are as follows:

- *Intratympanic steroids*: These can be useful when the tinnitus patient also complains of hearing loss or vertigo, or both.
- *Ginkgo biloba extracts*: Dried extracts of *G. biloba* leaves may enhance cochlear microperfusion but has exhibited variable clinical response.
- *Tricyclic antidepressants* like nortriptyline and amitriptyline may be useful in severe tinnitus with associated depression.
- *Alprazolam* may be tried in those who have no benefit with masking and TRT.

Other drugs have been tried in tinnitus like betahistine, lidocaine, gabapentin, naltrexone, sertraline, carbamazepine, benzodiazepine, melatonin, vitamins and dietary supplements, and acamprosate, with minimal or no therapeutic response. Most of these drugs have a nonspecific mechanism of action with considerable side effects, because of which pharmacotherapy is not an attractive option for tinnitus.

◼ Transcranial Stimulation

Therapeutic brain stimulation could lead to focal modulation of neuronal activity, a principle that has been explored for the elimination of abnormal neuronal activity in tinnitus. This can be done by *repetitive transcranial magnetic* stimulation (rTMS) and transcranial direct current stimulation (tDCS), which are currently in experimental stages. The dose and efficacy are yet to be established.

■ Miscellaneous Therapies

Laser treatment: On similar lines to chronic pain management, the use of low-energy laser has been described for tinnitus, although this approach has not found many takers.

Acupuncture: The complementary and alternative medicine methods have also been tried in tinnitus, with marginal success. This is primarily attributable to the relaxation provided to the agitated person rather than any direct effect on tinnitus.

Pearl

Typewriter tinnitus resembles that of a typewriter tapping. It may arise from vascular compression of cranial nerve VIII and mimics myoclonus. It responds well to carbamazepine.

Points to Ponder

- Tinnitus can be classified into subjective and objective tinnitus. The majority of cases fall into the subjective type.
- Subjective tinnitus is the perception of sound without any auditory stimulus.
- Objective tinnitus is when the examiner can also perceive the sound with the help of a stethoscope or a microphone in the ear.
- The exact cause of tinnitus is not known but is thought to be due to either loss of outer hair cells of the cochlea or abnormally activated neurons of the auditory pathway.
- Pulsatile tinnitus, when synchronous with the heartbeat, is caused by a vascular pathology.
- The key to subjective tinnitus treatment lies in behavioral and psychological therapy in the form of CBT and TRT.

Case-Based Questions

1. **A 45-year-old man presents with history of sudden hearing loss and tinnitus of the left ear that had been present for the past 1 year. This followed a viral infection. On examination, both ears appear to be normal with normal tympanic membranes.**

   a. What investigations should be carried out?

   b. What is the treatment you would prescribe for this patient?

   Answers

   a. Standard investigations include examination under the microscope to look for causes for tinnitus in the external auditory canal and over the tympanic membranes. Pure tone audiometry, tympanometry, brainstem evoked response audiometry (BERA) as well as EEG and event-related potentials (ERPs) can be carried out to map the type of hearing loss and the frequency of the tinnitus.

   b. Most cases of sudden hearing loss due to viral infection lasting for a year are due to sensorineural hearing loss leading to tinnitus. Tinnitus maskers can help drown out the sound of tinnitus, especially in quiet surroundings. Behavioral and psychological therapy like CBT and TRT are administered to help the patient adapt and accept the sound in the ear. There is no evidence to support the effectiveness of drug therapy on tinnitus.

Frequently Asked Questions

1. What is tinnitus and how will you classify it?
2. What are some common causes of objective tinnitus?
3. What is the etiopathogenesis of tinnitus?
4. How will you proceed to evaluate a patient presenting with tinnitus?
5. What is tinnitus retraining therapy or TRT?
6. What is a tinnitus masker?

Endnote

The term "tinnitus" is derived from the Latin verb "tinnire," meaning to ring. It is a common condition and up to 15% of the general population suffer from this condition. Famous personalities who have suffered from tinnitus include former presidents like Ronald Reagan and musicians like Ludwig van Beethoven. Beethoven described his tinnitus as a "roar" in his ears and the sound made it difficult to appreciate music and he would often withdraw from conversations. The cause for his tinnitus is unknown but is thought to be due to lead poisoning.

14 Myringotomy and Grommet Insertion

Kuldeep Moras

The competencies covered in this chapter are as follows:

EN4.10 Observe and describe the indications for and steps involved in myringotomy and myringoplasty.

AN40.5 Explain anatomical basis of myringotomy.

Introduction

Synonym: Tympanostomy

Myringotomy is a surgical procedure where an incision is made on the eardrum to drain the fluid from the middle ear or to provide ventilation into the middle ear. Myringotomy is often combined with placement of a middle ear ventilation tube called a "grommet" or "tympanostomy tube" that provides ventilation to the middle ear in cases of eustachian tube dysfunction.

Indications

The incisions given on the tympanic membrane for myringotomy are radial or curvilinear. *Radial incision* is given for the following conditions:

- Otitis media with effusion (serous otitis media).
- Persistent hemotympanum.
- Recurrent otitis media.
- Otitic barotrauma.
- Middle ear atelectasis.
- It is also given for intratympanic instillation of medications like dexamethasone and gentamicin.

It is required especially when placement of a grommet is indicated. Long-term or permanent ventilation tube is put when there is poor eustachian tube function especially in individuals like pilots who are exposed to frequent atmospheric pressure changes.

The curvilinear incision is given in acute otitis media, especially with severe pain or with impending complications like facial paralysis, labyrinthitis, and meningitis.

Procedure

It is done under general anesthesia in children and under local anesthesia in adults. It is performed using the operating microscope. It can also be performed using a nasal or oto-endoscope. The ear canal is cleaned of wax and debris by suctioning or by giving a saline wash. The tympanic membrane is examined. An incision is made with a myringotome (or sickle knife) in the anteroinferior quadrant (**Fig. 14.1a**) and the effusion or fluid is suctioned out. A counterincision in the posteroinferior quadrant allows air to enter the middle ear and helps in suctioning out the thick fluid. Any bleeding in the external canal can be controlled by cotton soaked in adrenaline or dilute hydrogen peroxide. A grommet is inserted in the opening such that it is partly in the middle ear and partly outside (**Fig. 14.1b**). Sterile cotton is placed in the external auditory canal. Incision for myringotomy and grommet in situ are shown in **Fig. 14.2**.

Postoperative Care

Oral antibiotics (penicillin or cephalosporins) may be given for a week. The patient has to avoid water entering the ear for a period of 6 months to 1 year, till the grommet gets extruded. This is achieved by placing a cotton ball smeared with vaseline or by using swimming ear plugs. Regular follow-up is needed to assess the status of the grommet.

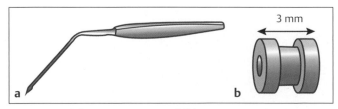

Fig. 14.1 **(a)** Myringotome and **(b)** grommet.

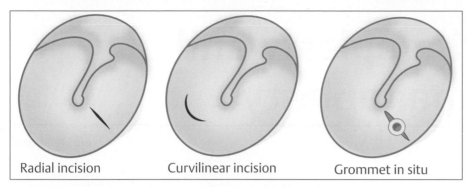

Fig. 14.2 Incisions for myringotomy and grommet in situ.

Radial incision   Curvilinear incision   Grommet in situ

Pearl

Radial incision allows the radial fibers of the eardrum to hold or hug the grommet and keep it in place. The grommet gets extruded due to the posterior epithelial migration of the squamous epithelium of the tympanic membrane, which gradually pushes out the grommet. This takes 6 to 12 months to occur.

Complications

- *Intraoperatively*, tympanostomy tube can be lost or migrate into the middle ear and injury to the middle ear ossicles (incudostapedial joint) can occur. There can be bleeding due to trauma to the canal or a high jugular bulb.

- *Postoperatively*, infection and otorrhea, residual perforation of the tympanic membrane after extrusion of the grommet, early extrusion of the grommet, myringosclerosis (hyalinization of the fibrous layer of the tympanic membrane), and blockage of the tube by debris can occur.

Points to Ponder

- Myringotomy is a useful procedure to let fluid out from the middle ear.
- It is also done in conditions where there is barotrauma due to eustachian tube dysfunction.
- Most grommets stay in place for 6 months to 1 year after placement.

Case-Based Question

1. **A 6-year-old girl with an 8-month history of hearing difficulty in the right ear was brought in by her mother to the ENT clinic. There was no history of ear trauma, pain in the ear, or discharge. It was a gradual hearing loss. Examination of the eardrum revealed a dull tympanic membrane and tympanometry showed a type B curve in that ear. What is the next step in the treatment?**

Answer

A type "B" tympanometry reveals fluid in the ear consistent with otitis media with effusion (OME). She will require a myringotomy with grommet insertion in the right ear. The incision commonly performed is a radial incision in the anteroinferior quadrant. Once the fluid is sucked out from the middle ear, the grommet is inserted. The hearing will improve immediately.

Frequently Asked Questions

1. What are the indications for myringotomy?
2. In which condition would you place a curvilinear incision on the tympanic membrane?
3. How long does the grommet stay in place after insertion?
4. What postoperative instructions will you advise the parents after a grommet insertion?
5. What are the complications associated with myringotomy and grommet insertion?

Endnote

Otitis media with effusion or glue ear is not a new disease. It was known even during the time of Hippocrates. In 400 BC, Hippocrates described how the ear can get filled with mucous and the treatment he recommended was incision of the eardrum. Although it was hypothesized that hearing will improve if the eardrum is perforated, the first intentional surgical procedure of myringotomy was carried out only in 1748. In those early days, without a microscope, there was damage to the middle ear structures also, like the ossicles, during the procedure!

15 Myringoplasty and Tympanoplasty

D. Deviprasad

The competency covered in this chapter is as follows:

EN4.10 Observe and describe the indications for and steps involved in myringotomy and myringoplasty.

Myringoplasty

■ Introduction

Myringa means tympanic membrane (TM) and plasty refers to a surgical procedure for the repair, restoration, or replacement. Myringoplasty is defined as the surgery to repair a perforation on the TM.

This procedure does not include clearance of the disease from the middle ear and correction of the ossicular chain defects, which are together termed tympanoplasty. Myringoplasty is carried out using an operating microscope, although some prefer to use an endoscope.

■ Indications

- Chronic otitis media: Mucosal type (tubotympanic disease) with a permanent perforation.
- Traumatic persistent perforation (after mechanical trauma/barotrauma/iatrogenic trauma).
- Persistent perforation after the extrusion of a grommet.

The objectives of myringoplasty are to prevent recurrent middle ear infections, improve hearing (conductive part), and facilitate usage of a hearing aid in patients with mixed hearing loss.

■ Contraindications

Myringoplasty is contraindicated in the following:

- The presence of cholesteatoma (squamosal type/atticoantral disease).
- When the contralateral ear is dead, that is, profound hearing loss (as there is a 1–2% chance of sensorineural hearing loss in the operated ear).
- Severe eustachian tube dysfunction (like in cleft palate).
- Children below the age of 7 years.
- Active infection in the external or middle ear.
- Active upper respiratory tract infection.
- Uncontrolled systemic disorders like diabetes and hypertension.

Pearl

Patch test

If the baseline audiogram has an air–bone gap of more than 40 dB, a paper patch, smeared with liquid paraffin or soframycin cream at the edges, is carefully placed over the perforated membrane under vision of a microscope.

On a repeat audiogram, if the *air–bone gap reduces*, the patient needs only myringoplasty.

If the air–bone gap remains the same, the patch may not have been applied properly or there may be ossicular fixity.

If the air–bone gap increases, there is an ossicular chain discontinuity and the patient will require a tympanoplasty. The air–bone gap increases because the sound that is directly transmitted to the oval window through the perforation is also cut off by the (temporary) intact membrane created by the patch and the sound is unable to transmit from the membrane to the oval window due to ossicular discontinuity.

■ Steps

The procedure can be done under local or general anesthesia depending on the following:

- Surgeon's preference.
- Preference of the patient.
- Age and general condition of the patient.
- Anatomical constraints of the ear to be operated upon.
- Extent of the disease.

The patient is positioned in the supine position with the head turned to the opposite side so that the ear to be operated on is directed upward.

The approach can be via the following:

- *Postauricular (William Wilde's) incision*, that is, 5 mm to 1 cm behind the postauricular grove (**Fig. 15.1**).
- *Endaural incision:*
  - *Lempert 1 incision*, that is, medial to the bony cartilaginous junction of the external auditory canal (EAC) from the 6 o'clock position to the 12 o'clock position.
  - *Lempert 2 incision*, that is, extension of Lempert 1 incision laterally into the incisura terminalis (**Fig. 15.2**).
- *Endomeatal (Rosen's) incision*, that is, 2 mm lateral to the annulus at the 12 o'clock position, extending inferiorly and laterally to about 6 mm lateral to annulus at the 9 o'clock position and then extend inferiorly and medially to the 6 o'clock position, ending 2 mm lateral to the annulus (**Fig. 15.3**).

The type of approach and incision depends on the surgeon's preference, diameter of the ear canal, and whether a microscope or an endoscope is used for magnification in the surgery.

The graft materials that can be used for myringoplasty are temporalis fascia, tragal perichondrium, tragal cartilage (sliced to 0.5-mm thickness), areolar tissue superficial to the temporalis fascia, fascia lata, vein, and periosteum.

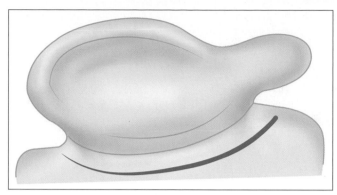

Fig. 15.1 Postauricular (William Wilde's) incision, 5 mm to 1 cm behind the postauricular grove.

Pearl

The temporalis fascia is the preferred graft material because of the following:

- It is accessible at the upper end of the postauricular or endaural incision.
- It is adequately large.
- It is easy and safe to harvest with minimal local morbidity.
- Its thickness is close to that of the TM.
- It has a low basal metabolic rate and can survive longer till blood supply is established.

Following the incision and harvesting of the graft, the margin of the perforation is freshened by incising and removing a rim of the epithelium along the edge of the perforation (**Fig. 15.4a**).

The skin of the bony meatus is elevated. A "vascular strip" is created between the tympanomastoid and tympanosquamous suture line, 3 to 4 mm from the posterior annulus, especially when the postauricular approach is used. The remaining skin is raised up to the annulus.

In *overlay* or onlay technique, this elevation is done along with the outer epithelial layer of the TM and part of the anterior canal skin 3 to 4 mm from the annulus (**Fig. 15.4b**).

The outer squamous epithelium of the TM is peeled off, the graft (*blue color*) is placed over the middle fibrous layer, and the squamous epithelium (preserved canal skin with the outer epithelium of the membrane; *brown color*) is replaced in the original position with a part of the epithelium on the margins of the graft.

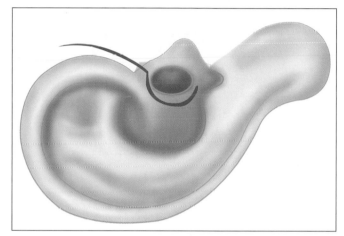

Fig. 15.2 Endaural or Lempert's incision.

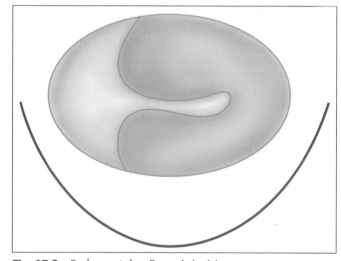

Fig. 15.3 Endomeatal or Rosen's incision.

In the *interlay technique*, the elevation is done along with the epithelium, annulus, and the fibrous layer of the TM (**Fig. 15.4c**, and in the *underlay* technique, the elevation is done along with the annulus and all the three layers of the TM (**Fig. 15.4d**). This step is called "raising the tympanomeatal flap."

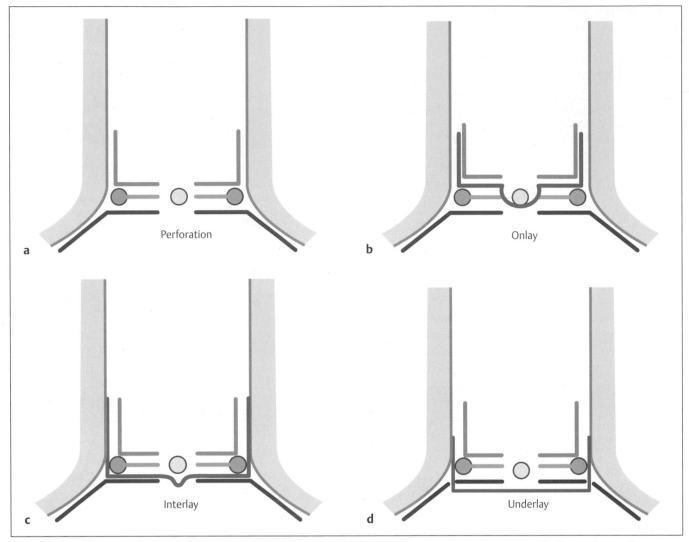

Fig. 15.4 **(a)** Tympanic membrane perforation. *Red* indicates middle ear mucosa, *green* indicates middle fibrous layer of tympanic membrane, *brown* indicates outer squamous epithelium, and *yellow* indicates the handle of malleus. **(b)** The onlay technique. *Blue* indicates the temporalis fascia graft. **(c)** The interlay technique. The graft (*blue color*) is placed between the middle fibrous layer and the mucosal layer of the middle ear. **(d)** The underlay technique. The graft (*blue color*) is placed under the mucosa of the middle ear.

To summarize:

- In the onlay technique, the graft is placed on the fibrous layer and the removed outer epithelium is placed on the margins of the graft.
- In interlay technique, the graft is placed between the fibrous and medial epithelial layers.
- In underlay technique, the graft is placed medial to the inner epithelial layer after scraping part of the inner layer, especially around the perforation.

The graft is placed medial to the handle of the malleus, often with the gelfoam pieces (± antibiotic drops) in the middle ear to support it and prevent it from getting medialized in the underlay technique.

The flap is repositioned. Complete coverage of the perforation by the graft is ensured. Gelfoam pieces (± antibiotic drops) are placed lateral to the drum in the bony ear canal

and the cartilaginous ear canal is packed with an antibiotic wick. Postaural or endaural incision is closed in layers. A mastoid dressing may be applied.

■ Complications

In the *overlay* technique, there may be blunting at the anterior tympanic sulcus, epithelial pearls, iatrogenic cholesteatoma, and lateralization of the TM.

In the *interlay* technique, there may be blunting at the anterior tympanic sulcus and lateralization of the membrane.

In the *underlay* technique, there may be medialization of the membrane leading to shallow middle ear cavity, residual perforation anteriorly (prevented by "anterior tucking"), and myringitis due to mucosalization of the lateral aspect of the newly formed membrane.

A residual perforation or re-perforation (usually within 1 year of the procedure) may happen in any technique.

Tympanoplasty

■ Introduction

Tympanum means the middle ear and plasty refers to a surgical procedure for the repair, restoration, or replacement. Tympanoplasty is defined as the surgery for the clearance of the disease from the middle ear (tympanum) and repairing the ossicular chain defects, ossiculoplasty if present, for restoring hearing mechanism with or without the repair of the TM.

■ Classification

There are five types of tympanoplasty:
- *Type I*: Perforation is repaired with a graft, after examination of the middle ear, and after ensuring that the ossicular chain is intact and mobile (**Fig. 15.5**).
- *Type II*: The malleus is partly eroded; and the graft is placed on the remnant of the malleus and the incus (**Fig. 15.6**).

- *Type III*: The malleus and long process of the incus are eroded; and the graft is placed on the stapes head. This is called *columellar tympanoplasty* or *myringostapediopexy* (**Fig. 15.7**).
- *Type IV*: The graft is placed on mobile footplate (when other ossicles are absent). A *cavum minor* is created, where the lower part of middle ear, from the eustachian tube anteriorly to the round window posteriorly, has an air column for shielding the round window from direct transmission of sound waves (**Fig. 15.8**).
- *Type V*: The footplate of the stapes is fixed (but the round window is mobile); a third window is created (*fenestration operation*) into the inner ear at the lateral semicircular canal and a graft is placed over it (**Fig. 15.9**).

The indications, contraindications, anesthesia, patient positioning, approaches to the middle ear, graft materials, and techniques essentially remain similar to that in myringoplasty. In addition, tympanoplasty may also be performed in cholesteatoma or squamosal type of chronic otitis media after ensuring complete clearance of the disease from the middle ear cleft. As the proper exposure of middle ear may necessitate elevation of the entire TM (all the three layers), underlay grafting is the most likely method used.

Ossiculoplasty may be done using various types of graft materials:
- *Autografts*, like tragal or conchal cartilage, bone of remodeled incus, or the lateral wall of the mastoid cortex, are easy to harvest and shape and are cost-effective. Residual disease must not be present on the bone.
- *Allografts* are mainly prosthesis made of teflon, titanium, glass isomer, polyethylene, and hydroxyapatite. They are

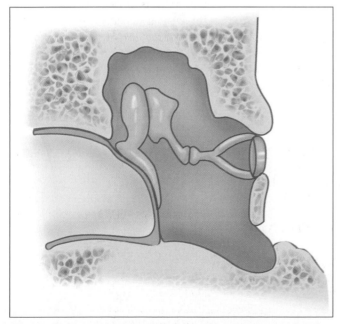

Fig. 15.5 Type I tympanoplasty: perforation repaired with a graft (*green*).

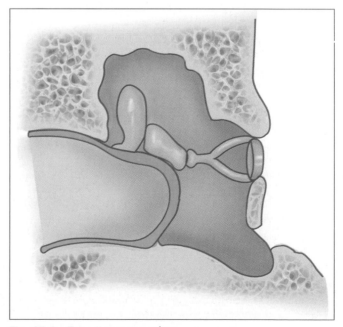

Fig. 15.6 Type II tympanoplasty.

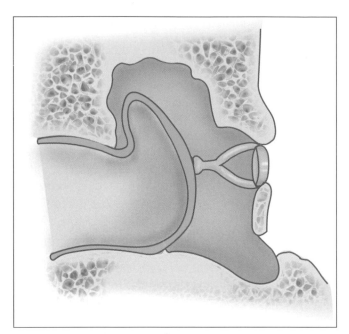

Fig. 15.7 Type III tympanoplasty.

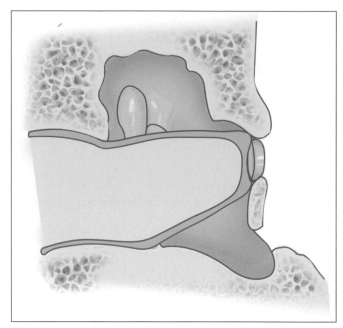

Fig. 15.8 Type IV tympanoplasty.

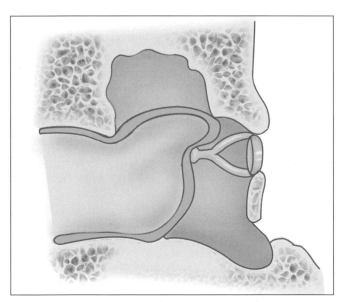

Fig. 15.9 Type V tympanoplasty.

ready to use with a long shelf life, but are expensive and have a higher chance of rejection and extrusion.

• *Homografts* like nasal septal, tragal, or conchal cartilages, cadaver dura, and ossicles with or without TM are harvested and preserved in 70% alcohol. They are economical and easy to shape but not easy to obtain, have ethical issues, and carry the risk of transmitting diseases of the donor.

• *Hetero (xeno) grafts* like serosa or vein of animals are economical but not easy to procure, have ethical issues, and carry risk of transmitting diseases of the donor.

The prosthesis used in allografts may be a partial ossicular reconstruction prosthesis (PORP), that is, from the head of

the stapes to the TM (incus is absent) or a total ossicular reconstruction prosthesis (TORP), that is, from the footplate of the stapes to the TM. An intervening cartilage is placed between the prosthesis and the TM to avoid extrusion. When the lenticular process of the incus is eroded, bone cement may be used to bridge the gap between the incus (long process) and the stapes head.

■ Complications

The prosthesis or graft can be rejected, absorbed, or extruded. There can be adhesions and granulation tissue formation. Disruption of the ossicular chain leading to worsening of conductive hearing loss and dislocation of the stapes footplate leading to perilymph leak and sensory hearing loss can occur. If only type I tympanoplasty is done, depending on the technique of laying of the graft, the patient may have complications similar to that of myringoplasty.

Points to Ponder

• Myringoplasty should be considered in patients with moderate to large central perforations, mucosal type.
• Small perforations may heal with chemical cauterization.
• The two commonly performed techniques of myringoplasty are overlay and underlay.
• The commonly used graft for covering the perforation is the temporalis fascia.
• Tympanoplasty includes inspection of the middle ear with ossicular reconstruction if required.
• There are five types of tympanoplasties.

Frequently Asked Questions

1. What are the different grafting materials used for TM repair?
2. How is a myringoplasty different from a tympanoplasty?
3. What are the different techniques of myringoplasty?
4. What are the disadvantages of the overlay type of myringoplasty?
5. What is type III tympanoplasty?

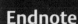

Endnote

Throughout history, different techniques were tried to promote TM healing.

William Wilde and D. B. Roosa used silver nitrate and trichloroacetic acid as chemical cautery on the margins of the perforated TM to promote healing. Berthold (1878) freshened or excised the perforation margin and used a full-thickness skin graft. He was the first to use the term myringoplasty. Zollner (1956) described the fascia lata, Heerman (1958) used the temporalis fascia, and Shea (1960) advocated vein as grafting materials to cover the defect of the membrane. A small dumbbell-shaped fat plug, harvested from the back of the ear lobule, can also be inserted through a small perforation after freshening its margin, as fat graft myringoplasty.

The term "tympanoplasty" was first coined by Wullstein in 1953. Wullstein and Zollner classified tympanoplasty in 1956.

16 Cortical Mastoidectomy

Andrews C. Joseph

The competency covered in this chapter is as follows:

EN4.11 Enumerate the indications, describe the steps, and observe a mastoidectomy.

Introduction

Synonyms: Simple mastoidectomy, Schwartz operation, conservative mastoidectomy, complete mastoidectomy

Mastoid antrum serves as a physiological buffer for the air pressure in the middle ear cleft. Clearance of disease from the mastoid antrum is essential for the normal functioning of middle ear cleft. Hearing preservation surgeries such as tympanoplasty often require this step. Cortical mastoidectomy aims at opening the mastoid antrum and air cells. The procedure is done with visualization under an operating microscope.

Definition

It is an operative procedure of the mastoid air cells and the antrum in which there is complete removal of all the accessible mastoid air cells, keeping the posterior wall of the external auditory canal intact.

Indications

Cortical mastoidectomy is done in the following conditions:
- Acute otitis media not responding to conservative therapy.
- Refractory secretory otitis media.
- Acute coalescent mastoiditis.
- Masked mastoiditis.
- Subperiosteal abscess and Bezold's abscess.
- It is done as an initial step to perform:
  - Radical or modified radical mastoidectomy.
  - Endolymphatic sac surgery.
  - Posterior tympanotomy.
  - Facial nerve decompression.
  - Translabyrinthine or retrolabyrinthine approach for acoustic neuroma.
- It can be done for otorrhea due to mastoid disease not responding to medical treatment.

Contraindications

Uncontrolled systemic diseases are relative contraindications.

Steps of Surgery

- *Anesthesia*: Can be done under local or general anesthesia.
- *Position of patient*: Supine position and head turned to opposite side with operating ear up.
- *Preparation*: *Infiltration and draping*
  - Infiltration.
    - *Dose: 5 to 10 mL of 2% lignocaine with 1 in 10,000 (of 1:2,00,000 concentration) adrenaline.*
  - Prepare the surgical site 2 fingerbreadth above and behind the ear (2 cm).
  - Parts are cleaned and draped.

■ Procedure

- Postaural (Wilde's) incision is placed 1 cm behind the postauricular sulcus from the root of helix to mastoid tip (**Fig. 16.1**).
- A modification of the incision is required in infants and children where the mastoid tip is not fully developed. The incision is deepened into subcutaneous tissue and muscle (**Fig. 16.2**).

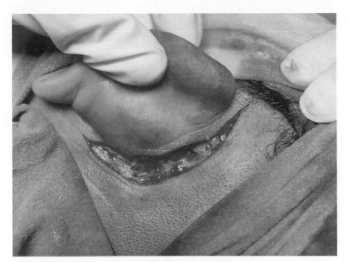

Fig. 16.1 Postauricular (Wilde's) incision.

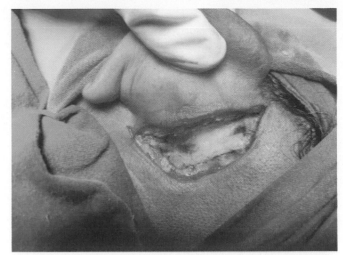

Fig. 16.2 Incision deepened.

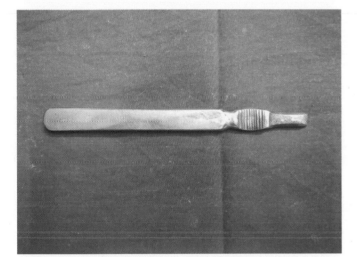

Fig. 16.3 Farabeuf mastoid periosteal elevator.

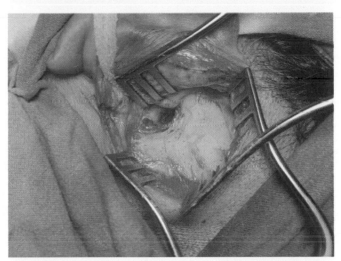

Fig. 16.4 Mollison's self-retaining hemostatic mastoid retractor.

- The periosteum is incised in T-, Y-, or U-shaped manner and elevated with the help of Farabeuf mastoid periosteal elevator (**Fig. 16.3**).
- The spine of Henle, MacEwen's triangle (bounded by superficial temporal line superiorly, posterosuperior segment of bony external canal anteriorly, and line drawn as a tangent to external canal posteriorly), and posterior bony margin of the meatus are visualized. The mastoid antrum lies 1.5 cm deep to MacEwen's triangle.
- Mollison's self-retaining hemostatic mastoid retractor is inserted to hold the soft tissues away from the underlying exposed bone (**Fig. 16.4**).
- The mastoid cortex over MacEwen's triangle is removed using a drill fitted with large cutting burr to reach the mastoid antrum. Drilling should be continued till the cortical bone is exposed (**Fig. 16.5**).
- The antrum is identified by confirming aditus using Dundas ball probe/cell seeker (**Fig. 16.6**).

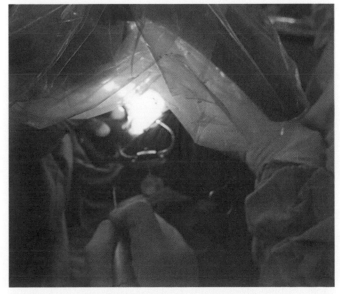

Fig. 16.5 Drilling in progress using microscope.

- Opening to the antrum is enlarged by removal of cells superiorly and posteriorly using a large curette or burr (**Fig. 16.7**).
- From the antrum, all the accessible mastoid air cells are followed up to their termination and exenterated. Saline irrigation and suctioning are done throughout the drilling. In the completed mastoid cavity, the structures left behind include the tegmen tympani above, sinus plate posteriorly, posterior meatal wall anteriorly, and shadow of short process of incus. The cavity is polished using a diamond burr (**Fig. 16.8**).

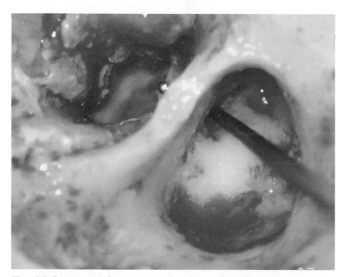

Fig. 16.6 Mastoid antrum with aditus identified.

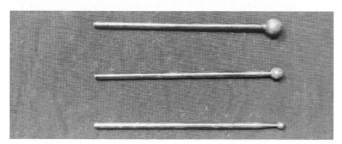

Fig. 16.7 Different types of burrs used while drilling the mastoid.

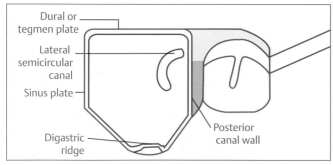

Fig. 16.8 The boundaries of a cortical mastoidectomy are outlined in red. Anteriorly–posterior wall of external auditory canal; superiorly–Tegmen plate; posteriorly–sinus plate; inferiorly–digastric ridge.

- The skin and periosteum are approximated by suturing in two layers, and a mastoid dressing is applied (**Fig. 16.9**).

Postoperative Care

- Appropriate antibiotic therapy.
- Analgesics, anti-inflammatory drugs, and decongestants.
- Mastoid dressing is removed on the 3rd postoperative day.
- Look for facial nerve function, nystagmus, vomiting, and vertigo.
- Tuning fork tests will reveal the hearing status after surgery.

Complications

- The facial nerve can be injured during infiltration, dissection, or by heat generated during drilling.
- The second genu and vertical segment are more prone to injury during drilling.
- Sigmoid sinus injury can lead to profuse bleeding and, occasionally, air embolism.
- Injury to lateral semicircular canal can cause vertigo.
- Cerebrospinal fluid (CSF) can leak due to injury to the dura.
- Dislocation or injury to the incus.
- Bony fixation of malleus and incus.
- Postoperative hematoma.

Pearl

Korner's septum is the persistence of the petrosquamous suture as a bony plate, separating superficial squamosal cells from deep petrosal cells. Surgical importance is that it may cause difficulty in locating antrum and deeper cells, which may lead to incomplete removal of disease in mastoidectomy.

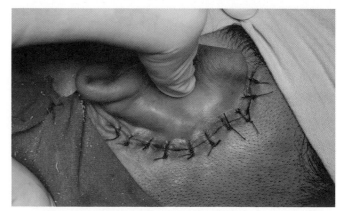

Fig. 16.9 Postauricular incision sutured.

Points to Ponder

- Cortical mastoidectomy is an operative procedure of the mastoid air cells and the antrum involving complete removal of all accessible mastoid air cells, keeping the posterior wall of the external auditory canal intact.
- Mastoid antrum is situated posterosuperior to the spine of Henle. Hence, during drilling, one should not go inferior to the spine of Henle.
- The second genu and vertical segment of the facial nerve are prone to injury during mastoid drilling.
- Trautmann's triangle: The triangle formed by the bony labyrinth (solid angle) anteriorly, sigmoid sinus posteriorly, and superior petrosal sinus superiorly. It is a bony partition which separates the posterior cranial fossa from the mastoid.
- MacEwen's triangle: It is a landmark for identifying mastoid antrum, bounded by superficial temporal line superiorly, posterosuperior segment of bony external auditory canal anteriorly, and line drawn as a tangent to external canal posteriorly.
- Solid angle is the angle formed by the three semicircular canals.

Case-Based Question

1. **A 14-year-old boy presented with ear pain, fever, and discharge from the left ear of 3 days duration. He said the symptoms started with ear pain following a cold. On examination, the pinna was protruding forwards with a red, tender, fluctuant swelling behind the ear over the mastoid region. What would be the diagnosis and how would you manage this condition?**

Answer

Ear pain following a cold signifies acute otitis media. Since the patient developed a swelling behind the ear with fever and the pinna is pushed forwards, a subperiosteal abscess may be a likely diagnosis. A computed tomography (CT) scan will reveal the extent of mastoid involvement, and the patient will have to undergo a cortical mastoidectomy to remove all the diseased air cells.

Frequently Asked Questions

1. What are the indications for cortical mastoidectomy?
2. What is the role of a mastoid retractor?
3. What is the name of the incision commonly used for mastoidectomy?
4. What are the likely complications of this procedure?
5. What is the surgical importance of the mastoid antrum?
6. What are the boundaries of a cortical mastoidectomy?
7. Which part of the facial nerve is commonly injured during this surgery?

Endnote

Mastoidectomy was developed as a surgical procedure to drain infected ears. The first documented case of mastoidectomy was by a French surgeon Ambroise Pare in the 16th century. In 1873, Hermann Schwartze published an article which detailed the indications for mastoidectomy and provided a step-by-step description of the surgery. For his contribution, the surgery has been named after him as Schwartze mastoidectomy.

17 Stapedotomy

Kuldeep Moras

The competency covered in this chapter is as follows:

EN3.5 Observe and describe the indications for and steps involved in the surgical procedures in ear, nose, and throat.

Introduction

Stapedotomy is the procedure wherein a hole is made in the footplate of the stapes for placement of a prosthesis. It is commonly done for otosclerosis (**Fig. 17.1**).

Indications

Stapedotomy is done in otosclerosis when there is conductive hearing loss of more than 30 to 40 dB in the speech frequencies (500, 1,000, and 2,000 Hz) and a good speech discrimination score (above 60–70%).

Contraindications

- The only hearing ear as there is a rare chance of causing sensorineural hearing loss or total deafness after the surgery.
- Otospongiosis (active stage of disease) with positive Schwartz's sign: surgery is delayed.
- Presence of coexisting Ménière's disease where there can be a distended saccule and there is a risk of developing a dead ear, if the saccule is punctured.
- Young children as eustachian tube dysfunction is common and can result in middle ear infection, otitis media, and labyrinthitis.
- In patients with preexisting tympanic membrane perforation and chronic suppurative otitis media (CSOM), the perforation is closed first by myringoplasty and stapedotomy is carried out at a later stage.
- Cochlear otosclerosis.
- Certain occupations involving high physical strain like lifting heavy weights or in construction workers as there is increased risk of perilymph fistula resulting in vertigo and sensorineural hearing loss.
- Pregnancy: surgeries done 6 to 12 months after delivery.

Surgical Procedure

■ Anesthesia

Surgery is usually done under local anesthesia as hearing can be assessed on the table immediately. General anesthesia is preferred in anxious patients and those who do not want local anesthesia.

■ Steps

The surgical steps of stapedotomy are illustrated in detail in **Fig. 17.2**.

1. It is usually done via the endomeatal (through the ear) approach. The postaural approach is used when the external auditory canal is very narrow.
2. Infiltration of the skin of the ear canal is done with lignocaine and adrenaline, which reduce bleeding during the surgery by causing vasoconstriction.

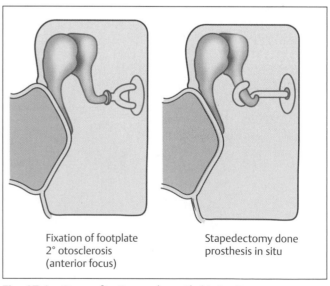

Fixation of footplate 2° otosclerosis (anterior focus)

Stapedectomy done prosthesis in situ

Fig. 17.1 Stapes fixation and prosthesis in situ.

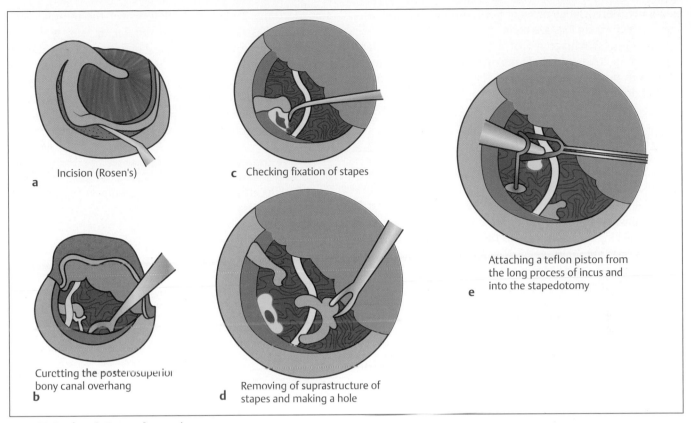

a Incision (Rosen's)

c Checking fixation of stapes

e Attaching a teflon piston from the long process of incus and into the stapedotomy

b Curetting the posterosuperior bony canal overhang

d Removing of suprastructure of stapes and making a hole

Fig. 17.2 (a–e) Steps of stapedotomy.

3. Rosen's endomeatal incision is given from the 6 o'clock position to the 12 o'clock position, 5 to 6 mm lateral to the annulus and the tympanomeatal flap is elevated like a door and the middle ear is opened.
4. The ossicles are visualized by curetting the postero-superior bony overhang of the ear canal at the level of the annulus.
5. The ossicular mobility is checked and stapedial fixation is confirmed.
6. The stapes suprastructure is fractured and removed.
7. A hole is made in the posterior half of the stapes footplate using a stapes perforator or laser.
8. A teflon piston or prosthesis is placed over the long process of the incus and the other end is inserted into the stapedotomy opening.
9. Minimal bleeding may occur during the procedure and this eventually forms a clot around the stapedotomy and gets converted into a seal around the piston, preventing leak of perilymph. Sometimes small pieces of gelfoam or fat from the ear lobule are placed around the piston at the stapedotomy site.
10. The tympanomeatal flap is repositioned back into place.
11. The patient is usually discharged on the postoperative day 2 and asked to take rest for 1 week.

> **Pearl**
>
> The use of endoscopes, instead of microscopes for stapedotomy, is popular among some surgeons. The posterosuperior deep meatus need not be curetted as the structures can be visualized by the angled endoscope. The disadvantage is that one hand is required to hold the scope unless a scope holder is used and the depth perception is different.

Complications

- Tympanomeatal flap tear or perforation of the tympanic membrane.
- Injury to the chorda tympani or the facial nerve.
- Dislocation of the incus.
- Perilymph fistula.
- Perilymph gusher.
- Floating or subluxation of the footplate.
- Vertigo is common postoperatively but usually subsides with medication. Severe vertigo may suggest labyrinthitis due to secondary infection.
- Sensorineural hearing loss is rare but can occur following the procedure.

Perilymph gusher is the sudden persistent flow of perilymph because of congenitally abnormal patent cochlear aqueduct. Here, the chances of perilymph fistula and sensorineural hearing loss are high.

Floating or subluxated footplate is when the footplate dips into the inner ear while making a fenestra in the footplate. The procedure may have to be technically modified or abandoned altogether.

Postoperative Advice

Oral antibiotics such as amoxicillin, cefixime, or cefpodoxime may be given for a week. Do not let water enter the ear for 1 month. It is advised not to have a head bath for 2 weeks. Bowing the nose is not advisable. Open the mouth while sneezing as it will reduce the sudden rise in middle ear pressure. Avoid traveling by air for 2 weeks. Avoid diving. However, the patient can swim 2 months after surgery. Avoid lifting heavy objects.

Stapedectomy

Prior to the advent of stapedotomy, the entire footplate or part of the footplate was removed. This was called stapedectomy. To cover the defect over the footplate, the temporalis fascia from behind the ear or vein graft harvested from the dorsum of the hand or fat from the ear lobule was used to seal the oval window and Teflon piston or prosthesis was placed over it. This procedure was later discontinued as stapedotomy gave better hearing results with less incidence of postoperative sensorineural hearing loss as compared to stapedectomy.

Points to Ponder

- Stapedotomy is the surgical procedure of choice for otosclerosis.
- It involves making a small opening into the footplate of the stapes for insertion of a prosthesis.
- Stapedectomy was the older technique where the entire footplate was removed.
- Stapedotomy gives very good hearing results postoperatively when there is only conductive hearing loss with an intact tympanic membrane.
- Patients should be made aware that sensorineural hearing loss is one of the dreaded complications of this procedure.

Case-Based Question

1. **A 35-year-old woman presented with a 5-year history of gradual hearing loss in the left ear. Audiometry showed a 45-dB conductive hearing loss with a dip at 2,000 Hz. A diagnosis of otosclerosis was made and she underwent stapedotomy in that ear. Postoperatively, she developed dizziness. What could be the cause of the dizziness?**

Answer

Vertigo or dizziness is a common complaint after stapedotomy. This is because an opening is made into the stapes footplate and during the procedure or after surgery, the perilymph can leak out from around the piston that has been inserted. To prevent this, a tight seal has to be obtained around the piston. This can be done with the help of a blood clot or fascia or fat from the ear lobule.

Frequently Asked Questions

1. What is the indication for stapedotomy?
2. What are the contraindications for this procedure?
3. Name three complications associated with this surgery.
4. What is the difference between stapedotomy and stapedectomy?

Endnote

Valsalva was the first person to describe stapes fixation caused by otosclerosis. It was Kessel who, in 1878, described a surgical procedure to overcome the deafness associated with otosclerosis. He outlined a technique in which the stapes was mobilized or manipulated so that it became mobile. This technique fell into disrepute until Rosen revived it in 1952. Stapes mobilization is not practiced now as re-fixation occurs.

18 Disorders of Eustachian Tube

Shama Shetty

The competency covered in this chapter is as follows:

AN40.2 Describe and demonstrate the boundaries, contents, relations, and functional anatomy of middle ear and auditory tube.

Introduction

The eustachian tube (ET) (*synonyms:* pharyngo-tympanic tube, auditory tube) is an important component of the middle ear cleft. The other components include the middle ear and the mastoid air cell system. Most inflammatory diseases of the middle ear are related to eustachian tube dysfunction (ETD). Due to the structure of the ET, inflammatory diseases of the middle ear are more common in children.

Embryology

The ET lumen develops from the first pharyngeal pouch. The endodermal lining of the first pharyngeal pouch extends laterally and makes contact with the ectoderm of the first pharyngeal cleft on either side. The distal part of the pouch becomes elongated and expanded to form the tubotympanic recess, which later forms the middle ear cavity. The proximal portion narrows to form the ET (**Fig. 18.1**).

Anatomy

The ET consists of a lumen with its mucosa, cartilage, surrounding soft tissue, paratubal muscles, and bony support (sphenoid sulcus and medial pterygoid plate). The length of tube in adults is 31 to 38 mm, average being 36 mm.

The ET can be divided into three portions:
* Cartilaginous.
* Junctional.
* Osseous.

The cartilaginous portion is proximal and opens into the lateral wall of nasopharynx at the level of inferior concha, and the osseous or bony portion is distal and opens into the anterior wall of the tympanic cavity (**Fig. 18.2**). The junctional portion is that constricted part of the tube at which

the cartilaginous and osseous portions connect, that is, the isthmus. The cartilage is firmly attached to the skull base by the lateral and medial suspensory ligaments, separated by the Ostmann's fat pad (**Fig. 18.3**).

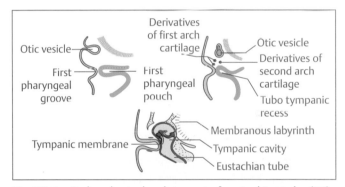

Fig. 18.1 Embryologic development of eustachian tube (ET).

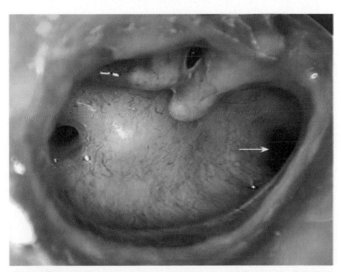

Fig. 18.2 Right tympanic membrane perforation through which the eustachian tube opening is visible anteriorly into the middle ear.

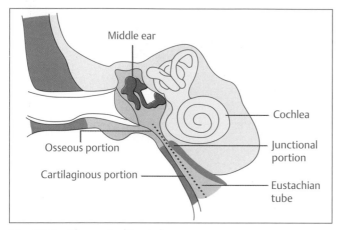

Fig. 18.3 The eustachian tube.

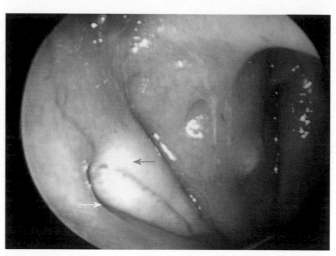

Fig. 18.4 Endoscopic picture of the nasopharynx showing right eustachian tube (ET) opening (*yellow arrow*) and torus tubarius (*blue arrow*).

■ Fibrocartilaginous Portion (Lateral Two-Third)

It protrudes into the nasopharynx; this protrusion is known as the torus tubarius (**Fig. 18.4**). Lymphoid collection over torus is called Gerlach's tubal tonsil.

Posterosuperior to the torus is the fossa of Rosenmuller. The cartilage of the tube is shaped like an inverted J in cross section (like a shepherd's crook). The remaining part is covered by a fibrous membrane. The salpingopharyngeal fascia attaches to the free edge. The fat tissue located in the inferolateral portion of the tube, termed *Ostmann's fat pad*, most likely aids in closing the tube (**Fig. 18.5**).

■ Osseous Portion (Medial One-Third)

It lies within the petrous portion of the temporal bone and is continuous with the anterior wall of the superior portion of the middle ear, that is, 4 mm from the floor of the middle ear. There are four muscles associated with the ET: the tensor veli palatini, the tensor tympani, the levator veli palatini, and the salpingopharyngeus.

Osseous portion is patent at all times when the middle ear cleft is healthy, in contrast to the fibrocartilaginous portion, which is closed at rest and opens during swallowing or when forced open, such as during Valsalva's maneuver. The lumen is lined with pseudostratified, ciliated type columnar epithelium of varying thickness in the cartilaginous part and the osseous part is lined by low columnar ciliated epithelium with goblet cells. The mucosa is continuous with the lining of the tympanic cavity at its distal end, as it is with the nasopharynx at its proximal end.

The ET in an infant is different anatomically and physiologically from that of an adult. The main differences between the two groups are pointed out in **Table 18.1**. The ET reaches its adult length and orientation by 7 years of age.

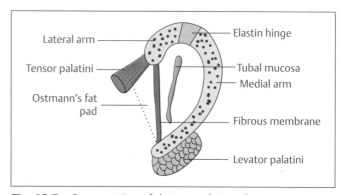

Fig. 18.5 Cross section of the eustachian tube.

Pearl

In infants and young children, the ET is shorter, wider, and less angulated at the isthmus. The ability to actively open is also less. This accounts for the increased risk of middle ear disease in that age group.

Physiology

Osseous portion is always open.
The fibrocartilaginous part is closed at rest and opens on:
- Swallowing.
- Yawning.
- Sneezing.
- Forceful inflation.

Contraction of the tensor veli palatini leads to active opening of the cartilaginous part of the ET while contraction of the levator veli palatini leads to passive opening of the tube. It closes by elastic recoil of elastin hinge along with

Table 18.1 Difference between eustachian tube in an infant and an adult

Characteristics	Infant	Adult
Length	13–18 mm at birth	31–38 mm
Angle of the tube to horizontal plane in degrees	10	45
Bony portion	Longer and wider	Bony part is one-third of total length
Cartilage	Flaccid	Comparatively rigid
Cartilage volume	Less	More
Ostmann's fat pad	Less in volume	Large and helps to keep tube closed
Density of elastin at the hinge	Less dense	More dense—helps to keep tube close by recoil of cartilage
Ventilatory function	Not well developed	Well developed

the deforming force of the Ostmann's fat pad. The sensory nerve endings in the middle ear may act as chemo- or baro-receptors, which can influence the opening of the ET.

There are three physiologic functions attributed to the ET:
- Pressure regulation and ventilation of the middle ear.
- Protection of the middle ear from nasopharyngeal sounds, pathogens, and secretions including reflux.
- Drainage of secretions produced within the middle ear into the nasopharynx by the mucociliary clearance mechanism.

Eustachian Tube Dysfunction

ETD is a poorly characterized clinical condition. It means impairment of ET function leading to a variety of symptoms.

It has traditionally been classified as acute ETD and chronic ETD depending upon the duration of the symptoms:
- Acute ETD is associated with upper respiratory tract infection like the common cold and allergic rhinitis. The symptoms are less than 3 months.
- Chronic ETD is due to obstruction along the length of the ET or due to a patulous ET and the duration of symptoms is usually more than 3 months.

An attempt has been made recently to reclassify ETD into the following categories. In the reclassification, there are three types of ETD:
- **Dilatory ETD:**
  - Anatomic obstruction.
  - Functional obstruction —the tube does not open.
  - Dynamic dysfunction (muscular failure).
- **Baro-challenge-induced ETD**.
- **Patulous ETD**.

■ Anatomic Obstruction

Anatomic obstruction can be:
- Intraluminal or within the lumen.
- Periluminal or around the lumen.
- Peritubal obstruction, around the ET.

Etiology

- *Obstruction of the lumen or within the periluminal tissues*:
  - Inflammation secondary to upper respiratory tract infection or allergy.
  - Congenital or acquired stenosis of the tube.
- *Peritubal obstruction*:
  - By a tumor or an adenoid mass.
- *Obstruction at the middle ear end of the tube*:
     Acute or chronic inflammation of the mucosal lining; may also be associated with polyps or cholesteatoma.
  - Congenital cholesteatoma.
- *Obstruction at the nasopharyngeal end of the tube*:
  - Adenoids, nasal packing, tumor.

■ Functional Obstruction

This occurs when the lumen of the cartilaginous portion of the tube fails to open during activities like swallowing. This may be due to a persistent collapse of the ET due to:
- Increased tubal compliance (e.g., lack of stiffness or the tube is too floppy),
- An inefficient active opening mechanism, or
- Both.

Examples:
- Cleft palate—chronic otitis media is common in these patients. Tensor veli palatini may not be well developed and does not have a proper insertion into the torus tubaris.

- Surgery of the palate or nasopharynx.
- Common in children with middle ear disease.
- Tumors involving the tensor veli palatini muscle.
- Floppy cartilage.
- Down's syndrome—tensor veli palatini muscle tone is poor and the shape of the nasopharynx is abnormal.

■ Treatment of Dilatory Dysfunction

Medical Management

- Treatment of upper respiratory allergy.
- Treatment of nasal or paranasal sinus infection.
- Antireflux medications.

The most common causes of ETD are those due to viral infections or allergy. Treatment includes:

- Systemic decongestants like pseudoephedrine, 60 mg orally every 6 hours.
- Topical nasal decongestants like oxymetazoline 0.05% thrice daily for 3 days.
- Autoinflation is not recommended to those with active nasal infection.
- Allergic patients may benefit from intranasal corticosteroids like fluticasone propionate.
- Air travel or diving should be avoided.

Surgical Management

- Removal of anatomical obstruction—adenoidectomy, septoplasty, functional endoscopic sinus surgery (FESS).
- Myringotomy and ventilation tube (grommet) insertion.
- Eustachian tuboplasty.
- Balloon dilatation of the ET.

■ Baro-Challenge-Induced Eustachian Tube Dysfunction

It is a condition resulting from failure of the ET to maintain middle ear pressure at ambient atmospheric level. The symptoms manifest during deep sea or scuba diving or on descent from an altitude.

The patient complains of aural fullness, popping or discomfort in the ear, or pain. Poor ET function, recent upper respiratory tract infection, and sleeping during the flight may predispose to otitic barotrauma. Patients are typically asymptomatic once they return to ground level.

In some cases, significant baro-challenge may cause temporary middle ear effusion or hemotympanum. This occurs when the atmospheric pressure is more than the middle ear pressure by 90 mm Hg and the ET gets blocked. This causes negative pressure in the middle ear which leads to tympanic membrane retraction and transudation or hemorrhage. In these cases, middle ear effusion or hemotympanum may be evident on otoscopy. Due to a bleed in the inner ear or rupture of intralabyrinthine membranes, there can be sensorineural hearing loss and vertigo.

Management

Patients are usually asymptomatic once they return to normal ground level pressure from a height or deep sea diving. In some cases, there may be temporary middle ear effusion or hemotympanum which can be managed conservatively.

■ Patulous Eustachian Tube Dysfunction

It is caused by an abnormally patent ET. In most cases, it is idiopathic. It may be precipitated by recent weight loss, pregnancy, and oral contraceptive use. The presenting symptoms are aural fullness and autophony (hearing one's own breath sounds). The symptoms may be better in the supine position and during upper respiratory tract infection. It may worsen during exercise. Some patients with patulous ET will habitually sniff. In this condition, pressure changes in the nasopharynx are easily transmitted to the middle ear. On otoscopic examination, the movements of the tympanic membrane can be seen with inspiration and expiration.

Management

Acute cases are usually self-limiting. The following conservative measures can be tried:

- Weight gain.
- Administration of normal saline drops.
- Topical administration of sodium iodide to induce mucosal edema.

For long-standing cases, the following surgical methods may be attempted:

- Intraluminal cauterization of the ET.
- Insertion of grommet into the tympanic membrane.
- Implantation of autologous cartilage around the ET.
- Plugging the tube.

Examination of Eustachian Tube

■ History

Due to tubal occlusion, there can be ear pain, sensation of fullness in the ear, decreased hearing, tinnitus or popping sensation in the ear, and imbalance/vertigo.

■ Clinical Examination

- Otoscopy shows retracted tympanic membrane, congestion along the handle of malleus and pars tensa, and transudate behind tympanic membrane.

- Postnasal examination—look for adenoid or any other nasopharyngeal mass.
- Rinne's and Weber's tuning fork tests—normal or conductive hearing loss.
- Pure tone audiometry: A mild or moderate conductive hearing loss may be found in patients with ETD.
- Tympanometry is performed to look for negative middle ear pressure.
- Endoscopic examination of the nose to visualize the nasal cavity, nasopharynx, and the opening of the ET.
- ET function tests include the following:
  - Valsalva maneuver.
  - Politzer test.
  - Toynbee maneuver.
  - Sonotubometry.

Valsalva Maneuver

In this positive pressure in the nasopharynx causes air to enter the middle ear through the ET. This results in a "popping sound." In a tympanic membrane perforation, a hissing sound may be heard. If there is discharge in the middle ear, a crackling sound is heard.

It is contraindicated in patients with atrophic scars of tympanic membrane. This can lead to rupture of the membrane. And it is also contraindicated where there is an upper respiratory tract infection as it can drive the infection in the middle ear.

Politzer Test

This is done in children who find it difficult to do the Valsalva maneuver. The tip of the Politzer bag is introduced into the nasal cavity of the test side while the other side is closed. The patient is asked to swallow while blowing air into the nose with the Politzer bag. On auscultation of the test ear, a hissing sound is heard. Alternatively, compressed air can be used. This maneuver can be used to ventilate the middle ear for the treatment of otitis media with effusion.

Toynbee's Test

This uses negative pressure, that is, the patient swallows while the nose is pinched. The air from the middle ear is drawn to the nasopharynx causing inward movement of tympanic membrane.

Sonotubometry

A microphone is placed in the ear canal and a sound source in the nose. Opening of the ET increases the sound pressure in the ear canal which can be documented.

- Imaging studies should be reserved for cases where additional or alternate pathology is suspected based upon history or examination.

Role of Eustachian Tube Dysfunction in Middle Ear Disease

Poor ET function in early life leads to poor pneumatization of the temporal bone. This can predispose to chronic middle ear disease. The middle ear is important for exchange of air while the mastoid bone with the air cells act as a reservoir for air. These are compromised in ETD.

Clinical Scenarios due to ETD

Several clinical conditions are produced by the poor functioning of the ET:

- *Acute otitis media occurs* commonly due to spread of upper respiratory infection through the ET. Stagnation of secretions in the middle ear due to poor clearance may be caused by edema of the ET mucosa.
- *Permanent perforation* of the tympanic membrane (chronic otitis media, mucosal disease). A poorly functioning ET plays a role in persisting permanent perforation of the tympanic membrane. If tympanoplasty is to be carried out in these conditions, for optimum success, it should be determined that the ET is functioning normally.
- *Otitis media with effusion* occurs due to ETD which isolates middle ear space from the outside environment. The dysfunction can occur due to:
  - Obstruction by adenoids or tumors.
  - Due to functional reasons such as cleft palate and in syndromic children.
  - Factors affecting the ET such as allergy, laryngopharyngeal reflux, and smoking (passive).
- *Retraction pockets and cholesteatoma*: They occur in conditions with long-standing, negative, middle ear pressure due to ETD. The retraction pockets on the tympanic membrane tend to form in the posterosuperior quadrant of the pars tensa and in the pars flaccida. A retraction pocket can eventually lead to a cholesteatoma.
- Other sequelae that can occur are tympanic membrane atelectasis, adhesive otitis media, tympanosclerosis, and cholesterol granuloma.

Pearl

The lining of the middle ear mucosa absorbs the trapped air creating negative pressure, as the partial pressure of gases in the middle ear is less than that of the blood stream. This causes retraction of the tympanic membrane. Swallowing causes air to enter the middle ear to equalize the pressure when the tube is normal or there is a partial obstruction.

Case-Based Question

1. **A 20-year-old student was traveling home after exams, by plane. As the plane was descending, he developed severe pain in the right ear. The pain disappeared after landing. On enquiry, he gave a history of an upper respiratory tract infection 3 days prior to travel by plane. On examination of the right ear, the tympanic membrane was not congested but retracted. The patient was not febrile.**

   a. What is the likely diagnosis?
   b. What is the pathophysiology of the pain on descent of the plane?
   c. What investigations would you order for this patient?
   d. How will you treat this condition?

   Answers
   a. ETD. The second possibility is acute otitis media (AOM), but since the tympanic membrane was not congested and the patient at the time of examination had neither ear pain or fever, it can be excluded.
   b. Since the patient had a prior history of upper respiratory tract infection which was resolving, there might have been edema of the mucosa of the ET. As the plane descends, the pressure of the air in the middle ear is less than the outer atmospheric pressure. The negative middle ear pressure causes the tympanic membrane to get retracted and the ET, due to dysfunction, gets locked by the higher outer external pressure. This leads to ear pain. The pain subsides a short time after landing.
   c. Otomicroscopy to look for any evidence of infection and retraction. Tympanometry will usually be a "C" type curve denoting negative middle ear pressure.
   d. Treatment consists of ways to improve ET patency. This includes systemic and topical nasal decongestants, steroid nasal sprays, and Valsalva maneuver if there is no nasal infection.

Frequently Asked Questions

1. What is the etiology of ETD?
2. What symptoms do patients with ETD present with?
3. Name the common investigations that can be ordered to diagnose ETD.
4. How will you manage ETD due to allergic rhinitis?
5. What are the clinical sequela of long-term ETD?
6. How will you perform Valsalva maneuver?
7. What finding will you expect in tympanometry in a patient with ETD?

Endnote

The first description of the ET was thought to be by Bartolomeo Eustachio, a sixteenth-century Italian anatomist, in 1563. He described it as a tube for draining pathological material from the middle ear. But the ancient Greeks had already described a tube which connected the air in the ear to the rest of the body.

Antonio Valsalva gave details of the cartilaginous, membranous, and osseous parts of the tube and described a muscle which helps to open the tube in 1704. His observations on the functions of the ET resulted in the Valsalva maneuver, which at that time was used to expel pus from the middle ear into the external auditory canal.

19 Tumors of the Ear

Navneeta Gangwar

> The competency covered in this chapter is as follows:
> EN2.11 Describe and identify malignant and premalignant ENT diseases by clinical examination.

Introduction

Tumors of the external ear can be classified into benign and malignant.

Common benign tumors of the external auditory canal include:

- Osteoma.
- Exostosis.

Malignant tumors of the temporal bone are uncommon. The etiological factors that have been proposed are:

- Chronic suppurative otitis media.
- Previous radiotherapy.
- Chronic exposure to ultraviolet rays.

Tumors of the Auricle

The tumors of auricle are uncommon and less known. Malignant tumors are more commonly encountered than their benign counterpart. **Table 19.1** outlines the benign and malignant tumors of the auricle.

■ Malignant Tumors of Auricle

The most common malignant tumor of auricle is squamous cell carcinoma (SCC). The second most common is basal cell carcinoma (BCC).

Squamous Cell Carcinoma

Figs. 19.2 and **19.3** show squamous cell carcinoma of pinna.

Etiology

- Prolonged exposure to ultraviolet radiation (SCC > BCC).
- Actinic keratosis (60% chances of SCC).
- Keratoacanthoma.

- Exposure to radiation.
- Immunosuppression (5- to 16-fold).

Treatment

For small lesions with no nodal metastasis, wide excision with 1 cm margin is sufficient.

In large tumors within 1 cm of the external auditory canal with nodal metastasis, en bloc resection of lateral temporal bone, superficial parotidectomy, and neck dissection followed by postoperative radiotherapy are performed. A prosthesis may be used for reconstruction of the pinna.

Basal Cell Carcinoma

BCC usually presents as a nodular ulcer with raised or beaded edge and central crust, which on removal results in bleeding (**Fig. 19.4**). It is common in elderly male of >50 years, and the usual sites are the helix and the tragus.

Treatment

Superficial skin lesions are treated with radiotherapy.

Lesions involving the cartilage require total amputation of the pinna with en bloc removal of the parotid gland.

Table 19.1 Benign and malignant tumors encountered on the pinna

Benign tumors	Malignant tumors
Papilloma Chondroma Hemangioma Fibroproliferative dermal tumor (Keloid) **(Fig. 19.1)** Schwannoma Angioleiomyoma	Squamous cell carcinoma Basal cell carcinoma Malignant melanoma

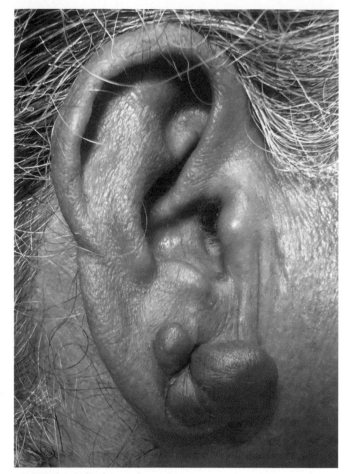

Fig. 19.1 Keloid over the right ear.

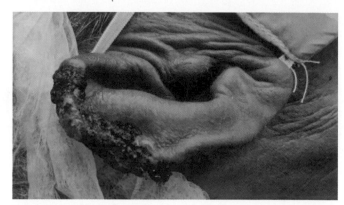

Fig. 19.2 Squamous cell carcinoma of the right pinna.

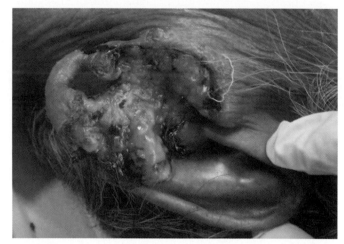

Fig. 19.3 Squamous cell carcinoma of the pinna, upper half.

Tumors of External Auditory Canal

Tumors of the external auditory canal can be benign or malignant (**Table 19.2**).

■ Malignant Tumors of the External Auditory Canal

Most malignancies of the temporal bone arise from the pinna because of chronic exposure to sunlight and they tend to be BCC or SCC. These tumors tend to extend into the external auditory canal.

Primary tumors of the external auditory canal tend to occur in ears with chronic inflammation such as those due to chronic otitis media with otorrhea and cholesteatoma.

Embryonal Rhabdomyosarcoma

This is a rare tumor of external auditory canal which arises from the embryonic muscles or tissue (pluripotent mesenchyme). It is more common in children.

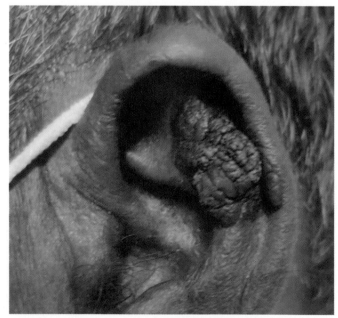

Fig. 19.4 Basal cell carcinoma of the left pinna.

Table 19.2 Benign and malignant tumors of the external auditory canal

Benign tumors	Malignant tumors
Papilloma (**Fig. 19.5**)	Squamous cell carcinoma
Fibroma	Basal cell carcinoma
Osteoma/exostosis	Adenoid cystic carcinoma
(**Fig. 19.6**)	Adenocarcinoma
Chondroma	Embryonal rhabdomyosarcoma
Angioma	Malignant melanoma
Adenoma	Carcinoid tumors

Clinical Features

- Early cases mimic chronic suppurative otitis media, and present with ear discharge, polyp, or granulations.
- Facial palsy occurs early.
- Swelling in the region of the ear.

Management

- Biopsy confirms the diagnosis.
- Treatment is a combination of radiotherapy and chemotherapy. Surgery is considered in select localized tumors.

Squamous Cell Carcinoma

This is commonly seen in the bony external auditory canal and presents with blood-stained ear discharge with an ulcerating mass (**Fig. 19.7**). It may spread to the middle ear and other parts of temporal bone, parotid gland, and skull base. In advanced cases, it can produce pain and facial nerve paralysis.

It may also present as refractory otitis externa (**Fig. 19.8**).

Investigations

- Punch biopsy to confirm the diagnosis.
- Contrast-enhanced computed tomography (CT) scan.
- Pure tone audiometry.

Treatment

- Radiotherapy has been tried for early malignancy.
- Surgery:
  - Lateral temporal bone resection in early cases.
  - Subtotal/total temporal bone resection in advanced cases.

There is a need to do a superficial or total parotidectomy in most cases with or without resection of the upper part of ramus and condyle of the mandible for clearance. Neck dissection is done when the lymph nodes in levels II, III, and Va are involved.

- Palliative radiotherapy or chemotherapy for inoperable cases.
- Postoperative radiotherapy with or without chemotherapy is given for advanced malignancy.

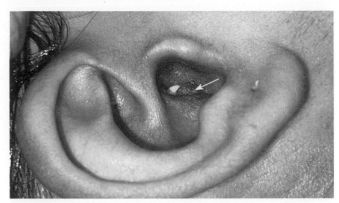

Fig. 19.5 Squamous papilloma of the external auditory canal.

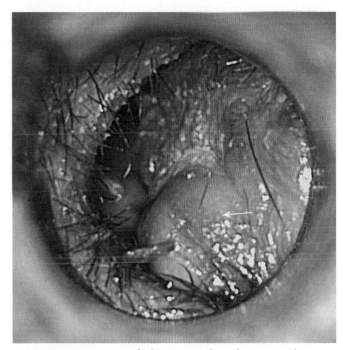

Fig. 19.6 Osteoma of the external auditory canal. Note: Exostosis and osteoma are covered in Chapter 7 "Diseases of the External Ear."

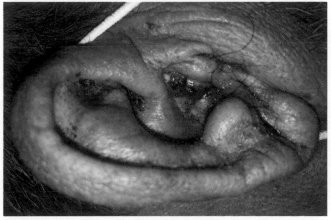

Fig. 19.7 Squamous cell carcinoma presenting as an ulceroproliferative mass in the external auditory canal.

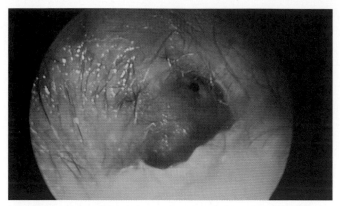

Fig. 19.8 Adenoid cystic carcinoma of the external auditory canal which presented as refractory otitis externa.

Tumors of Middle Ear

There is a wide range of middle ear tumors. The benign ones are more common than the malignant tumors. The classification is given in **Table 19.3.**

■ Temporal Bone Paragangliomas

Synonyms: Glomus tumors, nonchromaffin paraganglioma, chemodectoma

Paragangliomas are benign, slow-growing, locally invasive, highly vascular tumors which originate from cells of the neural crest.

In the temporal bone, they are present in relation to:
- The dome of jugular bulb.
- Ninth cranial nerve (Jacobson's nerve).
- Tenth cranial nerve (Arnold's nerve).

Based on their site of origin they are classified as:
- Jugular.
- Tympanic (over promontory).
- Jugulotympanic paragangliomas.

Other sites in the head and neck are in relation to the carotid bifurcation (carotid body tumors), along the vagus nerve (intravagale), and larynx.

Etiopathogenesis

Paragangliomas are the most common true neoplasms of the middle ear. Females are more commonly affected than males (6:1). The peak incidence is in the fifth decade of life. It is characterized by locally aggressive behavior with destruction of bone and soft tissues and can extend from the temporal bone intracranially or into the upper neck.

It may be hereditary (autosomal dominant) and is also associated with phakomatoses (Von Recklinghausen neurofibromatosis, Sturge-Weber syndrome, tuberous sclerosis, and von Hippel-Lindau disease) and multiple endocrine neoplasia type I (MEN I) syndrome. Of these glomus tumors, 10% can be multicentric.

Table 19.3 Classification of middle ear tumors

Benign tumors	Malignant tumors	
Paraganglioma Adenoma Osteoma Neurinoma Hemangioma	**Primary**	**Secondary**
	Squamous cell carcinoma Sarcoma Adenocarcinoma	Tumors of nasopharynx can extend into middle ear

Pearl

Phakomatoses are a broad group of congenital disorders affecting the brain, spine, and peripheral nerves and is also known as neurocutaneous syndromes.

Although the paraganglionic cells usually contain catecholamines (in the chromaffin cells) and are included in the diffuse neuroendocrine system (DNES), these tumors usually do not secrete hormone. They do not stain positive with chromium salts. But 1% of paragangliomas display functionally significant hormone secretion like catecholamines, metanephrine, etc.

Histopathology

- Paragangliomas are deep red, firm, rubbery masses that bleed profusely during manipulation.
- Microscopically they show clusters of chief cells (zellballen pattern), enclosed by fibrous septa and surrounding cells within a vascular network. Unmyelinated nerve fibers are also found scarcely.

Pearl

A zellballen is a small group of chromaffin cells with pale eosinophilic staining. These various groups are separated by fibrovascular stroma. A zellballen pattern is characteristic of paragangliomas.

Clinical Features

The symptoms are insidious in onset:
- Tinnitus is the commonest presenting symptom. It is pulsatile and reduces by compression over the jugular vein in the neck.
- Conductive hearing loss. Rarely, in advanced lesions, it may be mixed.
- Aural pain and aural fullness.
- Dizziness is uncommon and indicates extension into the inner ear.
- Large tumors can cause symptoms due to compression of cranial nerves VII, VIII, IX, X, XI, and XII.
- Otorrhea, when present, is usually blood-stained. Bleeding is common and may be profuse and unprovoked, especially after attempted manipulation.

Signs

- Tympanic membrane may have a bluish tinge.
- Pinkish mass can be seen behind intact tympanic membrane (*rising sun sign*).
- *Brown's sign*—blanching when positive pressure (with Siegel's speculum) is applied on the tympanic membrane.
- Polyp may be seen coming out through a perforation and extending into the external auditory canal.
- *Aquino's sign*—blanching of the tympanic membrane with gentle pressure on the ipsilateral carotid artery.
- Tachycardia, arrhythmias, flushing, or labile hypertension.
- Jugular foramen syndrome, that is, insidious onset of neuropathy of the lower cranial nerves (cranial nerves IX, X, and XI).
- Hypoglossal nerve paralysis (occipital extension).
- Horner's syndrome due to involvement of superior cervical ganglion (sympathetic).

Diagnosis

- Plain X-ray (jugular foramen view) shows expansion and erosion of the jugular foramen. It is not commonly done nowadays.

- Contrast-enhanced CT scan will show an enhancing lesion with loss of crest of bone between carotid canal and jugular foramen in glomus jugulare tumor. This is also known as *Phelp's sign*. The extent of the lesion can also be delineated (**Figs. 19.9** and **19.10**).
- Magnetic resonance imaging (MRI) with gadolinium contrast is the preferred imaging modality. The T1 image will show an avidly enhancing mass with a *salt and pepper pattern*.
- Carotid angiography will confirm the vascularity of the tumor and the feeding vessels, which can be selectively embolized (**Fig. 19.11**).
- Jugular venography.
- Impedance audiometry may show oscillations with the pulsations.
- Urinary vanillylmandelic acid (VMA) and serum catecholamine levels.

Fisch Classification of Glomus Tumors

Glomus tumors are classified into:
- *Type A:* Tumor confined to the middle ear.
- *Type B:* Tumor extending to the mastoid (tympanomastoid).

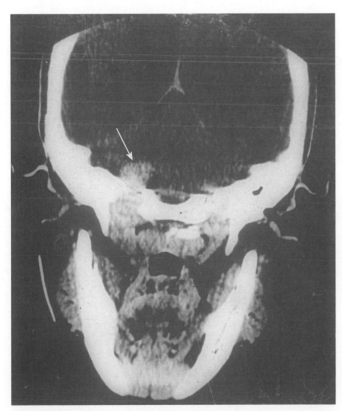

Fig. 19.9 Coronal computed tomography (CT) scan with contrast showing a jugular paraganglioma with intracranial extension.

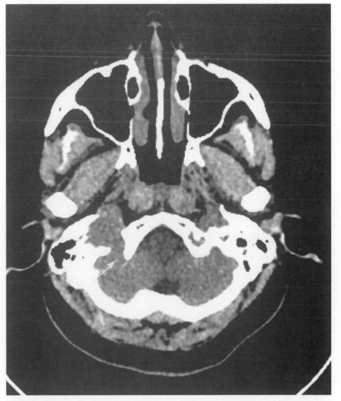

Fig. 19.10 Axial computed tomography (CT) scan showing spread intracranially.

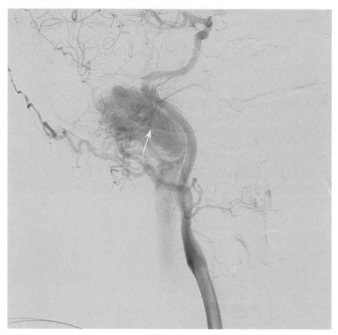

Fig. 19.11 Right side carotid angiography showing the tumor blush of the paraganglioma.

- **Type C**: Tumor with labyrinthine and infralabyrinthine spread extending up to the petrous apex:
  - *C1*: Limited involvement of the vertical portion of the carotid canal.
  - *C2*: Significant involvement of vertical portion.
  - *C3*: Invasion of the horizontal portion of the carotid canal.
- **Type D:** Intracranial extension:
  - *D1*: <2 cm in diameter.
  - *D2*: >2 cm in diameter.

Treatment

Observation

In patients with minimal symptoms, particularly older patients, serial MRI is done to assess the growth of the tumor and the patient is kept on regular follow-up.

Radiotherapy

This is used as a treatment for elderly patients with symptomatic tumors or for patients who are unwilling to undergo surgery. Stereotactic radiation may be used postoperatively in patients in whom the tumor could not be completely removed.

Surgery

Microsurgical removal of the tumor is the current treatment of choice especially in young patients. Preoperative embolization can be done to decrease the vascularity of the tumor. The tumor is supplied by multiple branches of the external carotid artery, more commonly the ascending pharyngeal artery. If internal carotid artery compromise is expected, a balloon occlusion or stenting is done preoperatively. The surgical approach varies according to type and extent of the tumor:

- Type A: Transmeatal tympanotomy approach.
- Type B: Extended facial recess approach.
- Type C: Fisch infratemporal approach.
- Type D: Skull base approach with posterior fossa craniotomy.

Tumors of the Inner Ear

■ Tumors of Inner Ear or Cerebellopontine Angle

Vestibular Schwannoma

Synonyms: Acoustic neuroma, neurilemmoma

It is a slow-growing, encapsulated benign tumor of the eighth cranial nerve which constitutes 80% of cerebellopontine tumors and 10% of brain tumors.

Pathology

It is composed of elongated spindle cells with rod-shaped nuclei lying in rows or palisades (Antoni A and Antoni B). Malignant transformation is very rare. Small tumors are pink/yellow and rubbery, whereas large ones are more yellow, mottled, and cystic. Neurofibromatosis type 2 can present with bilateral vestibular schwannoma.

Origin and Growth

It is usually seen in the 30 to 60 years age group with equal sex predilection. It arises from Schwann cells of vestibular nerve in the internal auditory meatus. It gradually grows into the cerebellopontine angle involving cranial nerve V anterosuperiorly and cranial nerves IX, X, and XI inferiorly. In the late stages, it displaces the brainstem and cerebellum and causes raised intracranial tension which can lead to death (**Fig. 19.12**).

Clinical Features

- Unilateral, progressive, sensorineural hearing loss with gross impairment of speech discrimination.
- High-pitched, continuous tinnitus.
- Vestibular symptoms are mostly imbalance as the tumor grows slowly and compensation occurs.
- Features of cranial nerve involvement includes:
  - Cranial nerve V: Numbness and paresthesia of face, reduced corneal sensitivity. It is the earliest to get involved.

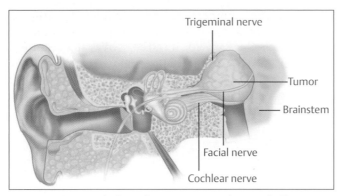

Fig. 19.12 Vestibular schwannoma in the cerebellopontine angle.

- – Cranial nerve VII: Sensory fibers are affected first leading to numbness of posterior aspect of meatus (*Hitzelberger's sign*), loss of taste of anterior two-thirds of tongue on electrogustometry, decreased lacrimation on Schirmer's test, and delayed blink reflex.
  - – Cranial nerves IX and X: Dysphagia, hoarseness, and nasal regurgitation due to pharyngeal, laryngeal, and palatal paralysis.
  - – Cranial nerves III, IV, VI, XI, and XII are involved by large tumors.
- Ataxia and imbalance (with nystagmus) are seen in cerebellar involvement.
- Weakness and numbness in limbs due to brainstem involvement.
- Headache, nausea, vomiting, blurring of vision, and diplopia in raised intracranial tension.

Investigations

- Pure tone audiometry shows unilateral sensorineural hearing loss, initially involving high frequencies.
- Speech discrimination score is diminished and disproportionate to pure tone hearing loss. Roll over phenomenon is present. (Roll over phenomenon is seen in retrocochlear pathology where the speech discrimination scores decrease as the sound intensity increases.)
- Recruitment is not present and stapedial reflex is absent. Threshold tone decay test is positive.
- Caloric test shows a diminished or absent response.
- Complete neurological evaluation and fundus examination are needed to rule out papilledema.
- MRI with gadolinium enhancement is the investigation of choice. It can detect small intracanalicular (internal acoustic meatus) tumors. Its relation to the surrounding structures including cerebellum and brainstem can be noted (**Fig. 19.13**).
- Contrast-enhanced CT scan can be done.
- Brainstem evoked response audiometry (BERA) is useful in retrocochlear lesions. A delay of >0.2 ms in "wave V" between the two ears is significant.

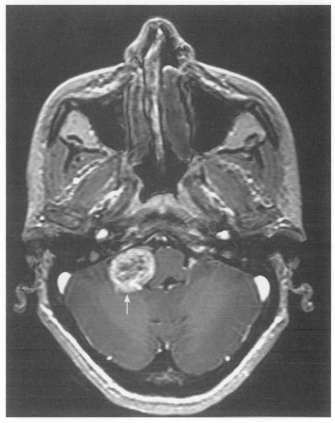

Fig. 19.13 Magnetic resonance imaging (MRI) with gadolinium contrast showing a vestibular schwannoma in the right cerebellopontine angle.

- Vestibular evoked myogenic potentials (VEMP) can help in identifying whether tumor is arising from superior or inferior division of the vestibular nerve.
- *Vertebral angiography* helps in differentiating cerebellopontine angle tumors.

Pearl

Unilateral, progressive, sensorineural hearing loss associated with poor speech discrimination, with or without tinnitus, warrants an MRI to rule out cerebellopontine angle tumors such as vestibular schwannoma.

Staging

Tumors are classified into following grades:
- Intracanalicular.
- Small (1.5 cm).
- Medium (1.5–4 cm).
- Large (4 cm).

Grading can also be done based on the hearing and speech discrimination score or based on the word recognition score which may help in deciding the treatment and surgical approach.

Differential Diagnosis

- Meningioma.
- Epidermoid cyst.
- Arachnoid cyst.
- Schwannoma.
- Lipomas.
- Cholesterol granulomas.
- Cholesteatoma.
- Aneurysm.
- Metastasis.

Treatment

- *Wait and watch policy* is for small tumors which do not show significant growth and in elderly patients in whom the symptoms are not pronounced.
- *Surgery* is the treatment of choice. The approach depends on the size and extent of the tumor, and on the hearing loss and speech discrimination:
  - Hearing preservation approaches (when the speech discrimination score is good) are the middle cranial fossa approach, the retrolabyrinthine approach, and the retrosigmoid approach.
  - In severe hearing loss with poor speech discrimination, the translabyrinthine approach is used. It avoids brain retraction and thereby, postoperative edema.
  - A combined translabyrinthine-suboccipital approach may be used for total removal of large tumors in contact with the brainstem.

- Stereotactic gamma irradiation therapy is helpful in reducing the size of tumor or altering the biology of the tumor to reduce growth. It can be used as an alternate to primary surgery or for residual tumors.
- When there is a bilateral tumor (as in neurofibromatosis type 2) which has been removed, a brainstem implant can be done for hearing rehabilitation.

Points to Ponder

- Malignancy of the pinna and external auditory canal are not common.
- External auditory canal malignancy can present as refractory otitis externa.
- Paragangliomas of the temporal bone are located in relation to the jugular bulb, Jacobson's nerve, or Arnold's nerve.
- Surgical approach to the paragangliomas depend on the extent of the lesion.
- Unilateral tinnitus with progressive sensorineural hearing loss, with or without imbalance, requires an MRI with contrast to rule out a vestibular schwannoma.
- Treatment of a vestibular schwannoma depends on the size and extent, and on the hearing loss and speech discrimination. Small tumors, especially in the elderly, can be kept on follow-up.

Case-Based Questions

1. **A 45-year-old woman presented with left-sided pulsatile tinnitus. Examination of the left tympanic membrane showed a pinkish red mass behind an intact tympanic membrane. The audiogram showed a conductive hearing loss on the left.**

   a. What is the possible diagnosis?
   b. What could happen with siegelization?
   c. What is the radiological investigation done and why?
   d. What is the role of angiography?

   Answers
   a. Left tympanic or jugulotympanic paraganglioma.
   b. Blanching of the tumor—Brown's sign.
   c. Contrast-enhanced CT scan or MRI. Highly enhancing mass is suggestive of a vascular tumor. MRI may show a salt and pepper appearance. The site and extent can be delineated.
   d. Angiography will confirm the vascular tumor (tumor blush) and the feeding vessels. The artery (feeding vessel) can be selectively embolized.

2. **A 54-year-old male presented with right-sided persistent tinnitus. There is progressive hearing loss over the last 8 months. A pure tone audiogram showed a right-sided severe sensorineural hearing loss. He had some imbalance while walking.**

   a. What is the most likely diagnosis?
   b. What is the radiological investigation of choice?
   c. What are the other audiological investigations that are done?
   d. If there was a bilateral lesion that has been removed, how can hearing rehabilitation be done?

   Answers
   a. Right vestibular schwannoma.
   b. MRI with contrast (with gadolinium).
   c. Brainstem evoked response audiometry and speech discrimination score. If the speech discrimination score is poor, a translabyrinthine approach can be used for tumor removal as the hearing preservation is not required.
   d. Brainstem implant.

Frequently Asked Questions

1. What is Brown's sign?

2. What is Phelp's sign?

3. What are the common sites of paragangliomas in the head and neck?

4. What is Hitzelberger's sign?

5. Enumerate the investigations that are done for a vestibular schwannoma.

6. What are paragangliomas of the temporal bone? What are the relevant investigations that should be carried out?

Endnote

Gamma knife surgery is not a traditional surgery but a form of radiation therapy. It uses computer-guided software to deliver highly focused radiation to a small, precise location in the brain. The radiation beam follows the contour of the tumor while sparing normal tissues. The indications for gamma knife surgery include benign and malignant tumors of the brain, vestibular schwannomas, arteriovenous malformations, tremors of Parkinson's disease, and trigeminal neuralgias. Since the 1990s, gamma knife radiosurgery has become popular and is widely used as the first line of treatment for small- to medium-sized vestibular schwannomas where there is no mass effect on the brain or hearing loss.

20 Anatomy of the Nose and Paranasal Sinuses

Suresh Pillai and Tulasi Karanth

The competencies covered in this chapter are as follows:

EN1.1 Describe the anatomy and physiology of the ear, nose, throat, head, and neck.

AN37.1 Describe and demonstrate the features of the nasal septum, lateral wall of the nose, and their blood and nerve supplies.

AN37.2 Describe the location and functional anatomy of the paranasal sinuses.

AN37.3 Describe the anatomical basis of sinusitis and maxillary sinus tumors.

External Framework of the Nose

The nose gives an aesthetic shape to the face (**Fig. 20.1a, b**). Its projection also makes it prone to trauma. The osseocartilaginous framework is formed by bones and cartilages with adjacent connective tissue. The bony vault is formed by the paired nasal bones medially and the frontal (ascending) process of the maxilla on either side. The nasal bones are thicker proximally and thinner distally.

The upper lateral cartilage attaches to the nasal bones cranially, the cartilaginous septum medially, and the lower lateral cartilage caudally. The lower lateral (alar) cartilage has a medial crus, intermediate crus, and lateral crus. Adjacent and lateral to the lateral crus of alar cartilage and the upper lateral cartilage are the sesamoid cartilages and fibrofatty connective tissue. The dorsal part of the cartilaginous nasal septum gives support to the cartilaginous external framework. The following are some pertinent points on the external nose:

- The *pyriform aperture* is formed by the caudal edge of the nasal bones and frontal process of the maxilla, along with the anterior ridge of the premaxilla up to the anterior nasal spine.
- The *nasion* is the deepest part of the curve between the glabella and the nasal dorsum (nasofrontal groove) where the frontal bone meets the two nasal bones.
- The *rhinion* is the site of attachment of the upper lateral cartilage to the tip of the nasal bones in the midline.
- The *scroll area* is the junction of the cephalic part of the lateral crus of the lower lateral cartilage with the caudal part of the upper lateral cartilage.

The external framework is covered by skin and subcutaneous tissue. The skin is thinner and more mobile in the upper half, and thicker, with sebaceous glands, and adherent in the upper part. The subcutaneous layer consists of a superficial fatty layer, subcutaneous musculoaponeurotic system, deep fatty layer, and the periosteum or perichondrium. The vessels and nerves traverse the deep fatty layer, and therefore care should be taken not to breach this layer, remaining deep to it, in the external rhinoplasty approach.

The arterial blood supply is from the branches of the facial and ophthalmic arteries and external nasal branches of the anterior ethmoidal and infraorbital arteries. The venous drainage is the facial and ophthalmic veins. The lymphatic drainage is to the submandibular and parotid group of lymph nodes.

Pearl

The facial vein communicates with the cavernous sinus via the ophthalmic vein through a valveless venous system. Infection from the nose (including the vestibule) and the upper lip (considered the *dangerous areas of the face*) can spread from these areas into the cavernous sinus (**Fig. 20.2**).

Nasal Cavity

The nasal cavity extends from the anterior nares to the choana through which it communicates with the nasopharynx. The anterior nares can have a varied shape and size depending on the columella and the alar rim. Each nasal

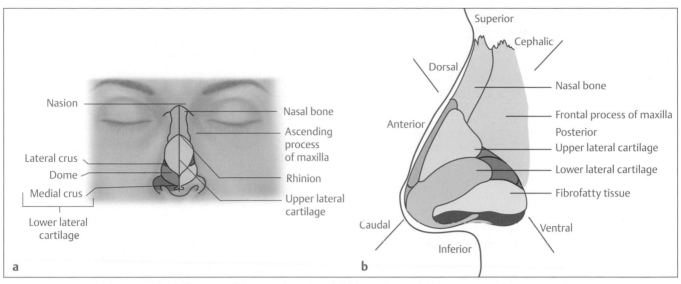

Fig. 20.1 External framework of the nose. **(a)** Frontal view and **(b)** lateral view (with anatomical orientation).

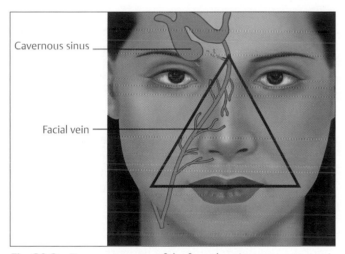

Fig. 20.2 Dangerous areas of the face showing an anastomosis between the facial vein and the cavernous sinus.

cavity has floor, lateral wall and roof with the nasal septum dividing the two sides. The floor is formed by the palatine process of the maxilla and the horizontal process of the palatine bone. The roof is formed from anterior to posterior by the nasal bones with adjacent frontal bone, the cribriform plate of the ethmoid bone and the sphenoid bone. The cribriform plate to sphenoid part slopes downwards from anterior to posterior.

Pearl

The roof of the nasal cavity in the region of the cribriform plate (the olfactory area) is considered the dangerous area of the nose as it is a route by which infection can spread intracranially from the nose.

■ Nasal Vestibule

It is at the entrance of the nasal cavity and is lined by skin with thick hair (vibrissae) and the sebaceous glands. It is bounded medially by membranous septum, caudal end of the cartilaginous septum and columella, and laterally by the ala. The vestibule ends at the limen nasi (lower end of the upper lateral cartilage), after which lies the respiratory epithelium. The external nasal valve is formed by the septum, alar rim (lateral crus of the lower lateral cartilage, with the sesamoid cartilages and fibrofatty tissue), and nasal sill (floor).

■ Nasal Septum

The nasal septum is an osseocartilaginous partition dividing the nasal cavity into right and left cavities. It also gives support to the dorsum and tip of the nose, and forms a part of the nasal valves.

Parts

It has three parts:
- Membranous.
- Cartilaginous.
- Osseous.

Relations with respect to the nasal septum are described in six directions: caudally (anteroinferiorly), cranially (posterosuperiorly), anteriorly, posteriorly, superiorly, and inferiorly.

Membranous Part

It is the part of the nasal septum lined by skin between the columella and the caudal end of the cartilaginous septum.

The caudal end of septal cartilage is covered by skin and it loosely inserts into the groove between the medial crura of the lower lateral cartilage. This insertion can be separated on palpation to leave a small region that is covered with skin on either side with no supportive structure in between. This part of the septum is called the membranous septum.

Pearls

- If the caudal end of the septal cartilage lies on either side of the medial crura, it is recognized on examination of the nasal vestibule as caudal dislocation. It is usually associated with an anterior deviated nasal septum to the opposite side.
- Freer's incision is an incision made over the part of the septal cartilage lined by skin during septoplasty. Incision here prevents mucosal tear during mucoperichondrial or mucoperiosteal flap elevation.

Cartilaginous Part

It is the anterior part of the septum formed by the septal cartilage (**Fig. 20.3**). The septal cartilage is a quadrangular-shaped cartilage with a tail-like extension posteriorly. Inferiorly, the septum lies in a groove called the maxillary crest. The maxillary crest supports the inferior portion of the septal cartilage with the anteroinferior part resting on the anterior nasal spine. Superiorly, the cartilage joins the upper lateral cartilage on either side. Cranially, the septal cartilage, along with the upper lateral cartilage, attaches to the nasal bones in a region called the *keystone area*. Posteriorly, the cartilage is attached to the perpendicular plate of the ethmoid (superiorly) and vomer (inferiorly). A part of the septal cartilage is continuous in a tail-like extension between the two bones. The septal cartilage is a support to the dorsum of the nose from the rhinion to the supratip area.

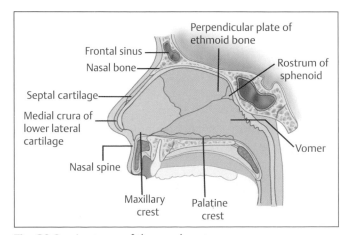

Fig. 20.3 Anatomy of the nasal septum.

The junction between the septal cartilage and the vomer can sometimes harbor an accessory olfactory epithelium called the *vomeronasal organ or Jacobson's organ*, which comprises tiny paired, blindly terminating channels. It is responsible for social and sexual behaviors in mammals, but the function is rudimentary in humans.

The *septal swell body* on the anterior part of the septum is a structure similar to the turbinate soft tissue consisting of venous sinusoids and glandular tissue, which can regulate airflow.

Pearls

- The *nasal spine* is a major support for the nasal dorsum and can cause external nasal deformity if removed.
- The *keystone area* is a site of attachment between the cartilaginous external nasal framework and the bony external nasal framework. Disruption of this region during surgery can lead to drooping of the tip and a dorsal hump.
- Subluxation of the septal cartilage from the maxillary crest results in a shelflike projection into the nasal cavity on that side with a groove on the crest on the opposite side.

Bony Part

It is the posterior part of the nasal septum. The superior part is formed by the perpendicular plate of the ethmoid. This is attached to the nasal bone and the frontal bone in its anterior end. It separates on either side of the olfactory groove as it runs posteriorly. In its posterior end, it is attached to the rostrum of the sphenoid. The inferior part is formed by the vomer, which is a quadrilateral bone lying on the maxillary crest anteriorly and the palatine crest posteriorly. The anterior border attaches to the septal cartilage and the perpendicular plate of the ethmoid. The posterior free border forms the posterior end of the septum, separating the choanae.

■ Lateral Wall of the Nose

The lateral wall of the nose is composed of the mucosa lined scroll-like structures named the superior, middle, and inferior turbinates (from above to below; **Fig. 20.4**). Spaces, covered by the scroll and lateral to it, are named as the respective meatus (superior meatus, middle meatus, and inferior meatus).

Parts

The parts of the lateral wall of the nose are the following: the external nasal valve, nasal vestibule, internal nasal valve, inferior turbinate and meatus, atrium, middle turbinate and middle meatus, and superior turbinate and meatus.

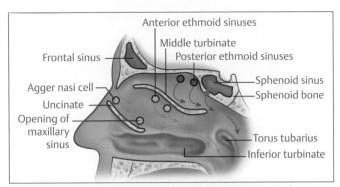

Fig. 20.4 Anatomy of the lateral wall of the nose. The *arrow* represents the direction of the mucociliary clearance pathway of the anterior (*green*) and posterior (*blue*) groups of sinuses.

The external nasal valve is at the most caudal part of the nasal orifice. The internal nasal valve is the area between the anterior end of the inferior turbinate laterally, caudal end of the upper lateral cartilage superiorly, and the corresponding portion of the septum medially.

Pearls

- The patency of the internal nasal valve can be tested by Cottle's test.
- Decreased fogging over a cold spatula improves with lateral retraction of skin overlying the nasolabial fold. Obstruction in the internal nasal valve requires functional rhinoplasty in addition to septoplasty to get symptomatic improvement for nasal block.

Inferior Turbinate

It is formed by the inferior concha bone, which is a scroll-like structure covered by the mucosa and the submucosal tissue. The bone articulates with the maxillary bone anteriorly and the perpendicular plate of the palatine bone posteriorly. The scroll increases resistance to inhaled air, thereby converting the turbulent inhaled air into laminar flow. The submucosal part of the inferior turbinate contains sinusoids, which have the capacity to swell up during parasympathetic activity and empty during sympathetic activity, thereby regulating nasal resistance and nasal cycle. The opening of the nasolacrimal duct is in the inferior meatus, 3 mm from the head of the inferior turbinate. The opening is controlled by Hasner's valve.

Pearl

Injudicious removal of the inferior turbinate during surgery should always be avoided. It may result in secondary atrophic rhinitis and empty nose syndrome.

Atrium of the Nose

It is the bony depression just anterior to the anterior end of the middle meatus.

Middle Turbinate

It is a part of the ethmoid bone. The anterior third attaches to the crista ethmoidalis of the maxilla (anterosuperior attachment) and superiorly to the lateral edge of the cribriform plate (and hence is oriented in the sagittal plane). It encloses the middle meatus formed mainly by the uncinate process, hiatus semilunaris, and bulla ethmoidalis. The second part of the middle turbinate (basal/ground lamella) slopes downward (oriented in the coronal plane) and attaches to the lamina papyracea, separating the anterior from posterior ethmoid sinuses. The third part is attached horizontally to the crista ethmoidalis of the perpendicular process of the palatine bone (oriented in the axial plane).

Middle Meatus

It contains mainly the uncinate process, hiatus semilunaris, and bulla ethmoidalis. The *uncinate process* is a sickle-shaped bony structure attached inferiorly to the inferior turbinate (horizontal part), and curves upward attaching to the lacrimal bone laterally (vertical part) and then runs superiorly. The superior attachment is variable. The superior attachment can be to the lamina papyracea laterally, the cribriform plate superiorly, or to the middle turbinate medially. This attachment decides the path of drainage of the frontal recess, that is, medial or lateral. The *hiatus semilunaris* is a space that drains the anterior group of the paranasal sinuses (maxillary, frontal, and anterior ethmoid sinuses).

The natural ostium of the maxillary sinus is usually situated deep into the pocket formed by the sickle-shaped uncinate (usually at the junction of its horizontal and vertical parts).

The frontal sinus drains into the anterosuperior aspect of the middle meatus at the frontal recess. The *frontal recess* is bounded by the agger nasi anteriorly, the bulla ethmoidalis posteriorly, the middle turbinate medially, and the lamina papyracea laterally. Its exact relation to the vertical part of the uncinate depends on the superior attachment of the uncinate process. The *bulla ethmoidalis* is the largest anterior ethmoidal air cell.

Superior Turbinate

It is also a part of the ethmoid bone, with the superior meatus lateral to it, into which drains the posterior ethmoid sinus. The sphenoid sinus drains into the sphenoethmoidal recess, which is between the nasal septum and the superior turbinate just above the choana.

Choana

It is the posterior aperture of the nasal cavity through which it communicates with the nasopharynx. It is bounded medially by the free edge of the vomer, inferiorly by the horizontal plate of the palatine bone, superiorly by the sphenoid body, and laterally by the medial pterygoid plates.

Blood Supply of the Nasal Cavity

The external and internal carotid systems contribute to the blood supply of the nasal cavity (**Fig. 20.5**).

Branches of the external carotid artery:

* The *sphenopalatine artery*, a branch from the maxillary artery, enters the nasal cavity through the posterior part of the middle meatus through the sphenopalatine foramen. The sphenopalatine artery branches into three to five branches just lateral to the foramen to supply the posterosuperior part of the lateral wall and the septum.
* The *greater palatine artery* enters the nasal cavity through the incisura foramen and supplies the inferior part of the nasal septum.
* The *superior labial artery* (septal branch) supplies the anteroinferior part of the septum.
* Branches of the facial artery supply the nasal vestibule, and nasal branches of the anterosuperior dental nerve supply part of the lateral wall of the nose.

Branches of the internal carotid artery:

* The *anterior ethmoidal artery* is a branch of the ophthalmic artery (which originates from the internal carotid artery). It originates in the orbit, enters the lateral lamella of the lamina cribrosa (supply to the meninges), and then reenters the nasal cavity to supply the septum.
* The *posterior ethmoidal artery* originates from the ophthalmic artery posterior to the anterior ethmoidal artery in the orbit and has a similar course to the anterior ethmoidal artery.

Venous Drainage of the Nasal Cavity

It occurs through veins with similar names as the arteries laterally and the ophthalmic veins superiorly, which in turn drain into the cavernous sinus. These veins are valveless and may contribute to spread of infection from one space to the other.

Pearl

Direction of blood flow from most of these arteries remains opposite to the direction of the inspired air. The flow is from posterior to anterior. This helps in warming and humidification through a process known as air conditioning.

Pearl

Kiesselbach's plexus (**Fig. 20.6**) is the arterial anastomosis between the four major vessels supplying the nasal septum (anterior ethmoidal artery of the internal carotid artery, posterior septal branch of the sphenopalatine artery, septal branch of the greater palatine artery, and septal branch of the superior labial artery, the latter three from the external carotid artery). This is seen in the anteroinferior part of the mucosa-lined cartilaginous septum. This region is also called Little's area and is a region prone to trauma, and a site for recurrent epistaxis.

Nerve Supply of the Nasal Cavity

The nerve supply to the nasal cavity can be divided into the following:

* Special senses (olfaction).
* Somatic nerve supply (through the branches of the trigeminal nerve).
* Autonomic nerve supply.

Olfaction is perceived in the olfactory area of the nose, which has an area of 2 to 5 cm² and comprises the cribriform plate area along with the adjoining parts of the nasal septum and the superior turbinate on either side. The olfactory cell bodies are situated in the olfactory epithelium. Twelve to 20 nerve fibers bundle together as filaments

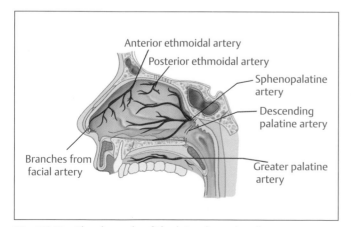

Fig. 20.5 Blood supply of the lateral nasal wall.

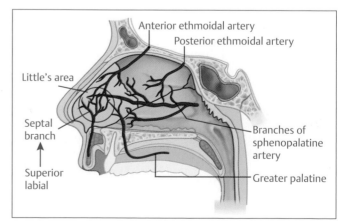

Fig. 20.6 Blood supply of the nasal septum showing Little's area (*black circle*).

and pass through the cribriform plate to the olfactory bulb where sensation is processed and signals are transmitted.

Somatic sensation or general sensory innervation to the nasal cavity is provided by ophthalmic and maxillary divisions of the trigeminal nerve through the following:

- Anterior ethmoidal nerve (anterosuperior part of the nasal septum and the lateral wall of the nose).
- Terminal branches of the greater palatine nerve (antero-inferior part of the nasal septum).
- Infraorbital nerve (vestibule).
- Sphenopalatine nerve (posterosuperior part of the nasal septum and the lateral wall of the nose).

Autonomic nerve supply has secretomotor and vasomotor actions, which are important for the functions of the nose.

- The sympathetic nerve supply (vasoconstriction) is provided by the postganglionic fibers of the T1 cervical sympathetic ganglion carried through the plexus covering the carotid arteries and its branches. This plexus branches off the carotid artery to form the deep petrosal nerve.
- The parasympathetic nerve supply (vasodilatation) is given off through the facial nerve, which leaves through its first genu to continue as the greater superficial petrosal nerve. The greater superficial petrosal nerve joins the deep petrosal nerve to form the vidian nerve. The vidian nerve traverses through the vidian canal to end in the sphenopalatine ganglion. Here, the postganglionic parasympathetic nerve fibers arise. The autonomic nerves join the sphenopalatine nerve to provide autonomic nerve supply to the nasal and paranasal cavities.

Pearl

Olfactory nerves may carry the meningeal layers with them as they traverse the cribriform plate. Injury to this region can result in cerebrospinal fluid (CSF) rhinorrhea, and possibly anosmia or hyposmia.

Anatomy of the Paranasal Sinus

Adjoining the nasal cavities are air-filled cavities called paranasal sinuses (**Fig. 20.7a, b**). The paranasal sinuses are divided into anterior and posterior groups based on their drainage pathway. The *anterior group of sinuses* are the following:

- Maxillary sinus.
- Frontal sinus.
- Anterior ethmoidal sinus.

All three drain into the middle meatus.

The *posterior group of sinuses* are the following:

- Posterior ethmoidal sinuses, which drain into the superior meatus.
- Sphenoid sinus, which drains into the sphenoethmoid recess.

■ Maxillary Sinus

It is also known as the antrum of Highmore, is a pyramidal-shaped sinus present in the body of the maxillary bone that has a capacity of 15 mL. The base of the pyramid is toward the lateral wall of the nose, while the apex is directed toward the zygomatic process. The bony medial

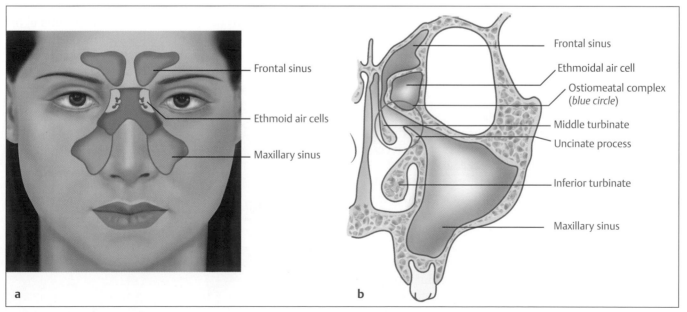

a

b

Fig. 20.7 **(a)** Position of the anterior group of sinuses in relation to the face and the orbit. **(b)** Paranasal sinuses of left side (coronalplane).

wall has a large (bony) dehiscence with a mucous membrane layer on either side (maxillary and nasal) with a small functional opening in the middle meatus. These two layers are called the fontanelle and are divided into anterior and posterior fontanelles based on its relation to the vertical part of the uncinate process. Accessory ostia (anterior in front of the uncinate process and posterior in the posterior part of the middle meatus) can form in these fontanelles. The posterior bony wall separates the maxillary sinus cavity from the pterygopalatine and infratemporal fossae. The superior bony wall forms the floor of the orbit. It houses a canal for the inferior orbital nerve. This canal may sometimes be dehiscent or hang into the sinus cavity with a mucosal mesentery. The floor is related to the maxillary teeth, mainly the second premolar and the first molar. The final shape and size of the maxillary sinus form after the secondary dentition. The ostium of the maxillary sinus opens in the superior part of the medial wall of the sinus, into the ethmoid infundibulum.

■ Frontal Sinuses

These are pneumatization in the frontal bone with a capacity of 4 to 7 mL. These are loculated with multiple incomplete septa. Inter-sinus septa is usually present and is usually oblique toward either side. The extent of pneumatization on either side is often variable and these are rarely symmetrical. It can be absent on one or both sides. The sinus drains through a small passage called the frontal recess. It is an hourglass-shaped conduit with the central constriction being formed by the frontal beak. These form after birth and are usually not seen on imaging till the age of 6 to 7 years. The floor forms a part of the roof of the orbit, and the posterior wall is related to the anterior cranial fossa.

■ Ethmoidal Air Cells

These are small multiple air cells in the ethmoidal bone or ethmoidal labyrinth on either side of the cribriform plate. These are divided into two main groups:
- The anterior ethmoidal air cells, comprising 10 to 15 cells, are the group of air cells anterior to the basal lamina (middle third of the middle turbinate as it curves downward) and drain into the middle meatus.
- The posterior ethmoidal air cells are the group of air cells posterior to the basal lamina and drain into the superior meatus.
- The *agger nasi air cell* is the anterior-most ethmoidal air cell present anterior to the frontal recess.
- The *bulla ethmoidalis* is the largest anterior ethmoidal air cell and is located posterior to the frontal recess.
- The *frontoethmoidal air cell* is the anterior ethmoidal air cell encroaching into the posterior table of the frontal bone.

- The *Haller cell* is the anterior ethmoidal air cell in the roof of the maxillary sinus adjacent to the maxillary ostium.
- The *Onodi cell* is an extension of the posterior ethmoidal air cell into the sphenoid sinus with the optic canal often within it.

■ Sphenoid Sinus

It occupies the body of the sphenoid (**Fig. 20.8**).

It develops after the age of 5 years and has a capacity of 0.5 to 3 mL. The extent of pneumatization within the sphenoid bone varies between individuals. The opening of the sphenoid is located in the anterior wall and the secretions drain into the sphenoethmoid recess, medial to the superior turbinate, and superior to the superior border of the choana.

Relations

- Superiorly is the anterior and middle cranial fossa, and it is related to the optic chiasm, optic nerve, and sella turcica with the pituitary gland. The endoscopic access for surgery to these structures can be through the sphenoid sinus.
- The lateral wall is related to the cavernous sinus, internal carotid artery, and the second to sixth cranial nerves. The optic canal and the internal carotid artery may lie dehiscent within the sinus. When the sphenoid is well pneumatized onto the optic nerve and internal carotid artery, the opticocarotid recess is present.
- The floor is related to the roof of the nasopharynx.

■ Ostiomeatal Complex

The ostiomeatal complex (OMC) is the functional unit of the paranasal sinuses (**Fig. 20.9**). It is the common pathway for ventilation and drainage. The anterior OMC refers to drainage of the anterior group of sinuses and the posterior OMC unit refers to drainage of the posterior group of sinuses.

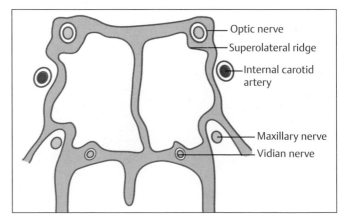

Fig. 20.8 Neurovascular relations of the sphenoid sinus.

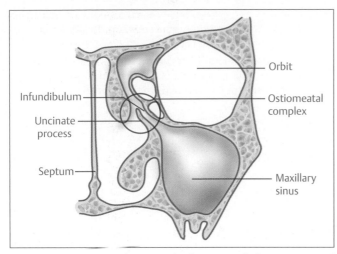

Fig. 20.9 Diagram showing the location of the ostiomeatal complex.

The anterior OMC consists of the maxillary ostium, the ethmoid infundibulum (drainage pathway for the maxillary and anterior ethmoid cells into the hiatus semilunaris), the ethmoid bulla, the uncinate process, frontal recess, and the hiatus semilunaris (between the ethmoid bulla and the uncinate process).

Anteriorly, the OMC communicates with the nasal cavity and is related to the atrium and the agger nasi.

Posteriorly and superiorly, it is limited by the basal lamella. Inferiorly, it communicates with the middle meatus. Medially, it is limited by the middle turbinate and laterally by the lamina papyracea.

Anatomical variations that can obstruct the anterior OMC are the following:

- Deviated nasal septum.
- *Middle turbinate variations:* The concha bullosa (pneumatized middle turbinate) and the paradoxically bent middle turbinate.

- *Uncinate process:* Anteriorly curved prominent uncinate process (gives a double middle turbinate appearance), pneumatized uncinate process, and lateralized uncinate process.
- *Ethmoid bulla:* Over-pneumatized, Haller's cell.
- *Frontal recess:* Prominent agger nasi cell, frontal cells (I–IV), and frontal bullar cell.

Pearl

The *silent sinus syndrome* (SSS) is due to unilateral maxillary sinus hypoplasia causing facial asymmetry, hypoglobus (inferior displacement of the eyeball in the orbit), and painless enophthalmos in which the uncinate process is more superior and lateral in position, in direct contact with the inferomedial wall of the orbit, occluding the OMC.

Points to Ponder

- The external nose is bony in the upper one-third of the dorsum of the nose and cartilaginous in the lower two-thirds.
- The dangerous area of the face denotes the region from where infection can travel to the cavernous sinus through a network of valveless veins.
- The nasal bones are thicker proximally and thinner distally and is one of the commonest bones to be fractured in the human body.
- The nasal septum is a midline structure that divides the nasal cavity into two halves. It is cartilaginous anteriorly and bony posteriorly.
- Little's area, located in the anteroinferior part of the cartilaginous septum, is one of the commonest sites for epistaxis because of Kiesselbach's plexus.
- The OMC is a drainage pathway for the anterior group of sinuses. Obstruction to this pathway can lead to sinusitis.

Case-Based Questions

1. **A middle-aged man came to the ear, nose, and throat (ENT) clinic with complains of left-side facial pain and headache. Examination with a nasal endoscope revealed a large mass in the left OMC.**

   a. What is the OMC?

   b. What sinuses will be affected by a mass in the OMC?

   c. What is the next step of management?

   Answers

   a. The OMC is a drainage pathway for the anterior group of sinuses. It consists of a frontal recess, ethmoidal infundibulum, hiatus semilunaris, uncinate process, bulla ethmoidalis, and maxillary sinus opening.

   b. It will affect the anterior group of sinuses including the frontal, anterior ethmoidal, and maxillary sinuses.

   c. Since a mass is present in the OMC leading to sinusitis, biopsy of the mass is the next step to determine whether it is benign or malignant.

2. **A 56-year-old man was brought into the emergency room (ER) after suffering facial injury following a road traffic accident. He was bleeding from the nose and on examination there was a bony crepitus over the nasal bones.**

   a. What is the commonest site for bleeding from the nose?

b. What is the reason for a bony crepitus over the dorsum of the nose?

c. What other important features should be ruled out in a patient with facial trauma?

Answers

a. Little's area is the commonest site of anterior epistaxis.

b. Fractures of the nasal bones lead to a bony crepitus. This is a grating sensation produced when the bony fractured ends rub against each other.

c. In all cases of nasal injury, especially to the upper part of the nose, CSF rhinorrhea should be ruled out. The commonest site for CSF leak is from the cribriform area.

Frequently Asked Questions

1. What are the parts of the bony septum?

2. Describe Kiesselbach's plexus.

3. What is the ostiomeatal complex?

4. By what age does the frontal sinus develop?

5. What is the importance of the Onodi air cell?

6. What are the lateral relations of the sphenoid sinus?

Endnote

Woodruff's plexus: This is a network of blood vessels located on the lateral nasal wall, posteriorly, below the inferior meatus. It was originally described by George H. Woodruff in 1949. This plexus has been frequently mentioned in the medical literature as one of the causes of posterior epistaxis. There was controversy as to whether this plexus of vessels is arterial or venous in nature. Studies of cadaveric specimens with microdissection conclusively proved that these vessels were large, thin-walled veins with poorly developed muscular walls. So these vessels have a greater tendency to bleed, leading to posterior epistaxis.

21 Physiology of the Nose and Paranasal Sinuses

Kailesh Pujary and Anusha Shashidhara Shetty

The competency covered in this chapter is as follows:

EN1.1 Describe the anatomy and physiology of ear, nose, throat, and head and neck.

Introduction

The nose, in addition to providing aesthetic value to the face, is a sensory and respiratory structure, and provides physical and immunological protection. The external nose and the sinonasal unit act as a gateway between the external environment and the human body. The inspired air is cleansed and humidified, and sampled for olfaction. Every structure within the sinonasal unit provides a defensive mechanism against the external environment.

There are five main functions of the nose:

- Respiration.
- Air conditioning (filtration, temperature control, and humidification).
- Protection of lower airway (vibrissae, mucociliary clearance, and sneeze reflex).
- Vocal resonance.
- Olfaction.

Respiration

- Human beings breathe naturally through their nose. Mouth breathing is not normal and is acquired at a later age. For example, in a newborn, bilateral choanal atresia, where the choanae are blocked, is a life-threatening condition as it could lead to death if the airway is not relieved immediately.
- Respiration occurs in two stages, namely, *quiet inspiration* and *expiration*:
  - In *quiet inspiration*, the inspired air enters the nasal cavity and encounters the inferior turbinate on either side. The shape and orientation of the turbinates streamline the inspired air posteriorly into the nasopharynx and provide sufficient resistance to change the airflow from laminar to a transitional pattern. In the mid-portion of the nasal cavity, there are laminar and turbulent flows which are important for the function of air exchange. Most of the air passes between the middle turbinate and the inferior turbinate. The turbinates (inferior, middle, and superior) contribute to the total surface area of the nasal cavity that aids in warming and humidifying the inspired air.
  - In *expiration*, the expired air re-enters the nasal cavity from the nasopharynx. It faces resistance from the internal nasal valve (angle between caudal border of upper lateral cartilages, septum, anterior end of inferior turbinates, and nasal floor) and changes the airflow into eddies which flow into the sinus ostia and ventilate the paranasal sinuses (**Figs. 21.1** and **21.2**). During expiration, the flow is less turbulent with less exchange of heat and metabolites which is important for recovery of the mucosa.

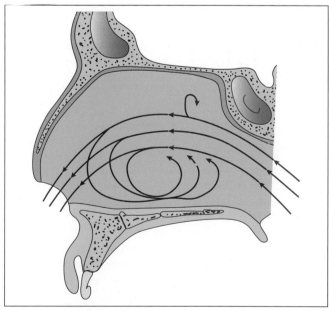

Fig. 21.1 Laminar airflow broken up into eddy currents in the internal nasal valve.

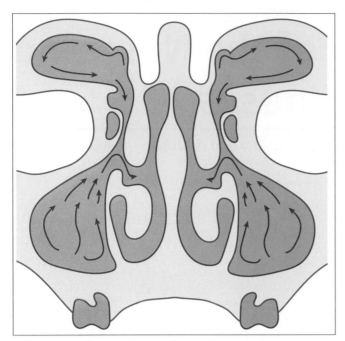

Fig. 21.2 Airflow ventilating the paranasal sinuses.

- The *anterior end of the inferior turbinate* is a dynamic structure as it increases and decreases in size to ensure that the air inspired can be warmed and humidified. Similar tissue on the anterior part of the nasal septum, the *septal swell body*, has the same function. The turbinates and the swell bodies contain arteries/arterioles (resistance vessels), and venules and sinusoids (capacitance vessels). The expansion and shrinkage affect the resistance and airflow. The nose contributes to approximately *50% of the airway resistance.*

Note: Complete nasal block can reduce pulmonary ventilation.

Pearl

The nasal resistance decreases during exercise and increases in facial palsy.

■ Nasal Cycle

- Even in a normal anatomical nasal airway, asymmetric airflow through the nose occurs due to changes in the volume of blood in the capacitance vessels. This is known as the *nasal cycle*. At any given time, only one side of the nasal airway is fully patent to airflow. The other nasal cavity is partially patent.
- A combination of neural and vasomotor input is responsible for the alternating engorgement and constriction of arterioles, precapillary sphincters, and venous sinusoids within the entire nasal mucosa.
- Rhinomanometry was used by investigators, and it was found that approximately 80% of normal individuals undergo this recurring process.

- The patency and congestion of the two sides alternate every 2 to 7 hours.
- Factors affecting nasal cycle:
  - Posture.
  - Infection.
  - Exercise.
  - Mucosal irritants.
  - Hormones.
  - Pregnancy.
  - Hypothyroidism and hyperthyroidism.
  - Temperature, humidity.
  - Drugs (topical, oral, parenteral).

Air Conditioning of Inspired Air

Humans inspire between 10,000 and 20,000 L of air per day. The inspired air is efficiently filtered, purified, humidified, and temperature-controlled before it enters the lungs:

- *Filtration and purification*: Inspired air first encounters the nasal *vibrissae* which are coarse hair follicles. They filter large aerosolized particulate matter. About 80% of the particles, 3 to 5 μm in diameter, and 60% of the particles, 2 μm in diameter, are filtered by the anterior part of the nose, either by getting trapped in the nasal vibrissae or by the mucous blanket. Turbulence helps in deposition of particles.
- *Temperature control*: Total surface area of the nasal cavity is increased by the turbinates which significantly contribute to warming and humidification of inspired air. At respiratory rates of up to 7 L/min, the nasal cavity can warm air to 37°C from ambient temperatures and can also cool the air to as low as 25°C. The humidity of inspired air is maintained at approximately 85%. This controlled humidity and temperature of air entering the lungs facilitates pulmonary alveolar gas exchange. Warm inspired air decreases the nasal airway resistance while cold air increases it.

Protection of Airway

This can occur through the following three mechanisms:
- Nasal vestibule vibrissae.
- Mucociliary mechanism.
- Sneeze reflex.

■ Nasal Vestibule Vibrissae

The vestibule of the nose is lined by stratified squamous epithelium containing sebaceous gland, sweat glands, and vibrissae, which act as a protective barrier. The vibrissae filter large particulate matter. The vestibule of the nose can sense the amount of airflow and hence regulate its entry with the help of the muscles.

■ Mucociliary Mechanism

Three factors contribute to the mucociliary mechanism (**Fig. 21.3**): (1) nasal mucosa, (2) mucus, and (3) cilia.

- *Nasal mucosa* from above downwards comprises epithelium bearing the goblet cells, basement membrane, lamina propria, and periosteum. Pseudostratified columnar epithelium lines the entire nasal cavity except the roof.
- Tiny hair-like projections referred to as cilia of length 1 to 2 μm arise from the superior surface of the columnar epithelium (respiratory epithelium). These cilia help to drain the mucus into the nasopharynx. The goblet cells, which are interspersed throughout the columnar epithelium, are responsible for mucus production.
- *Mucus* is produced by the goblet cells. It forms a blanket layer above the epithelium and traps the cellular debris and pathogens from the inspired air. The sinonasal mucosa produces approximately 600 to 1,800 mL of mucus. The mucus also contains proteins such as lactoferrin which aids in local immune defense. The IgA in the mucus prevents the adhesion of pathogens on the mucosa. The mucus also provides water for humidification. The turbulent airflow helps in deposition of particles on this mucous blanket.

Mucus consists of two layers (**Fig. 21.3**):
- – Gel phase: Viscous layer that ride along the tips of the cilia.
- – Sol phase: Present between the shafts of cilia and has lower viscosity as it is composed of water and electrolytes.

- *Cilia* are cylindrical organelles protruding from the surface of the respiratory epithelium. They beat in a coordinated to-and-fro manner in order to clear the mucous blanket containing pathogens and debris from upper and lower respiratory tract. Every epithelial cell bears around 50 to 200 cilia, measuring 5 to 7 μm in length. Each cilium has a rapid propulsive stroke and a slow recovery stroke. In the propulsive stroke, the cilia extend into the mucus and moves the mucous blanket in one direction toward the nasopharynx (**Fig. 21.4**). In the recovery stroke the cilia bend and travel back to their starting point. Hence, the mucociliary clearance is dependent on normal ciliary function and mucus composition.

In the paranasal sinuses, the mucociliary clearance is directed toward the ostium of that sinus (**Fig. 21.2**). It has a particular pattern; for example, in the maxillary sinus the pattern is stellate, starting from the floor, and is directed toward the maxillary ostium situated in the upper part of the medial wall.

Factors affecting the mucociliary mechanism:
- Primary ciliary dyskinesia (Kartagener's syndrome).
- Cystic fibrosis.
- Bacterial pathogens—*Hemophilus influenza, Streptococcus pneumonia, Staphylococcus aureus.*
- Viral pathogens.
- Age—reduces in elderly.
- Ciliary movement reduces when temperature is <32° C and >40° C.
- Medications—phenylephrine stimulates ciliary movement while benzalkonium chloride reduces it.

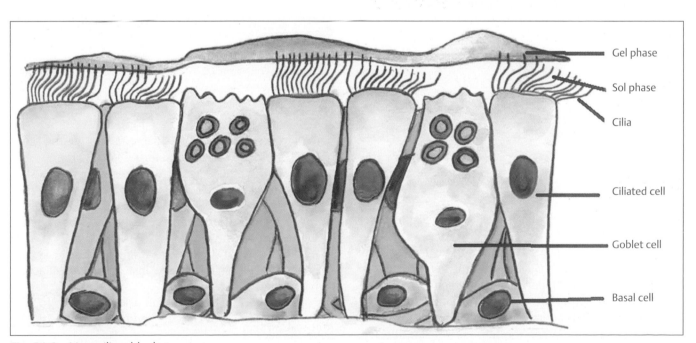

Fig. 21.3 Mucociliary blanket.

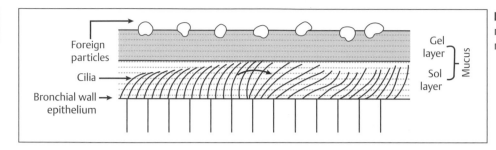

Fig. 21.4 Ciliary movement with rapid propulsive stroke and slow recovery stroke.

■ Sneeze Reflex

It is a protective mechanism that causes forceful nasal expulsion of air and secretions in response to a noxious stimulus. Three pathways (cranial and neural) are stimulated simultaneously (**Flowchart 21.1**).

Vocal Resonance

In phonation there are a few nasal consonants, M/N/NG, which pass through the nasopharyngeal isthmus and are emitted through the nose. Hence, the nose and nasopharynx act as a resonating chamber. When the nasal cavity and nasopharynx are blocked, consonants M/N/NG are uttered as B/D/G, respectively. This is termed as *rhinolalia clausa*.

The reverse uttering of consonants is true in velopharyngeal insufficiency, such as in cleft palate, where B/D/G are pronounced as M/N/NG. This is termed as *rhinolalia aperta*.

Pearl

Following are some of the nasal reflexes seen in humans:
- Submersion reflex: Due to nasal mucosal irritation there is apnea, bradycardia, glottic closure, and vasoconstriction.
- Nasal vasoconstriction due to cooling of the skin; warming of skin increases the nasal temperature.
- Nasobronchial reflex.

Olfaction

- Olfaction in humans is not as well developed as in other mammals.
- The sense of smell plays a vital role in the *quality of life (pleasure) and safety*. Quality of life is better when we enjoy the flavors of food we eat, have good social interactions, and appreciate our surroundings. Safety is in detecting noxious odors and sensing dangers like spoilt food and gas leak. When the sense of smell is affected, the taste sensation can also be affected as they are interrelated.
- The olfactory epithelium is situated in the olfactory cleft that comprises the roof of the nasal cavity which includes the cribriform plate, upper septum, and medial surface of superior turbinate.
- The epithelium consists of:
    - Olfactory mucosa (olfactory receptor neurons, sustentacular microvilli, and basal cells).
    - Lamina propria.
- The olfactory receptor neurons (ORNs) are bipolar neurons with dendrites extending to the epithelial surface and axons synapsing intracranially in the olfactory bulb. Odorants bind to the ORN and stimulate it by binding to a specific olfactory G protein.
- There are 350 different types of receptors; each receptor can detect around 100 similarly structured molecules.
- The molecule fits into the receptor like a lock and key, which releases a chemical cascade followed by an electrical signal sent to the center in the brain.
- Water and lipid soluble volatile substances can be smelt.

Pearl

The olfactory epithelium can regenerate within 100 days.

■ Olfactory Pathway and Smell Test

The olfactory pathway is outlined in **Fig. 21.5**. There are numerous commercial kits available for testing the sense of smell. These are mainly used for research purpose.

When performing simple bedside tests, observe the following principles:
- The substance tested should be aromatic. Example is coffee powder. There are scratch and sniff kits available for performing this.
- Avoid irritant substances like ammonia which can trigger the trigeminal pathway instead of the olfactory pathway.

For testing, block one nostril and ask the patient to sniff while keeping the eyes closed. Then repeat the test on the opposite side.

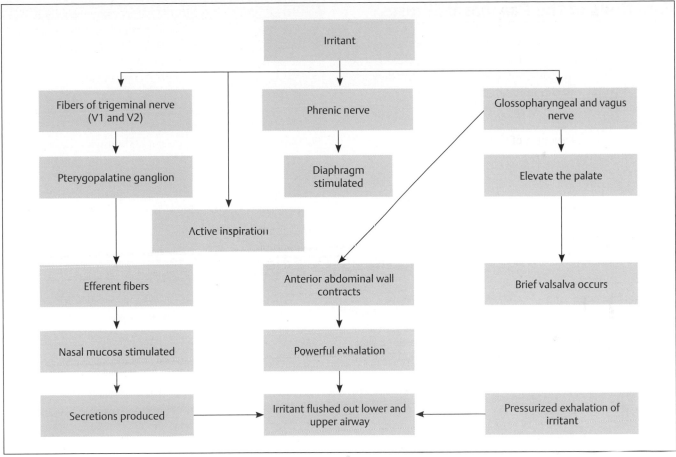

Flowchart 21.1 Three pathways involved in the sneeze reflex.

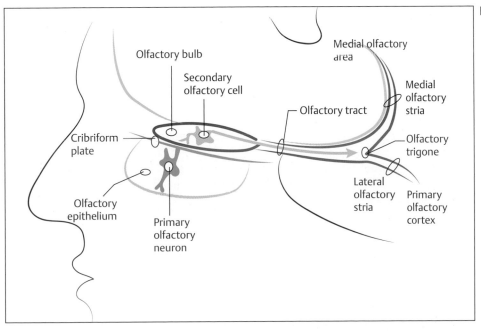

Fig. 21.5 Olfactory pathway.

Functions of the Paranasal Sinuses

The paranasal sinuses are air-filled spaces lined by respiratory epithelium present in the skull bones adjacent to the nasal cavities. Their functions are uncertain, but they are said to contribute to the following:

- Physical buffer against injury.
- Resonance of voice.
- Reduction of the weight of the skull.
- Humidification.
- Heat insulation.
- Air conditioning.
- Production of mucus.

Points to Ponder

- The nose is involved in five main functions: respiration, air conditioning, protection of lower airway, vocal resonance, and olfaction.
- Nasal cycle is physiological and occurs every 2 to 7 hours.
- Air conditioning involves filtration, humidification, and temperature regulation.
- Mucus is produced by goblet cells and has two layers, a gel phase and a sol phase.
- The sneeze reflex is a defense mechanism to expel foreign body and other noxious stimuli from the airway.

Case-Based Questions

1. **A middle-aged man came to the ear, nose, and throat (ENT) clinic with a history of alternating nasal obstruction of a few years duration. It varies with the position of the head. If he is sleeping on the right side, the right side would get blocked. He didn't suffer from any other symptoms. On examination of the nose, the septum was straight and there were no nasal masses. The right inferior turbinate was enlarged compared to the left.**

   a. What is the diagnosis?

   b. What is the explanation for this condition?

   c. What factors can abolish this?

   Answers

   a. Nasal cycle. It is physiological and normal. It is present in 80% of the population.
   b. Alternating congestion and decongestion of the turbinates is controlled by the autonomic nervous system.
   c. Exercise, drugs, hormones, infections, and posture.

Frequently Asked Questions

1. Enumerate the functions of the nose.
2. What are the functions of the paranasal sinuses?
3. What is mucociliary clearance, and what are the factors affecting it?
4. What is nasal cycle and, what are the factors affecting it?
5. Describe temperature regulation by the nasal cavity.

Endnote

Smell is closely related to memory and can trigger a strong emotional reaction. This link with memory is more intense when compared to the other senses. This is because olfaction is located in the same part of the brain that is responsible for regulating memory, emotions, and creativity. The olfactory neurons travel from the olfactory bulb to the amygdala and hippocampus. Impaired smell can be an early sign of cognitive decline and is seen in conditions like dementia and Parkinson's disease. Older people, unable to identify common odors, are twice as likely to develop dementia in 5 years when compared to those with normal sense of smell.

History Taking and Examination of Nose and Paranasal Sinuses

Meera Niranjan Khadilkar and Sushmitha Kabekkodu

The competencies covered in this chapter are as follows:

EN2.5 Demonstrate the correct technique of examination of the nose and paranasal sinuses including the use of nasal speculum.

PE28.12 Perform examination of the nose.

History Taking

- **Chief complaints**: List the presenting symptoms in chronological order.
- **History of presenting illness**: A detailed description of the presenting complaints regarding the onset, duration, progression, severity, aggravating and relieving factors, and other accompanying or related symptoms.
- **Past history**: Similar complaints in the past with any treatment taken, history of comorbidities such as diabetes, hypertension, asthma, coronary artery disease, bleeding disorders, and tuberculosis. History of surgeries in the past and history of allergy to medications, if any.
- **Personal history**: Patient's personal habits (smoking, alcohol consumption, chewing pan/tobacco), diet, sleep, bowel and bladder habits.
- **Family history**: Similar complaints in the family. The presence of genetic disorders in siblings and relatives.

Common Nasal Symptoms

■ Nasal Obstruction

It may be unilateral or bilateral (**Table 22.1**).

■ Nasal Discharge

This may be:
- *Clear*—early stage of viral rhinitis, cerebrospinal fluid (CSF) rhinorrhoea.
- *Mucoid*—allergic rhinitis, chronic inflammation.
- *Mucopurulent*—bacterial rhinosinusitis.
- *Purulent*—furuncle, foreign body.
- *Blood-stained*—foreign body, malignancy.

> **Pearl**
>
> *Reservoir sign* is seen in CSF rhinorrhoea. Trickling of CSF is noted when the patient switches from supine to sitting position with head bent forwards.

■ Postnasal Drip

It is a typical feature of sinusitis. There is a constant need to clear the throat (hawking), which is more pronounced on waking up in the morning. This is due to discharge passing from the nasal cavity to the nasopharynx and down into the oropharynx, along the posterior pharyngeal wall.

Table 22.1 Common causes of unilateral and bilateral nasal obstruction

Unilateral	Bilateral
C-shaped deviated nasal septum	S-shaped deviated nasal septum
Inferior turbinate hypertrophy	Bilateral inferior turbinate hypertrophy
Concha bullosa	Allergic rhinitis
Antrochoanal polyp	Ethmoidal polyps
Benign tumors	Septal hematoma
Malignancy	Lesions in the nasopharynx, e.g., adenoids
Foreign body of nose	

■ Crusting

It usually occurs due to a persistently dry nasal cavity, which is seen in atrophic rhinitis, rhinitis sicca, and nasal vestibulitis.

■ Sneezing

This is a feature of allergic rhinitis and vasomotor rhinitis. It is important to elicit history of diurnal and seasonal variation, and history of bronchial asthma in a patient with allergic rhinitis.

Pearl

Sternutation is the act of sneezing.

■ Itching

There may be itching of the nose or eyes as seen in allergic rhinitis.

Pearl

Cardinal symptoms of allergic rhinitis include:
- Nasal obstruction.
- Watery nasal discharge.
- Sneezing.
- Itching of nose.

■ Epistaxis

Bleeding from the nose may be unilateral or bilateral, anterior or posterior, mild/moderate/profuse, due to local, systemic, or idiopathic etiology (**Table 22.2**).

Pearl

Little's area: It is located in the anteroinferior part of the nasal septum where there is a network of blood vessels called *Kiesselbach's plexus*. It is formed by greater palatine artery, septal branch of sphenopalatine artery, septal branch of superior labial artery, and anterior ethmoidal artery.

Woodruff's plexus: It is also known as naso-nasopharyngeal plexus and is a network of veins. It is responsible for posterior epistaxis. It is located inferior to the posterior end of inferior turbinate.

Pearl

The sphenopalatine artery is also known as the artery of epistaxis. It is the terminal branch of the maxillary artery and has a major contribution in the blood supply to the nose. It is frequently involved in hypertensive epistaxis.

■ Anosmia/Hyposmia

Anosmia/hyposmia is absent or decreased smell perception. It may occur due to viral infections (influenza, COVID-19), nasal polyps, atrophic rhinitis, surgical trauma, head injury, olfactory neuroblastoma, and intracranial tumors.

■ Headache/Facial Pain

This is an associated symptom encountered in sinusitis.

Frontal Sinusitis

It presents with pain over the forehead, which is more pronounced during office hours. It starts on waking up in the morning and gradually increases during the day till noon and thereafter gradually subsides. Since it is present during working hours, it is also called office headache. This is because stasis of secretions occurs in the frontal sinus at night when the patient is supine. During the day, when the patient is upright, the sinus starts draining relieving the pressure and the pain.

Ethmoid Sinusitis

It produces pain between and behind the eyes, with or without periorbital swelling.

Maxillary Sinusitis

This causes facial pain or pain referred to the vertex of head with or without facial swelling. There may be pain along the maxillary teeth.

Sphenoid Sinusitis

It typically presents with deep-seated pain behind the eyes or pain radiating to the vertex or occipital region. It is also known as *occipital headache.*

Table 22.2 Common causes of epistaxis

Local causes	Systemic causes
Trauma to the nose and Little's area	Hypertension
Nasal malignancy	Bleeding disorders
Forceful blowing of nose, sneezing	Liver diseases
Juvenile nasopharyngeal angiofibroma	Vitamin K deficiency
Foreign body	Renal disease
Rhinosporidiosis	Leukemia
Granulomatous lesions in the nose	Use of anticoagulants

- There are many causes for headache. Migraine and tension headache are common. In migraine the symptoms are usually typical and includes unilateral throbbing headache with other symptoms like nausea and vomiting, and blurring of vision; certain trigger factors can precipitate it.
- Tension headache is like a tight band around the head. They may be part of the differential diagnosis or can be present along with sinusitis.

■ Snoring

It may occur due to nasal or nasopharyngeal obstruction.

■ Change in Voice

Patients may complain of hyponasal or hypernasal voice.

Hyponasality or Rhinolalia Clausa

This occurs when there is decreased airflow through the nose due to nasal or nasopharyngeal obstruction. Causes include deviated nasal septum, allergic rhinitis, common cold, nasal polyps, benign and malignant tumours of nose, and adenoid hypertrophy.

Hypernasality or Rhinolalia Aperta

This occurs due to increased nasal airflow. Causes include velopharyngeal insufficiency as a result of cleft palate, submucosal cleft, and adenoidectomy.

■ Hearing Loss

Patients with allergic rhinitis, sinusitis, and nasopharyngitis may experience eustachian tube obstruction or edema leading to otitis media with effusion (OME), which can result in conductive hearing loss.

Pearl

Unilateral serous otitis media in adults point toward nasopharyngeal tumor until proven otherwise. Examination of the nasopharynx by nasal endoscopy is mandatory.

■ Neck Swelling

Malignancy of nasopharynx may present with neck swelling as a result of cervical lymph nodal metastases in 70% of cases, typically in level II and level V lymph nodes. Maxillary sinus malignancy which spreads anteriorly to the soft tissues of the face may have a metastatic level I lymph node.

■ Cranial Nerve Palsy

Cranial nerves III, IV, V, etc., may be involved by malignant lesions of the nasopharynx and by inflammatory lesions which spread to the cavernous sinus.

Examination of the Nose and Paranasal Sinuses

The patient is seated upright in front of the examiner. Examination is performed using a head mirror to reflect light on the nose from a Bull's eye lamp which is placed on the left side of the patient at the level of the ear of the patient. Head light may also be used instead of Bull's eye lamp. There are eight aspects to be examined in the nose and paranasal sinuses. These include:
- External nasal framework.
- Tests of airway patency.
- Examination of columella and vestibule.
- Anterior rhinoscopy.
- Posterior rhinoscopy.
- Cottle's test for nasal obstruction.
- Tests of olfaction.
- Paranasal sinus tenderness.

■ External Nasal Framework

The general appearance of the nose is assessed by inspection and palpation:
- Inspection consists of observing for any changes in the skin and osseocartilaginous framework of the nose, such as saddle nose deformity, scars, sinuses, swelling, redness, or growth (**Fig. 22.1**). When assessing for an

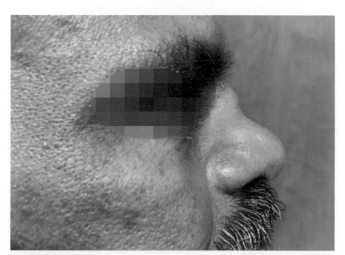

Fig. 22.1 Saddle nose deformity due to depression of the dorsum of nose.

external deformity the nose should be examined from the front, sides, and below.

- Palpation is done to look for change in temperature, tenderness, skin fixity, bony crepitation, step deformity, or fluctuation. This comprises of examination of:
  - The root of the nose.
  - The dorsum.
  - The alae.

Pearl

Clinical signs of nasal bone fracture include tenderness, crepitation, step deformity, edema around root of the nose or upper one-third of the dorsum, periorbital edema, and periorbital ecchymosis.

■ Tests of Nasal Airway Patency

Cold Spatula Test

A clean, cold, tongue depressor is held below the nostrils and the area of mist formed on the tongue depressor is noted during normal, quiet expiration. The size of the mist is reduced or absent on one side in case of unilateral obstruction, and may be reduced on both sides in case of bilateral obstruction. This is a subjective test (**Fig. 22.2**).

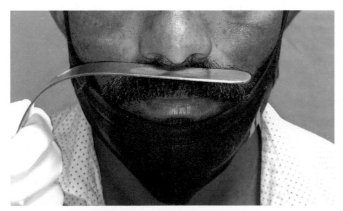

Fig. 22.2 Demonstration of cold spatula test.

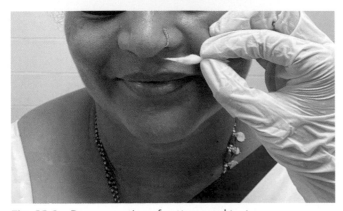

Fig. 22.3 Demonstration of cotton wool test.

Cotton Wool Test

A thin wisp of cotton is held below each nostril and movement is noted during inspiration and expiration. This is a subjective test (**Fig. 22.3**).

■ Examination of Columella and Vestibule without Nasal Speculum

Nasal vestibule is the entry point into the nasal cavity lined by squamous epithelium. Look for excoriation of the lining of the vestibule, crusts, furuncle, fissures, and squamous papilloma. Sometimes the caudal end of the septum is deviated to one side, called caudal deviation or dislocation (**Fig. 22.4**).

Tip Elevation Test

The nose is examined by elevating the tip of the nose by the thumb. Caudal dislocation of septum, lesions in the vestibule, polyp, nasal mass, or discharge, if present, is noted.

■ Anterior Rhinoscopy

The examiner sits facing the patient with the light focused on the nose. A nasal speculum is used to open the vestibule (**Fig. 22.5**). The speculum is held in the left hand (if right-handed) so that the light is not blocked during examination. The right hand is also free for using other instruments (**Figs. 22.6, 22.7,** and **22.8**). The speculum must be fully closed during insertion and partially open during withdrawal to avoid pulling the nasal vibrissae which is painful. *The following sites of the nasal cavity are examined*:

- Nasal septum: Look for the color of the septal mucosa. See if there is a deviated nasal septum, septal spur, septal hematoma, or septal perforation. If there is a deviation, determine the type, that is, C-shaped or S-shaped deviation, and site, that is, anterior/posterior, high/low.
- Floor of the nasal cavity: Look for discharge, growth, or defect such as an oronasal fistula.

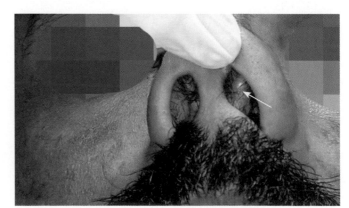

Fig. 22.4 Demonstration of tip elevation test. Caudal dislocation can be seen on the left side (*yellow arrow*).

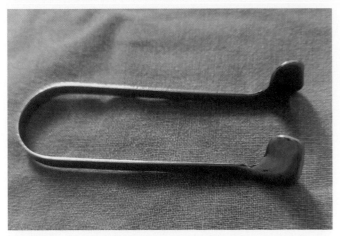

Fig. 22.5 Thudicum nasal speculum for anterior rhinoscopic examination of the nose.

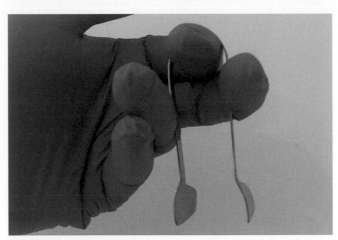

Fig. 22.6 Technique of holding the Thudicum nasal speculum.

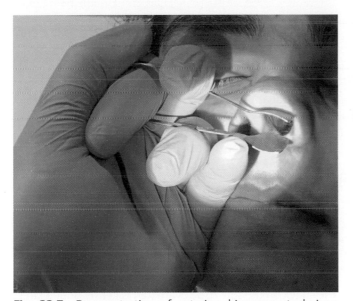

Fig. 22.7 Demonstration of anterior rhinoscopy technique with Thudicum speculum.

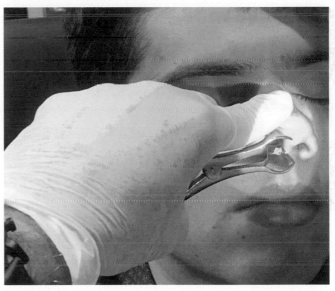

Fig. 22.8 Demonstration of anterior rhinoscopy with Vienna nasal speculum.

- Lateral wall of the nasal cavity:
  - Inferior turbinate: Size, that is, whether it is normal, hypertrophied, or atrophied. In allergic rhinitis it can be polypoidal or mulberry in appearance. The color can appear congested in infection, and pale in allergy. It may be edematous.
  - Inferior meatus: Look for discharge or mass.
  - Middle turbinate: Whether normal or hypertrophied or atrophied. It can be congested if there is associated sinusitis with pus discharge from the middle meatus. It can be pale and polypoidal as in allergic rhinitis.
  - Middle meatus: Look for discharge or mass such as polyps or tumors.
  - Superior turbinate is usually not visible except in conditions like atrophic rhinitis when there is a roomy nasal cavity.

Note: If there is discharge or polypi between the middle turbinate and septum, it is more likely to be from the superior meatus (posterior ethmoid sinus) (**Fig. 22.9**). Lesions arising from the roof of the nasal cavity (congenital such as meningocele or tumours such as olfactory neuroblastoma) also present between the septum and middle turbinate.

- *Roof of the nasal cavity* for any mass present such as a meningocele.
- *Appearance of the nasal mucosa*:
  - Normal.
  - Congested—common cold, sinusitis.
  - Pale—allergic rhinitis.

If there is a mass, describe the color, shape, and surface (smooth or granular). Probing of the mass will help assess the consistency (soft, firm, or hard), whether sessile or pedunculated, site of origin, and whether it is sensitive to

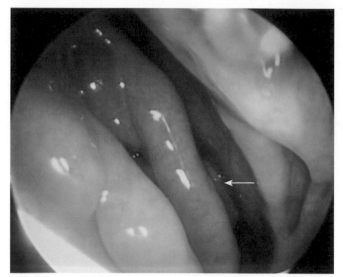

Fig. 22.9 Polyp from posterior ethmoid cells presenting between the middle turbinate and septum (*arrow*). An anterior turned uncinate process (double middle turbinate appearance) and a polyp in the middle meatus are also seen.

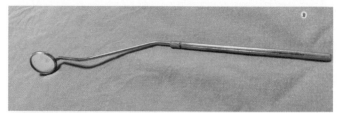

Fig. 22.10 St. Clair Thompson postnasal mirror.

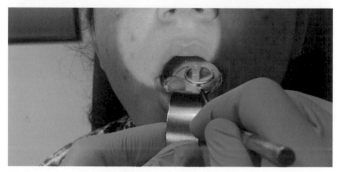

Fig. 22.11 Demonstration of posterior rhinoscopy technique.

touch or bleeds on touch. If it is a vascular tumor such as an angiofibroma, it is advisable not to probe as it can provoke profuse bleeding.

> **Pearl**
>
> Probe test helps distinguish nasal polyp from inferior turbinate. Polyps are insensitive to touch, avascular, soft, and mobile whereas a turbinate is sensitive to touch, vascular, and hard.

■ Posterior Rhinoscopy: For Examination of the Nasopharynx

The examiner sits facing the patient. The patient is instructed to breathe through the nose. The anterior one-third of the tongue is depressed using Lack's tongue depressor. St. Clair Thompson postnasal mirror is warmed (or dipped in anti-fog solution) and held like a pen (**Fig. 22.10**). It is then inserted along the dorsum of the tongue (if warmed, the mirror is touched against the dorsum of the hand to check the temperature before introducing into the patient's mouth) and guided further posteriorly behind the soft palate (**Fig. 22.11**). Care is taken to avoid stimulation of the gag reflex due to contact with the posterior pharyngeal wall or posterior third of tongue. The patient is asked to relax and breathe through the nose so as to prevent upward movement of the soft palate which would occlude the view of the nasopharynx. The following structures are visualized (**Figs. 22.12** and **22.13**):

- Choana.
- Posterior ends of the turbinates and septum.
- Adenoids.
- Nasopharyngeal aspect of soft palate and uvula.

- Eustachian tube orifice.
- Torus tubarius.
- Fossa of Rosenmuller.

Abnormalities noted include adenoid hypetrophy, discharge, crusting, antrochoanal polyp, tumors from the fossa of Rosenmuller, and choanal atresia.

> **Pearl**
>
> Fossa of Rosenmuller is the commonest site of origin of nasopharyngeal carcinoma.

■ Cottle's Test

The cheek on the side to be evaluated is gently pulled laterally with one or two fingers. This test is used to determine if the most significant site of obstruction is at the level of the internal nasal valve. If the patient says the airway has improved then it is said to be positive (**Fig. 22.14**).

> **Pearl**
>
> Modified Cottle's test: Nasal patency at the external nasal valve and internal nasal valve is assessed by intranasally by lifting the lateral crus of the lower lateral cartilage and the upper lateral cartilage, respectively, with a probe.

■ Tests of Olfaction

The patient is asked to close the eyes and identify the smell of a substance held in front of each nostril with the other nostril closed. Commonly used substances include coffee, rose essence, peppermint, etc. Ammonia is not used for this test as it stimulates the fifth cranial nerve.

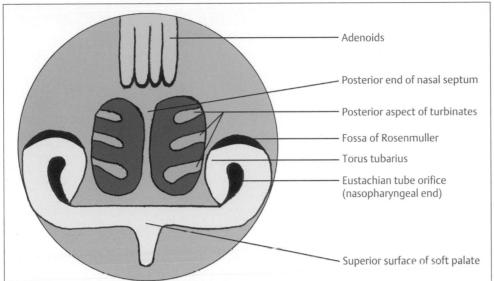

Fig. 22.12 Diagrammatic representation of posterior rhinoscopy.

Adenoids

Posterior end of nasal septum

Posterior aspect of turbinates

Fossa of Rosenmuller

Torus tubarius

Eustachian tube orifice (nasopharyngeal end)

Superior surface of soft palate

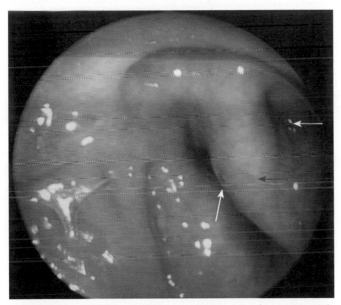

Fig. 22.13 Lateral wall of left nasopharynx (endoscopic view). *Yellow arrow* shows eustachian tube orifice. *Red arrow* shows torus tubarius. *White arrow* shows fossa of Rosenmuller.

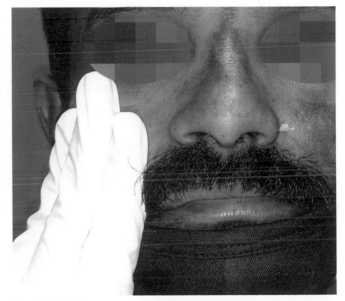

Fig. 22.14 Demonstration of Cottle's test.

Pearl

Amoore's seven primary odors are minty, musky, putrid, pungent, ethereal, camphor, and floral.

Pearls

- *Hyposmia* is decreased perception of smell.
- *Anosmia* is complete loss of perception of smell.
- *Hyperosmia* is increased perception of smell.
- *Phantosmia* is olfactory hallucination.
- *Parosmia* is distorted perception of smell.
- *Cacosmia* is foul smell.

■ Examination of the Paranasal Sinuses

Sinus tenderness is a sign of acute sinusitis or acute exacerbation of chronic sinusitis. Absence of sinus tenderness does not preclude the presence of sinus infection. The tenderness should be elicited one sinus and one side at a time, not simultaneously.

Frontal Sinus Tenderness

This is elicited by upward pressure on the area just beneath the medial end of the eyebrows, corresponding to the floor of the frontal sinus. Pressing laterally is avoided due to the presence of the supraorbital and supratrochlear nerves as it may simulate sinus tenderness (**Fig. 22.15**). The floor of the frontal sinus is the dependent area and is thinner. Tapping over the anterior wall may also be done but it is a thicker wall compared to the floor.

Ethmoid Sinus Tenderness

This is tested by pressure medial and slightly deep to the medial canthus (**Fig. 22.16**).

Maxillary Sinus Tenderness

This is elicited by pressure on the canine fossa. Also, tapping on the upper teeth using a tongue depressor may produce pain in maxillary sinusitis (**Fig. 22.17**).

There exists no test to elicit sphenoid sinus tenderness. Sphenoiditis may be suspected based on the clinical history of retro-orbital pain, or pain radiating to the vertex or occipital region.

Pearl

Boundaries of canine fossa:
- Superior—infraorbital ridge.
- Inferior—alveolar ridge.
- Medial—canine eminence.
- Lateral—root of zygoma.

Examination of the following areas must be performed to determine the extent of sinus disease:
- Orbit, orbital contents, vision (in sinonasal tumors and in complications of sinusitis).
- Oral cavity—vestibule, teeth, palate, upper alveolus (in sinonasal tumors and as a source of infection to the sinuses).
- Oropharynx—for postnasal drip and prominent lateral pharyngeal bands (**Video 22.1**).

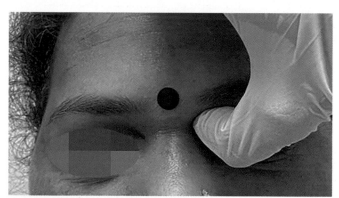

Fig. 22.15 Demonstration of frontal sinus tenderness.

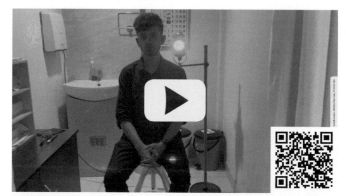

Video 22.1 Examination of nose and paranasal sinuses.

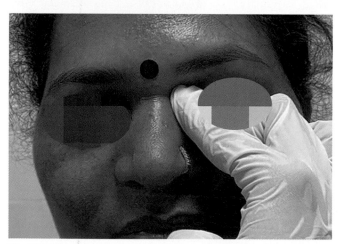

Fig. 22.16 Demonstration of ethmoid sinus tenderness.

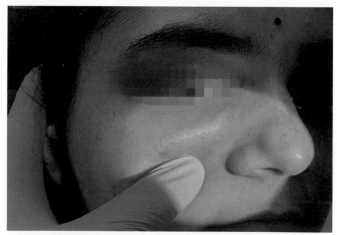

Fig. 22.17 Demonstration of maxillary sinus tenderness.

Points to Ponder

- Taking an accurate, detailed history can help in making a diagnosis. Most patients present with six major nasal complaints, namely, nasal obstruction, discharge, bleeding from the nose, sneezing, itching, and loss of smell.
- Sneezing, nasal obstruction, watery nasal discharge, and itching of nose point to allergic rhinitis.
- Nasal speculum is not used for examining the nasal vestibule and columella.
- Be systematic when examining the nasal cavity. Each cavity is examined separately. Start from the medial wall (septum), then go onto the floor, lateral wall, and roof.
- Cottle's test is positive when the nasal obstruction is at the level of the internal nasal valve.
- Sinus tenderness should always be elicited through the thinnest wall of the sinus.

Case-Based Questions

1. **A 50-year-old male presented with bleeding from the right nostril of 1 week duration. It was unprovoked bleeding and profuse in quantity.**

   a. How would you proceed to examine this patient?

   a. What are the likely sites of bleeding?

   Answers

   a. Ideally a thorough nasal examination is required from the external nasal framework to the posterior rhinoscopic examination. The vestibule should be examined without a speculum to look for any lesion in that region. Bleeding at this site can be due to vestibulitis or hemangioma or granulation tissue. Anterior rhinoscopic examination should be performed to assess the septum, the floor, the lateral wall, and any mass in the nasal cavity. Posterior rhinoscopic examination will rule out malignancy or benign tumors of the nasopharynx.

   b. The commonest site anteriorly is Little's area which is located on the anteroinferior part of the nasal septurm. A total of four arteries anastomose here under the mucosa to form the Kiesselbach's plexus which can be easily traumatized.

   Posterior bleeding is usually from sphenopalatine artery or Woodruff's plexus.

2. **A 25-year-old female presented with nasal obstruction of 5 years duration on the right side. It was a constant obstruction. Examination revealed a deviated nasal septum to the right. Cottle's test was positive. What is the inference?**

   Answers

   If Cottle's test is positive then the nasal obstruction was relieved on pulling the cheek laterally. Therefore, the obstruction is at the level of the internal nasal valve, which is the narrowest portion of the nasal cavity. The boundaries of the internal nasal valve include:

   - Medially—dorsal part of the nasal septum.
   - Laterally—caudal margin of the upper lateral cartilage.
   - Inferiorly—head of the inferior turbinate.

Frequently Asked Questions

1. What conditions produce watery nasal discharge?
2. How do you palpate for frontal sinus tenderness?
3. What are the boundaries of the canine fossa?
4. How do you perform a posterior rhinoscopic examination?
5. What is the importance of Little's area?

Endnote

Maurice H. Cottle (1898–1981) is considered the father of rhinology. He established the American Rhinologic Society in 1954 and was its first president. He is credited with performing the first septoplasty procedure in 1948. A number of tests, procedures, and anatomical areas are named after him. They include: Cottle's test, Cottle's areas, Cottle's line, Cottle's technique of septoplasty, Cottle's incision, Cottle's nasal speculum, and Cottle's classification of deviated nasal septum.

Introduction

Nose and paranasal sinus (PNS) diseases are very common in otolaryngology practice. Nasal endoscopes and imaging modalities give a better understanding of the basic anatomy, its variants, and the area of involved in the disease. They are an important aid to the diagnosis and treatment of sinonasal diseases.

Diagnostic Nasal Endoscopy

It is a routine investigative procedure for assessment of diseases of the nose and PNS. It has both a diagnostic and a therapeutic role. Fiberoptic endoscopes, although smaller in diameter, which allows better maneuverability, has the disadvantage of less visual clarity and the need for both hands for manipulation. The diameters of the rigid nasal endoscope commonly available are 2.7 and 4 mm, and the tip angle can be 0 degrees for end-on view and angled endoscopes at 30, 45, and 70 degrees.

■ Advantages

- Good illumination.
- Angled views.
- Meatuses (inferior, middle, and superior) and posterior parts of the nasal cavities can be visualized better.
- Nasopharyngeal assessment.
- Guided visualization beyond a deviation or lesion.
- For teaching and documentation purpose. For this, a camera with a monitor is needed.

■ Indications

- Evaluation of nasal obstruction, hyposmia/anosmia, and obstructive sleep apnea.
- Evaluation of headache.
- To diagnose nose and PNS diseases including sinusitis.
- Guided biopsy of the masses in the nasal cavity/nasopharynx.
- Localize the site of bleeding in epistaxis and site of leak in cerebrospinal fluid (CSF) leak/rhinorrhea.
- Guided collection of a swab for bacterial and fungal culture, a potassium hydroxide (KOH) wet mount, and nasal smear.
- Follow-up evaluation following treatment of inflammatory conditions and tumors of the nose and PNS; inspect for residual/recurrent disease.

During the diagnostic nasal endoscopy (DNE), the following procedures may be done:
- Bipolar cautery in epistaxis.
- Postendoscopic sinus surgery for removal of blood clots, crusts and discharge, and release of synechiae.
- Instillation of medications in the nose and PNS, for example, steroids in chronic rhinosinusitis, antifungal in fungal sinusitis, and topical decongestant and anesthetic in acute sinusitis (reduces the edema, which may facilitate drainage and reduce pain).
- Removal of crusts in atrophic rhinitis.
- Removal of foreign body, maggots.
- To aid in nasal irrigation for chronic nasal diseases.

■ Procedure

Anesthesia

Topical anesthesia can be applied as a nasal spray from an atomizer or nasal packing with cotton pledgets soaked in one of the following agents placed in the nasal cavity for 10 minutes:
- 4% Xylocaine + 0.1% xylometazoline drops (vasoconstrictor).
- 4% Xylocaine + 1:1,000 adrenaline.

The procedure may be difficult to perform in children and anxious individuals in whom general anesthesia may be required.

Position

The patient is positioned supine with a 30-degree head-end elevation or the patient in the sitting position.

Instrumentation

- Rigid endoscope: 4-mm 0- and 30-degree nasal endoscopes, and 2.7-mm 0-degree endoscope.
- Freer's elevator, nasal suction tips, Luc's forceps, Tilley's nasal dressing forceps, Blakesley's forceps, antifogging solution for endoscope, light source, and light cable/carrier.

- Camera and monitor (for magnified view and demonstration).

Technique

After adequate nasal decongestion, endoscopy is performed using 0-degree endoscope using three passes:

- *First pass* (examination of the floor of the nasal cavity, nasopharynx, and inferior meatus): The endoscope is passed gently along the floor of the nasal cavity between the nasal septum and the inferior turbinate toward the choanae (**Fig. 23.1a**). It helps view the entire nasal cavity and inspect for any septal deviation, discharge, color of the mucosa, or any mass. In the nasopharynx, one can inspect the roof, the walls of the nasopharynx, eustachian tube opening, and the nasopharyngeal

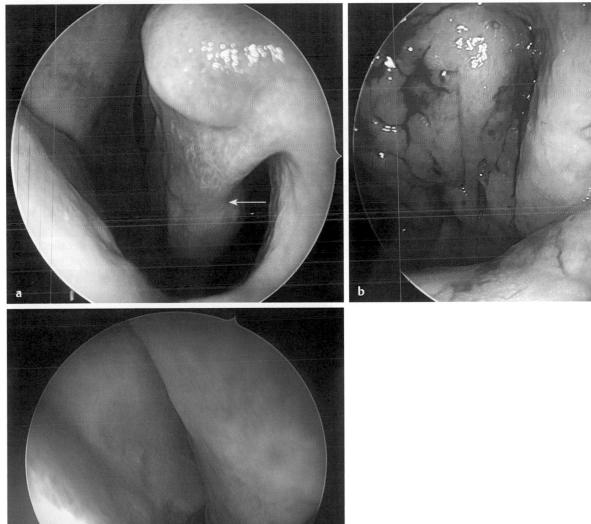

Fig. 23.1 (a) Diagnostic nasal endoscopy showing the nasal cavity and inferior turbinate (*yellow arrow*) of the left side. (b) Diagnostic nasal endoscopy showing the nasopharynx with the eustachian tube orifice (*yellow arrow*) on the left side. (c) Right inferior meatus.

Case-Based Questions

1. **A 58-year-old man came to the ear, nose, and throat (ENT) clinic with a 2-month history of right-sided nasal obstruction and blood-stained discharge from the right nostril. Although he had consulted a local physician, he did not get any relief. In the past 1 week, facial pain developed on the right side. Clinical evaluation revealed an ulcero-proliferative mass in the right nasal cavity.**

   a. What relevant investigations are required in this case and why?

   Answer

   Any elderly patient presenting with nasal obstruction, blood-stained nasal discharge, and facial pain of long duration should be evaluated for malignancy, especially if there is a nasal mass that has an ulcero-proliferative appearance.

   Relevant investigations include the following:

   - DNE to note the characteristics of the tumor (size, shape, surface, bleeding on touch, consistency, etc.), as well as the extent of the tumor.
   - Radiological investigations: CT scan with contrast will show the presence of bony erosion or expansion, sinus involvement, and vascularity of the tumor. MRI should be done if required to see intracranial and orbital complication, perineural spread, etc.
   - Biopsy for histopathological diagnosis.

2. **A patient with allergic rhinitis wishes to know what he is allergic to.**

   a. What test would you do?

   b. What is the interpretation?

   Answers

   a. The skin prick test in which different allergens are introduced into the skin of the forearm with a lancet should be done.

   b. Common allergens like house dust mite, animal dander, and pollen are introduced into the skin. Controls are normal saline and histamine. The skin reactions produced are graded from 0 to 4+, the latter being the maximum. Once the allergens are known, the patient can be prescribed immunotherapy for symptomatic relief of allergic rhinitis.

Frequently Asked Questions

1. What are the passes in DNE?
2. What is the role of CT scan in sinusitis?
3. What are the tests done to detect allergens in allergic rhinitis?
4. Why is a biopsy taken in atrophic rhinitis?
5. What are the X-ray views taken in sinusitis?
6. What are the advantages of CT scan over X-rays?
7. What is rhinomanometry?
8. In which conditions would you prefer an MRI?
9. What is the skin prick test?

Endnote

PNSs were known from ancient times. The human brain was thought to produce mucous and the PNS provided the pathway to drain out the mucous. The ancient Egyptians made use of the sinuses to enter the cranial cavity to scoop out the brain for the mummification process. The first reliable medical drawing of the PNS was by Leonardo da Vinci, an artist, inventor, and scientist. It was not until 1660 that it was discovered that it is not the brain but the mucosae of the nose and PNS that produce mucous.

24 Diseases of the External Nose and Vestibule

Ashish Chandra Agarwal

Introduction

The nose is a prominent feature of the face. Lesions over the nose cause concern due to medical and cosmetic reasons (**Fig. 24.1**). The disorders affecting the nose may also be part of an underlying systemic disease. This chapter provides an overview of the common conditions encountered by the medical student while examining the external nose.

Congenital Conditions

■ Nasal Dermoid

It is an epithelial lined cyst consisting of mesodermal structures such as hair follicles, sebaceous glands, and sweat glands. It presents as a midline cystic lesion under the skin of the dorsum of the nose. Sometimes an associated sinus tract may be present having an external opening in the form of a pit on the nasal dorsum with or without tufts of hair. Rarely, the dermoid can have an intracranial, extradural

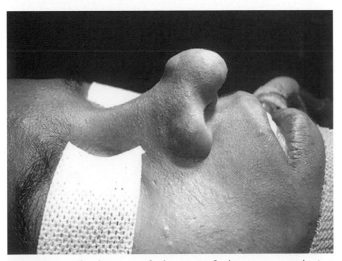

Fig. 24.1 Fibrolipoma of the tip of the nose producing cosmetic deformity.

communication. Magnetic resonance imaging (MRI) is mandatory to rule out the presence of a tract intracranially. Treatment consists of surgical excision of the cyst and its tract. The approaches may be lateral rhinotomy, external rhinoplasty, or a midline vertical incision. In patients with intracranial extension, an additional frontal craniotomy may be required.

■ Nasal Glioma

These are benign, neuroglial tissues that have lost connection with the cranial glial tissue during embryonic development. Nasal glioma may be intranasal or external nasal. The external nasal lesion presents as a noncompressible, subcutaneous swelling either in the midline or on one side of the nasal dorsum. The intranasal lesion may mimic a polyp and present with nasal obstruction. Investigations include diagnostic nasal endoscopy and computed tomography (CT) scan to see the extent of the lesion and whether bony margins are eroded. MRI will rule out any intracranial extension. Treatment is surgical excision. For an external nasal lesion, the following approaches can be used: lateral rhinotomy, external rhinoplasty, or midline nasal. An endoscopic approach is preferred for an intranasal lesion.

■ Nasal Encephalocele and Meningoencephalocele

This condition arises as a result of herniation of meninges alone (meningocele), or meninges along with brain tissue (meningoencephalocele), through a congenital, bony, skull base defect. Nasal meningoceles can be classified as frontoethmoidal or basal types. The frontoethmoidal masses present as a pulsatile swelling either in the midline, on one side of the nasal dorsum, or adjacent to the medial canthus.

Basal meningoceles arise as a result of defects in the cribriform plate and sphenoid regions and present as an intranasal mass with nasal obstruction. The swelling increases in size during coughing, crying, or straining. They may be reducible and transilluminate. Furstenberg's sign (increase in size or pulsation with compression of the ipsilateral jugular vein) may be positive.

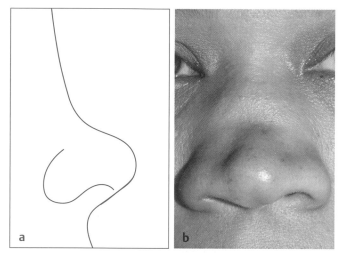

Fig. 24.5 (a, b) Saddle nose deformity.

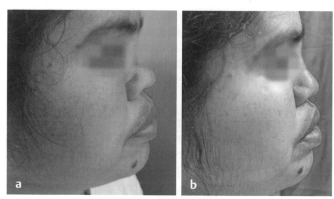

Fig. 24.6 (a) Saddle nose deformity. **(b)** External nose after correction.

Synthetic materials have a high rate of infection and extrusion, so they are used only if necessary.

Hump Nose

Excess bone or cartilage on the dorsum of the nose is called a hump (**Fig. 24.7a, b**). It can involve either the bony or cartilaginous framework or both. The deformity can be present from birth. If the defect is minor and is of no cosmetic concern to the patient, then it can be left alone. If surgical correction is required, then reduction rhinoplasty can be performed. In this procedure, the hump is rasped or shaved after lifting up the skin of the dorsum of the nose. This technique requires an internal (intercartilaginous) or external rhinoplasty approach.

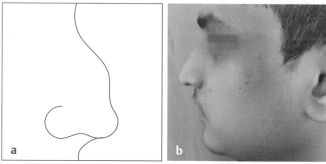

Fig. 24.7 (a) Hump nose. **(b)** Patient with hump on the dorsum of the nose.

Crooked Nose and Deviated Nose

In a crooked nose, the nasal dorsum, extending from the frontonasal angle to the tip, is curved in a "C"- or a "S"-shaped manner (**Fig. 24.8a**). The condition is usually due to a trauma sustained during birth or in the later years. Often these cases may have a deviated nasal septum and the correction will have to be functional and cosmetic. The deformity can be corrected surgically by a septorhinoplasty (**Fig. 24.8b**).

If the dorsum of the nose is deviated to one side in a straight line, it is said to be a deviated nose.

Neoplasms of the External Nose

Rhinophyma

It is a benign, slow-growing lesion arising due to hyperplasia of the sebaceous glands and the underlying connective tissue. It is also known by other names such as potato tumor

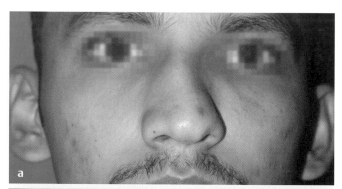

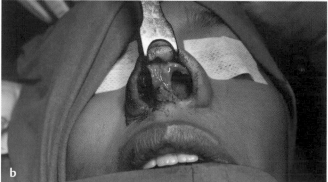

Fig. 24.8 (a) C-shaped deviation of external nose (crooked nose). **(b)** External rhinoplasty incision and elevation of the skin of the dorsum of the nose.

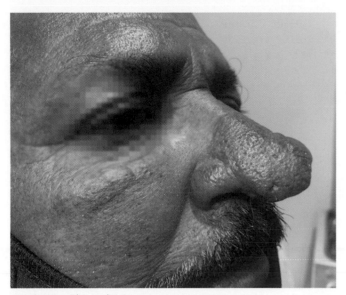

Fig. 24.9 Rhinophyma or potato tumor.

and elephantiasis of nose (**Fig. 24.9**). It is seen in individuals having long standing acne rosacea. Middle aged men are usually affected. The patient presents with a pink, irregular thickening of the skin of the lower two-thirds of the nose. It has an unsightly appearance. There may be obstruction in breathing. Medical treatment consists of oral isotretinoin and oral or topical antibiotics like tetracycline and metronidazole. Surgical treatment involves shaving the bulk of the lesion with scalpel, ultrasonic scalpel, dermabrasion, or laser. After excision, the site can be either left to re-epithelialize or a skin graft is placed over the raw area.

■ Basal Cell Carcinoma

It is a slow growing malignant tumor arising due to neoplastic proliferation of cells that resemble basal cells of the epidermis. The lesion is locally invasive and rarely metastasize. Both, elderly males and females are equally affected. Light skin color, exposure to solar radiation, arsenic, and immunodeficiency syndromes make an individual prone to develop this condition. The patient will give a long history of exposure to sunlight. Some individuals may have a genetic predisposition. The entity is also known as rodent ulcer or basaloma. The presentation can be in the form of a papule with pearly border, an ulcer with rolled edges or an erythematous papule. Surgical excision with a 3- to 5-mm margin of skin around the palpable border is the treatment of choice. If primary closure is not possible then local flaps, regional flaps, free grafts, or a prosthesis may be required.

■ Squamous Cell Carcinoma

It is a neoplastic condition resulting from malignant change in the epidermal keratinocyte. The predisposing factors are the same as that of a basal cell carcinoma. Areas of active chronic keratosis and Bowen's disease are recognized sites

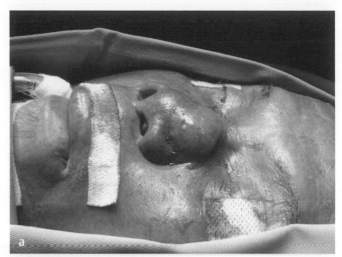

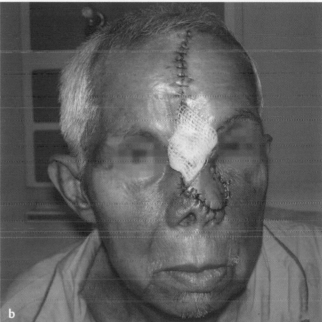

Fig. 24.10 **(a)** Malignant tumor over the dorsum of the nose. **(b)** Postoperative picture of the forehead flap used to correct the defect after excision.

for the potential development of this malignancy. The presentation can be in the form of an erythematous plaque, verrucous growth, or a nodule with induration of the surrounding tissue (**Fig. 24.10a**). Metastasis to the regional lymph nodes is common, either to the parotid or submandibular lymph nodes. Surgical resection of the lesion with adequate margins along with reconstruction of the defect with or without neck dissection followed by postoperative radiotherapy is the treatment of choice (**Fig. 24.10b**).

■ Malignant Melanoma

Melanomas are aggressive tumors that arise from melanocytes. It is characterized by malignant melanocytes invading the dermis. Growth of this lesion takes place in both horizontal and vertical planes. Depth of the lesion is the main prognostic indicator, the deeper the depth of invasion, the worse the prognosis. Among the several varieties, the superficial spreading variant is the commonest to involve the face. It usually starts as a brown macule, which on close inspection reveals a variety of colors within the lesion, namely, black, blue, brown, and white. Pruritus and bleeding from the lesion are the other clinical features. Treatment is by surgical excision with a clear circumferential margin ranging from a few millimeters to few centimeters depending on the size of the tumor.

Points to Ponder

- Clinical examination of the nose starts with evaluation of the external nose. It is therefore essential to have a thorough knowledge of the various conditions that can affect this region.

- Patients can present in any age group with lesions of the external nose due to medical or cosmetic reasons.
- Radiological evaluation, either CT or MRI or both, is required in children with congenital conditions like dermoid cysts to rule out intracranial extension.
- A furuncle of the nose which lies in the dangerous area of the face should never be taken lightly as it can lead to cavernous sinus thrombosis.
- The commonest cause for saddle nose deformity is trauma.
- Nose is a common site for "actinic" cutaneous changes due to exposure to ultraviolet (UV) light from the sun in people who work outdoors. A small percentage of such lesions proceed to develop frank malignancy.
- In malignant melanoma, the vertical growth is associated with poorer prognosis.

Case-Based Questions

1. A 50-year-old male patient, on immunosuppressant drugs for kidney transplant, developed a furuncle of the right nostril with inflammation of the skin of the dorsum of the nose. After 3 days, there was proptosis of the right eye. What is the probable etiology for this proptosis?

Answer

A furuncle in the nasal vestibule occupies the dangerous area of the face. Since the patient was on immunosuppressant drugs, the infection flared up and spread through the valveless facial veins and superior ophthalmic vein to the cavernous sinus leading to cavernous sinus thrombosis and proptosis of the right eye. This is a serious condition which presents with ophthalmoplegia, headache, fever, and proptosis due to retrobulbar pressure. Treatment consists of high dose intravenous antibiotics and anticoagulants like heparin and steroids.

2. A 35-year-old male came to the ENT outpatient department with complains of a crooked nose and nasal obstruction on the right side. A nasal examination revealed a C-shaped deviation of the dorsum of the nose to the right side with a deviated nasal septum also on the right side. How will you manage this patient?

Answer

A combination of external deformity of the nose with a nasal deviation requires surgery for cosmetic and functional reasons. After counseling the patient and obtaining consent, the patient can be posted for septorhinoplasty during which the external deviation of the dorsum is corrected (rhinoplasty) along with the septal deviation (septoplasty). Rhinoplasty can be performed through an internal approach or external approach.

Frequently Asked Questions

1. What are the congenital causes of unilateral nasal obstruction?
2. What is Frustenberg's sign?
3. What are the causes for "saddle-nose" deformity?
4. What is the procedure and approaches for correction of external nasal deformity?
5. Write a note on Rhinophyma.

Endnote

The father of rhinoplasty was an Indian surgeon who was born 2600 years ago. His name was Sushruta. He is also considered to be the father of plastic surgery. During that period punishment for crimes consisted of amputation of the nose. He developed a technique of rhinoplasty where the cheek was rotated to cover the defect over the nose. This was stitched in place with cotton threads. He went on to write the Sushruta Samhita which described the practice of surgery during that period.

25 Diseases of the Nasal Septum and Nasal Obstruction

Mahesh Bhat T. and Cimona Dsouza

The competencies covered in this chapter are as follows:

EN4.23 Describe the clinical features, investigations, and principles of management of deviated nasal septum.

EN4.22 Elicit, document, and present a correct history; demonstrate and describe the clinical features; choose the correct investigations; and describe the principles of management of nasal obstruction.

Deviated Nasal Septum

■ Introduction

A deviated nasal septum (DNS) is common. It is present in 80% of the population. The majority of the people with a DNS do not have symptoms. The commonest symptom associated with a DNS is nasal obstruction. A surgical correction of a DNS, septoplasty, is the third most common surgery performed in the head and neck.

The nasal septum separates the two nasal cavities and gives support to the dorsum of the nose as well as the columella and tip. Deviation of the septum is a common condition noted in rhinology practice and is often asymptomatic. It may cause nasal obstruction and chronic sinus disease and contribute to cosmetic deformity. The resultant impaired airflow can reduce the olfaction, humidification, filtration, and oxygen inflow.

■ Etiology

Septal deviation can be divided into congenital or acquired deviation. Trauma and developmental errors are the main factors for a septal deviation.

- *Acquired septal deviation* is usually caused by trauma. Trauma can be any of the following:
  - Accidents like falling down with external injury. (Injuries to the nose occur during childhood but are often ignored.)
  - Personal assault as in a fist fight or with weapons.
  - Iatrogenic due to surgery or a procedure performed on the nose.
- *Congenital septal deviation* etiology has not been completely elucidated, but the following factors play a role:

- It is thought to result from external pressures on the nose in utero due to uterine contractions.
- The position of the infant during the birthing process can affect the incidence of septal deviation. It is more in the occipitoposterior position.
- During the delivery process, trauma to the external nose can occur due to the use of forceps for delivery in obstructed labor.
- Unequal growth between the palate and the skull base may cause nasal septum buckling.
- DNS is noted in patients with cleft lip or palate or in those with dental abnormalities.
- *Chronic pressure* from mass effect (e.g., inflammatory polyp or neoplasm) may gradually push the septum to the opposite side. This is sometimes referred to as a secondary DNS.

■ Classification

Multiple classifications have been suggested in the literature for nasal septal deviations:

- *Cottle* proposed a simple classification based on the degree of nasal obstruction:
  - *Simple deviation*: This type of septal deviation does not cause symptoms of nasal obstruction and does not require any intervention.
  - *Obstruction*: This type of septal deviation produces symptoms of nasal obstruction due to contact of the nasal septum with the lateral nasal wall but is relieved on application of a vasoconstrictor.
  - *Impaction*: This type of septal deviation produces symptoms of nasal obstruction due to contact of the nasal septum with the lateral nasal wall and is not relieved on application of a vasoconstrictor agent.

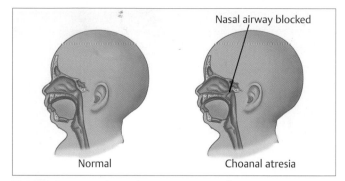

Fig. 25.6 Bony choanal atresia.

choana, retarded growth, genitourinary abnormalities, and ear defects including deafness.
- The patient may have a narrow nasopharynx with a mediatized lateral wall of the nose, high-arched palate, and a wide vomer.

■ Investigations

Diagnosis requires a high degree of suspicion:
- An attempt should be made to pass a small feeding tube or red rubber catheter into the nasal cavity to see if it reaches the oropharynx.
- Contrast X-rays.
- CT scan is the investigation of choice as it will show not only the atresia but also the type: whether it is bony, membranous or mixed, unilateral or bilateral, complete or incomplete, and other associated changes in the surrounding structures.

■ Treatment

- Immediate treatment of bilateral atresia is placement of a McGovern nipple or an oral airway so that the patient can breathe through the mouth.
- Surgical repair can be done by the transpalatal approach, endoscopically, or a combined transnasal–transoral approach. When using an endoscope, micro-debriders and lasers (CO_2 or KTP-532) are useful to open up the blocked or narrowed areas in the choana. Temporary stents are placed after surgery to keep the choana patent in revision cases and cases when stenosis is anticipated.
- Bilateral choanal atresia is an emergency and needs to be managed as early as possible. Unilateral choanal atresia can be done when the child is older.

Nasal Obstruction

■ Introduction

Nasal obstruction is a symptom and not a disease. It is caused by diseases or lesions that result in narrowing of the airway or blockage of the nasal cavity.

■ Clinical Presentation

Patients with nose block typically report a sensation of stuffiness in the nasal cavity.

From the history, the side, duration, whether recurrent/intermittent/continuous, seasonal variation, and aggravating and relieving factors should be elicited. When experienced at night, it can adversely affect the quality of sleep, and could result in excessive daytime sleepiness, lethargy, and fatigue. Prior history of trauma or nasal surgery should be documented.

Other associated symptoms may include the following:
- *Rhinorrhea*: Clear rhinorrhea could be associated with allergic rhinitis. Unilateral clear rhinorrhea raises the suspicion of cerebrospinal fluid (CSF) leak. Purulent rhinorrhea may indicate an infective cause.
- *Postnasal drip.*
- *Facial pain occurs* usually due to secondary sinusitis.
- Alteration in the *sense of smell and taste.*
- *Atopic features*—pruritus, epiphora, and sneezing—are more prominent in allergic rhinitis. A history of asthma or dermatitis is more likely in the context of allergic rhinitis.
- *Epistaxis* may be present due to the presence of infection or tumors.

■ Clinical Assessment

Differential Diagnoses

The differential diagnoses for nasal obstruction are presented in **Table 25.1**.

History

When assessing a patient with nasal obstruction, the following factors should be taken into consideration:
- Is it unilateral or bilateral? Alternating nasal obstruction generally indicates mucosal inflammation manifesting in the normal nasal cycle.
- Are symptoms seasonal or diurnal?
- Are there specific triggers (e.g., exposure to smoke or pets)?
- Aggravating and relieving factors.
- Are there factors suggestive of infection? Purulent rhinorrheas with facial pain and fever are seen in the case of acute sinusitis.
- Are there factors suggestive of neoplasia? Unilateral nasal obstruction with epistaxis raises the possibility of a neoplastic process. In this case, it is important to enquire about ear symptoms as a postnasal space mass may impair eustachian tube function and result in a unilateral middle ear effusion. Other factors suggestive of neoplasia include paresthesia, diplopia, and trismus, which are related to local extension of tumor into adjacent structures.

Table 25.1 Differential diagnosis for nasal obstruction

	Unilateral	Bilateral
Congenital	Choanal atresia Nasal glioma, meningocele, encephalocele	Choanal atresia Pyriform aperture stenosis
Inflammatory: Acute Chronic	Sinusitis: Viral, bacterial, fungal Sinusitis: Bacterial, fungal	Sinusitis, coryza Chronic rhinitis, atrophic rhinitis, granulomatous conditions, sinusitis
Traumatic	Septal fracture, hematoma, abscess	Septal fracture, hematoma, abscess
Anatomical	Deviated nasal septum: *C*-shaped deviation Turbinate enlargement	Deviated nasal septum: *S*-shaped deviation
Neoplasms: Benign Malignant	Inverted papilloma, juvenile nasopharyngeal angiofibroma Sinonasal malignancies	Olfactory neuroblastoma
Miscellaneous	Rhinolith, antrochoanal polyp Foreign body	Allergic rhinitis, rhinitis medicamentosa, non-allergic rhinitis, ethmoidal polyposis, adenoid hypertrophy

- Is there a medical history of atopy, asthma, aspirin sensitivity, and coexisting inflammatory conditions?
- Is there a history of sinonasal surgery for septal deviation, nasal polyposis (risk of recurrence), or tumor?
- Is there a history of facial/nasal trauma?
- What medications are being used?
- Is there a social history of note? Smoking can impair mucociliary clearance and is a risk factor for malignancy. Alcohol is a vasodilator and may cause mucosal congestion. A history of illicit drug use is important; for example, nasal administration of cocaine can lead to septal perforation. Exposure to hard wood dust (carpenters, wood turners) can predispose to sinonasal adenocarcinoma.

Examination

The examination should take into consideration airflow dynamics and areas where increased resistance can occur. A useful method is to commence with external examination of the nose followed by examination of the internal anatomy.

External examination should mainly focus on deformities of the bony and cartilaginous structures of the nose, as well as the adjacent tissues. Nasal tip depression, if present, should be noted as it can contribute to nasal obstruction. Examine the airflow during normal and deep inspiration and assess for collapse of the nasal valve. The internal nasal valve provides the greatest resistance to airflow; hence, even minor narrowing can cause nasal obstruction.

Cottle's Maneuver

In this maneuver, the cheek is pulled laterally to prevent collapse of the internal nasal valve and the patient is asked to breathe through their nose to assess for improved flow.

If this maneuver improves the patient's symptoms, the cause is likely to be related to this valve.

Modified Cottle's test utilizes a probe to lift the alar cartilage or upper lateral cartilage to assess the site of block. The airway will improve on lifting the structures in alar collapse if the site of obstruction is at the level of the external nasal valve. The airway will improve on lifting the structures at the level of the upper lateral cartilage if the site of obstruction is at the internal nasal valve.

If the diagnosis remains unclear, the patient may need fiberoptic or rigid *nasal endoscopy* to examine the more posterior aspects of the nasal cavity. This is usually performed after the nasal cavity is prepared topically with a combination of decongestant and local anesthetic spray.

When specific diagnosis is required of a lesion, a biopsy is taken for histopathological examination. This is usually done after imaging.

The patient's neck should be examined for lymphadenopathy, and the ears for middle ear effusion, especially when a sinonasal/nasopharyngeal neoplasm is included in the differential diagnosis.

The above history and examination will identify most causes of nasal obstruction; however, in patients in whom the cause is uncertain, the condition persists despite medical therapy, or where neoplasm is suspected, further investigation is warranted.

Imaging

CT is the preferred imaging modality for the nose and paranasal sinuses. In most cases, it allows for appropriate imaging of the sinuses and their drainage pathways and also investigates for extra nasal extension of disease, such as into the orbit or intracranial cavity. Contrast is required when a tumor or a complication of sinonasal infection is suspected.

Clinical Features

Symptoms

- Nasal obstruction.
- Nasal discharge.
- Hyposmia or anosmia.
- Facial pain.

Signs

- Purulent discharge.
- Cheesy debris present in the nasal cavity.

Diagnosis

- CT of nose and paranasal sinus. There will be:
  - Focal areas of hyperattenuation.
  - Bony erosions.
  - Sinus expansion.
- Diagnostic nasal endoscopy:
  - Demonstrates polyposis and cheesy debris.

Differential Diagnosis

- Allergic fungal rhinosinusitis.

Treatment

- Functional endoscopic sinus surgery with removal of polypi, cheesy material, and establishment of sinus aeration.

■ Rhinitis Medicamentosa

Synonym: Rebound rhinitis.

Inflammation or congestion of nasal mucosa caused by overuse of topical nasal decongestants. It can be considered as a subset of drug-induced rhinitis.

The patients are typically cases of nasal obstruction of varying etiology who were prescribed nasal decongestants. Prolonged use of these nasal decongestants beyond 2 weeks may result in rebound vessel dilatation, increased vascular permeability, and increased mucosal congestion due to an altered vasomotor tone caused by a secondary decrease in endogenous norepinephrine.

Clinical Features

Symptoms

- Nasal obstruction, which initially resolved with decongestant and now needs increased use for achieving the same effect or is unresponsive. The decongestant would have been prescribed for a short duration but continued by the patient due to the relief, especially at night.

- Snoring may be present.
- Mucoid rhinorrhea.

Signs

- Boggy nasal mucosa.
- Erythematous and granular appearance of mucosa or it may be pale.
- In the later stages the mucosal changes can lead to turbinate hyperplasia and chronic rhinosinusitis.

Diagnosis

- Clinical history.
- Diagnostic nasal endoscopy to rule out other causes of nasal obstruction.

Differential Diagnosis

- Allergic rhinitis.
- Rhinosinusitis.
- Nonallergic rhinitis.

Treatment

- Patient counseling while prescribing the topical decongestant and on when to limit the use.
- Stop nasal decongestant usage.
- Intranasal (topical) corticosteroid spray.
- Short course of oral steroids is useful in severe cases till the topical steroids start acting.
- Saline nasal douches.
- Antihistamines for a short period.

Granulomatous Diseases of the Nose

A granuloma is an organized collection of specialized macrophages, known as epithelioid cells, which fuse to form multinucleated giant cells. Granuloma formation may be seen in infectious, inflammatory, and neoplastic conditions as well as in various vasculitides (**Table 26.1**).

■ Rhinoscleroma

It is a chronic granulomatous disease caused by the gram-negative coccobacillus *Klebsiella rhinoscleromatis (Frisch bacillus)*. It is contracted by direct inhalation of droplets or contaminated material. The disease begins in areas of epithelial transition like the vestibule of the nose, the subglottis, and the area between the nasopharynx and oropharynx and progresses to involve the nasal cavity, paranasal sinuses, nasopharynx, oral cavity, larynx, and trachea. It is seen in patients belonging to lower socioeconomic classes and is endemic in Africa, Southeast Asia, South America, and Mexico.

Table 26.1 Etiology of granulomatous diseases of the nose

Infective	Inflammatory	Neoplastic
Bacterial	Sarcoidosis	Extranodal natural killer (NK)/T-cell lymphoma
Tuberculosis Leprosy Syphilis Rhinoscleroma Actinomyces	Wegener's granulomatosis (granulomatosis with polyangiitis)	
	Churg-Strauss (eosinophilic granulomatosis with polyangiitis)	
	Cocaine-induced	
Fungal	Lupus vulgaris Giant cell granuloma Cholesterol granuloma	
Aspergillus Mucormycosis Coccidiomycosis Blastomycosis Histoplasmosis		
Protozoan		
Rhinosporidiosis Leishmaniasis		

Stages

Catarrhal: Foul-smelling nasal discharge and crusting mimicking atrophic rhinitis.

Granulomatous: Painless, granulomatous nodules develop in the nasal mucosa. Subepidermal infiltration of inflammatory cells lends a woody feel to the soft tissue of the external nose (*Hebra nose*) and the lips.

Sclerotic: Characterized by fibrosis, resulting in deformities of the upper lip, nasal adhesions, and choanal stenosis. There may be adhesions in the nasopharynx or oropharynx. Laryngeal disease is characterized by subglottic stenosis.

Clinical Features

- Nasal obstruction.
- Nasal discharge.
- Epistaxis.
- Anosmia.
- Nasal deformity.
- Dysphagia.
- Progressive dyspnea and stridor (with subglottic involvement).

Diagnosis

Nasal Endoscopy

Endoscopic examination may reveal a small intranasal nodule or polyp adherent to the nasal septum. As the disease progresses, it may grow into an exophytic mass.

Adhesions may be seen between the septum and the lateral nasal wall.

Biopsy

Histopathological examination shows infiltration of the submucosa with plasma cells, lymphocytes, and eosinophils. *Mikulicz cells*, which are macrophages with a central nucleus, clear cytoplasm, and large vacuoles containing bacilli, and *Russell bodies*, which are eosinophilic inclusions seen in plasma cells, are characteristic of the disease.

Imaging

CT scan may show homogenous, nonenhancing, soft tissue masses in the nasal cavity or nasopharynx and concentric narrowing of the airway. CT/MRI may be required to rule out malignancy in cases of extensive disease.

Treatment

Long-term antibiotic therapy with third-generation cephalosporins, clindamycin, rifampicin, or ciprofloxacin for 4 to 6 weeks. Tetracycline is the drug of choice. The duration of antibiotic therapy may be guided by repeated biopsies and cultures. Treatment is stopped only when two consecutive biopsies are negative. Steroids may also be given to decrease inflammation and formation of adhesions. For local application, 2% acriflavine solution may be used.

Surgical excision of cicatricial lesions may be combined with rhinoplasty for the management of deformities. Tracheostomy may be required for patients with subglottic involvement, presenting with airway compromise and stridor.

Patients need follow-up as relapses are known to occur.

■ Syphilis

Syphilis is an infectious granulomatous disease caused by the spirochete *Treponema pallidum.* In the postantibiotic era, syphilitic lesions of the nose are rarely seen. It is characterized by perivascular cuffing and endarteritis. Syphilis may be congenital or acquired.

Acquired Syphilis

- *Primary acquired*—primary chancre, a hard, painless ulcerated papule in the vestibule which disappears in 6 to 10 weeks.
- *Secondary acquired*—most infectious stage that occurs 6 to 10 weeks after inoculation. It presents as rhinitis with fissuring of the vestibule. There may be concomitant systemic signs such as fever, generalized lymphadenopathy, roseolar and papular rash, and mucosal patches of the pharynx.
- *Tertiary acquired*—gumma of the nasal septum, which may later cause septal perforation. Characteristically, septal perforation may involve the bony and cartilaginous septum and may result in the collapse of the nasal bridge, resulting in a saddle nose deformity. Offensive nasal discharge with crusts may be seen. Palatal perforations, nasal stenosis, atrophic rhinitis, and intracranial complications are also known to occur.

Congenital Syphilis

- *Early congenital*: There is nasal discharge, fissuring, and excoriation of the vestibule and the upper lip. It is also known as "snuffles" as it is typically seen in the first 3 months of life.
- *Late congenital*: Around puberty, the patient presents with gumma which may destroy the nasal architecture. Stigmata of congenital syphilis like corneal opacities, Hutchinson's teeth, and deafness may also be seen.

Diagnosis

Dark ground illumination microscopy may be done to look for spirochetes. Serological tests such as venereal disease research laboratory (VDRL) test, treponemal hemagglutination test (TPHA), and fluorescent treponemal antibody absorption test (FTA-ABS) offer 90% sensitivity.

Treatment

The drug of choice is penicillin. Injection benzathine penicillin 2.4 million units is given weekly for 3 weeks. Nasal douching with alkaline solution helps to remove crusts. Cosmetic deformities may be corrected once the disease becomes inactive.

■ Tuberculosis of the Nose

TB of the nose almost always occurs secondary to pulmonary TB. Primary sinonasal TB is rare. It presents as bright, red, nodular thickening with or without ulceration. The most commonly involved sites are the anterior aspect of the septum and the anterior end of the inferior turbinate. It may cause perforation of the cartilaginous septum. Diagnosis is confirmed by biopsy. Ziehl-Neelsen stain shows acid-fast bacilli while histopathology reveals evidence of caseating granulomas with Langerhans giant cells. Treatment is with antitubercular drugs.

■ Lupus Vulgaris

Lupus vulgaris is an indolent, chronic form of tubercular infection that affects the skin and mucous membranes. The most affected site is the mucocutaneous junction of the nasal septum. It can also affect the skin of the face. It presents as a reddish, firm nodule which on diascopy has the appearance of apple jelly. Hence, these nodules are referred to as apple jelly nodules. Rarely, there may be extensive involvement of the nasal floor and turbinates. Diagnosis is by histopathology and these lesions are managed with antitubercular drugs.

> **Pearl**
>
> Diascopy is a test in which pressure is applied to the skin of the face by applying a clear glass or plastic slide. The observer looks at the lesion under pressure. In lupus vulgaris, the lesions look like apply jelly nodules.

■ Leprosy

Leprosy is a granulomatous infection caused by the bacterium *Mycobacterium leprae*. The nose is often the first site affected by the disease and nasal involvement is seen more commonly in lepromatous leprosy than in tuberculoid leprosy. Leprosy affects the anterior septum and the anterior end of the inferior turbinate. It is characterized by nodular lesions of mucous membrane associated with nasal discharge, crusting, and bleeding. These nodules may ulcerate and cause perforation of the septal cartilage. There may be periostitis of the nasal bones, inferior turbinates, and anterior nasal spine leading to nasal deformity. Diagnosis is confirmed by microscopic examination of nasal scrapings and biopsy. Acid-fast bacilli may be seen in foamy histiocytes called lepra cells. Leprosy is treated with rifampicin, dapsone, and isoniazid. Deformities may require surgical correction once the disease is inactive.

■ Rhinosporidiosis

Rhinosporidiosis is a chronic, granulomatous disease caused by *Rhinosporidium seeberi*. It is commonly seen in South India, Pakistan, and Sri Lanka. It is acquired through contaminated water in ponds frequented by animals. *Rhinosporidium seeberi* was initially considered to be a fungus but has since been reclassified as a protozoan belonging to the class Mesomycetozoa.

Life Cycle of *Rhinosporidium seeberi*

Fig. 26.10 shows the life cycle of *Rhinosporidium seeberi*. The initial stage is the juvenile sporangium represented by **A**. It has a single nucleus with a cytoplasm which is granular. Further development takes place where the sporangia pass through the stages of immature sporangia (**B** and **C**), intermediate sporangia (**D** and **E**), and mature sporangia (**F**), through which mature endospores burst out. **G** represents the free endospores with a tail of mucoid material behind them called comet of Beattie. **H** and **J** represent the infective spores called electron dense bodies or EDB.

Clinical Features

The patient complains of nose block, blood-stained nasal discharge, and may even present with frank epistaxis.

It presents as a friable, pink-purple, strawberry-like leafy mass attached to the nasal septum or the lateral wall of the nasal cavity (**Fig. 26.11**). It is vascular and bleeds on touch with an irregular surface with white dots representing sporangia. The lesion may have a small attachment (pedunculated) or may be diffuse, that is, multiple (sessile), especially in recurrent cases. In certain cases, it may extend to the nasopharynx and may be attached to the soft palate. It commonly affects the nasal cavity and the nasopharynx but other mucosal surfaces such as palate, conjunctiva, epiglottis, larynx, trachea, bronchi, vulva, and vagina may also be affected.

Diagnosis

Diagnosis is confirmed by histopathology which shows an intact epithelial layer and numerous sporangia in a background of chronic inflammation characterized by neutrophils, lymphocytes, plasma cells, and multinucleated giant cells. The culture of *Rhinosporidium seeberi* is not possible at present.

Treatment

Treatment is surgical with complete excision of the mass with cauterization of the base. Recurrences are known to occur after surgery. Antifungals are not effective. Dapsone is the only drug shown to have any benefit in the treatment of rhinosporidiosis.

■ Wegener's Granulomatosis or Granulomatosis with Polyangiitis

Wegener's granulomatosis or granulomatosis with polyangiitis (GPA) is an autoimmune, necrotizing vasculitis affecting small and medium-sized vessels. It primarily involves the upper respiratory tract, lungs, kidneys, and skin.

Clinical Features

Wegener's granulomatosis is characterized by systemic symptoms such as anemia, malaise, fatigue, and migratory arthralgia.

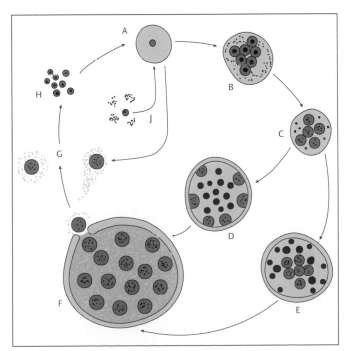

Fig. 26.10 Life cycle of *Rhinosporidium seeberi*.

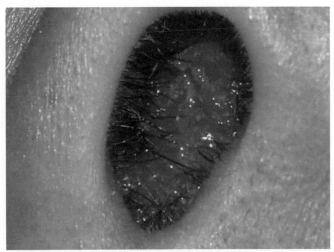

Fig. 26.11 Rhinosporidiosis presenting as a friable, red mass in the right nasal cavity.

Patients may complain of nasal discharge, nasal obstruction, crusting, epistaxis, and facial pain. There may be extensive destruction of the septum, turbinates, and sinuses resulting in a roomy cavity, septal perforation, and collapse of the dorsum of the nose.

The disease generally progresses to involve the kidneys in the form of focal or diffuse glomerulonephritis, and renal failure is usually the cause of death in these patients.

Diagnosis

Nasal biopsy shows epithelioid granulomas with necrotizing vasculitis. ESR is raised and enzyme-linked immunosorbent assay (ELISA) is positive for antineutrophilic cytoplasmic antibodies (cANCA). Urine analysis may show red blood cells (RBCs), casts, and albumin. Serum creatinine may be raised. Chest X-ray may show nodules, cavities, and fibrosis.

Treatment

Treatment consists of immunomodulators such as cyclophosphamide, azathioprine, and methotrexate. High-dose steroids may also be given.

Points to Ponder

- The commonest viral infection in man is acute viral rhinitis caused by the rhinovirus.
- It is a self-limiting condition, and treatment is aimed at symptomatic relief.
- Chronic rhinitis is classified into allergic rhinitis and nonallergic rhinitis.
- Allergic rhinitis is immunoglobulin E-mediated condition, whereas chronic nonallergic rhinitis is not mediated by IgE.
- The most common organism implicated in atrophic rhinitis is *Klebsiella ozaena*.
- Rhinitis sicca produces dryness and crusting (greyish white) in the anterior part of the nose while atrophic rhinitis produces crusting (greenish) in the posterior part.
- Rhinitis medicamentosa is the result of prolonged use of topical decongestant like xylometazoline.
- Rhinoscleroma passes through three stages: catarrhal, granulomatous, and sclerotic.
- Rhinosporidiosis often presents with nasal obstruction and epistaxis.

Case-Based Questions

1. **A 23-year-old female presented with a history of nasal obstruction and anosmia. She said that her relatives complained of foul smell emanating from her. She also had a sensation of something moving inside her nose. On anterior rhinoscopy, the nasal cavities were roomy and there were greenish crusts seen posteriorly.**

   a. What is the possible diagnosis?

   b. What are the secondary causes for this condition?

   c. Why does this patient have nasal obstruction and anosmia?

   d. What is the medical treatment of this condition?

   e. What is the commonest surgical procedure done for this condition?

   Answers

   a. Atrophic rhinitis.

   b. Secondary causes include granulomatous conditions like TB, rhinoscleroma, post-radiotherapy, occupational (phosphorite dust), and extensive resection during surgery in sinonasal region.

   c. Nasal obstruction is due to decreased sensation, large crusts, and altered airflow. Anosmia is due to atrophy of the olfactory epithelium or nerve endings or epithelium and large crusts or disrupted airflow.

   d. Nasal douching, 25% glucose in glycerine nasal drops, and nutritional supplements.

   e. Modified Young's operation.

2. **A 32-year-old male patient presented with epistaxis and nasal obstruction. His nose had a woody feel. He also complained of breathing difficulty and was noted to have mild stridor. Biopsy from the nasal mucosa revealed macrophages with a central nucleus and clear cytoplasm which had vacuoles containing bacilli; Russel bodies were also noted along with plasma cells and lymphocytes.**

   a. What is the possible diagnosis?

   b. What are the macrophages described called?

   c. Why does this patient have stridor?

   d. What is the medical treatment for this condition?

   Answers

   a. Rhinoscleroma.

   b. Mikulicz cells.

   c. Subglottic involvement with narrowing.

   d. Tetracycline is the drug of choice. Rifampicin can be used. Duration of treatment depends on sequential negative biopsies.

Frequently Asked Questions

1. How does modified Young's procedure help in atrophic rhinitis?

2. What is the mode of action of 25% glucose in glycerine in atrophic rhinitis?

3. What is the mode of infection, appearance, and treatment of rhinosporidiosis?

4. Define rhinitis medicamentosa and outline its treatment.

5. What are snuffles? In which disease do you encounter this condition?

6. What is the etiology of rhinitis sicca? How does the clinical appearance differ from atrophic rhinitis?

Endnote

Rhinosporidiosis is an interesting disease which was initially noticed in 1900. The first description of this condition was given by an Argentinian named Guillermo Seeber. He proposed a fungal infection as the cause, and the organism was isolated by Ashworth in 1923 and he named it Rhinosporidium seeberi. This disease is mainly concentrated in hot tropical climates like Sri Lanka and South India, and there is a history of bathing in stagnant ponds. Polymerase chain reaction (PCR) tests revealed that the organism is actually a protozoan parasite that infects fish and amphibians and not a fungus as was originally believed.

Shrinath D. Kamath P.

Th competencies covered in this chapter are as follows:

EN4.27 Elicit, document, and present a correct history; demonstrate and describe the clinical features; choose the correct investigations; and describe the management of allergic rhinitis.

PE31.1 Describe the etiopathogenesis, management, and prevention of allergic rhinitis in children.

Introduction

Allergic rhinitis is an immunoglobulin E (IgE)-mediated hypersensitivity reaction involving the mucosal lining of the nasal cavity (**Fig. 27.1**). It is prevalent in 20 to 30% of the Indian population. It is commonly seen in children younger than 10 years and peak symptoms have been observed at 10 to 40 years. The prevalence is increasing due to a more urban lifestyle and the condition is underdiagnosed especially in children. In the concept of "one airway, one disease," when symptoms are present in the upper airway, the lower airway is most likely to be involved as well.

Etiopathogenesis

When a patient with allergic rhinitis is exposed to an allergen, the reaction develops in two phases (**Fig. 27.2**):
- **Early phase:** Symptoms develop within 30 minutes. Early phase reaction is a type 1 hypersensitivity reaction

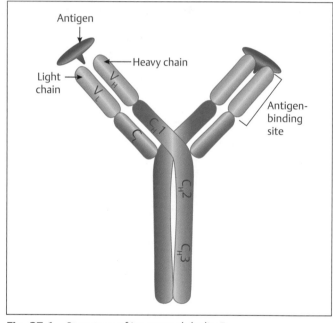

Fig. 27.1 Structure of immunoglobulin E.

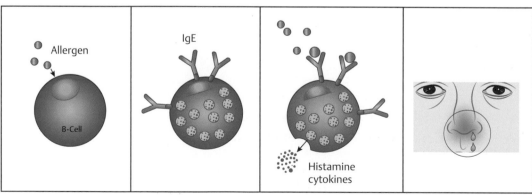

Fig. 27.2 Mechanism of allergic rhinitis.

| Exposure to allergen | IgE production, attach to mast cell | Allergen attachment, mast cell release histamine | Allergic |

due to the release of chemical mediators of inflammation at the affected site. The phase occurs within minutes (**Flowchart 27.1**).

- **Late phase:** Symptoms develop after 6 hours. Late phase reaction, however, is due to the release of cytokines, chemokines, and growth factors. These are released more slowly and symptoms may take hours to develop (**Flowchart 27.2**).

Classification

■ Traditional Classification of Allergic Rhinitis

Occupational exposure to wood dust, flour, animals, and latex can predispose to allergic rhinitis (**Table 27.1**). There has been a genetic correlation and allergic disease can run in families. Smoking, occupational irritants, and food preservatives are some of the irritants that can act as a trigger.

One of the commonest causes of perennial or persistent allergic rhinitis is the house dust mites or *Dermatophagoides pteronyssinus* (**Fig. 27.3**). They feed on the squamous epithelium of the human skin, which is shed regularly and is present on the bedsheets and pillow covers. After feeding on the epithelia, the mites shed protease enzymes in high amounts in fecal pellets, which are the antigens causing allergy in humans.

■ Current Classification Based on ARIA

According to the Allergic Rhinitis and its Impact on Asthma (ARIA) guidelines, the symptoms of allergic rhinitis can be classified as mild and moderate to severe (**Table 27.2**).

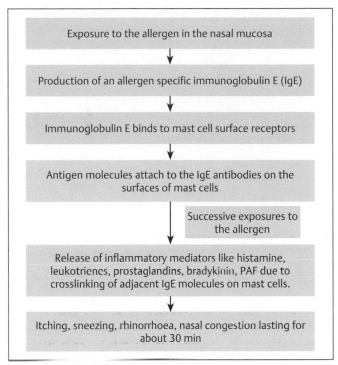

Flowchart 27.1 Etiopathogenesis—early phase reaction.

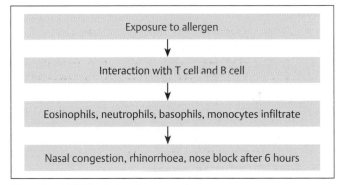

Flowchart 27.2 Late phase reaction.

Table 27.1 Traditional classification of allergic rhinitis

Seasonal allergic rhinitis	Perennial allergic rhinitis	Episodic allergic rhinitis
Occurs due to exposure to seasonal allergens. In tropical countries, some of these allergens are present throughout the year	Nasal symptoms are present for >2 h a day, 9 mo a year	Occurs due to allergens not common in patient's environment
Examples • Ragweed • Grasses • Outdoor molds • Pollen	*Examples* • House dust mite • Indoor molds • Animal dander • Cockroach	*Example* • Cat allergy following exposure at a friend's house

Table 27.2 Current classification of allergic rhinitis

Intermittent allergic rhinitis	Persistent allergic rhinitis
Symptoms present for <4 d a week or for <4 consecutive weeks	Symptoms present for >4 d a week and for >4 consecutive weeks

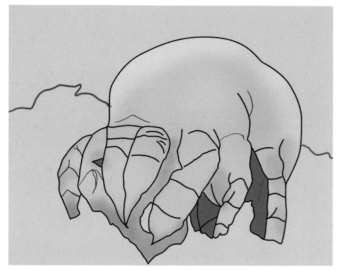

Fig. 27.3 House dust mite or *Dermatophagoides pteronyssinus*.

Mild allergic rhinitis is when all of the following symptoms are present:
- No troublesome symptoms.
- No impairment of daily activities.
- No impairment at work or school.
- Normal sleep.

Moderate or severe is when one or more of the following symptoms are present:
- Troublesome symptoms.
- Impairment of daily activities.
- Impairment at work or school.
- Disturbed sleep.

Clinical Features

■ Intermittent or (Seasonal) Allergic Rhinitis

Symptoms

- There will be recurrent episodes of the following:
  - Sneezing.
  - Itching of the nose.
  - Watery nasal discharge.
  - Nasal congestion.
  - Watering from the eyes.
- There may be wheezing, tightness of chest, eczema, and urticarial after exposure to the allergen.
- The sneezing bouts are recurrent, immediately after the exposure to the allergen.
- The patient with anterior rhinorrhea has sniffing and nose blowing and those with posterior rhinorrhea might have snorting, throat clearing, and a postnasal drip.

- The itching may involve the nose, eyes, ears, palate, and throat.
- The nasal obstruction is usually bilateral, and occasionally alternating. In case of a persistent unilateral nasal obstruction, coexisting mechanical causes such as septal deviation may be present.
- Anosmia, if present, is secondary to obstruction of airflow into the olfactory cleft due to inflammation or edema. It may also manifest as loss of taste.

Eye symptoms such as itching, epiphora, and redness of conjunctiva are often associated with allergic rhinitis. Eustachian tube dysfunction may manifest with ear block or mild hearing loss. The systemic symptoms associated with allergic rhinitis are general malaise, fatigue, irritability, snoring, and sleep problems. Some patients may experience dysphonia.

■ Persistent or (Perennial) Allergic Rhinitis

Symptoms

In addition to sneezing, patients may have viscid rhinorrhea, loss of smell, loss of taste, sinusitis, eustachian tube dysfunction, nasal block, and postnasal drip. Some patients may have dry cough.

> **Pearl**
>
> *Samter's triad* refers to a condition consisting of asthma, aspirin sensitivity, and nasal polyps. It is also known as aspirin exacerbated respiratory disease (AERD). Along with nasal stuffiness and sneezing, patients will have wheezing and tightness of chest. Treatment is by avoidance of aspirin and other cross-reacting nonsteroidal anti-inflammatory drugs (NSAIDs), and by aspirin desensitization.

Signs of Allergic Rhinitis

- On anterior rhinoscopy, the mucosa on the lateral nasal wall and the turbinates may appear pale or bluish, edematous, and may be coated with thin clear secretions (**Fig. 27.4**). There may be mucoid strands between the turbinates and septum. In addition, patients with chronicity will have polyps, especially in the middle meatus.
- On examination of the face, there may be puffiness of the eyelids and darkening of the lower eyelids, referred to as *allergic shiner* (**Fig. 27.5**). This occurs due to venous stasis of the lower eyelids secondary to edema of the nasal mucosa. The stasis and resultant hypoxia may result in spasm of the tarsal muscle and edema, which can result in the characteristic *Dennie–Morgan* lines in the lower eyelid.

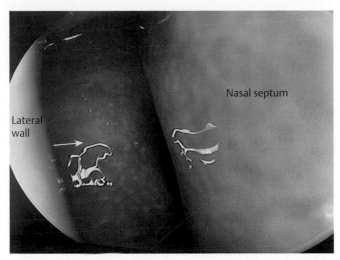

Fig. 27.4 Anterior rhinoscopy showing pale, edematous middle turbinate (*yellow arrow*) with mucoid discharge (*red arrow*) in the right nasal cavity.

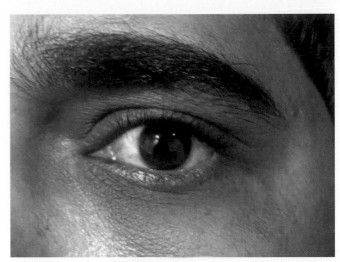

Fig. 27.5 Allergic Shiners: Vasocongestion of the left lower eyelid.

- Children with chronic allergic rhinitis may develop adenoid facies due to long-standing nasal obstruction.
- Due to frequent upward pushing of the nasal tip with the palm (*allergic salute*), a supratip crease called an *allergic crease* may form in the region of the upper lateral cartilage and alar cartilage.
- During rhinorrhea, older children may prefer to move their nose tip side to side (*bunny nose*) or sniff on one side with associated movement of the ipsilateral angle of the mouth upward and laterally (*allergic grimace*).
- Ear examination may show features of eustachian tube catarrh or otitis media with effusion.

Nasal endoscopy may demonstrate the classical features of nasal mucosa in allergic rhinitis as described earlier, and may also reveal the presence of nasal polyposis.

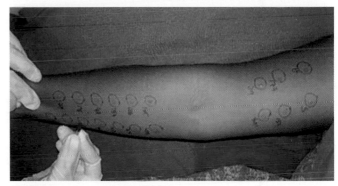

Fig. 27.6 Skin prick testing.

Pearls

- Allergic march or atopic march is the sequential development of allergy, which is IgE mediated, from early childhood to adult life with change in symptomatology with age, based on the type of antibody response. There may be remission.
- Some authors refer to it as allergic dermatitis, and food allergies that start in childhood, and the development later of allergic rhinitis and bronchial asthma in sequence.

Diagnostic Tests

Skin prick testing (SPT): It is done by introducing antigen extracts under the epidermis of the skin of the forearm using lancets. The allergen (antigen extract) combines with IgE-sensitized mast cells to produce degranulation. Saline and histamine solutions are used as controls. After 15 to 20 minutes, a positive reaction is when the wheal measures ≥3 mm more than the negative control. The commonly used allergens are grass pollen, house dust mite, cat and dog fur, cockroach, and certain fungi. Antihistamines need to be stopped 10 to 14 days prior to the test and there should be no dermographism (**Fig. 27.6**).

Intradermal testing (IDT): Allergen extract is injected into the superficial dermis. After 10 minutes, the wheal is examined and measured. A positive wheal measures ≥7 mm, with a width 2 mm more than the negative control.

In vitro testing includes the serum IgE level, serum antigen–specific IgE, and nasal-specific IgE estimation.

Nasal provocation testing (NPT): Allergen is applied on the nasal mucosa and the response is measured using a combination of subjective symptom scores and objective measures such as acoustic rhinometry, rhinomanometry, peak inspiratory flow, and testing of nasal secretions for inflammatory markers.

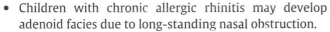

Radioallergosorbent test or RAST: It is a blood test to detect specific IgE antibodies in order to find out what the patient is allergic to. The advantage is that it is an in vitro test, does not get affected by medications, and more antigens can be tested.

Pulmonary function tests are done to find out any associated lung pathology such as asthma.

Treatment

Prevention by *avoiding* the known allergen can be effective. Multiple strategies to avoid the common allergens have been advocated like removing a pet from the house, covering the pillows and mattresses, washing the bed covers in hot water, no carpets, not keeping plants inside the house, and vacuum cleaning the sofas, mattresses, and pillows. Breastfeeding especially in the first 3 months of infancy may be protective and reduce the incidence of allergy in children.

Antihistamines: Second-generation H1 antihistamines like loratadine, fexofenadine, cetirizine, and levocetirizine are commonly prescribed medications. These do not easily cross the blood–brain barrier as these are less lipophilic. Thus, the sedative and anticholinergic effects are low. Except nasal congestion, the histamine-mediated symptoms such as sneezing, itching, rhinorrhea, and ocular symptoms are reduced. Topical azelastine nasal sprays can be used instead of oral antihistamine in seasonal allergic rhinitis.

Azelastine is a second-generation antihistamine and can be used in the form of a nasal spray. It blocks the H1 receptors on the nasal mucosa and has a fast onset of action, within 15 minutes. The effect can last for 12 hours.

Decongestants (topical and systemic) have an α-adrenergic action. These act by vasoconstriction. Thereby, the volume of blood in the sinusoids and nasal blood flow are reduced. Commonly used decongestants are *phenylephrine* (catecholamine derivative) and *xylometazoline or oxymetazoline* (imidazoline derivatives). The onset of action is rapid with better efficacy than systemic decongestants. But the usage of decongestants should be restricted to short period as prolonged usage may result in rhinitis medicamentosa. These drugs may help open up the nasal cavity so that topical steroid nasal sprays can be useful. Systemic decongestants like pseudoephedrine and phenylephrine may be effective in reducing the nasal congestion.

Anticholinergic drugs like ipratropium bromide used intranasally reduce the perennial allergic and nonallergic rhinitis symptoms of clear anterior rhinorrhea.

Four percent cromolyn sodium in the form of intranasal spray is effective in the treatment of seasonal allergic rhinitis. It is safe in children and pregnant women.

Leukotriene receptor antagonists like montelukast have been used in seasonal allergic rhinitis.

Intranasal corticosteroids are the first-line treatment in moderate to severe allergic rhinitis. These inhibit the release of early- and late-phase mediators. Examples of topical steroid sprays are fluticasone and mometasone.

Systemic corticosteroids are useful when the symptoms are severe and not reducing with other medications.

Omalizumab is a recombinant, humanized, monoclonal anti-IgE antibody. By forming complexes with free IgE, the interaction with mast cells and basophils is blocked. Currently, it is approved only for severe asthma with or without allergic rhinitis.

Saline nasal douches can be used to clear the secretions, allergens, and inflammatory mediators; the tonicity may improve mucociliary clearance.

Combination therapy of topical steroid and topical antihistamine is used when some symptoms are persistent. Topical steroids with oral antihistamines and, in addition, saline nasal douches are also advocated.

Immunotherapy or desensitization is repeated exposure to antigens with increasing doses, where the antigens can be presented subcutaneously or sublingually. It is used when the symptoms are poorly controlled with medications, and the patient wants to avoid long-term pharmacotherapy and its side effects.

The disadvantages of immunotherapy are the following:
- It is effective when the number of antigens the patient is allergic to is limited.
- It has poor compliance to treatment due to long duration of therapy. It may take up to 1.5 years for full desensitization.
- It is expensive.

Role of surgery in allergic rhinitis is limited to relieving nasal obstruction. It may also allow access for topical steroids.

Points to Ponder

- Allergic rhinitis is an extremely common condition and affects 15% of patients coming to the ear, nose, and throat (ENT) clinic.
- There are two types of allergic rhinitis, seasonal and perennial, or the more currently accepted classification of intermittent and persistent.
- From the pathogenesis point of view, there is an early phase and a late phase.
- The four cardinal symptoms of allergic rhinitis include sneezing, itching of the nose, watery nasal discharge, and blocked nose.
- Symptoms of allergy can be controlled by drugs but to get complete and permanent relief, immunotherapy can be tried.

Case-Based Questions

1. A 28-year-old male patient presented with a 2-year history of recurrent sneezing and nasal discharge associated with itching of the eyes and nose. Two years back, he got a cat as a pet. Recently, he has developed wheezing and chest tightness.

a. What is the condition he is suffering from?

b. What are allergic shiner and allergic salute?

c. What tests can help confirm the allergen?

d. What is the topical medication of choice for the treatment of the nasal symptoms?

Answers

a. Allergic rhinitis with bronchial asthma.

b. Allergic shiners are dark discoloration of the lower eyelid due to venous stasis and extravasation of hemosiderin. Allergic salute is the upward rubbing of the nose, which when done repeatedly forms the allergic crease.

c. Allergic skin prick test and RAST.

d. Steroid nasal spray for the allergic rhinitis.

2. A 35-year-old woman presented with symptoms of allergic rhinitis. She had repeated bouts of sneezing and itching of the nose with watery nasal discharge. She also developed bilateral nasal obstruction.

a. What is the reason for nasal obstruction?

b. How will you proceed to treat this patient?

Answers

a. Nasal obstruction occurs during the late phase of an allergic reaction where the inferior turbinates undergo hypertrophy due to increased vascularity. It can also be due to mucosal edema or the formation of nasal polyps.

b. Management is mainly medical rather than surgical.

The first-line drug is a topical steroid nasal spray, either fluticasone or mometasone. It can be combined with an oral histamine.

Frequently Asked Questions

1. What are the symptoms and signs of allergic rhinitis?

2. What is the skin prick test?

3. What are the types of allergic rhinitis?

4. What is the treatment of allergic rhinitis?

5. What is Samter's triad?

6. How will you classify antihistamines?

Endnote The word "allergy" was coined by an Austrian pediatrician named Clemens Von Pirquet (1874–1929). He noticed that patients who had a previous injection of horse's serum had a more severe reaction when given a second injection. He called this phenomenon allergy.

Charles Mantoux expanded on this idea of allergy and injected tuberculin into the skin of patients to diagnose tuberculosis. This led to the Mantoux test.

28 Vasomotor Rhinitis

Vadisha Bhat

The competency covered in this chapter is as follows:

EN4.28 Elicit, document, and present a correct history; demonstrate and describe the clinical features; choose the correct investigations; and describe the principles of management of vasomotor rhinitis.

Introduction

Rhinitis can be classified as allergic rhinitis or nonallergic rhinitis. Allergic rhinitis is immunoglobulin E (IgE) mediated inflammation, whereas a diagnosis of nonallergic rhinitis is made after ruling out allergic or IgE-mediated disease.

Nonallergic Rhinitis

It includes the following:
- Infectious rhinitis.
- Vasomotor rhinitis.
- Occupational rhinitis.
- Hormonal rhinitis.
- Drug-induced rhinitis.
- Gustatory rhinitis.
- Nonallergic rhinitis with eosinophilia syndrome (NARES).

Vasomotor rhinitis is a form of nonallergic, noninfectious rhinitis causing nasal obstruction and nasal discharge. It is also called intrinsic rhinitis, as the factors within one's body cause this condition. Some authors have suggested the term "intrinsic rhinopathy," as the suffix "itis" means inflammation, and vasomotor rhinitis does not have pathological evidence of inflammation.

■ Etiopathogenesis

The exact etiology of vasomotor rhinitis is poorly understood. It is believed to be caused by the imbalance between parasympathetic and sympathetic innervations to the nasal mucosa. The nasal mucosa is innervated by the autonomous nervous system, which controls the blood vessels and the nasal glands. The parasympathetic innervation is through the vidian nerve (nerve of the pterygoid canal), formed by the greater superficial petrosal nerve, which is a branch from the facial nerve, and the deep petrosal nerve, which is formed by the fibers over the internal carotid artery. The parasympathetic system is the secretomotor to the nasal glands, whereas sympathetic stimulation causes vasoconstriction of the nasal blood vessels. Parasympathetic overactivity causes increased nasal congestion and increased secretions from the nasal glands, causing symptoms of vasomotor rhinitis.

Patients may be "*runners*" with mainly nasal discharge or "*blockers*" with mainly nasal obstruction. Rhinorrhea is due to an increased cholinergic response, while nasal obstruction is due to an increased response of nociceptive neurons to harmless stimuli.

■ Precipitating Factors

Vasomotor rhinitis is precipitated by some nonspecific irritants such as cold air, dry air, smoke, perfumes (strong odors), or alcoholic beverages. Exaggerated response of the nociceptive neurons in the nasal mucosa to the innocuous stimuli causes nasal congestion and obstruction. Emotional factors like stress and sexual arousal are also known to precipitate the symptoms due to autonomic stimulation.

After laryngectomy, there is no significant nasal airflow, and hence the turbinates become swollen due to loss of vasomotor control. This is termed nonairflow rhinitis.

■ Clinical Features

Symptoms

Nasal obstruction, nasal discharge, and postnasal discharge are the predominant symptoms of vasomotor rhinitis. The nasal block may be alternating between the two sides. The nasal discharge is usually seromucinous and there may be postnasal drip. The symptoms usually start in adulthood. There will not be a history of seasonal variation of the symptoms. Unlike allergic rhinitis, sneezing and itching are not significant symptoms but can occur.

Signs

Nasal mucosa appears edematous because of the vasodilatation with hypertrophy of the turbinates, which may appear boggy due to the edema (**Fig. 28.1**). There may be watery or mucoid nasal discharge in the nasal cavity.

> ### Pearl
>
> The prevalence of nonallergic rhinitis in the general population is as high as 25%. Unlike allergic rhinitis, there is no specific test to diagnose nonallergic rhinitis. This condition is mainly diagnosed through clinical features like rhinorrhea, nose block, sneezing, and postnasal drip. A patient can reasonably be diagnosed as having nonallergic rhinitis if he or she has two or more of the above symptoms for more than 9 months in a year.

Management

■ Investigations

There are no specific tests for the diagnosis of vasomotor rhinitis. Diagnosis is made based on the history and clinical examination without any identifiable nasal allergy, sinonasal infections, or structural abnormalities like deviated

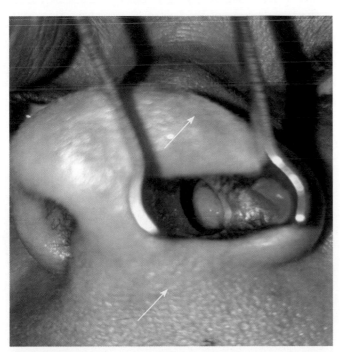

Fig. 28.1 Anterior rhinoscopy showing hypertrophied inferior turbinate. (This image is provided courtesy of Dr. P. Thirunavukarasu, Chennai.)

nasal septum. The skin prick test (refer to Fig. 27.6), if done, will be negative. The IgE levels will be normal, and there will not be eosinophils in the nasal smears. Diagnostic nasal endoscopy helps complete examination of the nasal cavity. Computed tomography (CT) scan of the paranasal sinuses may be required in some cases to rule out chronic sinusitis and sinonasal polyposis.

The *differential diagnosis* of vasomotor rhinitis includes allergic rhinitis and infective rhinitis.

■ Treatment

Treatment aims to relieve nasal obstruction and reduce nasal secretions.

Medical

Avoidance of factors that trigger the episodes is ideal but not always possible.

The drugs that can be used are the following:

- *Anticholinergic drugs* like ipratropium bromide nasal spray are helpful in reducing the nasal secretions. These are useful for patients in whom the main symptom is rhinorrhea.
- *Intranasal steroid sprays* help reduce the local inflammatory response and relieve nasal obstruction, secretions, and sneezing symptoms, if present. The action may not start immediately, and the spray needs to be taken for a long duration.
- *Antihistamines* reduce nasal secretions and sneezing and thus show some benefit. These are the commonly prescribed medications for most patients during the initial course, as differentiation of this condition from allergic rhinitis is difficult in many cases. Oral or topical (azelastine) antihistamines may be used.
- *Nasal decongestants* like pseudoephedrine (taken orally) and oxymetazoline/xylometazoline nasal drops (used topically) improve the nasal patency. Prolonged use of topical decongestants may lead to a condition called *rhinitis medicamentosa* due to the rebound phenomena.

Surgical

Surgery is indicated in patients with severe symptoms who do not respond to medical treatment.

Vidian neurectomy: This involves sectioning of the vidian nerve, which disrupts the sympathetic and parasympathetic innervations to the mucosa. This reduces nasal secretions. Vidian neurectomy should be reserved for patients with severe rhinorrhea and those not responding to medical treatment. The surgery can be performed endoscopically or via the transantral approach.

Posterior nasal nerve neurectomy may significantly reduce rhinorrhea, nasal block, and sneezing. Selective transection of the parasympathetic branches to the nasal cavity is done with sparing of branches to the lacrimal gland and palate. This avoids the complications of vidian neurectomy like dry eye and palatal numbness.

Reduction of the inferior turbinate (turbinoplasty) can be done by various different methods, including chemical cautery with silver nitrate, or using bipolar cautery, submucosal diathermy, cryotherapy, laser, microdebrider, or coblation. A submucosal resection or partial inferior turbinectomy can be done. However, excess removal of the inferior turbinate should be avoided as it may cause secondary atrophic rhinitis or may compromise the functions of the nose.

Points to Ponder

- Vasomotor rhinitis is a nonallergic, noninfective rhinitis and usually starts in adulthood.
- The proposed pathogenesis is the imbalance in the sympathetic and parasympathetic innervations to the nasal mucosa, that is, parasympathetic overactivity.
- Unlike allergic rhinitis, sneezing and itching are less common symptoms.
- Diagnosis is mainly based on the history, clinical examination, and exclusion of allergic rhinitis. Treatment is primarily medical. Surgery is reserved for persistent symptoms.

Case-Based Questions

1. **A 37-year-old woman presents with a 2-year history of runny nose and bilateral nose block. Along with this, she had postnasal drip, which was causing throat irritation. She said smoke and strong perfumes aggravated her condition. On examination, there was bilateral hypertrophied inferior turbinates with mucoid nasal discharge. There was no history suggestive of any nasal allergy.**

   a. What is the diagnosis?
   b. How will you proceed to treat this patient?

   Answers

   a. Vasomotor rhinitis.
   b. The patient is advised to avoid any inciting factors like smoke and strong perfume. Antihistamines combined with oral decongestants will help in alleviating the nasal secretions and nose block. Topical steroid nasal sprays like fluticasone will help reduce the symptoms when taken long term. If medical management does not alleviate the nose block, turbinoplasty surgery can be considered.

2. **A patient presents with refractory vasomotor rhinitis for which the medications prescribed did not help in reducing the symptoms. Is there any surgery that may be of benefit?**

   Answer

   Vidian neurectomy or cutting the vidian nerve. This can be done endoscopically. The vidian nerve, along with the vidian artery, runs along the pterygoid canal, which is located on the lateral aspect of the floor of the sphenoid sinus. The parasympathetic fibers from the greater superficial petrosal nerve and the sympathetic fibers from the deep petrosal nerve from the internal carotid artery plexus, together, form the vidian nerve.

Frequently Asked Questions

1. What is nonallergic rhinitis?
2. What is the etiology of vasomotor rhinitis?
3. What is the medical management of vasomotor rhinitis?
4. What is the differential diagnosis for vasomotor rhinitis?
5. What surgeries can be performed to alleviate the symptoms of vasomotor rhinitis?

Endnote

Studies have shown that a normal person sneezes up to four times a day and blows his or her nose four times a day. So if a person sneezes or blows the nose more than four times a day, it could possibly indicate rhinitis. The speed of a human sneeze has been calculated as air traveling over 160 km/h, which is almost double the speed of a cough.

29 Acute and Chronic Sinusitis Including Fungal Sinusitis

Bini Faizal

The competencies covered in this chapter are as follows:

AN37.3 Describe the anatomical basis of sinusitis.

EN4.33 Elicit, document, and present a correct history; demonstrate and describe the clinical features; choose the correct investigations; and describe the principles of management of acute and chronic sinusitis.

Introduction

Sinusitis is defined as an inflammation of the paranasal sinus mucosa. The term *rhinosinusitis* is preferred as the lining mucosa of the nasal cavity is continuous with that of the paranasal sinuses. The diagnosis is based on the presence of specific subjective and objective findings (**Table 29.1**). The signs include findings on nasal endoscopy and on imaging:

- *Acute sinusitis* is infection in the paranasal sinuses lasting up to 4 weeks.
- *Subacute sinusitis* is when the patient presents with symptoms between 4 and 12 weeks.
- *Chronic sinusitis* is when the symptoms are present for more than 12 weeks.
- *Recurrent acute sinusitis* is when there are three or more episodes in a year with the absence of symptoms in the intervening period.
- *Acute exacerbation of chronic sinusitis* is when a patient with persisting chronic sinusitis develops acute symptoms.

Acute Sinusitis

The presence of symptoms of nasal block or discharge with facial pain or olfactory dysfunction lasting more than 10 days but less than 4 weeks are included under acute sinusitis. The components of subjective and objective criteria for diagnosis are given in **Table 29.1**.

■ Etiology

- *Viral infection* that usually subsides in 7 to 10 days. When there is secondary bacterial infection, the symptoms persist or worsen.
- *Anatomical factors* that block the ostiomeatal complex (OMC) like deviated nasal septum, tumors of nasal cavity, and anatomical variations like concha bullosa may contribute to the obstruction of the drainage of the sinuses facilitating secondary infection.
- *Allergic rhinitis* causes edema of the mucosa, which affects the drainage through the ostia.
- *Dental caries* of the root of the maxillary teeth (especially the premolars, first, and second molars). They are

---

Table 29.1 Subjective and objective criteria for diagnosis of sinusitis

Diagnostic criteria	Symptoms/signs
Primary symptom	Nasal block/discharge
Additional symptoms	Facial pain and olfactory dysfunction
Duration	More than 10 d and less than 4 wk
Nasal endoscopy	Polyps, discharge, and edema
Computed tomography scan	Mucosal edema

Note: Either a single sinus or multiple sinuses can be involved. If all the sinuses are involved on one side, it is termed *pansinusitis*.

related to the floor of the maxillary sinus and the roots may lie within the sinus cavity without a bony covering. This allows an infection like root abscess to extend into the sinus. The presence of an oroantral fistula may also lead to acute, recurrent, or chronic infection of the maxillary sinus.

- *Trauma* leading to fracture of the facial bones in relation to the paranasal sinuses may facilitate sinus infection.
- *Barotrauma* during deep sea diving or flying causes change in pressure, which can lead to fluid accumulation in the sinuses.
- *Swimming* in contaminated water can affect the nose and paranasal sinuses.
- *Adenoid hypertrophy* in children can impair the drainage of mucous from the nose, leading to stagnation in the nasal cavity. From there, the infection can spread into the sinuses.
- *Immunocompromised states* like diabetes, malnutrition, immunodeficiencies, and prolonged use of corticosteroids can make an individual more prone to sinusitis.
- *Genetic disorders or congenital conditions* like cystic fibrosis and primary ciliary dyskinesia.
- *Infectious/inflammatory conditions* like tuberculosis.
- *Immune mediated conditions* like Churg–Strauss syndrome, and *immunosuppression*.
- *Other predisposing factors* would be environment pollution, smoking, laryngopharyngeal reflux, and endocrine conditions like hypothyroidism and pregnancy.

Causative Organisms

Most cases of acute sinusitis start as a viral upper respiratory tract infection commonly caused by *rhinovirus*. Influenza and parainfluenza viruses, adenovirus, respiratory syncytial virus, and enterovirus are other viruses implicated.

Around 90% of patients with viral upper respiratory infections also have sinus involvement. A diagnosis of bacterial sinusitis is made if the symptoms persist beyond 10 days or worsen after initial improvement. The bacteria get deposited in the sinuses from the nasal cavity when the patient sneezes, coughs, or through direct entry. The bacteria commonly implicated are *Streptococcus pneumoniae*, *Haemophilus influenzae*, and *Moraxella catarrhalis*. Less commonly seen are *S. pyogenes* and *Staphylococcus aureus*.

Maxillary sinusitis due to dental origin is caused by anaerobic organisms or is a mixed infection ascending through maxillary premolars or molars into the sinus.

Pseudomonas aeruginosa is noted in nosocomial infections, in immunocompromised individuals, and in cystic fibrosis.

Pathology of Sinusitis

The frontal sinus, maxillary sinus, and anterior ethmoidal cells drain into a potential space called infundibulum and from there the secretions drain into the middle meatus through hiatus semilunaris. Blockage of the OMC plays a major role in sinusitis.

The posterior ethmoid sinus drains into the superior meatus and the sphenoid sinus drains into the sphenoethmoid recess. An isolated involvement of the posterior group of sinuses is less common and more often are involved as part of pansinusitis (**Fig. 29.1**).

Cilia in the mucosa of the sinuses always beat toward the sinus ostia. This allows the sinus secretions to drain into the nasal cavity. An isolated sinus disease can develop into pansinusitis by involving the infundibulum (**Fig. 29.2**).

Any obstruction to this mucociliary mechanism as caused by a deviated nasal septum, allergy, polyps, hypertrophied turbinates, benign or malignant neoplasms and mucociliary dysfunction will interfere with the normal ventilation and drainage of the sinuses, causing stasis of secretions. Initially, the exudate is serous and later may become mucopurulent or purulent. Severe infections cause destruction of mucosal lining and also affect the cilia. The viscosity of the fluid changes, becoming thicker, which also

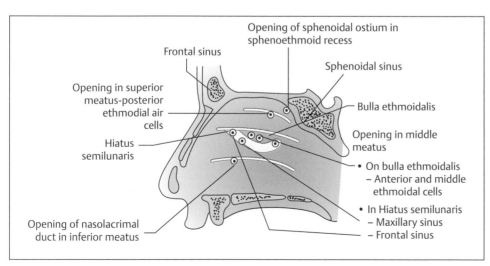

Fig. 29.1 Lateral wall of nasal cavity with sinus openings.

Frontal sinus

Opening of sphenoidal ostium in sphenoethmoid recess

Sphenoidal sinus

Opening in superior meatus-posterior ethmodial air cells

Bulla ethmoidalis

Hiatus semilunaris

Opening in middle meatus

Opening of nasolacrimal duct in inferior meatus

- On bulla ethmoidalis
  – Anterior and middle ethmoidal cells
- In Hiatus semilunaris
  – Maxillary sinus
  – Frontal sinus

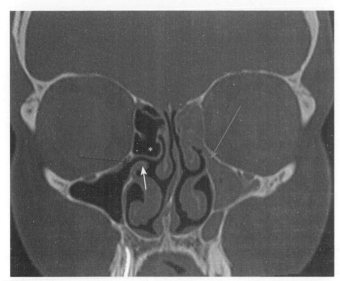

Fig. 29.2 Patent right infundibulum and blocked left infundibulum (*orange arrow*: infundibulum; *white arrow*: uncinate process; *blue arrow*: blocked OMC; *white star*: bulla ethmoidalis).

affects the clearance by the cilia. Failure of the drainage from the sinus due to ostial obstruction and ciliary dysfunction results in empyema of the sinus. Persistence of the disease can lead to a chronic infection, and destruction of the bony walls of the sinuses leads to complications.

Pearl

OMC plays a key role in the pathogenesis of sinusitis. An isolated sinusitis may develop into pansinusitis when the OMC is blocked.

■ Clinical Features

Symptoms

The general symptoms of all sinusitis are common except for region-specific pain and tenderness:
- *Constitutional symptoms* consist of fever, general malaise, and body ache.
- *Headache and pain*:
  - In *frontal sinusitis*, pain is over the forehead. This headache is referred to as morning headache or office headache. The pain can radiate to the vertex of the head.
  - In *maxillary sinusitis*, the pain is over the cheek and may be in the frontal region as well. There may be pain along the ipsilateral upper teeth related to the maxillary sinus, which may be the initial presenting symptom for which the patient may go to the dentist. The patient develops headache toward afternoon with a headache-free morning since the sinuses drain better in the lying down position.

- In *ethmoid sinusitis*, pain is between the eyes or behind the eyes.
- In *sphenoid sinusitis*, the pain is retro-orbital, in the vertex or in the occipital region. This is also called occipital headache.

Headache or heaviness of the head in sinusitis is aggravated on bending forward and on moving the head. There may be associated ear pain or fullness.
- Younger children present with cough, halitosis, low-grade fever, and purulent nasal discharge. Older children have headache and nasal congestion.
- *Olfactory disturbances* like hyposmia or anosmia may be present.

Pearl

Office headache

The patient wakes up with a headache that gradually increases during the day, reaches a peak by noon, and then diminishes. The upright position during the day helps in the gravity-dependent drainage of the sinus. It is called office headache because of the timing, similar to office hours.

Ice cream headache

A brief episode of headache over the frontal region when taking a cold item such as ice cream. It is also known as cold stimulus headache or brain freeze. It is thought to be due to intense vasoconstriction of the blood vessels as the cold item passes over the hard palate. The sensation is carried by the trigeminal nerve.

Signs

- *Tenderness*:
  - Pressure over the canine fossa produces pain in maxillary sinusitis.
  - In frontal sinusitis, palpation at the superomedial part of the roof of the orbit (the floor of the frontal sinus) elicits tenderness.
  - Tenderness on the side of the nose adjacent to the medial canthus is diagnostic of ethmoiditis.
- *Redness and edema of the cheek* is seen in children.
- The eyelids may become puffy. Frontal sinusitis with osteomyelitis of the anterior wall of frontal sinus results in redness and bulge over the frontal bone referred to as *Pott's puffy tumor.*
- *Nasal discharge*: Anterior rhinoscopy or nasal endoscopy shows pus or mucopus in the middle meatus. Pus in the superior meatus (between the middle turbinate and the septum) is suggestive of infection in the posterior ethmoid cells. Mucosa of the middle meatus and turbinate may appear red and swollen. Decongestion with a vasoconstrictor may have to be performed if the middle meatus is not seen clearly.
- *Postnasal discharge.*

Pearl

Ethmoiditis is the most common sinus infection seen in children since the development of other sinuses is incomplete at birth.

Investigations

Diagnostic Nasal Endoscopy

This is done under topical anesthesia to assess the condition of the mucosa, type of discharge, and lesions obstructing the drainage pathway (**Fig. 29.3**). A swab for culture and sensitivity can be taken especially in persistent or recurrent infection. The nasal endoscopy, though diagnostic, can be partially therapeutic when a decongestant is used in the middle meatus as it improves drainage and may reduce the severity of the symptoms.

A decongestant is a vasoconstrictor agent, like adrenaline, which, when added to a cotton pledget, shrinks the nasal mucosa and clears the nasal obstruction in the middle meatus.

X-Ray of the Paranasal Sinuses

Waters' view (occipitomental view) will show either an opacity or a fluid level in the involved sinus (**Fig. 29.4**). X-rays are not routinely done for sinusitis, except for screening or when the diagnosis is in doubt.

Computed Tomography Scan

It is the preferred imaging modality of the sinuses to diagnose sinusitis. Imaging is done in acute sinusitis if the patient is not responding to the medical management or has developed complications (**Fig. 29.2**).

Ultrasound (A Mode)

It may be helpful in pregnancy and in an intensive care setting.

Treatment

Medical Treatment

- *Antimicrobial drugs*: Antibiotics are given if there is fever, purulent nasal discharge, and increased total blood count. Ampicillin and amoxicillin are quite effective and cover a wide range of organisms. Erythromycin, doxycycline, or cotrimoxazole are equally effective and can be used in those who are allergic to penicillin. β-lactamase producing strains of *H. influenzae* and *M. catarrhalis* may necessitate the use of amoxicillin with clavulanic acid or cefuroxime axetil. Treatment is given for 10 to 14 days.

Pearl

Antibiotics should not be given when there is a suspected viral infection. The proper use of antibiotics will avoid resistant strains.

- *Nasal decongestant drops* like oxymetazoline 0.05% and xylometazoline 0.1% are used as nasal drops or sprays to decongest sinus ostium and encourage drainage. Drops have to be instilled in the lateral wall of the nose with the head hanging from the side of the bed, the Mygind position, or the Mecca position. The patient is encouraged to

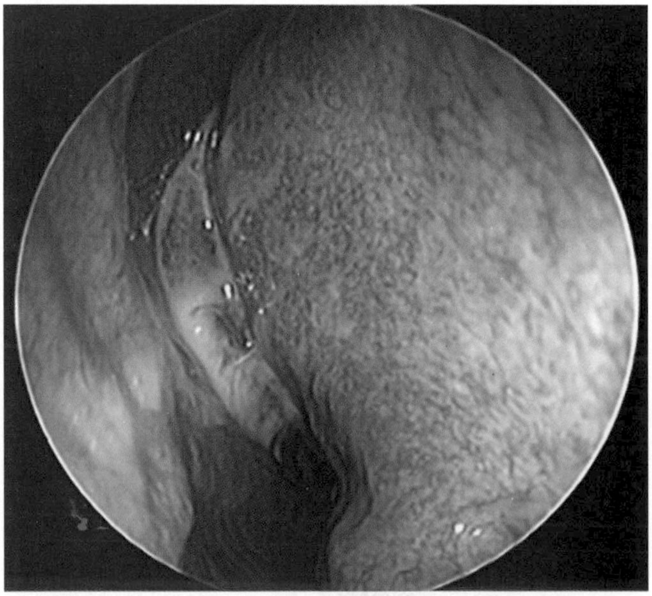

Fig. 29.3 Purulent discharge in the middle meatus.

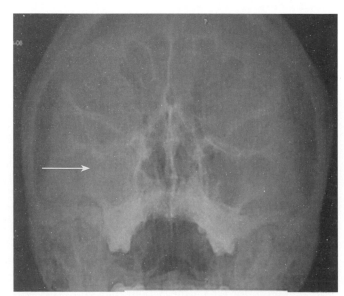

Fig. 29.4 Right maxillary sinusitis in modified Waters' view (*open mouth*).

do intermittent pinching of the nose and sniffing, after instilling drops.

- *Saline nasal douching* with warm saline is beneficial as it clears the secretions in the nasal cavity and encourages ciliary activity.
- *Mucolytics* like guaifenesin will cause thinning of the mucous, which will facilitate mucociliary clearance.
- *Analgesics* like paracetamol or other nonsteroidal anti-inflammatory drugs should be given for relief of pain and headache.
- *Steam inhalation* and *hot fomentation* (local heat) to the affected sinus is often soothing and may provide symptomatic relief. Inhalation should be given 15 to 20 minutes after nasal decongestion for better penetration. The use of these methods is debatable as some discourage steam inhalation unless it is in a controlled setting.
- *Vaccination*, which has been given for *H. influenzae* type A and *S. pneumoniae*, has shown to reduce the incidence and severity of sinusitis.

Surgical Treatment

Most cases of acute sinusitis respond to medical treatment. Failure of medical treatment and development of complications are treated surgically through functional endoscopic sinus surgery (FESS). Antral lavage of the maxillary sinus is rarely necessary and is outdated. Similarly, trephining done for draining the frontal sinus by drilling a hole into the floor of the frontal sinus is also rarely practiced. These procedures are replaced by endoscopic sinus surgery.

■ Complications of Acute Sinusitis

When a patient develops high-grade fever, severe headache, visual changes, orbital involvement, or altered sensorium, investigations to rule out complications have to be done. A contrast-enhanced computed tomography (CECT) scan of the brain or magnetic resonance imaging (MRI) is required.

The common complications of acute sinusitis are the following:

- Chronic sinusitis.
- *Osteitis or osteomyelitis*: This includes Pott's puffy tumor (subperiosteal abscess of frontal sinus) and empyema of the maxilla.
- *Orbital cellulitis or abscess*: Infection spreads to the orbit either directly from the roof of the maxillary sinus, through the lamina papyracea after involvement of ethmoid sinuses, or from the floor of the frontal sinus.
- Meningitis, extradural abscess, subdural empyema, or frontal lobe abscess occurs if infection spreads through the posterior wall of the frontal sinus, the roof of the ethmoid sinus, or the sphenoid sinus.
- Visual deterioration and blindness due to involvement of the optic nerve in ethmoiditis and sphenoid sinusitis.
- Cavernous sinus thrombosis.

Chronic Rhinosinusitis

Sinus infection lasting for more than 12 weeks is called chronic sinusitis. The most common cause of chronic sinusitis is failure of the acute infection to resolve. It can be classified as chronic rhinosinusitis with polyps (CRSwNP) and chronic rhinosinusitis without polyps (CRSsNP; **Figs. 29.5** and **29.6**).

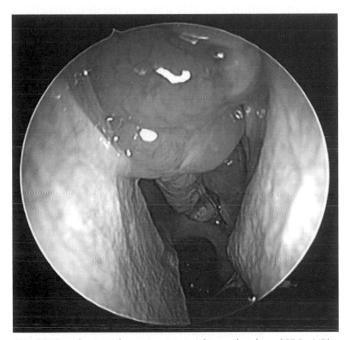

Fig. 29.5　Chronic rhinosinusitis with nasal polyps (CRSwNP).

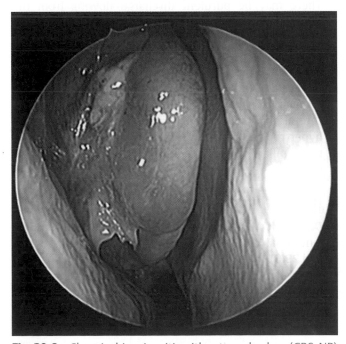

Fig. 29.6　Chronic rhinosinusitis without nasal polyps (CRSsNP).

adolescents because of their thinner, more porous bony septa and sinus walls, open suture lines, and larger vascular foramina. It is more common with frontal sinus and ethmoidal sinus infections. In young children, the ethmoids are commonly involved and so they tend to develop orbital complications. In older children due to involvement of the frontal sinus, intracranial complications can occur.

The spread of infection occurs directly through an osteomyelitic bone or bony defects. It can also occur via retrograde thrombophlebitis. The infection is usually polymicrobial.

Complications of rhinosinusitis are classified as orbital, intracranial, descending infections, or focal infections. Complications may be caused by either local spread through lamina papyracea or bone erosion or by distant spread through valveless diploic veins. The complete blood picture will show leucocytosis. Blood culture may be done. In case of suspected intracranial involvement, an imaging should be done prior to considering a lumbar puncture to avoid deterioration.

■ Complications of Paranasal Sinus Infection

- *Local*:
  - Mucocele/mucopyocele.
  - Mucous retention cyst.
  - Osteomyelitis.
- *Orbital* (based on the orbital septum: preseptal and postseptal):
  - Preseptal: inflammatory edema of lids, cellulitis, and abscess.
  - Postseptal:
    o Subperiosteal abscess.
    o Orbital cellulitis.
    o Orbital abscess.
    o Superior orbital fissure syndrome.
    o Orbital apex syndrome.
    o Cavernous sinus thrombosis.
- *Intracranial*:
  - Meningitis.

  - Extradural abscess.
  - Subdural empyema.
  - Brain abscess (frontal lobe or frontoparietal region).
- *Descending infections* like otitis media, pharyngitis, lower respiratory tract infection, and exacerbation of asthma.
- *Focal infections* like flare-up of arthritis and synovitis.

Direct spread to frontal bone in acute frontal sinusitis through the outer table of the skull cause osteomyelitis and a boggy subperiosteal abscess (**Figs. 29.9** and **29.10**). This condition is commonly referred to as Pott's puffy tumor, described by Sir Percival Pott.

■ Orbital Complications

The orbit, being closely related to the paranasal sinuses, can be involved in sinus infections. The ethmoids are separated from the orbit by a thin lamina papyracea and is the commonest site for spread. Congenital or acquired dehiscences in the lamina papyracea can facilitate the spread. Infection spreads from sinuses either by osteitis or through retrograde thrombophlebitis of the valveless, diploic veins.

Orbital complications include the following:

Preseptal Cellulitis

It involves preseptal space with intact orbital septum and no pus formation. Eyeball movements and vision are normal. Generally, the upper lid is swollen in frontal sinusitis (**Fig. 29.11**), the lower lid in maxillary sinusitis, and both the upper and lower lids in ethmoid sinusitis.

Subperiosteal Abscess

A subperiosteal abscess from ethmoiditis forms adjacent to the medial wall of the orbit and displaces the eyeball forward, downward, and laterally (**Fig. 29.12**). There may be impaired extraocular muscle movement. From frontal sinusitis, the abscess is situated just above the medial canthus and displaces the eyeball downward and laterally. Abscess from maxillary sinusitis (not common) forms on

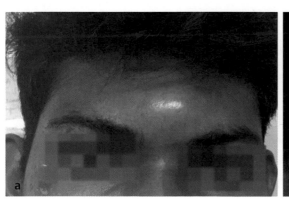
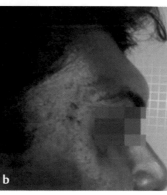

Fig. 29.9 **(a, b)** Pott's puffy tumor.

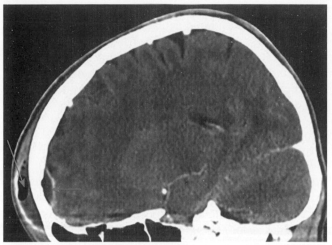

Fig. 29.10 Contrast-enhanced computed tomography (CT) scan showing a frontal subperiosteal abscess (*blue arrow*) with an extradural abscess (*green arrow*).

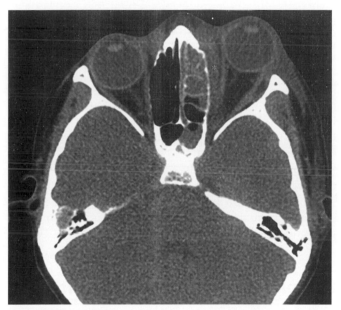

Fig. 29.12 Sphenoethmoiditis with subperiosteal abscess (*orange star*).

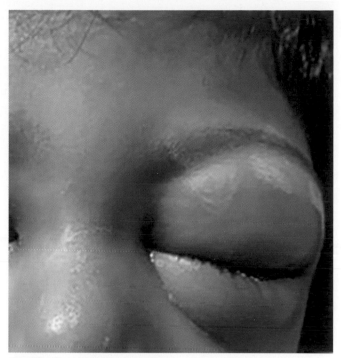

Fig. 29.11 Preseptal cellulitis.

Orbital Abscess

The clinical picture is similar to that of orbital cellulitis. There may be ophthalmoplegia. The diagnosis can be confirmed by a CECT scan or MRI.

Superior Orbital Fissure Syndrome

Infection of the sphenoid sinus or spread of infection from the posterior orbit can rarely affect the structures of the superior orbital fissure. Symptoms consist of deep orbital pain, frontal headache, and progressive paralysis of cranial nerves III, IV, and VI.

Orbital Apex Syndrome

It consists of features of the superior orbital fissure syndrome with additional involvement of the optic nerve. Exophthalmos is always present and the pain is localized to the orbit or the forehead. Some may complain of headache in the occipital region or the vertex.

Cavernous Sinus Thrombosis

Etiology

Infection of the paranasal sinuses, especially ethmoid and sphenoid sinuses and less commonly the frontal. Orbital complications from these sinus infections can cause thrombophlebitis of the cavernous sinuses. The valveless nature of the veins connecting the cavernous sinus leads to easy spread of infection (**Fig. 29.13**).

the floor of the orbit and displaces the eyeball upward and forward.

Orbital Cellulitis

When pus breaks through the periosteum into the orbit, it spreads between the orbital fat, extraocular muscles, vessels, and nerves. The clinical features will include edema of lids, exophthalmos, chemosis of conjunctiva, and restricted movements of the eyeball. Vision is affected with partial or total loss and is sometimes permanent. The patient may run a high fever. Orbital cellulitis is potentially dangerous because of the risk of meningitis and cavernous sinus thrombosis.

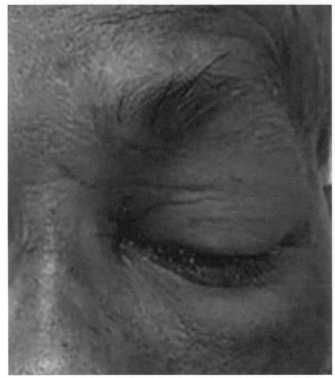

Fig. 29.13 Proptosis with swelling and ptosis of the left eye lid in cavernous sinus thrombosis

Clinical Features

The onset of cavernous sinus thrombophlebitis is abrupt with chills and rigors. The patient is acutely ill. The eyelids get swollen. There is chemosis of the conjunctiva and proptosis of the eyeball. Cranial nerves III, IV, and VI, which are related to the cavernous sinus, get involved individually and sequentially causing total ophthalmoplegia. The pupil becomes dilated and fixed. The optic disc shows congestion and edema and there is diminution of vision. The sensation in the distribution of V_1 (ophthalmic division of cranial nerve V) is diminished. The cerebrospinal fluid (CSF) is usually normal. This condition needs to be differentiated from orbital cellulitis.

Pearl

Orbital complications following sinusitis can endanger the vision and hence has to be treated aggressively.

■ Intracranial Complications

They usually present with fever, headache, and altered sensorium:

- *Extradural abscess* will also have local tenderness.

- *Subdural empyema* will have focal neurological deficits and lethargy with rapid deterioration.
- *Brain abscess* usually involve the frontal lobe or the frontoparietal region. There will be vomiting, focal neurological deficits, and behavioral and mood changes. Prior to doing a lumbar puncture, a CECT scan or MRI has to be done for evaluation to avoid coning.

■ Management of Complications of Sinusitis

When a complication of sinusitis is suspected, a complete ear, nose, and throat (ENT), ophthalmology, and neurological evaluation should be done. The visual acuity, eye movements, color vision, and fundus should be checked repeatedly in case of orbital involvement. Lumbar puncture for CSF analysis is done in case of intracranial complications. Blood cultures are sent. CECT scan of the sinuses show the bony and soft-tissue involvement. The involvement of the dura, cavernous sinus, orbital apex, and brain is better seen on MRI with contrast.

Acute complications are treated with intravenous broad-spectrum antibiotics. If there is no response, or there is worsening of symptoms within 24 hours, sinus surgery is done at the earliest along with drainage of the abscess, if present. Intravenous antibiotics are given for 2 weeks followed by oral antibiotics for 2 weeks. The patient has to be followed up regularly. The surgery required for acute complications of rhinosinusitis is often similar to that used for managing chronic rhinosinusitis. Ideally intracranial complications are treated and stabilized before doing sinus surgery, although in some cases these are managed simultaneously. Orbital complications like abscess are drained in the same sitting as the sinus surgery.

Complications of Chronic Sinusitis

■ Mucocele

A mucocele by definition is an epithelium-lined mucus-filled sac within the paranasal sinus with expansion of the sinus cavity and remodeling of the sinus walls. It occurs due to obstruction of the outflow tract of the involved sinus. At a site of bony erosion, the epithelium of the mucocele is often fused with the dura or the orbital periosteum. The frontal, ethmoidal, maxillary, and sphenoid sinuses are involved in descending order of frequency. Frontal sinus mucoceles are probably more common because of the complex and narrow drainage pathway of the frontal sinus that is easily obstructed. They present in the superomedial part of the orbit often displacing the eye forward, downward, and laterally (**Fig. 29.14**). Mucocele of the ethmoidal sinus displaces the eye laterally, whereas a sphenoid mucocele may cause axial proptosis. The symptoms may be mild. Diplopia and headache may be present. Eggshell crackling may be elicited on palpation.

X-ray shows an expanded frontal sinus with absence of the scalloping. CECT or MRI with contrast is required to assess for dural involvement. Surgical drainage (marsupialization) is done endoscopically. In case of extensive erosion of the posterior table of the frontal sinus, obliteration of the frontal sinus through an osteoplastic procedure is planned.

Points to Ponder

- Diagnosis of sinusitis is based on the symptoms and signs.
- CT scan is the investigation of choice when diagnosis is in doubt and when there are recurrent or persistent symptoms or complications as it can outline the bony walls better.
- For complications, MRI will help in detecting soft-tissue involvement beyond the sinuses.
- Medical treatment with amoxycillin is generally sufficient in uncomplicated sinusitis.

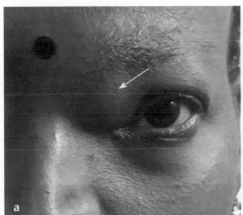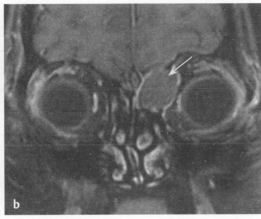

Fig. 29.14 **(a, b)** Frontal sinus mucocele.

Case-Based Questions

1. A 5-year-old girl presented with a 4-day history of left-sided, purulent rhinorrhea, cough, and a painful swelling of the ipsilateral eyelids. There was fever and the child was irritable. The eye movements and vision were normal and there was no chemosis.

   a. What is the diagnosis?

   b. How did the spread to the eye occur?

   c. How would you investigate?

   d. What is the treatment?

   Answers

   a. Acute bacterial sinusitis with preseptal orbital cellulitis.

   b. Spread occurs through the lamina papyracea or sometimes through venous thrombophlebitis.

   c. CECT scan or MRI. Swab from the middle meatus (pus) may be sent for culture and sensitivity.

   d. Intravenous broad-spectrum antibiotics. Endoscopic sinus surgery is reserved for increasing or worsening of symptoms or no improvement with 48 hours of antibiotics.

2. A 36-year-old man presented with nasal stuffiness, hyposmia, and cough for 5 months. There was a history of facial trauma 1 year back. Diagnostic nasal endoscopy showed purulent discharge in the right middle meatus with edematous mucosa.

   a. What is the diagnosis?

   b. What are the anatomical variations that can cause this condition?

   c. What are the investigations to be done?

   d. What is the treatment?

   Answers

   a. Chronic rhinosinusitis without polyposis.

   b. Any change that obstructs the ostiomeatal complex, like a deviated nasal septum, concha bullosa, Haller's cell, and pneumatized uncinated process.

   c. In addition to a diagnostic nasal endoscopy, a CT scan of the paranasal sinuses and a swab for culture and sensitivity from the right middle meatus can be performed.

The CT scan is usually done after 3 to 4 weeks of medical treatment.

d. Treatment is with oral antibiotics, saline nasal douches, and a steroid nasal spray for 3 weeks. Endoscopic sinus surgery should be considered if there is persistence of symptoms/disease.

3. **A 55-year-old man presented with left-sided nasal stuffiness and facial pain. On anterior rhinoscopy, there was blackish discoloration of the left middle turbinate. The patient tested positive for COVID-19 a month back and is a known diabetic on irregular treatment.**

a. What is the possible diagnosis?
b. What are the investigations required for diagnosis?
c. What is the treatment?

Answers

a. Left sinonasal mucormycosis (acute invasive fungal sinusitis).
b. Tissue for fungal stains and KOH mount, tissue biopsy for histopathological examination, and a contrast MRI are done.
c. Endoscopic debridement, antifungal medication such as amphotericin B, and control of diabetes.

Frequently Asked Questions

1. What is the etiology for acute sinusitis?
2. What are the signs and symptoms of acute sinusitis?
3. What is the treatment of chronic sinusitis?
4. What are the orbital complications of sinusitis?

5. What is a frontal mucocele?
6. Write a short note on allergic fungal sinusitis.
7. Describe the clinical features of acute invasive fungal sinusitis.

Endnote

Sir Percivall Pott (1714–1788) was an English surgeon and the first scientist to link cancer with occupational exposure. In 1775, he observed that chimney sweepers who were exposed to soot had a high incidence of scrotal cancer. This was the first time an etiological agent had been linked to malignancy. This discovery led to the Chimney Sweeper's Act of 1788. In ENT, his name is connected to osteomyelitis of the frontal bone or Pott's puffy tumor. His name is also linked to other diseases such as Pott's disease or tuberculosis of the spine and Pott's fracture.

30 Nasal Polyps

Suresh Pillai

> **The competency covered in this chapter is as follows:**
>
> EN4.25 Elicit, document, and present a correct history; demonstrate and describe the clinical features; choose the correct investigations; and describe the principles of management of nasal polyps.

Introduction

Nasal polyps are soft, pale masses that originate from the nasal mucosa or from the mucosa of the paranasal sinuses due to chronic inflammation of the sinonasal tract that leads to chronic rhinosinusitis (CRS). CRS is defined as an inflammation that persists for more than 12 weeks in the nose and paranasal sinuses. It is divided into two subtypes depending on the presence or absence of polyps: CRS with polyps (CRSwNP) and CRS without nasal polyps (CRSsNP). This chapter will deal with nasal polyps due to chronic inflammation or CRSwNP.

Nasal polyps are pale, edematous, masses arising from the middle meatus of the lateral wall of the nose of one side or both nasal cavities.

The prevalence of nasal polyps in the general adult population is between 1 and 4%, decreasing after 60 years of age. It is less common among the pediatric population, the prevalence being 0.1% in children.

Etiology

The etiology of nasal polyps is chronic inflammation of the nasal or sinus mucosa. These polyps can be multiple or single and can arise from different sinuses of one side or both sides.

The different causes for nasal polyps are the following: Allergic rhinitis, bacterial infection, asthma, allergic fungal rhinosinusitis (AFRS), aspirin-exacerbated respiratory disease (AERD), cystic fibrosis, Kartagener's syndrome, Young's syndrome, and eosinophilic granulomatosis with polyangiitis (EGPA).

■ Allergic Rhinitis

Nasal polyps are commonly found in people with allergic rhinitis. The prevalence is between 10 and 64%. These patients have an elevated level of immunoglobulin E and a positive skin prick test.

■ Bacterial Infection

CRS due to bacteria, especially *Staphylococcus aureus*, can lead to the formation of nasal polyps due to the release of enterotoxins. These enterotoxins behave as "superantigens," leading to T-cell activation and cytokine release.

■ Asthma

There is a direct link between nasal polyps and asthma. It has been estimated that 30 to 70% of patients with nasal polyps have coexisting bronchial asthma. This can be explained by the fact that the mucosal lining of the upper and lower respiratory tract is similar, consisting of pseudostratified ciliated, columnar epithelium. When nasal polyps are treated, asthma usually improves.

■ Allergic Fungal Rhinosinusitis

This is caused by a type 1 hypersensitivity reaction to a fungal antigen. Approximately 80% of patients with AFRS will have nasal polyps. Treatment for this condition is surgery.

■ Aspirin-Exacerbated Respiratory Disease

This is part of a triad called *Samter's triad*, which consists of nasal polyposis, bronchial asthma, and aspirin sensitivity. Aspirin and other nonsteroidal anti-inflammatory drugs

On palpation with a probe, these are insensitive to touch and do not bleed on touch. If a cotton wool carrier is used to decongest the nose, these will be seen to arise from the middle meatus. Long-standing cases are often associated with sinusitis. The polyps may be reddish with mucopurulent discharge in the nasal cavity when infected.

> **Pearl**
>
> To distinguish a polypoidal middle turbinate from a polyp, probe the mass. A polyp will be soft and mobile, whereas in the middle turbinate, the hard bone will be felt underneath.

Long-standing bilateral ethmoidal polyps can lead to a flattening and broadening of the bridge of the nose with telecanthus. This is called a frog face deformity.

The cold spatula test (CST) will show decreased fogging on both sides.

■ Investigations

Diagnostic Nasal Endoscopy

This will enable a close-up view of the polyps and to judge whether these are multiple and also the site of origin can be determined. In elderly people, polyps may be a sign of underlying malignancy, so an endoscopy can facilitate a biopsy.

Radiology

Waters' view or the occipitomental (OM) view of the paranasal sinuses will not reveal as much information as a CT scan, but can be used to determine the site and extent of sinus involvement in those who cannot afford a CT scan. The involved sinuses show opacification.

A CT scan of the paranasal sinuses is the investigation of choice. It will show the extent of disease, the sinuses involved, and whether there is bony erosion or bony expansion. It also helps outline the anatomy, anatomical variants, and vital structures before surgery.

A magnetic resonance imaging (MRI) is required to differentiate secretions from tumors and to see if there is suspected intracranial extension. In children, CT scan and MRI can help differentiate a polyp from a nasal glioma or meningocele.

Treatment

■ Medical

There should be a trial of medical therapy first to decrease the symptoms and improve the airway in case of ethmoidal polyps before planning for surgery. Medical therapy is also indicated in patients who refuse surgery or are not fit for surgery.

Medical treatment consists of topical and systemic corticosteroids depending upon the severity of the polyps. They exert an anti-inflammatory effect by reducing the activity of eosinophils and decreasing the secretion of cytokines. The use of oral steroids is sometimes referred to as medical polypectomy.

Topical intranasal corticosteroids (INCS) reduce the polyp size and recurrence after surgery. Examples of INCS include mometasone and fluticasone. These sprays are given once daily. If the polyps are large and completely filling the nasal cavity, oral corticosteroids can be given like prednisolone, 0.5 mg/kg body weight, once a day for 7 days. Antihistamines can be added if there is an allergic component. Leukotriene inhibitors like montelukast can be used if there is coexisting bronchial asthma or aspirin sensitivity.

■ Surgical

This is to be considered for those with extensive nasal polyps or for those in whom medication has not helped.

Throughout the course of the last century, various methods have been tried like simple polypectomy, intranasal ethmoidectomy, and external ethmoidectomy for removal of polyps. But with the advent of nasal endoscopes, with better illumination and magnification and clarity, the choice of surgery is functional endoscopic sinus surgery (FESS).

In FESS, nasal endoscopes (0 and 30 degrees), along with specialized nasal surgical instruments, are used to remove polyps and to open the sinuses under direct vision. This will minimize complications. Instruments like microdebriders are used as a vacuum aspirator to remove the polyps and blood from the surgical field so that there is better visualization. The aim of the surgery is to clear the airway for nasal breathing and also to allow the topical medication to reach the sinus mucosa. Postoperatively, the patients should be put on INCS to reduce the recurrence rate of polyps, which is commonly seen after surgery.

Antrochoanal Polyp or (Killian's Polyp)

■ Introduction

These are unilateral, solitary, polyps that arise from the mucosa of the maxillary antrum and enter the nasal cavity through the middle meatus. They are usually seen in children and young adults. They form 5% of all sinonasal polyps. They were first described by Gustav Killian in 1906.

■ Etiopathology

The exact etiology of antrochoanal polyps is still not known. Inflammation due to chronic sinusitis in the maxillary antrum may be responsible. The inflammation can cause edema of the maxillary sinus mucosa resulting in the formation of a retention cyst, which enlarges and protrudes out into the nasal cavity through the accessory maxillary ostium or natural maxillary ostium. Once it reaches the nasal cavity, it enlarges posteriorly toward the choana and the nasopharynx (**Fig. 30.5**).

■ Symptoms

Unilateral nasal obstruction is the main presenting symptom. It can be bilateral sometimes if the antrochoanal polyp is big and obstructs the nasopharynx, posteriorly. Other symptoms include unilateral nasal discharge and features of maxillary sinusitis on the affected side like facial pain and postnasal drip. Patients may also have loss of smell, snoring, headache, and epistaxis.

■ Signs

On examination during anterior rhinoscopy, a smooth, whitish or grayish mass with a stalk may be visible arising from the middle meatus. If this mass is extending toward the choana and nasopharynx, it is better visualized on posterior rhinoscopy. The mass may extend down into the oropharynx behind the soft palate and uvula (**Figs. 30.6** and **30.7**). It is soft, smooth, and insensitive on touch. If it is pink or reddish, it may be infected.

■ Investigation

Nasal endoscopic examination can be done to confirm the findings of the anterior rhinoscopy.

■ Radiology

Plain X-ray does not reveal as much information as CT scan. An occipitomental view (Waters' view) shows unilateral opacification of the maxillary sinus with a corresponding mass in the nasal cavity. A lateral view shows the mass extending into the nasopharynx with the typical "crescent sign" or (Dodd's sign) due to the presence of air between the soft-tissue mass and the junction of the roof and the posterior wall of the nasopharynx (**Fig. 30.8**). This is absent in the case of adenoids.

CT scan of the nose and paranasal sinuses shows the bony outlines more clearly. A mass is seen arising from the maxillary sinus and extending into the nasal cavity. There is no bony destruction. A contrast-enhanced CT scan is not required, unless an underlying tumor is suspected, especially in the older age group.

■ Treatment

Historically, a Krause nasal snare was used to avulse the polyp through the nose. But this led to recurrence because the maxillary sinus component was not addressed. The choice of treatment now is FESS, where nasal endoscopes are used to visualize the polyp as it enters the nasal cavity through the accessory maxillary sinus ostium. The ostium

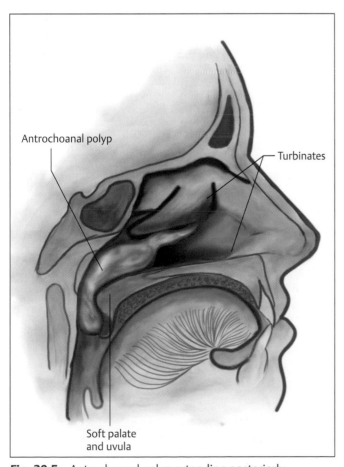

Antrochoanal polyp

Turbinates

Soft palate and uvula

Fig. 30.5 Antrochoanal polyp extending posteriorly.

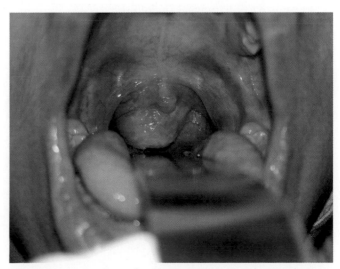

Fig. 30.6 Antrochoanal polyp extending into the oropharynx.

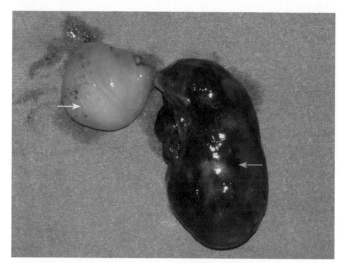

Fig. 30.7 Antrochoanal polyp after removal showing the antral part (*yellow*) and the choanal part (*blue*).

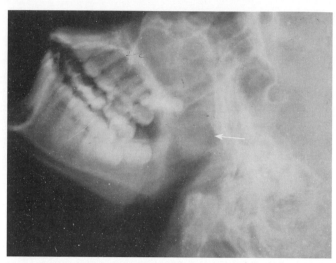

Fig. 30.8 Lateral X-ray of the nasopharynx showing the "crescent sign." This is an air shadow between the antrochoanal polyp and the nasopharyngeal wall.

is widened (middle meatal antrostomy), allowing for complete removal from the maxillary sinus (endoscopic polypectomy). Biopsy is required if a benign tumor or malignancy is suspected. If indicated, remnants, especially in the anterolateral wall, can be removed by visualizing through the middle meatal antrostomy and inserting a microdebrider through a separate opening made in the inferior meatus to shave off the polyp in the sinus.

Previously a Caldwell–Luc operation was performed to remove the maxillary component, but now due to the advent of endoscopic surgery, this is not usually required.

■ Differential Diagnosis of Unilateral Nasal Mass

- Antrochoanal polyp.
- Sphenochoanal polyp.
- Inverted papilloma.
- Juvenile nasopharyngeal angiofibroma (JNA).
- Hypertrophied middle turbinate.
- Granulomatous conditions like rhinosporidiosis.
- Malignant tumors of the sinonasal region.
- Meningocele and encephalocele.

Pearl

MRI will help distinguish nasal polyps from meningocele and encephaloceles entering the nasal cavity from the cranial cavity.

Ethmoidal polyps and antrochoanal polyps are the common nasal polyps encountered in the nose. These are different entities and of different etiologies. Ethmoidal polyps are

Box 30.1 Reasons why antrochoanal polyp expands posteriorly

- The maxillary sinus opening is directed more posteriorly
- The floor of the nasal cavity slopes downward posteriorly
- Inspiratory airflow pushes it posteriorly
- The posterior choanal opening is larger than the opening of the anterior nares
- The mucociliary blanket moves from an anterior to posterior direction
- The negative effect of swallowing may pull it backward
- The posterior accessory ostium is situated in the posterior part of the middle meatus

seen more anteriorly and are well visualized on anterior rhinoscopy. Antrochoanal polyps are better seen on posterior rhinoscopy. The reasons why an antrochoanal polyp expands in a posterior direction are outlined in **Box 30.1**. The other differences between these two types of polyps are explained in **Table 30.1**.

Points to Ponder

- Nasal polyps are the result of chronic inflammation due to multiple causes.
- Clinically, ethmoidal polyps can be distinguished from antrochoanal polyps.
- Ethmoidal polyps can be treated medically and surgically.
- Antrochoanal polyps require surgical intervention.
- A unilateral mass in an adult must be biopsied to rule out sinonasal tumors.

Table 30.1 Differences between ethmoidal polyps and antrochoanal polyps

	Ethmoidal polyps	Antrochoanal polyp
Age	Adults	Children and young adults
Etiology	Allergy and chronic inflammation	Infection
Side	Bilateral	Unilateral
Number (**Fig. 30.9**)	Multiple	Single
Extension	Usually anteriorly	Usually posteriorly
Origin	Ethmoid sinuses	Maxillary antrum
Shape	Multiple, grapelike masses	Single, dumbbell-shaped mass, connected by a stalk
Recurrence	Prone to recurrence; requires long-term medical treatment after surgery	No recurrence if completely removed

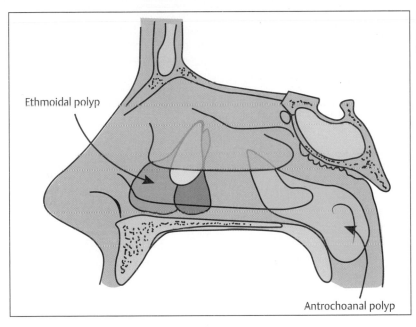

Ethmoidal polyp

Antrochoanal polyp

Fig. 30.9 Diagram showing that the ethmoidal polyps are multiple and seen more anteriorly compared to the antrochoanal polyp.

Case-Based Questions

1. **A 42-year-old man with a history of allergic rhinitis presented to the clinic with a 5-year history of bilateral nasal obstruction. On anterior rhinoscopy, he was found to have multiple grapelike masses in both nasal cavities. How will you manage this patient?**

Answer

The diagnosis is bilateral ethmoidal polyps. Ideally, a CT scan of the nose and paranasal sinuses should be taken to see the extent of involvement of the other sinuses. If the polyps are extensive and all sinuses show opacification due to involvement by the mass or infection, it is better to counsel the patient for surgery (FESS). But if the disease is not extensive, the patient can undergo a short course of oral steroids along with INCS before considering surgery.

2. **A 12-year-old boy was brought to the OPD with complaints of unilateral right-sided nasal discharge and right-sided nose block of 6 months' duration. On examination, there was tenderness over the canine fossa of the right side and reduced fogging of the right side while doing the cold spatula test. Anterior rhinoscopy revealed mucopurulent discharge. No mass was visible. What do these clinical signs point to? What is the next step in the management?**

Answer

Tenderness of the canine fossa is a sign of maxillary sinusitis. Unilateral, reduced fogging or misting on performing the CST is a sign of nasal obstruction. This could be due to a deviated nasal septum or a nasal mass. Diagnostic nasal endoscopy (DNE) needs to be performed. Suctioning out the nasal discharge from the right nasal cavity may reveal the cause of the nasal obstruction. A CT scan will reveal if there is an antrochoanal polyp in the right maxillary sinus causing sinusitis and the choanal part of the polyp causing nasal obstruction. Treatment is FESS (endoscopic polypectomy), after a course of antibiotics to treat the sinusitis, if it is diagnosed as an antrochoanal polyp.

Frequently Asked Questions

1. What is the etiology of ethmoidal polyps?
2. What are the clinical features of ethmoidal polyps on anterior rhinoscopy?
3. What are the reasons an antrochoanal polyp expands posteriorly?
4. What is the crescent sign?
5. What is the management of ethmoidal polyps?
6. Describe the differences between an antrochoanal polyp and an ethmoidal polyps.

Endnote

Description of a nasal polyp and its removal have been found in the literature since the days of ancient Egypt and Greece. Hippocrates (460–370 BC) developed a technique for removal of polyps, called the sponge method. He would take a piece of sponge and tie three to four strings to it. The other end of the strings was tied to a metal probe, which was passed through the nose and into the pharynx where he would loosen the strings from the probe. Then by pulling on the strings through the mouth, the large sponge would travel along the nasal cavity posteriorly, avulsing the polyps as it went along!

31 Epistaxis

Navneet Kumar and Sunil Varghese

The competency covered in this chapter is as follows:

EN4.30 Elicit, document, and present a correct history; demonstrate and describe the clinical features; choose the correct investigations; and describe the principles of management of epistaxis.

Introduction

Epistaxis, commonly known as nosebleeds, is not an infrequent condition among adults, affecting nearly 60% of the population. It accounts for 0.5% of all emergency department visits. There is no gross gender preponderance. It can affect individuals across all age groups, but increased incidence is seen in children below 10 years and in the elderly. Nosebleeds in children are usually due to digital (fingernail) trauma over the anterior septum. In the elderly, posterior epistaxis is more common.

Vascular Anatomy

The nose has a rich vascular supply from both the internal and external carotid arteries. There is also a good anastomotic network between the terminal branches of the right and left sides.

The majority of the epistaxis originates from a vascular plexus at the anteroinferior part of the nasal septum (Little's area), known as Kiesselbach's plexus. This vascular plexus is the confluence of the distal branches of the anterior ethmoidal artery, greater palatine artery, sphenopalatine artery, and superior labial artery (**Fig. 31.1**).

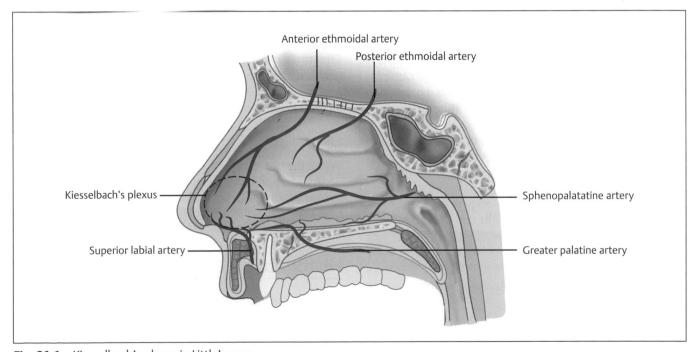

Fig. 31.1 Kiesselbach's plexus in Little's area.

(anterior ethmoidal artery), posterior part of the lateral wall adjacent to the posterior attachment of the middle turbinate (sphenopalatine artery), and occasionally the site may be in the inferior meatus or the floor of the nasal cavity anteriorly.

■ Cauterization

Cautery is done by applying a chemical agent such as silver nitrate or trichloroacetic acid over the bleeding site. This is usually done for anterior epistaxis and the chemical is put with the help of a cotton-tipped probe around the bleeding point rather than on the bleeding point directly. Electrocautery can also be used to cauterize the bleeding site. The common sites accessible for bipolar cauterization are Little's area (anteriorly), branches of the sphenopalatine artery (posteriorly), and branch of the anterior ethmoidal artery (on the septum adjacent to the anterior attachment of the middle turbinate). Anesthesia is achieved by topical lignocaine (spray or a cottonoid soaked in 4% solution) or by injecting 2% lignocaine locally. It is also beneficial to apply vasoconstrictor topically prior to cauterization to allow nosebleed control as well as to help in accurately identifying the bleeding site. Any method of cautery is more effective than nasal packing when a bleeding site is identified. Bipolar electrocautery is efficient, cost-effective, and comfortable when compared with other methods. It is better to avoid bilateral septal cauterization in the same sitting to prevent septal perforation. Other complications include injury of adjacent normal nasal mucosa and synechiae formation.

■ Nasal Packing

Nasal packing is done for patients in whom active nasal bleed is not resolved with digital compression or when bleeding is so profuse or diffuse that it becomes difficult to locate the bleeding site for cauterization and in failure of nasal cauterization. Nasal packs are broadly classified into resorbable and nonresorbable packs.

Resorbable packs are generally preferred in patients with a suspected bleeding disorder, vascular abnormalities like HHT, or when the patient is on antiplatelet and anticoagulation medication. In these cases, a rebleed can occur on removal of a conventional nonresorbable pack by causing mucosal abrasions or detaching eschar. Resorbable packs are also preferred in pediatric patients in whom pack removal can be difficult.

Nonresorbable packs include conventional ribbon gauze (impregnated with ointment or bismuth iodoparaffin paste), polyvinyl acetate sponge, and inflatable balloon devices.

Nasal packing is of two types depending on the site of bleeding: anterior nasal packing and posterior nasal packing.

For anterior nasal bleeds, anterior nasal packing with ribbon gauze is either layered in the nasal cavity oriented in a posterior to anterior direction or vertically stacked in an inferior to superior direction (**Fig. 31.2**). Anterior nasal packing can be done with multiple resorbable and nonresorbable materials and devices (**Box 31.2**).

Posterior nasal packing is done with nonresorbable packs only. Historically, tagged gauze packs ("Bellocq" packs) and tonsil packs were used to control bleeding. Polyvinyl acetate sponges (Merocel) and balloon catheters are commonly used to control posterior epistaxis. Foley's catheter can also be used if these devices are not available but are more difficult to use. A number 12 or 14 Foley's catheter is passed along the floor of the nose till the nasopharynx is reached and inflated with 15 mL of water and pulled forward to engage the posterior choana (**Fig. 31.3**). An anterior nasal pack is then inserted (**Fig. 31.4**).

Nonresorbable anterior nasal packs are placed in the nasal cavity for 48 to 72 hours and preferably under the cover of systemic antibiotics effective against *Staphylococcus*. When the pack is in situ, the patient may experience headache, facial pressure, tearing of eyes, or hyposmia.

Complications due to nasal packing are the following:
- Airway obstruction (due to a dislodged nasal pack, which can be life-threatening).
- Myocardial infarction (especially in the older age group).
- Sinusitis.
- Nasal septal perforation.
- Synechiae.

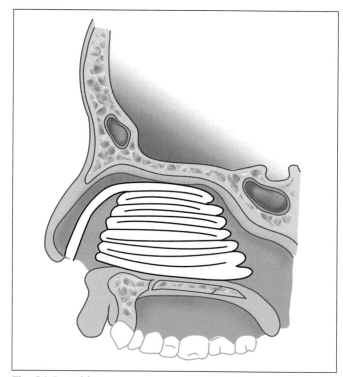

Fig. 31.2 Ribbon gauze anterior nasal packing.

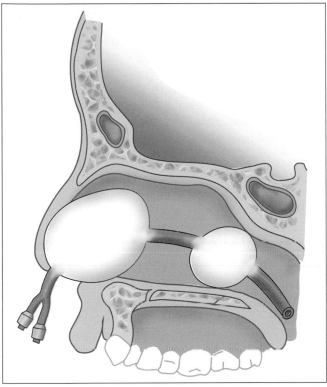

Fig. 31.3 Balloon catheter used for posterior and anterior epistaxis.

Box 31.2 Nasal packing material

Resorbable packing materials
- Oxidized regenerated cellulose (Surgicel)
- Hemostatic gelatin thrombin matrices (Floseal)
- Synthetic polyurethane sponge (nasopore)
- Chitosan-based polymers (posisep)
- Purified porcine skin and gelatin USP granules (gelfoam)
- Hyaluronic acid (merogel)
- Carboxymethyl cellulose (nasastent)

Nonresorbable materials
- Ribbon gauze
- Polyvinyl acetate sponge (merocel)
- Inflatable balloon and hydrocolloid fabric (rapid rhino)
- Inflatable two-balloon catheter (Epistat)
- Balloon epistaxis catheter with a suction irrigation port (post-stop)
- Foley's urinary catheter

After nasal packing, the cardiovascular system and respiration should be monitored especially in the elderly and in those with comorbidities. Rebleeds are seen in 40% of cases and the majority of them occur in first week after pack removal.

Floseal, which is based on gelatin granules and human thrombin, can be applied directly over the area to control the bleeding.

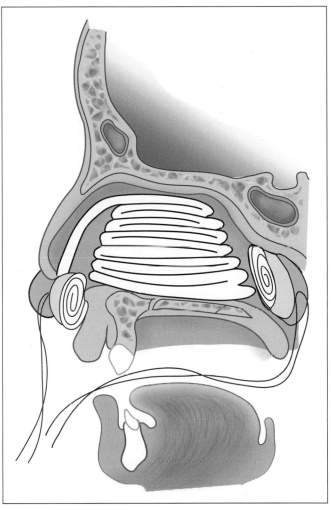

Fig. 31.4 Technique of anterior and postnasal packing using ribbon gauze for anterior nasal packing and gauze and thread for postnasal packing.

Note: Traditional postnasal pack consisted of a gauze bolster with silk threads tied at either end and in the middle. Red rubber catheters are passed through both nasal cavities and brought out through the mouth. The side threads of the gauze bolster are tied to the catheters and the catheters are gently pulled so as to engage the gauze in the nasopharynx against the choanae. An anterior nasal packing is then done. The threads brought out through the nose are tied in the region of the columella with an intervening gauze to avoid trauma to the columella. The middle thread of the gauze is used to remove the gauze bolster through the mouth when the pack is to be removed (**Fig. 31.5**).

■ Topical Agents

Topical saline gels, petroleum jelly, and antibiotic ointment have been used in recurrent epistaxis where the bleeds may be attributed to the atmospheric conditions, that is, in dry, hot, low-humidity climate or in winter. Also, in the

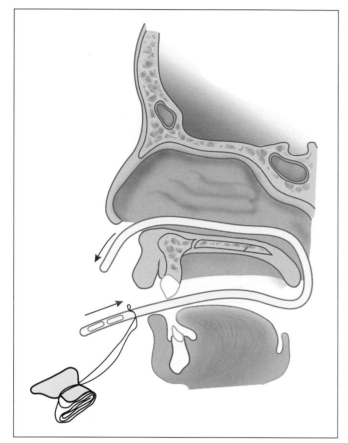

Fig. 31.5 Technique of postnasal packing using gauze and thread.

absence of active epistaxis, and when the bleeding site has been positively identified, topical application of emollient cream, lubricants, antibiotic cream, topical vasoconstriction, saline irrigation, and topical tranexamic acid can be used to prevent further episodes of nosebleeds.

■ Ligation of Arteries

Transnasal endoscopic sphenopalatine artery ligation (TESPAL) has replaced conventional external transantral (Caldwell-Luc) approach to the sphenopalatine artery or the internal maxillary artery. Around 6% of cases of epistaxis will require a more invasive procedure for intractable or recurrent epistaxis in spite of nasal cauterization and nasal packing. TESPAL has a success rate of 98% and a complication rate of 3.4%. The common complications are sinusitis and nasal crusting.

Anterior and posterior ethmoidal artery ligations are done via an external approach along the medial wall of the orbit. The posterior ethmoidal artery is usually not ligated due to its close proximity with the optic nerve and the risk of causing blindness. The anterior ethmoidal artery can be ligated under nasal endoscopic guidance in select cases but carries the risk of orbital injury and cerebrospinal fluid (CSF) leak.

Internal maxillary artery ligation can be done via an external sublabial (Caldwell-Luc) approach or a combined sublabial and endoscopic approach. The posterior wall of the maxillary sinus is removed and the internal maxillary artery is identified in the pterygopalatine fossa where it is clipped and/or cauterized with bipolar cautery. This procedure has a success rate of 89% and is usually undertaken when control of bleeding from the sphenopalatine artery is not achieved by TESPAL.

External carotid artery ligation is done under local or general anesthesia using either a transverse skin crease incision or longitudinal incision along the anterior border of the sternocleidomastoid muscle at the level of the hyoid bone. The carotid bifurcation is located and the external carotid artery is identified by its arterial branches in the neck and ligated. The superior thyroid artery is the first branch of the external carotid artery and is spared.

Septal surgery is done if the bleeding site is located behind a prominent septal deviation or on a septal spur. The bleeding area gets sealed off by fibrosis during healing. Septoplasty may be required to access the bleeding point for cauterization. Septodermoplasty is a procedure done for hereditary hemorrhagic telangiectasia wherein the mucosa is removed on both sides and replaced by a skin graft.

Endovascular embolization is indicated in intractable and recurrent epistaxis not controlled with conservative treatment. It is performed by an intervention radiologists where bilateral sphenopalatine arteries or distal internal maxillary arteries are embolized. Gelfoam particles or polyvinyl alcohol particles can be used for embolization. Embolization of anterior and posterior ethmoidal arteries is not done due to the high risk of occluding the ophthalmic artery and causing blindness. Complications of endovascular embolization of the bilateral sphenopalatine arteries are transient nasal ischemia, temporofacial pain, headache, swelling, jaw claudication, and trismus seen in 20% of cases. Major complications like skin/nasal necrosis, permanent facial paralysis, monocular blindness, and stroke are not common.

Anticoagulation and antiplatelet medications use have a high risk of large-volume blood loss and hospitalization for blood transfusion. In these patients, the next dose of antiplatelets or anticoagulants has to be skipped. If the bleeding is severe (posterior nasal bleed or hypovolemia or more than 2 units of packed red blood cells [RBCs] are transfused or a drop in hemoglobin >2 g%), appropriate local measures to control bleeding have to be taken and appropriate reversal agents will have to be administered to optimize the bleeding parameters. If the bleeding is not severe, local measures to control bleeding and oral or IV vitamin K will suffice.

The algorithm in **Flowchart 31.1** simplifies the management of epistaxis.

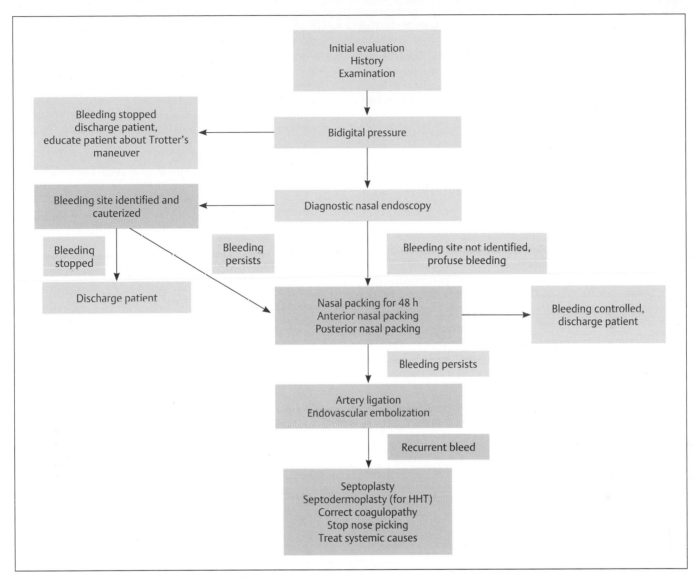

Flowchart 31.1 Management algorithm of epistaxis.

Points to Ponder

- Anterior epistaxis is more common than posterior epistaxis.
- In children, anterior epistaxis is more common. It may be due to the trauma of nose-picking or dry atmospheric conditions. These are self-limiting but can be recurrent.
- In the older age group, epistaxis is usually due to hypertension, and the bleed is commonly from the sphenopalatine artery.
- It is important to acquire an IV access and record the vitals while controlling the epistaxis.
- Trotter's method can be tried for 5 minutes in mild to moderate epistaxis before attempting other methods.
- For a bleeding mass, biopsy when required should be done in the controlled setting of the operating room with the required instrumentation.
- Avoid bilateral septal cauterization in the same sitting so as to avoid a septal perforation.

Case-Based Questions

1. **A 45-year-old lady comes to the casualty department with profuse left-sided anterior epistaxis of 2 hours. She gives a history of multiple episodes of epistaxis from the past 1 week on blowing the nose. The episodes had scanty bleeds and were self-limiting.**

   a. What will be the initial management of this patient?

   b. What would be the next appropriate step after control of the epistaxis?

   c. What will be the treatment if a hemorrhagic nodule is seen on the left side of Little's area?

   Answers

   a. Pinch the nose and put ice on the dorsum. Start an IV line for IV fluids. Blood must be sent for investigations (complete blood count, blood grouping and cross-matching, serum creatinine level). The pulse and blood pressure must be monitored, and an anterior nasal pack is inserted.

   b. Antibiotics are started as the pack is in situ. The pack is removed after 48 hours and a diagnostic nasal endoscopy is done for assessment.

   c. The lesion can be cauterized with bipolar cautery.

2. **A 60-year-old gentleman, known case of hypertension on irregular medication, presented in the emergency department with severe epistaxis. The blood pressure was 190/100 mm Hg and the pulse rate was 100 beats per minute. The epistaxis is not controlled with Trotter's method and application of ice over the dorsum.**

   a. What is the most likely site for epistaxis in this case?

   b. What is the next appropriate step for controlling epistaxis?

   Answers

   a. Sphenopalatine artery.

   b. Give an antihypertensive. Start an intravenous line and send blood for investigations. Monitor the blood pressure and pulse rate. A posterior nasal pack may be required. If there is provision, in persistent bleed, an endoscopic cauterization or a TESPAL can be performed, which will often require general anesthesia.

Frequently Asked Questions

1. What are the local causes of epistaxis?

2. What are the systemic causes of epistaxis?

3. Describe the types of nasal packing for epistaxis.

4. Describe the method of posterior nasal packing.

5. What is Kiesselbach's plexus and what is its clinical significance?

6. What is Little's area? What vessels anastomose at this site?

Endnote

Epistaxis and its management have been well documented throughout the history of medicine. Scribonius Largus was the physician to the Roman emperor Claudius. He described inserting a hollow reed surrounded by cotton into the nose of a patient with epistaxis so that there is pressure exerted and the patient can breathe. Other remedies during the ages included application of "cranial moss" or fungus from the skulls of hanged corpses into the nose to stop bleeding. It was J.L. Little in the United States and W. Kiesselbach in Germany, in the late 1800s, who came to the conclusion that the anterior part of the nasal septum was one of the most frequent sites for epistaxis.

32 | Foreign Bodies in the Nose

Rejee Ebenezer R. and Avinash Mohan

The competency covered in this chapters is as follows:

EN3.4 Observe and describe the indications for and steps involved in the removal of foreign bodies from the ear, nose, and throat.

Introduction

A foreign body is any object, living or nonliving, organic or inorganic, which originates from outside the body. In humans, the nose is a common site for the lodgment of foreign bodies. Foreign bodies in the nose are common in children due to their inherent curiosity and in adults with mental retardation and psychiatric illness.

Etiology

Foreign bodies can be classified as follows:
* *Organic matter*:
  - Inanimate objects such as vegetable seeds and nuts.
  - Animate beings such as insects, maggots, leeches, and round worm.
* *Inorganic matter*:
  - Materials such as plastic, cell battery, plastic toy, paper, cloth piece, chalk, eraser, jewelry, and pebble.

Foreign bodies in the nose can also be iatrogenic such as cotton pledgets, which are accidentally left behind after a surgical procedure.

After trauma, especially after a road traffic accident, there can be foreign bodies like glass pieces in the nose.

Pathology

Foreign bodies usually enter the nose through the anterior nares. They are either put by the patient or enter inadvertently (as in trauma), or put by someone else (children while playing and iatrogenic). Sometimes, food particles can enter through the choana while vomiting/regurgitation. Organic foreign bodies can irritate the nasal mucosa and elicit local inflammation, edema, and granulations. Organic foreign bodies such as plant matter are hygroscopic and swell up if they remain for a long time. Inorganic foreign bodies can stay in the nose for a long time without any local reaction. An exception is cell batteries, which can leak alkali and cause necrosis of the nasal mucosa within a short span of time.

Clinical Features

■ Symptoms

The characteristic symptom in a child is unilateral, purulent, foul-smelling nasal discharge that is occasionally blood stained. The patient can also have intractable sneezing and nasal obstruction. Other symptoms are facial pain, headache, whistling sound, and postnasal drip. There may be a prior history of foreign body in the ear, nose, or throat.

■ Signs

The foreign body may be visible on anterior rhinoscopy. Occasionally, the foreign body may be visible only after suctioning, which clears the secretions and purulent discharge. The most common site of lodgment of nasal foreign bodies is in the anterior part of the nasal cavity between the septum and the inferior and middle turbinates. There may be edema, congestion, ulceration, or granulation tissue. Rarely, there can be ulceration of the soft and hard palate.

Other sites like the ear, throat, and bronchus should be assessed for a foreign body as children tend to put multiple foreign bodies. The airway, breathing, and circulation should be assessed. The chest should be auscultated.

Investigations

* The diagnosis is often based on the medical history of the patient. It becomes easier when the incident is witnessed by someone else.

- Diagnostic nasal endoscopy (DNE) is done to inspect the nasal cavity in suspected cases where the foreign bodies are not visible on anterior rhinoscopy. The foreign body is removed in the same sitting.
- Paranasal sinus X-ray and lateral view of the nasopharynx X-ray will help detect a radio-opaque foreign body. In some cases, a computed tomography (CT) scan may be required especially when diagnosis is in doubt and anatomical abnormalities are suspected such as choanal atresia and meningocele.

■ Treatment

Most nasal foreign bodies are not acute emergencies as they get lodged between the turbinates and septum. But special care must be taken in the following situations:

- When the foreign body consists of a small battery, which can lead to corrosive action.
- Bilateral foreign bodies in infants who are obligate nasal breathers.
- Hygroscopic foreign bodies that swell up, and trauma to the nasal mucosa can occur while removing.
- Posteriorly located foreign bodies that can be aspirated.

The following instruments may be required for removal of a foreign body and should be kept in the instrument tray: a nasal speculum, bayonet forceps, alligator forceps, Hartmann forceps, blunt hook (**Fig. 32.1**), Rosen's eustachian tube catheter, suction, decongestant agent, Foley's catheter, head light, and nasal endoscopes.

Most nasal foreign bodies can be removed without anesthesia. General anesthesia is required for impacted and posteriorly located foreign bodies, or when there is risk of bleeding or aspiration, and in uncooperative patients. Prior to removal, explain the procedure and the possibility of minimal bleeding after removal to the patient or parent.

- Removal of inanimate, round, or solid foreign bodies is done by passing a eustachian tube catheter past the foreign body and gently dragging it along the floor of the nose. Alternately, a Foley catheter can be passed along the floor and the bulb inflated just beyond the foreign body and the catheter is gently pulled forward.

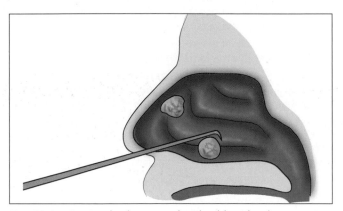

Fig. 32.1 Foreign body removal with a blunt hook.

- Small pieces of paper, cloth, or cotton can be removed using forceps.
- Forceps can be used for foreign bodies with visible edges, which can be grasped.
- An insect should be killed or immobilized before removal.
- Nasal endoscopy provides good visualization and is useful for removal of a foreign body.

After removal, an assessment has to be carried out regarding the condition of the nasal mucosa at the site of the foreign body impaction and to look for a second foreign body or remnant of the first foreign body.

Saline or decongestant nasal drops can be given for 3 to 5 days.

Complications

- Retained or neglected foreign body or its remnant can lead to chronic sinusitis or rhinolith formation.
- The child may aspirate the foreign body into the tracheobronchial tree.
- Other complications include cellulitis, septal abscess, and synechiae.

Pearls

- Nasal foreign body has to be ruled out in a child who presents with unilateral, foul-smelling, purulent, or blood-stained nasal discharge.
- "One leads to another": Always rule out a second foreign body in the opposite nasal cavity.
- DNE is a valuable investigation that helps detect foreign bodies that are not visible on anterior rhinoscopy and also remove foreign bodies that are situated posteriorly in the nasal cavity.

Rhinolith

A rhinolith forms due to deposition of calcium and magnesium phosphate and carbonate, in layers, on a foreign body or inspissated mucous or blood clot. This calcareous mass in the nasal cavity may be asymptomatic, and noted as an incidental finding on imaging or endoscopy.

A rhinolith can present with nasal block and nasal discharge. Occasionally, there may be nasal pain and epistaxis. On anterior rhinoscopy or DNE, there will be a gray–white or brownish mass that is more commonly seen on the floor of the nose between the septum and the turbinates. On probing, it is hard and gritty. It can cause pressure necrosis of the nasal septum.

It is seen as a radio-opaque mass on X-ray and CT scan. Removal often requires general anesthesia (**Fig. 32.2**).

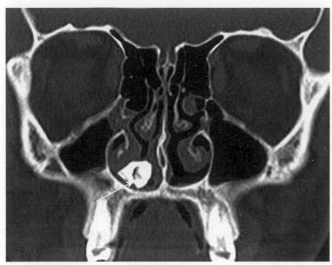

Fig. 32.2 Computed tomography (CT) scan, coronal view, showing rhinolith in the right nasal cavity.

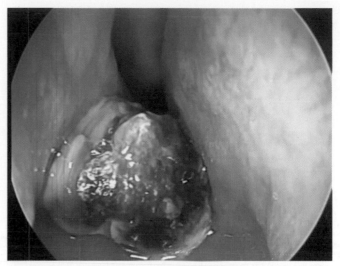

Fig. 32.3 Endoscopic picture of rhinolith in the right nasal cavity.

Endoscopic removal can be done in toto or piecemeal (**Figs. 32.3** and **32.4**). Rarely, an external (lateral rhinotomy) incision may be required to remove the rhinolith.

Nasal Myiasis (Maggots)

Myiasis can be classified into two types:
- Furuncular myiasis occurs in the subcutaneous layer (skin), and is seen in Mexico, Central and South America, and tropical Africa.
- Secondary myiasis occurs in open cavities or wounds. The flies lay eggs in open wounds usually when the person is asleep. Maggots (larva) of the house fly *Chrysomya* is common in the Indian subcontinent, south-east Asia, tropical and subtropical Africa, Malaysia, and the Philippines. They feed on infected or dead tissues in the host. The larva requires warm temperature to incubate and is seen in hot, humid conditions.

Nasal myiasis commonly occurs in patients with atrophic rhinitis and tumors especially in the lower socioeconomic group and those with poor hygiene.

■ Clinical Features

Symptoms

Symptoms include nasal block, severe pain, foul smell, blood-stained nasal discharge, epistaxis, and headache. Formication (sensation of insect crawling inside) will be present.

Signs

There can be associated edema and cellulitis of the nose, face, and eyelids. There can be erosion of the nasal septum

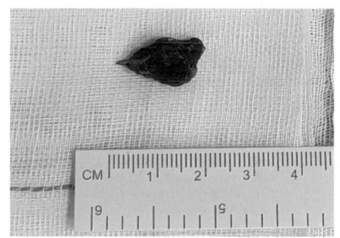

Fig. 32.4 Rhinolith after removal.

and palate, and orbital complications. Aspiration of the maggots into the lower airway can occur. Rarely, septicemia and meningitis can develop. On examination inside the nasal cavity, the larva will be seen moving in the tissues, usually away from light (**Fig. 32.5**).

■ Management

Nasal myiasis can be prevented by covering the sleeping area with a net.

The maggots are removed using a headlight or endoscope for visualization and nasal dressing forceps. For ease of removal, chloroform, ether, ethylene chloride, or lidocaine may be used. Turpentine oil (dilute) is an irritant that helps bring out the maggots from the deeper tissues. Single dose of oral ivermectin has been advocated. Tetanus toxoid injection should be given. Antibiotics are given for secondary infection. The primary condition in the nose that led to myiasis should be treated.

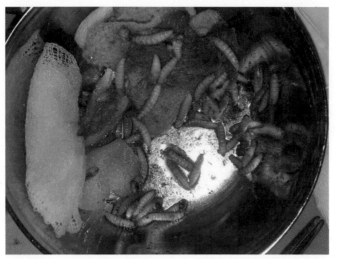

Fig. 32.5 Maggots in a bowl after removal.

Points to Ponder

- Foreign bodies can be organic or inorganic. Different instruments are available for ease of removal of foreign bodies depending on their size, shape, and surface.
- Long-standing, unilateral, nasal discharge in a child should be investigated for a foreign body.
- Rhinolith may have to be removed under anesthesia in the operation theater because of its size and removal can lead to bleeding due to granulation tissue surrounding it.
- Turpentine, an irritant, is commonly used to bring out the maggots buried deep in the tissues.

Case-Based Questions

1. **A 4-year-old boy is brought to the ear, nose, and throat (ENT) clinic with a 3-month history of nasal discharge from the right side. On examination, a large, smooth, white bead is seen impacted in the anterior nasal cavity.**

   a. What is the next step in the management?

   b. What are the complications during removal?

   Answers

   a. A smooth foreign body, such as a bead, may be difficult to grasp with serrated forceps. If a curved instrument such as a eustachian tube catheter is available, it can be inserted beyond the bead and it can be gently pulled anteriorly to bring the bead out.

   b. Complications include inadvertent slippage of the bead posteriorly into the nasopharynx. This can lead to aspiration by the child. Granulations around the foreign body can lead to bleeding from the nose while attempting to remove it.

2. **A 75-year-old man is brought to the emergency room complaining of facial pain and redness over the cheek of 1-week duration. He has a history of having undergone maxillectomy and radiotherapy for carcinoma of the maxillary sinus. On endoscopic examination, maggots can be seen crawling in the nasal cavity. What is the next step in the management?**

   Answer

   A large cavity, after surgery and radiotherapy in an elderly person, can lead to the presence of necrotic tissue, which is a good medium for the larva of the fly to grow, leading to nasal myiasis. This would have led to facial cellulitis. It is important to admit the patient, remove all maggots using irritants such as dilute turpentine, and debride the nasal cavity of all dead, necrotic tissue. The nasal cavity can be irrigated with normal saline, and facial cellulitis can be treated with antibiotics.

Frequently Asked Questions

1. What are the common foreign bodies seen in the nose?
2. What are the instruments available for removal of foreign bodies?
3. What is the etiopathology of rhinolith formation?
4. What is nasal myiasis? How will you manage this condition?

Endnote

Most foreign bodies are seen in the right nasal cavity because most people are right-handed. The commonest location within the nasal cavity for a foreign body to get lodged is either anterior to the middle turbinate or under the inferior turbinate. Only when it is large does it get impacted between the inferior turbinate and the septum.

33 Benign and Malignant Tumors of the Nose and Paranasal Sinuses

Ajay Bhandarkar

The competencies covered in this chapter are as follows:

AN37.3 Describe the anatomical basis of the maxillary sinus tumor.

EN4.34 Describe the clinical features, investigations, and principles of management of tumors of the maxilla.

EN2.11 Describe and identify by clinical examination the malignant and premalignant ear, nose, and throat (ENT) diseases.

Introduction

Sinonasal tumors are a diverse group of tumors responsible for less than 1% of all neoplasms. The symptoms produced by these tumors are often confused with those of rhinosinusitis, so the diagnosis is often delayed. The average delay between the first symptom and diagnosis is almost 6 months. By the time diagnosis is made, there is bony destruction of the facial bones and infiltration of the nerves, leading to facial pain.

Tumors of the maxillary sinus are a rare entity. The peculiarity of tumors arising within the paranasal sinuses is their late presentation. Tumors of the maxillary sinus can be benign or malignant. Classification of the tumors is based on the tissue of origin (**Table 33.1**).

Pertaining to the competency to be addressed, the benign tumor, that is, inverted papilloma and malignancy of the maxilla will be discussed. Olfactory neuroblastoma has been covered in this chapter as additional reading.

Inverted Papilloma

■ Synonyms

Synonyms of the inverted papilloma are Schneiderian papilloma, Ringertz's tumor, epithelial papilloma, transitional cell papilloma, cylindrical cell papilloma, and fungiform papilloma.

Sinonasal papillomas are benign, potentially premalignant tumor with slow local advancement and commonly

Table 33.1 Classification of tumors of the maxillary sinus and nasal cavity

Tissue of origin	Benign	Malignant
Epithelial	Squamous papilloma Inverted papilloma Minor salivary gland tumors	Squamous cell carcinoma Adenocarcinoma Adenoid cystic carcinoma Sinonasal undifferentiated carcinoma
Neuroectodermal	Meningioma Paraganglioma	
Mesenchymal	Capillary hemangioma Fibrous histiocytoma Osteoma Lipoma Fibrous dysplasia Hemangiopericytoma Hemangioendothelioma Chondroma	Olfactory neuroblastoma Angiosarcoma Mucosal melanoma Non-Hodgkin's lymphoma Chondrosarcoma
		Metastatic carcinoma

arising from the lateral nasal wall. They are divided into three subtypes, namely, columnar, exophytic, and inverted. The inverted papilloma is the most common of the three subtypes.

■ Etiology

The etiology of the inverted papilloma is unknown. However, an association has been noted with human papillomavirus 6, 11, 16, and 18.

■ Histopathology

The peculiarity of the tumor lies in the tumor spread. The epithelium is thickened due to hyperplasia of the basal cells with an intact basement membrane which projects into the underlying stroma.

■ Symptoms

- Unilateral nasal obstruction.
- Epistaxis.

Locally advanced tumor may present with the following:
- Facial swelling.
- Proptosis, diplopia, and epiphora (due to orbital involvement).

■ Signs

- A friable, reddish, solitary, granular mass arising from the lateral nasal wall is a sign of inverted papilloma (**Fig. 33.1**). The mass is sensitive to touch and bleeds on touch.
- The tumors may mimic a polyp.

■ Staging

Krouse proposed the following staging system for inverted papillomas:
- Stage I: The tumor is confined to the lateral nasal wall.
- Stage II: The tumor involves the ethmoid sinus and the medial and superior walls of the maxillary sinus.
- Stage III: The tumor involves the frontal or sphenoid sinus and the lateral or inferior wall of the maxillary sinus.
- Stage IV: The tumor extends beyond the confines of the sinonasal region or associated malignancy.

■ Investigations

The radiological extent is noted before taking a biopsy. This rule applies to all tumors.

Radiological Investigations

- Contrast-enhanced computed tomography (CECT) scan: A soft-tissue mass may be noted, which shows heterogenous contrast enhancement in the initial stages. Bone erosion is noted in advanced stages when the tumor extends beyond the confines of the sinus (**Fig. 33.2**).
- Contrast-enhanced magnetic resonance imaging (MRI): An isointense to hyperintense mass is noted in T1-weighted (T1W) imaging. A heterogenous hyperintense mass is noted on T2-weighted (T2W) imaging.

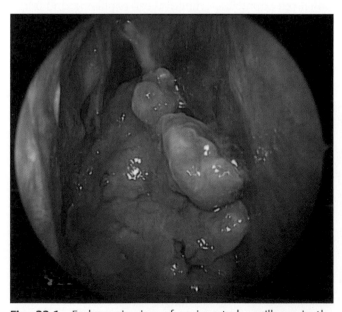

Fig. 33.1 Endoscopic view of an inverted papilloma in the right nasal cavity.

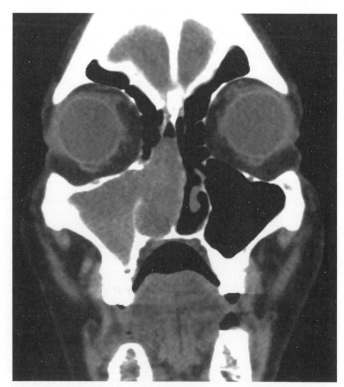

Fig. 33.2 Computed tomography (CT) scan showing an inverted papilloma involving the right nasal cavity and extending into the maxillary sinus.

On administration of contrast, the tumor shows a convoluted cerebriform pattern or a curvilinear pattern of enhancement.

Nonradiological Investigations

Diagnostic nasal endoscopy and biopsy: Deep biopsy on diagnostic nasal endoscopy will confirm the diagnosis of an inverted papilloma.

■ Treatment

Endoscopic wide excision of the tumor is the treatment of choice in inverted papillomas. Endoscopic medial maxillectomy is the most common surgical procedure performed in an inverted papilloma.

An external approach (lateral rhinotomy) with Moure's incision is carried out in case the tumor cannot be resected endoscopically. However, the surgical resection may vary depending on the extent of involvement.

■ Prognosis and Recurrence

With adequate tumor clearance, the prognosis is good. However, chances of recurrence exist with inadequate clearance. In 10% of cases, there is a potential for malignant transformation. This can occur simultaneously with the primary tumor or a few years later. Hence, follow-up is important.

Esthesioneuroblastoma (Olfactory Neuroblastoma)

This malignant tumor arises from the neural elements located in the cribriform plate of the ethmoid bone. This tumor has a bimodal age distribution with presentation in the second and sixth decades of life. There is no gender predilection to esthesioneuroblastoma.

■ Etiology

The etiology of the esthesioneuroblastoma is unknown.

■ Symptoms

- *Nasal obstruction*: Involvement of the cribriform plate and extension into the nasal cavity presents with either unilateral or bilateral obstruction.
- Epistaxis.
- *Hyposmia or anosmia* due to the origin and involvement of the olfactory neural filaments.

Usually, these tumors present in an advanced stage, due to the site of the lesion. The early stages are usually asymptomatic. Advanced tumors with intracranial involvement may present with headache and vomiting due to intracranial extension. Due to local spread, there can be involvement of the orbit in addition to involvement of the paranasal sinuses.

■ Signs

- A friable mass that is sensitive to touch and bleeds on touch may be noted on the second pass of diagnostic nasal endoscopy.
- Neck node metastasis.

■ Staging System

Kadish proposed a staging system for olfactory neuroblastoma:
- Stage A: The tumor is confined to the nasal cavity.
- Stage B: The tumor extends into the sinuses.
- Stage C: The tumor extends beyond the paranasal sinuses.
- Stage D: There is involvement of the neck node or distant metastasis.

■ Investigations

Radiological Investigations

- *CECT scan of the paranasal sinuses and neck*: A heterogenous, contrast-enhancing mass may be noted in the olfactory region with extension of the tumor depending on the stage. Neck node involvement may be evident on the neck scan.
- *MRI of the brain and paranasal sinuses*: Hyperintense signal intensity on T2W imaging with contrast enhancement is noted. It is required to assess the extent of soft-tissue involvement in the orbit and intracranial region.
- Chest X-ray is done to rule out lung metastasis.
- Bone scan/positron emission tomography CT (PET-CT) can be done to determine tumor extent and metastasis.

Nonradiological Investigations

- Diagnostic nasal endoscopy and biopsy.
- Urinary vanillylmandelic acid (VMA) is used to rule out the presence of coexistent neuroendocrine tumors.

■ Treatment

Surgical resection (anterior craniofacial resection), followed by intensity-modulated radiation therapy is the treatment of choice. For stage C and D tumors, additional chemotherapy with vincristine and cyclophosphamide is preferred.

Malignancy of the Maxillary Sinus

Malignancies of the maxillary sinus account for less than 1% of head and neck malignancies.

■ Etiology

Occupational exposure to chemicals is the prime etiological factor in malignancy of the maxillary sinus.

- *Woodworkers*: Hardwood and softwood dust exposure is associated with elevated relative risk of development of adenocarcinoma and squamous cell carcinoma, respectively.
- Exposure to leather dust and chemicals in shoe manufacturing industry.
- Exposure to textile dust and asbestos.
- Exposure to isopropyl alcohol during production.
- Exposure to chrome pigment and nickel during production and refining.

Apart from dust, the other suspected carcinogens in the manufacturing industry are tar, chromium, tannins, aldehydes, aflatoxins, chromates, oil, and dyes.

Smoking and alcohol have limited role in the development of paranasal sinus malignancies when compared to other regions of the upper aerodigestive tract. Majority of the maxillary sinus tumors are seen in the sixth and seventh decades of life with a male-to-female ratio of 2:1.

> ### Pearl
>
> Wood dust is one of the etiological agents for the development of carcinoma of the sinuses. Soft wood dust exposure leads to the development of squamous cell carcinoma, while hard wood dust exposure is more commonly associated with adenocarcinoma. The most carcinogenic hard wood is African mahogany. This is often used by the Bantu tribe of South Africa and they have the highest incidence of malignancy of the maxillary sinus in the world.

■ Histopathology

Squamous cell carcinoma and adenocarcinoma are the most common histological cancer subtypes noted in the maxillary sinus. Adenoid cystic carcinoma is the third most common histological subtype.

■ Symptoms and Signs

Often maxillary sinus malignancy presents as a locally advanced disease because the cavity of the maxillary sinus gets involved before it spreads to neighboring structures and presents symptomatically. The symptoms and signs have been presented based on the direction of spread of the tumor.

Medial Spread (into the Nasal Cavity)

Symptoms:
- *Unprovoked, painless epistaxis*: The friable nature of the tumor may present with this manifestation on its extension into the nasal cavity.
- *Nasal obstruction*: Usually this is unilateral due to occlusion of the nasal cavity by the mass. This may progress to bilateral obstruction following locoregional spread.
- *Anosmia* due to olfactory area obstruction by the tumor.

Signs:
- A friable mass may be noted in the nasal cavity.

Superior Spread (into the Orbit)

- Symptoms:
- *Epiphora and eyelid edema*: Defective lacrimal drainage pathway may produce epiphora and lymphatic obstruction around the eyelids may produce lid edema.
- *Proptosis* due to mass effect of the tumor.
- Diplopia.

Signs:
- Proptosis.
- Ophthalmoplegia due to orbital content involvement by the tumor.
- Reduced vision and absent light reflex due to involvement of the orbital contents by the tumor.

Anterolateral Spread (into the Skin of the Cheek)

Symptoms and signs (**Fig. 33.3**):
- *Paresthesia of the cheek skin*: This is due to involvement of the infraorbital nerve.
- *Swelling of cheek* due to tumor erosion through the anterolateral wall of the maxillary sinus. There may be fullness in the upper gingivolabial sulcus.

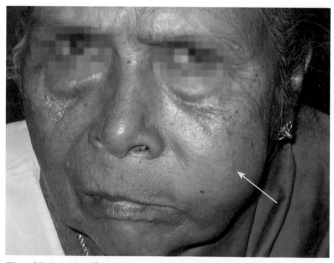

Fig. 33.3 Maxillary sinus malignancy extending to the left cheek. Fullness is seen over the region.

Inferior Spread (into the Palate)

Symptoms (**Fig. 33.4**):

- Ill-fitting dentures or loose teeth.
- Paresthesia around the upper premolars and molars.

Signs:

- Swelling on the hard palate, which may be hard on palpation.
- Oroantral fistula may be noted when the tumor erodes through the mucosa covering the hard palate.
- Loose teeth.

Posterior Spread (into the Pterygopalatine Fossa and the Infratemporal Fossa)

Symptoms:

- *Difficulty in opening the mouth* due to involvement of muscles of mastication in the infratemporal fossa.
- *Pain* due to involvement of the maxillary division of the trigeminal nerve.
- *Hearing loss (rare)* due to otitis media with effusion caused by involvement of the eustachian tube.

Signs:

- Trismus.
- *Swelling in the infratemporal fossa region*: A hard, non-tender swelling may be noted on clinical examination.

Metastasis

- *Lymph nodes*: Only 10% of maxillary sinus malignancies present with neck node metastasis due to paucity of lymphatics pertaining to the paranasal sinuses. However, neck node metastasis becomes evident due to locoregional spread of tumor into lymphatic-rich areas. The most common metastatic lymph nodes due

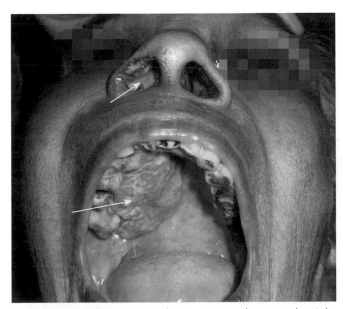

Fig. 33.4 Maxillary sinus malignancy extending into the right nasal cavity and right hard palate.

to locoregional spread are level 1B (due to extension into soft tissue of the face), level 2, and retropharyngeal group of lymph nodes, which are usually associated with a poor prognostic outcome.

- *Cranial nerve palsy*: Due to extensive involvement of the orbital apex and the cavernous sinus, patients may present with palsies of cranial nerve II to VI.
- *Lung metastasis*: Although uncommon, it may present with cough and hemoptysis.
- *Spine metastasis*: This is uncommon and may present with back pain.

■ Classification and Staging

Ohngren's and Lederman's classifications were widely used earlier to assess the treatment prognosis in patients with paranasal sinus tumors. However, currently, the TNM staging system is considered the gold standard for staging of paranasal sinus carcinoma.

TNM Classification

- T = tumor; N = node; and M = distant metastasis.
  - Tx: Tumor cannot be assessed.
  - Tis: Carcinoma in situ.
  - T1: The tumor is limited to the maxillary sinus mucosa.
  - T2 (medial and inferior extension of the tumor): Tumor extension into the middle meatus and/or hard palate with bone erosion.
  - T3 (superior, anterior, and posterior extension of tumor): Tumor extension into the medial and inferior walls of the orbit, ethmoid sinus, posterior wall of the maxillary sinus and pterygoid fossa, and subcutaneous tissue.
  - T4a (involvement of contents beyond the superior, anterior, and posterior walls): Tumor invading orbital contents, frontal and sphenoid sinuses, cribriform plate, cheek skin, pterygoid plates, and infratemporal fossa.
  - T4b (involvement of critical structures): Tumor invades the dura, orbital apex, brain, middle cranial fossa, nasopharynx, clivus, and cranial nerves (other than V2 of the fifth cranial nerve).
- N = node:
  - Nx: Lymph nodes cannot be assessed.
  - N0: No lymph node involvement.
  - N1: Involvement of a single ipsilateral lymph node with no extranodal extension ≤3 cm.
  - N2a: Involvement of a single ipsilateral node with no extranodal extension of size between 3 and 6 cm.
  - N2b: Involvement of multiple ipsilateral nodes without extranodal extension of size between 3 and 6 cm.
  - N2c: Involvement of bilateral or contralateral lymph nodes, none more than 6 cm without extra nodal extension.

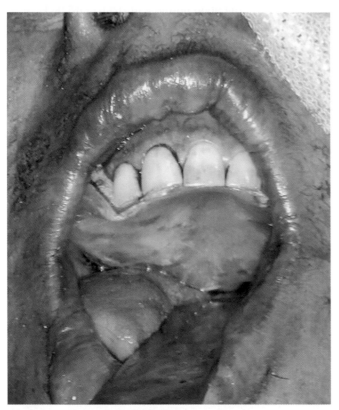

Fig. 33.9 Placement of the obturator after surgery.

■ Prognosis

It depends on the local spread and control of disease. Stage I and II tumors have a 5-year survival rate of more than 80%. Stage III and IV tumors have a 5-year survival rate of less than 40%.

Points to Ponder

- Maxillary tumors are rare and present late.
- Unilateral nasal obstruction is the most common presenting symptom in inverted papillomas.
- Inverted papillomas are benign, locally aggressive tumors with a small percentage having associated malignancy.
- Imaging of tumors should always be done prior to biopsy.
- The etiology of maxillary malignancy is linked to wood dust.
- Maxillary sinus malignancy can spread from the sinus in all directions, leading to orbital, nasal, cranial, and oral presentations.
- Combined modality of treatment (surgery followed by radiation therapy ± chemotherapy) is the ideal management policy for carcinoma of the maxillary sinus.

Case-Based Questions

1. A 45-year-old woman presented to the outpatient department with loose teeth and epistaxis of 2 months' duration of the left side. The patient did not give a history of paresthesia over the cheek, reduced ocular motility, or trismus. On examination, there was no involvement of the cheek of the same side, but there was a mass over the hard palate.

   a. What is the T staging of the tumor?
   b. What is the treatment of choice for this patient?

   Answers
   a. T2 because the nasal cavity tumor has extended into the hard palate.
   b. Total maxillectomy with removal of the hard palate followed by radiotherapy.

2. A 45-year-old man presented with right nasal obstruction of 10 months' duration. On examination, there was a reddish, friable, granular mass over the lateral wall of the right nasal cavity. The histopathology showed hyperplasia of the basal layer with projection into the underlying stroma.

   a. What relevant investigations have to be performed for this patient?
   b. What is the diagnosis?
   c. What is the treatment?

   Answers
   a. To confirm the diagnosis, a nasal endoscopic examination has to be performed and a biopsy is to be taken from the mass.

      A CT with contrast will help determine the extent of the tumor.
   b. Inverted papilloma.
   c. Since it is a benign lesion and is confined to the lateral wall, an endoscopic medial maxillectomy is the ideal surgical treatment. There is no medical treatment for this condition.

Frequently Asked Questions

1. What are the clinical features of a patient presenting with inverted papilloma?

2. What are the relevant investigations to be performed to arrive at a treatment plan for inverted papilloma?

3. What is the etiology of maxillary sinus malignancy?

4. What are the routes of spread of the malignancy from the maxillary sinus?

5. What is the "T" stage of the sinus malignancy if the skin over the maxillary sinus is involved?

6. What is the treatment of the sinus malignancy if there is intracranial extension through the cribriform plate?

Endnote

Maxillectomy is performed for removal of tumors from the maxilla. The concept of maxillectomy was first described by Lazars in 1826, but the first successful maxillectomy was performed by Syme 2 years later. It was a difficult surgery to perform because of excessive blood loss, infection, and disfigurement of the face. The high complication rate led to radiation being preferred as the sole treatment of maxillary sinus malignancy till the 1950s. Thereafter with the advancement in anesthesia, blood transfusion, and surgical techniques like the Weber–Fergusson incision, radical maxillectomy gained more popularity.

34 Septoplasty

Vijendra Shenoy S. and Kshithi K.

The competency covered in this chapter is as follows:
EN4.24 Enumerate the indications for, observe, and describe the steps in a septoplasty.

Introduction

Septoplasty is a conservative procedure commonly performed for correction of a deviated nasal septum causing symptoms. It can also be performed as part of other surgical procedures like rhinoplasty. There are various methods of doing a septoplasty. The commonly performed technique is called Cottle's premaxilla-maxilla technique.

Indications

Septoplasty is indicated in the following conditions:
- Nasal obstruction, which may be unilateral or bilateral. Bilateral is due to an "S"-shaped deviation or associated compensatory hypertrophy of the contralateral inferior turbinate.
- Sluder's neuralgia, which is headache due to septal spur impinging on the lateral wall (anterior ethmoidal nerve syndrome; **Fig. 34.1**).

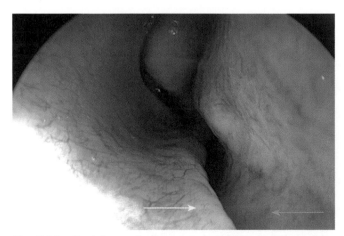

Fig. 34.1 Septal spur (*yellow arrow*). Inferior turbinate (*blue arrow*).

- In sleep apnea and snoring, it is done along with other procedures, or to facilitate use of the continuous positive airway pressure (CPAP) machine.
- Recurrent epistaxis from an area of septal spur or area adjacent to deviation. Elevation of the mucoperichondrium at the site of epistaxis heals by fibrosis, which can seal off the vessel.
- Recurrent sinusitis due to obstruction to ventilation or compressing the middle turbinate, which affects the drainage of the anterior group of sinuses.
- External deformity is corrected by septorhinoplasty. This procedure involves a cosmetic and functional correction.

It can be done for access to other procedures like the following:
- Functional endoscopic sinus surgery (FESS).
- Endoscopic dacryocystorhinostomy.
- Transseptal, transsphenoidal hypophysectomy.
- Sinonasal or orbital tumor removal.

In addition to creating space for surgery, it facilitates postoperative care and assessment. Temporarily deflecting the septum to one side or creating a septal window is also done in some cases to allow for additional instrumentation.

Contraindications

Septoplasty is not done when there are acute nasal and paranasal sinus infections, uncontrolled systemic conditions like hypertension, diabetes, and in bleeding diathesis.

Procedure

The procedure can be performed under general or local anesthesia. The patient is positioned supine with 15-degree elevation of the head end of the table and the patient's

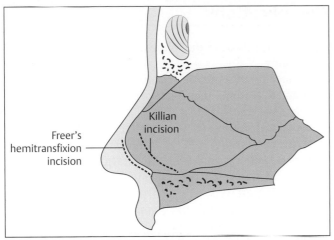

Fig. 34.2 Freer's hemitransfixion incision for septoplasty. Killian's incision is for submucous resection.

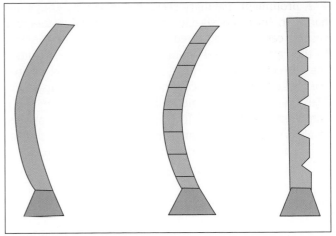

Fig. 34.3 Depiction of the straightening of septal cartilage after placing cross-hatching incision over the concave surface of the cartilage.

head turned 30 degrees to the right. The operating surgeon stands to the right side of the patient wearing a headlight.

The nasal cavities are packed with cottonoids soaked in 4% Xylocaine with 1:10,000 adrenaline for 10 minutes to achieve surface anesthesia and vasoconstriction. Infiltration with 2% Xylocaine with 1:100,000 adrenaline given over the caudal end of the septum and on either side of the septum from an anterior to posterior direction.

A Freer hemitransfixion incision is performed with a no. 15 scalpel at the caudal end of the septum while stabilizing it between the two prongs of the nasal speculum (**Fig. 34.2**). This incision is given on the concave side of the septum and is deepened up to the mucoperichondrium. The mucoperichondrium is raised from the underlying septal cartilage using a Freer elevator from anterior to posterior (caudal to cephalad) direction by sweeping the elevator in a superior to inferior direction. This constitutes the anterior tunnel.

While elevating the flap, a long-bladed Killian speculum is used to maintain the plane between the flap and septum and for visualization. An inferior tunnel is made by separating the mucoperiosteum from the maxillary crest. A posterior tunnel is also created by raising the mucoperiosteum from the perpendicular plate of the ethmoid bone and vomer. The bony cartilaginous junction is dislocated and the mucoperiosteum is elevated off the opposite side of the bony septum over the deviation.

The deviated septal cartilage and bone are now straightened by removing or repositioning the deviated parts. Cross-hatching by crisscross incisions eliminates the spring action and helps maintain the straightened position of the septum (**Figs. 34.3** and **34.4**). Scoring, shaving, and wedge excision of the cartilage may be done to make it straight. Bony deviation is removed by grasping with Irwin Moore forceps and twisting it to fracture the bone, before removal. Care should be taken in the superior part adjacent to cribriform plate to avoid trauma because it can result in cerebrospinal fluid (CSF) leak and anosmia.

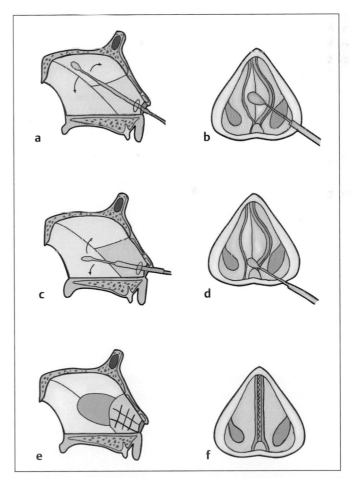

Fig. 34.4 Sagittal and coronal images depicting steps of septoplasty. **(a, b)** Elevation of mucoperichondrium and mucoperiosteum over septal cartilage and perpendicular plate of ethmoid (anterior and posterior tunnels). **(c, d)** Elevation of mucoperiosteum over the maxillary crest and vomer (inferior tunnel). **(e, f)** Final result after removal of deviated portion of the bony septum and cross-hatching incision over the septal cartilage.

A prominent maxillary crest is removed by gouge and hammer. Once repositioned and straightened, transseptal sutures can be placed if required to approximate the flaps to the cartilage. Nasal splints may be placed to maintain the corrected position for a few days. The nasal cavities are packed with either commercially available packs (e.g., Merocel, Nasopore, Rapid rhino) or ribbon gauze lubricated with petroleum jelly. An external bolster is applied to absorb any blood. Some surgeons prefer to avoid using nasal packing to reduce the postoperative discomfort.

Postoperative Care

The patient is placed in a 30-degree head end elevated position. The posterior pharyngeal wall is inspected to look for evidence of any fresh bleed. Antibiotics and analgesics are given for 5 to 7 days. Nasal packs are removed after 24 to 48 hours. Decongestant nasal drops are started. Saline nasal drops or sprays are given to avoid drying and crusting. Nasal splints, if placed, are removed after 7 days.

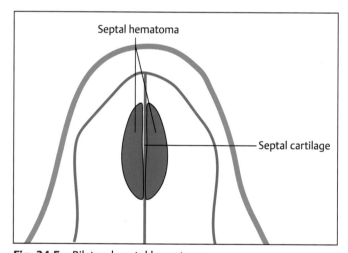

Fig. 34.5 Bilateral septal hematoma.

Complications

The complications are the following:
- Bleeding.
- Persistence of septal deviation.
- Septal hematoma (**Fig. 34.5**).
- Septal abscess.
- Septal perforation (if the mucoperichondrial flaps are torn on both sides at the same level).
- Supratip depression, columellar retraction, and saddle nose deformity may occur due to excess removal of cartilage (**Fig. 34.6**).
- Synechiae form when there are raw areas in the septum and adjoining lateral wall.
- CSF rhinorrhea occurs if the cribriform plate is injured while operating on the perpendicular plate of ethmoid.
- Toxic shock syndrome can occur if the nasal packs are not removed in time or if antibiotic coverage is inadequate.

Complications are usually less common in septoplasty as compared to submucosal resection (SMR) surgery.

The differences between septoplasty and SMR are presented in **Table 34.1**.

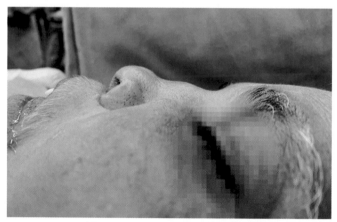

Fig. 34.6 Saddle nose deformity due to excess cartilage removal.

Table 34.1 Contrast between septoplasty and submucosal resection

Submucosal resection	Septoplasty
Killian's incision	Freer's incision
Mucoperichondrial and mucoperiosteal flaps are elevated on both sides	Mucoperichondrial flap elevated on one side
Removal of entire cartilage preserving only the L-strut (caudal 1 cm and dorsal 1 cm preserved)	Only the deviated portion of the septum is addressed
Caudal deviation cannot be corrected	It can be used for correction of caudal septal deviation
It is not performed in individuals younger than 17 y	It can be performed in children when indicated
Higher risk of complications	There is less chance of complications
Flappy septum due to lack of support that usually resolves with time due to fibrosis	It usually does not occur
Revision surgery is difficult	Revision surgery is comparatively easier

Cottle's line is an imaginary vertical line from the nasal process of the frontal bone to the anterior nasal spine. For deviations anterior to the line, septoplasty, and for deviations posterior to the line, SMR can be considered (**Fig. 34.7**).

■ Endoscopic Septoplasty

When the procedure is done under endoscopic guidance using a 0-degree nasal endoscope, it is called endoscopic septoplasty. It is ideal for removal of a spur but can be used for other deviations except caudal dislocation. It allows for good visualization and documentation, and is an aid for teaching.

■ Extracorporeal Septoplasty

In this process, the whole septum (bony and cartilaginous parts) is removed and reshaped or reoriented and then re-placed in position. It is done by the external rhinoplasty approach.

■ Pediatric Septoplasty

It can be done for severe breathing problem usually related to congenital anomalies and trauma, preferably above the age of 6 years. It should be conservative, although current evidence shows that the procedure does not affect midfacial growth.

■ Functional Rhinoplasty

This is done to improve the nasal airway. A spreader graft is placed between the upper lateral cartilage and the cartilaginous septum on the dorsum to increase Cottle's angle or a batten graft is placed to prevent collapse of the ala.

Turbinate Reduction or Turbinoplasty

At times, reduction of the size of the turbinates or turbinoplasty is performed along with septoplasty in order to improve the airway and relieve the nasal obstruction. This combined procedure is often referred to as septoturbinoplasty.

There are various methods to reduce the size of the turbinates. For the middle turbinate, it is done for a concha bullosa wherein the lateral part of the turbinate is removed. Turbinate reduction is more commonly done for the inferior turbinate in compensatory hypertrophy, allergic rhinitis, and vasomotor rhinitis.

There are the various methods used for turbinate reduction:

- A *partial turbinectomy* may be done. A total turbinectomy compromises the function of the inferior turbinate and may lead to an *empty nose syndrome* wherein the patient may still complain of nasal obstruction due to lack of sensation of the airflow through the nose.
- In *SMR*, a flap is created by giving an incision in the inferior margin and the excess bone and soft tissue are removed.

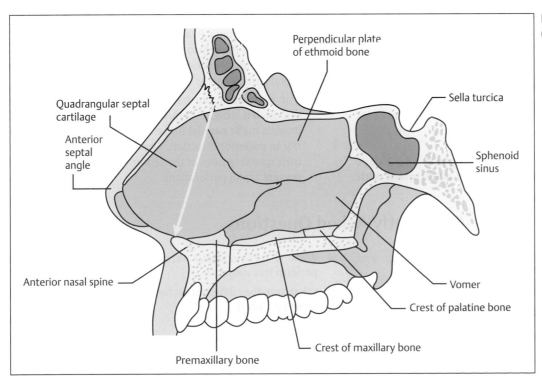

Fig. 34.7 Cottle's line (*yellow arrow*).

Perpendicular plate of ethmoid bone

Quadrangular septal cartilage

Anterior septal angle

Sella turcica

Sphenoid sinus

Anterior nasal spine

Vomer

Crest of palatine bone

Crest of maxillary bone

Premaxillary bone

35 Functional Endoscopic Sinus Surgery

Krishna Koirala

The competencies covered in this chapter are as follows:

EN3.5 Observe and describe the indications for and steps involved in the surgical procedures in ear, nose, and throat.

EN4.25 Elicit document and present a proper history; demonstrate and describe the clinical features; choose the correct investigations; and describe the principles of management of nasal polyps.

EN4.33 Elicit document and present a proper history; demonstrate and describe the clinical features; choose the correct investigations; and describe the principles of management of acute and chronic sinusitis.

Introduction

Functional endoscopic sinus surgery (FESS) is a minimally invasive surgical technique used to restore sinus ventilation and drainage. This technology has significantly advanced in recent years with improvements in instrumentation, radiology, and simulation, and the use of navigation. The procedure has revolutionized surgical treatment of nasal and sinus disease.

The changes in the sinonasal mucociliary clearance play a role in the pathogenesis of sinusitis. The aims of FESS in the treatment of sinusitis are the following:
- To improve aeration and ventilation by enlarging the sinus ostia (with mucosal preservation where feasible).
- To improving mucociliary transport.
- To provide an adequate route for topical medications.

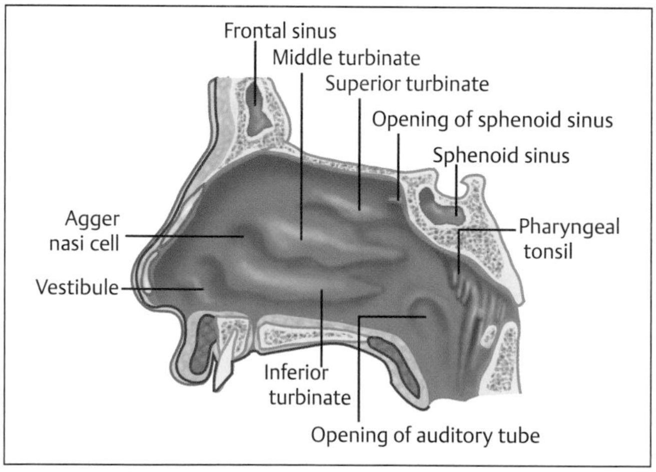

FESS is considered the gold standard in the surgical management of sinonasal pathology including chronic rhinosinusitis. Endoscopic sinus surgery is also useful in the management of sinonasal tumors and in pathologies beyond the sinuses.

A detailed understanding of the anatomy of the nose and paranasal sinus is required for adequate disease clearance and avoiding complications (**Figs. 35.1** and **35.2**). The anatomy of the paranasal sinuses varies from person to person and may also be different on each side in an individual. Therefore, performing computed tomography scan (1-mm axial, coronal, and sagittal cuts) is mandatory prior to the surgery.

Pearl

Understanding the anatomy of the nose and paranasal sinuses is key to performing FESS.

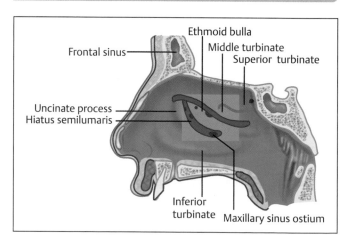

Fig. 35.1 Anatomy of the lateral wall of the nose.

Fig. 35.2 Lateral wall of nose showing structures in the middle meatus including the opening of the sinuses.

Indications

- Chronic rhinosinusitis refractory to medical treatment.
- Recurrent sinusitis.
- Nasal polyps (ethmoidal and antrochoanal).
- Invasive and noninvasive fungal sinusitis.
- Complications of acute and chronic rhinosinusitis including mucocele.

■ Indications for Endoscopic-Assisted Naso-Sinus Surgeries (Extended Indications)

- Closure of cerebrospinal fluid (CSF) leaks.
- Orbital and optic nerve decompression.
- Excision of localized benign and malignant sinonasal tumors.
- As an approach to pituitary tumors, anterior skull base lesions, pterygomaxillary fossa, and the petrous apex.
- In dacryocystorhinostomy (DCR), choanal atresia repair, foreign body removal, and control of epistaxis.

Note: The nasal endoscope is used for other procedures like removal of foreign bodies and rhinolith, septoplasty, turbinoplasty, and adenoidectomy.

Contraindications

- Patients not tolerating general or local anesthesia.
- Nasal lesions or pathologies extending into the lateral recesses of the frontal sinus, palate, into or above the orbit, and advanced intracranial involvement of the disease.

> **Pearl**
>
> Chronic rhinosinusitis refractory to medical treatment is the commonest indication of FESS.

Preparation

The patient lies on the operating table in the reverse Trendelenburg position (the head end elevated by 15 degrees). The endotracheal tube is secured to the corner of the patient's mouth, preferably on the left side.

The patient's eyes are either covered with a transparent tape or left open to look for any orbital complications during the procedure.

Both nasal cavities are initially packed with adrenaline (1:1,000) and oxymetazoline-soaked cotton for decongestion.

Technique

A detailed nasal endoscopy is performed using a 30-degree endoscope. The anatomy of the lateral nasal wall is assessed for any anatomical variations, and to identify the extent of the disease. The uncinate process and the region of the axilla of the middle turbinate are infiltrated with 1% lignocaine with 1:200,000 adrenaline using a 3-mL syringe with a 26-gauge needle. Then, adrenaline (1:1,000) or oxymetazoline-soaked cottonoid patties are placed in the middle meatus to decongest it.

Although there is no hard and fast rule to which side to operate on first, the side with more burden of disease or the side that is wider is to be operated on first. In a grossly deviated nasal septum, septoplasty can be performed for creating a roomy nasal cavity, for ease of instrumentation, better surgical field, and to facilitate better postoperative care.

Steps of Surgery

Figs. 35.3 and **35.4** illustrate the endoscopic anatomy:
- Uncinectomy (infundibulotomy).
- Middle meatal antrostomy (MMA).
- Anterior ethmoidectomy.
- Perforation of basal lamella.

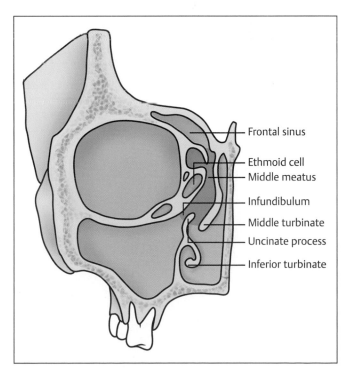

Fig. 35.3 Coronal view of endoscopic anatomy of the nose.

- Posterior ethmoidectomy.
- Sphenoid sinus exploration.
- Skull base disease clearance.
- Frontal recess exploration.

Pearl

Performing FESS stepwise reduces the chances of complications of FESS, and helps minimize the chances of recurrence.

Uncinectomy

Using a Freer elevator, the middle turbinate is gently displaced medially to access the uncinate process. A sickle knife or the sharp edge of a Freer elevator is used to incise

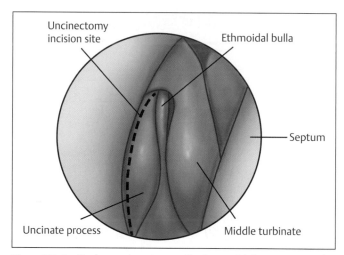

Fig. 35.4 Endoscopic view of the middle meatus for uncinectomy.

the lateral and inferior border of the uncinate process. It can also be performed by using a ball probe or back-biting forceps. Then the uncinate is removed with the help of Blakesley forceps, back-biting instruments, or microdebrider until the maxillary ostium is widely visualized. Occasionally the concha bullosa also needs to be excised to get a wider view of the middle meatus if it is present (**Fig. 35.5**).

Maxillary Antrostomy

On removal of the uncinate process, the natural ostium of the maxillary sinus can be visualized. It is in relation to the lower part of the infundibulum. The natural maxillary sinus ostium when required can be widened using thru-cut forceps, punch forceps, or microdebrider. The ostium is enlarged posteroinferiorly as superiorly it is related to the orbit and anteriorly to the nasolacrimal duct (these structures can be breached during uncinectomy). If there is an accessory ostium, it is joined with the natural ostium.

Excision of the Ethmoid Bulla and Ethmoidectomy

The ethmoid bulla is the largest and most consistent cell of the anterior ethmoid sinus (**Fig. 35.6**). It is the first cell to be encountered in the ethmoid sinus. This cell is penetrated inferomedially using curette, punch forceps, or microdebrider. Further dissection is done posteriorly till the basal (ground) lamella is reached. Basal lamella is penetrated inferomedially to access the posterior ethmoid cells. Complete dissection of the ethmoid cells is performed from medially to the lamina papyracea and superiorly to the

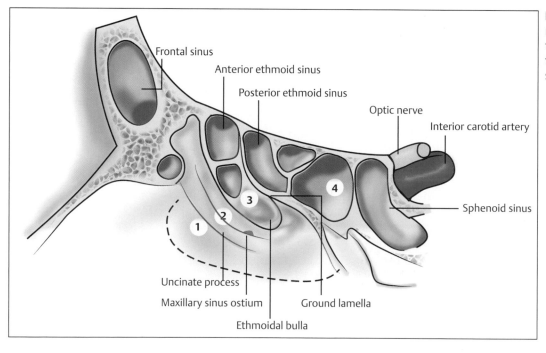

Fig. 35.5 Lateral wall of nose showing the sinuses to be opened during functional endoscopic sinus surgery (FESS).

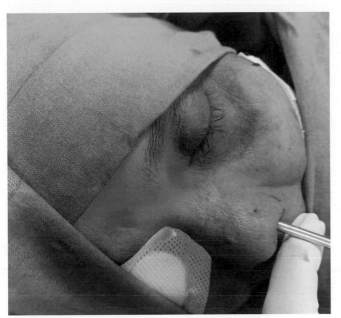

Fig. 35.6 Frontal sinus opened during functional endoscopic sinus surgery (FESS) revealing a "frontal glow" on the left side.

skull base. Any dehiscence in the lamina papyracea, site of the anterior ethmoidal artery, and slope of the skull base should be identified. One should not dissect medial to the superior attachment of the middle turbinate to avoid penetrating the fovea ethmoidalis and the vertical part of the cribriform plate.

■ Sphenoidotomy

The sphenoid ostium can be approached directly, that is, between the middle turbinate and the septum posteriorly or via the transethmoidal route. The sphenoid ostium is inferomedial to the posterior ethmoid. Resection of the inferior part of the superior turbinate allows better visualization of the sphenoethmoidal recess and sphenoid ostium. The ostium is enlarged inferiorly using a curette or Kerrison punch or microdebrider. The direction of entry to the sphenoid from the posterior ethmoid is inferior and medial as superiorly the skull base slopes downward from anterior to posterior, and laterally there are important structures (optic nerve and internal carotid artery) related to the lateral wall of the sphenoid sinus.

■ Frontal Sinusotomy

The frontal sinus is cleared toward the later part of the surgery after the skull base (fovea ethmoidalis) has been identified. It has a complex anatomy compared to other sinuses. A 45- or 70-degree scope allows for better visualization of this sinus. The posterior wall of the agger nasi cells needs to be carefully dissected to relieve the obstruction to the frontal sinus outflow. Frontal sinus drainage can be

variable depending on the different superior attachments of the uncinate process. Different probes, curved curettes, giraffe forceps, 45- to 90-degree forceps, and mushroom punch are used to dissect the cells related to the frontal sinus, and clear the frontal recess (**Fig. 35.6**). The frontal recess can also be approached between the agger nasi cells anteriorly and the bulla ethmoidalis posteriorly (the intact bulla technique).

At the end of the procedure, any mucosal tags, bony chips, and septations left are removed, and hemostasis is obtained. A merocel nasal pack can be placed for 24 to 48 hours if there is possibility of persistent oozing.

An endoscopic surgeon must respect the mucosa to avoid adhesions and scarring. The middle turbinate should be preserved as a landmark if revision surgery is required. The middle turbinate should not be destabilized. A lateralized middle turbinate can cause scarring and obstruction of the sinus drainage.

Complications

The paranasal sinuses are closely related to critical structures like the orbit, internal carotid artery, and brain, which when breached can lead to major complications during FESS (**Table 35.1**).

Postoperative Care

Meticulous postoperative care is required to avoid recurrence of the disease especially in chronic rhinosinusitis. Postsurgery medical treatment with saline nasal douches, topical or oral corticosteroids, and antibiotics helps in reducing inflammation and recurrence. Regular follow-up and nasal cleaning are also important to improve the postoperative outcome of FESS.

Points to Ponder

- FESS is the commonest surgical procedure performed for chronic sinusitis.
- CT scan of the nose and paranasal sinuses and detailed nasal endoscopy before surgery are the basic prerequisites for FESS.
- Oral and topical steroids for 2 weeks before surgery are indicated in CRS with nasal polyps.
- Understanding the basic anatomy and identifying the landmarks and anatomical variations lead to a good surgical outcome.
- Due to the complex anatomy of the nose and paranasal sinuses, major complications like blindness and CSF leak can occur, if not careful.

Table 35.1 Complications of FESS

Major (1%) complications	Minor (7%) complications
• Major epistaxis—from sphenopalatine branches and anterior ethmoidal artery • Orbital hematoma • Retrobulbar hemorrhage (anterior ethmoidal artery injury) • Diplopia (injury to the medial rectus) • Blindness/decreased visual acuity (optic nerve injury, retrobulbar hemorrhage) • Internal carotid injury • Intracranial hemorrhage • CSF leak/meningitis • Pneumocephalus • Anosmia • Nasolacrimal duct trauma	• Minor epistaxis • Hyposmia • Adhesions (synechiae) • Headache • Breach of orbital periosteum with fat prolapse • Periorbital emphysema • Periorbital ecchymosis • Periorbital hematoma • Dental/facial pain

Abbreviations: CSF, cerebrospinal fluid; FESS, functional endoscopic sinus surgery.

Case-Based Question

1. **A 38-year-old man presented with bilateral nasal obstruction. He was diagnosed with bilateral ethmoidal polyps. He was advised surgery in the form of FESS to remove the polyps.**

   a. What are the steps involved in this surgery?

   b. What complications should be explained to the patient?

   Answers

   a. FESS consists of a series of steps, carefully executed so that the polyps are removed and all the sinuses are opened up. Even though ethmoidal polyps are mainly confined to the ethmoidal air cells, the other sinuses can be involved with

   disease due to secondary sinusitis. It is important to ask for a CT scan of the nose and paranasal sinuses before surgery.

   The steps of FESS include uncinectomy, MMA, ethmoidal air cell exenteration, sphenoid sinus clearance, and, finally, frontal sinus recess clearance.

   b. In the case of ethmoidal polyps, the disease can always recur. This should be explained to the patient. Though FESS is a relatively safe surgery, if the surgeon does not have a thorough understanding of the anatomy, complications can occur.

   The major complications include those related to the eye and brain like orbital hematoma, blindness, diplopia, hemorrhage, and CSF leak and meningitis.

Frequently Asked Questions

1. What is FESS and what are its advantages over the traditional external approaches to the sinuses?

2. What are the indications for endoscopic sinus surgery?

3. What are the basic steps for this surgery?

4. What are the complications of FESS?

Endnote

The technique of FESS that is normally performed is called Messerklinger's technique in which dissection is carried out from an anterior to posterior direction. The opposite is Wigand's technique in which the surgical steps are carried out from a posterior to anterior direction. The man credited with developing FESS and introducing it for the treatment of chronic inflammation of the sinuses is Walter Messerklinger, a surgeon from Graz, Austria. Since Messerklinger did not speak English, it was left to his assistant Dr. Heinz Stammberger to popularize this around the world in the 1980s.

36 Anatomy of the Oral Cavity and the Salivary Glands

Meera Niranjan Khadilkar

Introduction

The oral cavity serves as the first part of the digestive tract.

The oral cavity extends from the lips anteriorly to the oropharyngeal isthmus posteriorly. The oropharyngeal isthmus is bound by the junction of the hard palate and soft palate superiorly, the anterior tonsillar pillars laterally, and the junction of the anterior two-thirds and posterior one-third of the tongue inferiorly.

The oral cavity is further divided into the oral vestibule and the oral cavity proper. The oral vestibule is the region bounded by the lips, buccal mucosa, and the occluded teeth (**Box 36.1**).

Lips

The lips are muscular folds forming the oral fissure (**Fig. 36.1**). The upper and lower lips are connected at the oral commissure (angle of the mouth). They have an external surface lined by skin and an internal surface lined by the mucosa. The surfaces merge at the vermilion border.

Pearl

Deviation of the angle of the mouth is an early sign of facial nerve palsy.

Box 36.1   Subsites of the oral cavity

Lips
Anterior tongue
Floor of the mouth
Buccal mucosa
Upper alveolar ridge
Lower alveolar ridge
Hard palate
Retromolar trigone

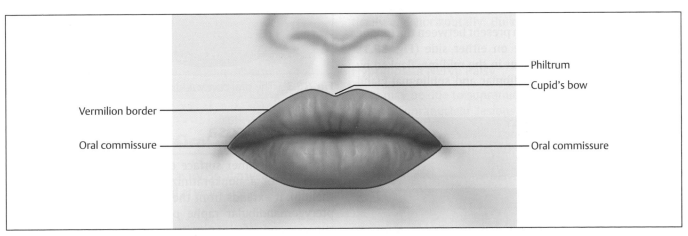

Fig. 36.1   The lips and parts of the lips.

Table 36.1 Lymphatic drainage of the oral cavity

Part	Subparts	Lymphatic drainage
Lips	Upper lip	Preauricular, intraparotid, and submandibular nodes
	Lower lip	Central part: Submental nodes Lateral part: Submandibular nodes
Anterior tongue	Tip	Submental nodes
	Lateral border	Ipsilateral submandibular and deep cervical nodes
	Central part	Bilateral deep cervical nodes
Floor of the mouth	Anterior part	Submental and bilateral submandibular nodes
	Posterior part	Upper deep cervical nodes
Buccal mucosa		Submental, submandibular, and deep cervical nodes
Upper alveolar ridge	Buccal surface	Submandibular nodes
	Lingual surface	Indirectly via the lateral retropharyngeal nodes or directly to the upper deep cervical nodes
Lower alveolar ridge	Buccal surface	Central part: Submental nodes Lateral part: Submandibular nodes
	Lingual surface	Central part: Submental nodes Lateral part: Submandibular nodes
Hard palate	Anterior part	Submandibular nodes
	Posterior part	Indirectly via the lateral retropharyngeal nodes or directly to the upper deep cervical nodes

infection, radiation therapy, stroke, pseudobulbar palsy, amyotrophic lateral sclerosis, and carotid endarterectomy.

Physiology of Oral Cavity

- The oral cavity is responsible for the oral phase of deglutition, that is, accommodation of ingested bolus by depression of the mandible, opening of the oral fissure, and depression of the tongue. This is followed by mastication, which is brought about by the combined action of the teeth, buccal mucosa, tongue, hard palate, and saliva to produce a bolus of desired consistency, size, and shape. Next, the tongue comes in contact with the hard palate to propel the bolus into the oropharynx.
- Saliva production occurs in the acinar cells of the salivary glands as isotonic extracellular fluid. This passes through the salivary ductal system and is converted to the final saliva, which is hypotonic. Saliva protects the oral cavity and teeth, has antimicrobial action, provides lubrication, acts as a buffer, promotes wound healing and regeneration, aids in digestion due to salivary amylase, and helps in taste sensation.
- The tongue is a chemosensory organ responsible for gustation (taste sensation). The chemoreceptors or taste buds are connected to nerve fibers, which carry impulses to the higher cerebral cortex.

- The oral cavity functions as a secondary respiratory channel.
- It contributes to resonance by amplification and modification of voice produced at the level of the glottis.
- It is responsible for the articulation of voice to produce recognizable speech by the action of the tongue, palate, and lips.
- It aids in behavioral expression.

Muscles of Mastication

These comprise the masseter, temporalis, medial pterygoid, and lateral pterygoid muscles. These are supplied by the mandibular division of the trigeminal nerve.

> **Pearl**
>
> Trismus (lockjaw) can occur as a result of spasm of the muscles of mastication.

Salivary Glands

They are exocrine glands responsible for saliva production. There are three pairs of major salivary glands (parotid, submandibular, and sublingual), and numerous minor salivary glands.

■ Parotid Gland

It is the largest salivary gland and is located below the external auditory canal (**Fig. 36.4**). It is bound anteromedially by the mandibular ramus and posteriorly by the sternocleidomastoid muscle and the mastoid. It is lined by a derivative of deep cervical fascia called the parotid fascia. It is divided into a superficial lobe and a deep lobe by the facial nerve. The parotid duct (Stensen's duct) is 5 cm long and runs over the masseter till its anterior border, traverses the buccinator, and finally opens into the buccal mucosa at the level of the upper second molar tooth.

Pearl

Curtain sign: The superior attachment of the parotid fascia to the zygomatic arch prevents upward spread of tumors.

Pearl

The faciovenous plane of Patey represents the demarcation between the two lobes of the parotid, aiding in parotid surgery without facial nerve injury.

■ Submandibular Gland

It is the second largest salivary gland and is located in the submandibular triangle, below the mandible. It is lined by a derivative of the superficial layer of the deep cervical fascia.

It is divided into a superficial lobe and a deep lobe by the mylohyoid muscle. The submandibular duct (Wharton's duct) is 5 cm long and arises from the deep lobe, traverses around the posterior part of the mylohyoid, crosses the lingual nerve, and finally opens in the floor of the mouth via the submandibular papillae on either side of the lingual frenulum (**Fig. 36.5**).

Pearl

The marginal mandibular branch of the facial nerve is at risk of injury during submandibular gland excision due to its proximity.

Pearl

Sialolithiasis is more common in the submandibular gland than in the parotid gland due to nondependent drainage, viscous secretion, angulation of the duct at the edge of the mylohyoid, and higher calcium and phosphate content in the submandibular gland.

■ Sublingual Gland

It is the smallest major salivary gland, situated between the mandible laterally and the geniohyoid, mylohyoid, and hyoglossus muscles medially. A group of ducts (ducts of Rivinus) drain the sublingual gland, the largest being Bartholin's duct, which joins the submandibular duct and opens on either side of the lingual frenulum.

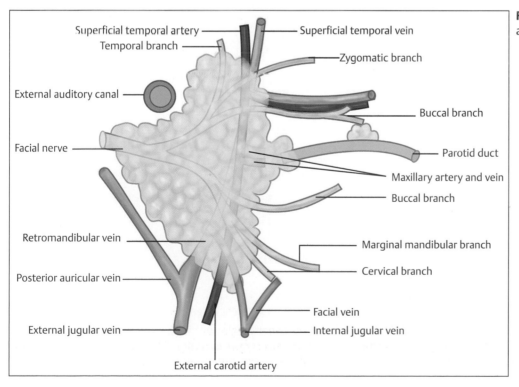

Fig. 36.4 The parotid gland and its relations.

Superficial temporal artery
Temporal branch
Superficial temporal vein
Zygomatic branch
External auditory canal
Buccal branch
Facial nerve
Parotid duct
Maxillary artery and vein
Buccal branch
Retromandibular vein
Marginal mandibular branch
Cervical branch
Posterior auricular vein
Facial vein
External jugular vein
Internal jugular vein
External carotid artery

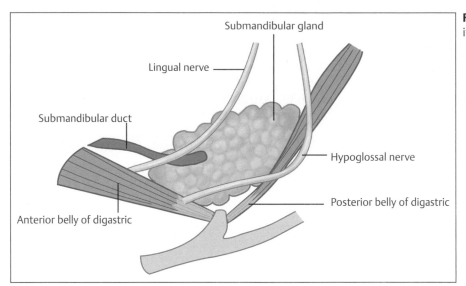

Fig. 36.5 The submandibular gland with its relations.

Minor Salivary Glands

There are around 800 to 1,000 minor salivary glands distributed all through the submucosa of the oral cavity, pharynx, sinonasal tract, larynx, trachea, lungs, and middle ear.

Pearl

About 90% of the minor salivary gland tumors are malignant.

Blood Supply

The parotid gland is supplied by the superficial temporal and maxillary branches of the external carotid artery and is drained by the retromandibular vein terminating into the external jugular vein.

The submandibular and sublingual glands are supplied by the branches of the facial and lingual arteries and are drained by common facial and sublingual veins terminating into the internal jugular vein.

Lymphatic Drainage

The parotid gland drains into intraparotid nodes, whereas the submandibular and sublingual glands drain into submandibular nodes.

Nerve Supply

The parotid gland receives sympathetic vasomotor supply from the plexus around the external carotid artery and parasympathetic secretomotor supply from the auriculotemporal nerve. The submandibular gland receives sympathetic supply from the superior cervical ganglion and parasympathetic secretomotor supply from the chorda tympani nerve via the submandibular ganglion.

Points to Ponder

- The oral cavity extends from the lips to the oropharyngeal isthmus.
- Subsites include the lips, anterior tongue, the floor of the mouth, buccal mucosa, upper and lower alveolar ridges, hard palate, and retromolar trigone.
- The oral cavity helps in deglutition, salivation, gustation, speech production, and respiration.
- Hypoglossal nerve palsy leads to deviation of the tongue with nuclear and infranuclear lesion.
- Major salivary glands (parotid, submandibular, and sublingual) and minor salivary glands are responsible for saliva production.

Case-Based Questions

1. **A 40-year-old man, a tobacco chewer, presented with a 2 × 2 cm ulcerative lesion in the right buccal mucosa of 5 months' duration with difficulty in opening the mouth. The right submandibular and upper deep cervical lymph nodes are enlarged and hard but mobile.**

   a. What is the most likely diagnosis?

   b. How should this case be managed?

Answers

a. The most likely diagnosis is oral cavity (buccal mucosa) malignancy.

b. Contrast-enhanced computed tomography (CECT) followed by biopsy of the lesion and fine-needle aspiration cytology (FNAC) of the enlarged lymph node will confirm the diagnosis. Surgical treatment includes wide excision of the lesion in the buccal mucosa with neck dissection.

2. **A 30-year-old lady presented with intermittent painful swelling below the mandible, with an increase in size during me als. The patient is afebrile.**

   a. What is the most likely diagnosis?

   b. How should this case be managed?

   Answers

   a. The patient is probably suffering from submandibular duct sialolithiasis or stone formation in the gland. The typical history is that of increase in size of the gland during meals.

   b. Ultrasound imaging or X-ray (occlusal view) aids in diagnosis. Treatment includes sialogogues to improve salivary outflow and removal of stones by lithotripsy, or sialendoscopy, or by transoral removal.

3. **A 53-year-old male patient with uncontrolled diabetes was treated for a right parapharyngeal abscess by** broad-spectrum antibiotics and incision and drainage via a neck incision at the level of the hyoid bone. The patient was noted postoperatively to have deviation of the tongue to the right side. After 4 months, there was no improvement in the condition and there was fasciculations noted over the right side of the tongue.

   a. Why is there a deviation of the tongue to the right side?

   b. What was the possible cause?

   c. What is the morbidity for the patient?

   Answers

   a. Right hypoglossal palsy.

   b. The nerve could have been involved due to the abscess or due to the procedure of incision and drainage.

   c. The swallowing and speech of the patient will be affected. That side of the tongue can undergo atrophy.

Frequently Asked Questions

1. Enumerate the subsites of the oral cavity.

2. What are the functions of the oral cavity?

3. Describe the lymphatic drainage of the oral cavity.

4. Enumerate the muscles of mastication.

5. Briefly describe the anatomy of the salivary glands.

6. Write a note on hypoglossal palsy.

7. What is the importance of the retromolar trigone in malignancies of the oral cavity?

Endnote

Anatomically, the submandibular gland is like a hook. It hooks around the mylohyoid muscles forming a superficial and a deep part. Excision of the submandibular gland is a common procedure for conditions such as tumors and calculi. The gland has a relationship with three important nerves and all three nerves must be identified and protected during surgery. They include the lingual nerve, hypoglossal nerve, and the marginal mandibular branch of the facial nerve.

37 Anatomy of the Pharynx

Arun Alexander and Soorya Pradeep

The competencies covered in this chapter are as follows:

EN1.1 Describe the anatomy and physiology of ear, nose, throat, and head and neck

AN36.1 Describe the (1) morphology, relations, blood supply, and applied anatomy of palatine tonsil, (2) composition of soft palate.

AN36.2 Describe the composition and functions of Waldeyer's ring.

AN36.3 Describe the boundaries and clinical significance of pyriform fossa.

AN36.5 Describe the clinical significance of Killian's dehiscence.

Introduction

The pharynx is a fibromuscular tube that extends from the skull base to the inferior border of the cricoid cartilage and forms a part of the upper aerodigestive tract. It is 12- to 14-cm long, extends till the level of the C6 vertebra, and is continuous with the esophagus inferiorly.

Based on its anterior relations, the pharynx consists of three regions (**Fig. 37.1**):
- Nasopharynx: Posterior to the nasal choanae.
- Oropharynx: Posterior to the oral cavity.
- Hypopharynx or laryngopharynx: Posterior to the larynx.

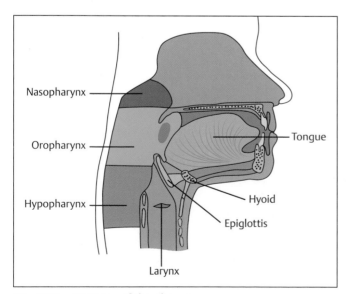

Fig. 37.1 Divisions of the pharynx.

Structure of the Pharynx

Skeletal Framework

The pharynx is attached superiorly to the base of the skull and the posterior walls merge in the midline to form a vertical cordlike ligament known as the pharyngeal raphe. Anteriorly, the lateral pharyngeal wall is attached to the medial plate of the pterygoid process and the pterygoid hamulus, the pterygomandibular raphe, the stylohyoid ligament, the greater horn of the hyoid, the superior tubercle of the thyroid, and the oblique line till the inferior tubercle.

Pharyngeal Wall

The pharyngeal wall has five distinct layers (**Fig. 37.2**):
- Mucosa: The mucosa of the nasopharynx consists of the ciliated pseudostratified columnar epithelium, whereas the rest of the pharyngeal mucosa consists of the non-keratinized stratified squamous epithelium.
- Submucosa: The submucosa is composed of elastic connective tissue with aggregates of lymphoid tissue, which forms the Waldeyer's ring.
- Pharyngobasilar fascia: It is a thick fascial layer firmly adherent to the base of the skull and is continuous with the buccopharyngeal fascia superiorly. These fascial layers reinforce the pharyngeal walls at sites where the muscular layer is deficient.
- Muscular layer: The muscles of the pharyngeal wall are grouped in two based on the orientation of the muscle fibers: the inner longitudinal muscles and the outer constrictors. The constrictor muscles are arranged as

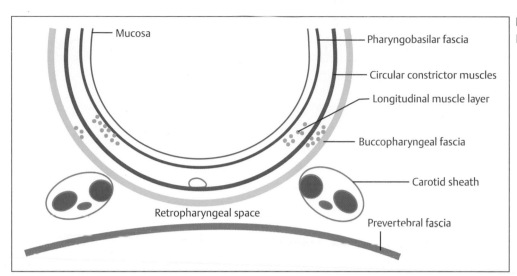

Fig. 37.2 Layers of the pharyngeal wall.

Labels: Mucosa, Pharyngobasilar fascia, Circular constrictor muscles, Longitudinal muscle layer, Buccopharyngeal fascia, Carotid sheath, Retropharyngeal space, Prevertebral fascia

Table 37.1 Muscles of the pharyngeal wall: Origin, insertion, action, and nerve supply

Muscle	Origin	Insertion	Action	Nerve supply
Superior constrictor	Pterygoid hamulus, pterygomandibular raphe, and adjacent bone of the mandible	Pharyngeal raphe	Constricts the pharynx	Pharyngeal branch of the vagus nerve
Middle constrictor	Stylohyoid ligament, the lesser horn of the hyoid bone, and the upper surface of the greater horn of the hyoid			
Inferior constrictor	Oblique line of the thyroid cartilage and cricoid cartilage			
Stylopharyngeus	Medial side of the base of the styloid process	Pharyngeal wall	Elevate the pharynx	Glossopharyngeal nerve
Salpingopharyngeus	Inferior aspect of the pharyngeal end of the pharyngotympanic tube			Vagus nerve
Palatopharyngeus	Upper surface of the palatine aponeurosis			Vagus nerve

interlocking cones with each layer overlapping the next (**Table 37.1**).

- Buccopharyngeal fascia: It is a thin layer of areolar tissue lining the muscular layer, which contains the pharyngeal plexus of veins and nerves. It is continuous with the pretracheal layer of the cervical fascia.

Pearl

The retropharyngeal space is a potential space between the buccopharyngeal fascia and the prevertebral fascia. It extends from the skull base to the upper mediastinum, whereas the prevertebral space extends from the skull base to the coccyx. The retropharyngeal space contains lymph nodes, which can suppurate and form a retropharyngeal abscess.

Gaps between the muscles are reinforced by the fascia and provide routes for structures to pass through the wall (**Table 37.2**).

Nasopharynx

The nasopharynx (postnasal space or epipharynx) is the uppermost part of the pharynx, which lies posterior to the nasal cavity and extends from the base of the skull to the soft palate.

The roof of the nasopharynx is formed by the basisphenoid and the basiocciput, while the floor is formed by the soft palate anteriorly and is deficient posteriorly where it becomes continuous with the oropharynx. It is anteriorly bounded by the choana and the posterior end of the septum and posteriorly by the arch of the atlas covered by the prevertebral muscles and the fascia.

The lateral wall of the nasopharynx contains the orifice for the cartilaginous eustachian tube, located 1 to 1.5 cm posterior to the posterior end of the inferior turbinate. The eustachian tube orifice is bounded superiorly and posteriorly by a mucosa-covered prominence known as the torus tubarius. Posterior to the torus, there is a recess known as

Table 37.2 Structures passing through gaps between the muscles

Gaps in the fascia	Structures traversing the gaps
Above the superior constrictor (sinus of Morgagni)	Cartilaginous eustachian tube, tensor and levator palatini, and palatine branch of the ascending pharyngeal artery
Between the superior and middle constrictors	Stylopharyngeus, styloglossus, glossopharyngeal, and lingual nerve
Through the thyrohyoid membrane	Internal laryngeal nerve and superior laryngeal vessels
Below cricopharyngeus	Recurrent laryngeal nerve and inferior thyroid artery

the fossa of Rosenmuller which is a hidden area and is the most common site for nasopharyngeal malignancies.

Adenoids (Luschka's tonsil, nasopharyngeal tonsil) are a subepithelial collection of the lymphoid tissue at the junction of the roof and the posterior wall of the nasopharynx. The overlying mucosa has pseudostratified ciliated columnar epithelium and is thrown into radiating folds. It increases in size between 2 and 6 years of life and then gradually atrophies.

The *nasopharyngeal bursa* is an epithelium-lined median recess within the adenoid mass extending from the pharyngeal mucosa to the periosteum of the basiocciput. It represents the attachment of the primitive notochord to the pharyngeal endoderm. If infected, it may cause persistent postnasal discharge and crusting. Rarely, it may develop into an abscess known as Thornwaldt's cyst.

The *tubal tonsil* is a collection of lymphoid tissue located posterior to the torus tubarius, in the fossa of Rosenmuller (pharyngeal recess). These are also called eustachian tonsils or Gerlach's tonsils.

Rathke's pouch is a remnant of the buccal mucosal invagination to form the adenohypophysis. It is represented clinically by a dimple above the adenoids.

The palatopharyngeus forms an important fold in the overlying mucosa called the palatopharyngeal arch or *Passavant's ridge*. It closes off the pharyngeal isthmus between the nasopharynx and the oropharynx during deglutition and speech

■ Role of Nasopharynx

- It acts as a conduit for warmed and humidified air.
- It ventilates the middle ear and equalizes air pressure between the pharynx and the middle ear through the eustachian tube.
- It provides resonance to voice.
- It acts as a drainage channel for the mucus secreted by the nasal and nasopharyngeal glands, and the middle ear.

■ The Waldeyer's Ring

The Waldeyer's inner ring consists of a collection of subepithelial lymphoid tissue at the entrance of the aerodigestive tract (**Fig. 37.3**). It consists of the following:
- Adenoids.

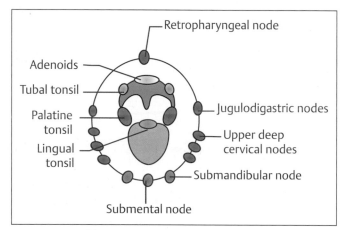

Fig. 37.3 Waldeyer's ring.

- Tubal tonsils.
- Lateral pharyngeal bands.
- Palatine tonsils.
- Submucosal lymphoid nodules in the posterior pharyngeal wall.
- Lingual tonsils on the base of the tongue.

The Waldeyer's outer ring comprises the lymph nodes of the head and neck region, namely, the following:
- Superficial cervical nodes.
- Submental and submandibular lymph nodes.
- Upper, middle, and lower deep cervical lymph nodes.
- Preauricular and intraparotid lymph nodes.
- Postauricular lymph nodes.
- Occipital lymph nodes.

The Waldeyer's ring plays an important role in local immunity:
- The B lymphocytes in the germinal centers of these lymphoid follicles help in immunoglobulin A (IgA) antibody formation.
- The immunoglobulin M (IgM) and immunoglobulin G (IgG) produced by plasma cells act on the pathogens that enter these lymphoid aggregations.
- The T lymphocytes provide cell-mediated immunity against various viruses, bacteria, and fungi.
- These act as sentinels at the portal of the aerodigestive tract and continuously monitor against a variety of infective agents in the incoming air and food via "immunological memory."

Oropharynx

The oropharynx lies posterior to the oral cavity, superiorly from the soft palate till the level of the hyoid bone inferiorly. The palatoglossal folds are mucosal folds overlying the palatoglossal muscles and form the anterior boundary of the oropharynx along with the soft palate and the posterior one-third of the tongue inferiorly. The oropharyngeal isthmus lies between the palatoglossal folds. The posterior boundary consists of the superior and the middle pharyngeal constrictor muscles and their overlying mucosa.

The subsites of the oropharynx include the following:
- Soft palate.
- Tonsils.
- Base of the tongue.
- Pharyngeal wall.

■ Soft Palate

It separates the oral cavity from the oropharynx and the oropharynx from the nasopharynx.

The tensor veli palatini, levator veli palatini, palatoglossus, and palatopharyngeus muscles form the musculature of the soft palate along with the muscularis uvulae, which form the uvula (**Fig. 37.4**).

When the oral cavity is filled with liquids or solids, the oropharyngeal isthmus is closed off by the depression of the soft palate, elevation of the back of the tongue, and movement toward the midline of the palatoglossal and palatopharyngeal folds. This allows us to breathe while chewing. On swallowing, the oropharyngeal isthmus is opened, the palate is elevated, the laryngeal cavity is closed, and the food is directed into the esophagus. A person cannot breathe and swallow at the same time because the airway is closed at two sites, the pharyngeal isthmus and the larynx.

Sensations from the palate are carried by the glossopharyngeal and lesser palatine nerves.

All the palatal muscles are supplied by the pharyngeal plexus except for the tensor veli palatini, which is supplied by the mandibular branch of the trigeminal nerve.

The descending palatine branch of the maxillary artery provides the major arterial supply, while venous drainage is via the pterygoid and tonsillar plexus of veins.

Lymphatics from the soft palate drain to level II and retropharyngeal lymph nodes.

■ Tonsillar Fossa

The boundaries of the tonsillar fossa are formed by the anterior tonsillar pillar, which consists of the palatoglossus muscle, and the posterior pillar, which is formed by the palatopharyngeus muscle. It contains the palatine tonsils, which are large ovoid collections of lymphoid tissue in the mucosa lining the superior constrictor muscle.

The sensory supply to the tonsillar fossa is carried by the maxillary and glossopharyngeal nerves.

The main arterial supply to the tonsils is via the tonsillar branch of facial artery, ascending pharyngeal, lingual arteries, and branches from the ascending and descending palatine arteries, while venous drainage is to the pharyngeal plexus.

Lymphatics from the tonsillar fossa drain into the jugulodigastric and upper deep cervical nodes.

■ Base of Tongue

It extends from the circumvallate papilla and sulcus terminalis to the vallecula posteriorly. The valleculae are a pair of mucosal depressions between the base of the tongue and the epiglottis. These lie on either side of a median mucosal fold (median glossoepiglottic fold), and between two lateral mucosal folds (lateral glossoepiglottic folds), connecting the tongue and the epiglottis. Laterally the base of the tongue extends between the tonsillolingual sulcus and consists of the intrinsic muscles of the tongue.

All the muscles of the tongue are supplied by the hypoglossal nerve except the palatoglossus, which is supplied by the pharyngeal branch of the vagus nerve, while sensations are carried by the glossopharyngeal nerve. Arterial supply is by the lingual artery and lymphatics drain to level II to IV lymph nodes.

■ Pharyngeal Wall

It is from the level of the hard palate to the level of the hyoid bone or the floor of the vallecula inferiorly. It extends from the posterior pillar of one tonsil to the other.

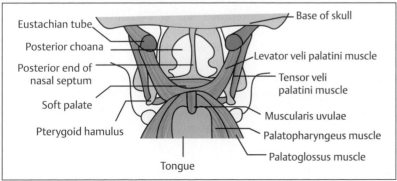

Fig. 37.4 Muscles of the soft palate (posterior view).

Eustachian tube
Posterior choana
Posterior end of nasal septum
Soft palate
Pterygoid hamulus
Tongue

Base of skull
Levator veli palatini muscle
Tensor veli palatini muscle
Muscularis uvulae
Palatopharyngeus muscle
Palatoglossus muscle

Hypopharynx

The hypopharynx is a space extending from the level of the hyoid bone above to the lower border of the cricoid cartilage. It is also known as the laryngopharynx.

It is divided into three parts:
- Pyriform fossa.
- Posterior pharyngeal wall.
- Post cricoid region.

Pyriform Fossa

The pyriform fossae are a pair of mucosal recesses created by the invagination of the larynx into the hypopharynx. Each recess is in the shape of an inverted pyramid with a broad base superiorly and apex inferiorly. Medially, it is bound by the aryepiglottic fold and the arytenoids and laterally by the thyroid cartilage and the thyrohyoid membrane. The upper limit is the pharyngoepiglottic fold.

The pyriform fossae form channels that direct solids and liquids from the oral cavity around the raised laryngeal inlet and into the esophagus.

Posterior Pharyngeal Wall

It extends from the superior level of the hyoid bone to the inferior border of the cricoid cartilage.

Postcricoid Region

It extends from the level of the arytenoids and connecting folds to the inferior border of the lamina of the cricoid cartilage, thus forming the anterior wall of the hypopharynx.

Pearl

Laryngeal crepitus: When the larynx is held by the examiner and moved from side to side, a crepitus or grating sensation is felt. This is due to the laryngeal cartilage rubbing against the cervical vertebra behind and this is normal. When the crepitus is absent, it indicates a mass in the postcricoid region (may be a malignancy) or a retropharyngeal abscess. Absence of this laryngeal crepitus is known as *Bocca's sign.*

Lymphatic Drainage

The hypopharynx has drainage into an abundant lymphatic network (**Table 37.3**).

This is the reason why 50% of patients harboring these malignant tumors present with nodal involvement as the first noticeable clinical symptom.

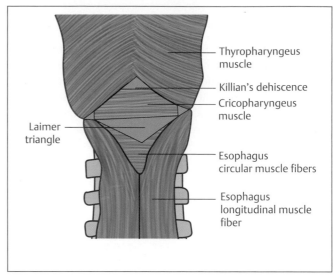

Fig. 37.5 Killian's dehiscence between the thyropharyngeus and cricopharyngeus muscles of the inferior constrictor.

Table 37.3 Lymphatic drainage of the hypopharynx

Pyriform fossa	Levels II–IV
Posterior pharyngeal wall	Retropharyngeal nodes Deep cervical nodes
Postcricoid area	Levels IV and VI Retropharyngeal nodes

Bilateral nodal metastasis is commonly seen in tumors crossing the midline.

Killian's Dehiscence

Killian's dehiscence (**Fig. 37.5**) is a potential weak spot in the posterior wall of the pharynx. Anatomically, it is a triangular space between the oblique fibers of the inferior constrictor (thyropharyngeus) and the circular fibers (cricopharyngeus). This area may be weakened in older people due to generalized muscle wasting. It is also called "gateway of tears" as it is a common site for accidental perforation of the esophagus during esophagoscopy.

In some patients, a diverticulum, which is an abnormal outpouching of mucosa and surrounding tissue, may form through Killian's dehiscence. This condition is called Zenker's diverticulum and the patient may present with dysphagia or with halitosis and regurgitation of collected food particles. Killian's diverticulum, if symptomatic, needs surgical resection, which may be done endoscopically using specially designed rigid esophagoscopes.

Points to Ponder

- The pharynx is divided into the nasopharynx, oropharynx, and hypopharynx.
- The function of the pharynx is to correctly channel air and food to the airway and digestive tract and prevent aspiration into the airway.
- The Waldeyer's ring is a set of submucosal lymphatic aggregates that surround the pharynx and is responsible for providing surface immunity against ingested as well as airborne pathogens.
- Waldeyer's ring has both an inner ring and an outer ring.
- The pharynx is rich in lymphatic supply and malignancies of the pharynx spread rapidly to the lymph nodes. Midline malignancies can cause bilateral lymph node involvement.
- The retropharyngeal space is a common site for abscess formation.
- Killian's dehiscence is a potential gap between the two parts of the inferior constrictor. Killian's diverticulum arises from this region.

Case-Based Questions

1. **A 60-year-old male patient, a smoker for the past 20 years, presented with gradual onset of throat discomfort and difficulty in swallowing. Examination of the neck revealed hard, bilateral neck nodes.**

   a. What is the probable diagnosis?

   b. What is the surgical importance of Waldeyer's ring?

   c. What is the primary function of the soft palate?

   Answers

   a. Malignancy of the oropharynx/hypopharynx.

   b. The Waldeyer's ring is a set of submucosal lymphatic aggregates that surround the pharynx and is responsible for providing surface immunity against ingested and inhaled pathogens.

   c. The soft palate helps prevent oral secretions and food from entering the nasal cavity.

2. **A 2-year-old child was brought to the pediatrics clinic with history of fever and difficulty in swallowing following a severe upper respiratory tract infection.**

   Examination of the throat revealed a bulge over the posterior pharyngeal wall slightly to the left of the midline.

   a. What is the most likely diagnosis?

   b. What investigations would you order?

   c. What are the boundaries of the retropharyngeal space?

   Answers

   a. Retropharyngeal abscess. This is seen in children who experience an upper respiratory tract infection leading to suppuration of the lymph nodes in the retropharyngeal space. These nodes are known as the nodes of Rouviere.

   b. A plain X-ray will reveal prevertebral widening. A more accurate assessment can be made with a contrast-enhanced CT scan.

   c. Boundaries of the retropharyngeal space are the following: anteriorly, the buccopharyngeal fascia; laterally, the carotid sheaths; and posteriorly, the prevertebral fascia.

Frequently Asked Questions

1. Describe the Waldeyer's ring and write a note on its surgical importance.

2. Write a note on Killian's dehiscence and its surgical importance.

3. What are the boundaries of the retropharyngeal space?

4. What are the subsites of the hypopharynx?

5. What is the importance of the laryngeal crepitus?

Endnote

William Waldeyer (1836–1921) was a German anatomist who became famous for his discoveries of Waldeyer's ring, Waldeyer's glands of the eyelids, and Waldeyer's fascia. He was also famous for his research into neuroscience and was responsible for coining the terms "neuron" and "chromosome" in 1888. He had more than 270 publications over a 40-year period and was known as an excellent teacher. His lectures were always "filled to the brim" by eager students.

38 Physiology of Pharynx

Sushmitha Kabekkodu

The competency covered in this chapter is as follows:

EN1.1 Describe the anatomy and physiology of the ear, nose, throat, and head and neck.

Introduction

The nasopharynx, oropharynx, and hypopharynx participate in various functions of the head and neck. The general functions of pharynx are the following:

- Deglutition.
- Respiration.
- Providing resonance to voice.
- Secretion of mucus for lubrication.
- Pathway of drainage.

Functions of the Nasopharynx

The nasopharynx acts as a conduit for the passage of air from the nasal cavity through the oropharynx to the lungs. It also acts as a resonating chamber for voice production. The eustachian tube orifice, which is located in the lateral wall of the nasopharynx, maintains the middle ear pressure and helps in ventilation of the middle air. The secretions from the nasal cavity drains through the nasopharynx. The nasopharyngeal isthmus closes during the deglutition, which helps in preventing nasal regurgitation.

Clinical significance:

- Eustachian tube dysfunction is one of the common causes of middle ear disease.
- A mass in the nasopharynx (adenoids and nasopharyngeal carcinoma) can cause hyponasal voice due to the absence of resonance function.
- Neurological palsy of the soft palate may lead to faulty closure of the nasopharyngeal isthmus, leading to nasal regurgitation.

Pearl

The movements and position of the soft palate are determined by the function of five muscles: tensor veli palatini, levator veli palatini, palatoglossus, palatopharyngeus, and musculus uvulae. All the muscles are innervated by the pharyngeal plexus except for the tensor veli palatini, which is supplied by the mandibular division of the trigeminal nerve.

Functions of the Oropharynx

The oropharynx acts as a conduit for the passage of air from the nasal cavity toward the larynx and lower airway, and food from the oral cavity to the esophagus. The oropharynx also plays an important role in deglutition. Resonance during voice production is aided by the oropharynx. The components of Waldeyer's ring play an important role in providing local immunity.

Clinical significance:

- A mass in the oropharynx can cause dysphagia.
- A large mass in the oropharynx may lead to breathing difficulty.
- A large mass in the oropharynx (like tonsillar malignancy and peritonsillar abscess) can lead to a "hot potato" voice.

Functions of the Adenoids and Tonsils

Adenoids and tonsils form a part of the Waldeyer's ring, which help in providing local immunity against bacteria and virus. T lymphocytes in these structures help in providing defense. Immunoglobulin A (IgA) production also helps in providing immunity.

Clinical significance:

- Physiological enlargement of the tonsils and adenoid occurs in the first 5 years of life. If it is symptomatic due to frequent infection or enlargement, surgical removal may be required.

Functions of the Hypopharynx

The hypopharynx acts as a common conduit for air and food passage. Like the nasopharynx and oropharynx, the hypopharynx also helps in providing vocal resonance during voice production. It also plays an important role in deglutition.

Clinical significance:

- A mass in the pyriform fossa or postcricoid region may lead to dysphagia with or without aspiration.
- It is adjacent to the larynx. Lesions from the hypopharynx can extend to the larynx causing change in voice and airway compromise.
- The hypopharyngeal mucosa (neopharynx) helps in voice production, in postlaryngectomy patients. This can be utilized for voice rehabilitation.

Deglutition

Deglutition is the process of propulsion of food bolus from the oral cavity to the stomach. This is controlled by neuromuscular activity of the pharyngeal muscles and nerves. The swallowing center is located in the medulla near the nucleus of the vagus nerve.

The phases in deglutition are the following:

- Oral phase—voluntary: 1 second.
- Pharyngeal phase—both voluntary and involuntary: 1 second.
- Esophageal phase—involuntary: 8 to 20 seconds.

■ Oral Phase

This is the voluntary phase starting from the chewing of food. The food will be mixed with saliva and converted to bolus. The bolus of food will be held between the tongue and the palate. The tongue later elevates against the palate, propelling the food into the oropharynx.

■ Pharyngeal Phase

This phase includes both voluntary and involuntary activities. The first activity that occurs is closure of the nasopharyngeal isthmus (soft palate raising against the Passavant ridge), followed by closure of the oropharyngeal isthmus aided by the palatoglossus and togue muscles. The rhythmic contraction of the pharyngeal constrictors pushes the bolus of food toward the cricopharyngeal sphincter. This is followed by closure of the laryngeal inlet (three-tier closure: epiglottis, aryepiglottic fold, and true and false vocal cord). When the food bolus reaches the cricopharynx, the sphincter relaxes, allowing food into the esophagus.

■ Esophageal Phase

This phase is involuntary starting from the closure of the cricopharyngeal sphincter. Peristalsis (primary) is a process that involves contraction of the circular muscles of the esophagus and propels the food bolus toward the stomach. Once the food reaches the lower end of the esophagus, the gastroesophageal sphincter relaxes, leading to transportation of food into the stomach.

Neural control during deglutition:

- Cranial nerves V and XII are responsible for mastication and tongue movement.
- Cranial nerve VII provides taste sensation in the anterior two-thirds of the tongue (chorda tympani) and provides motor supply to the orbicularis oris.
- Cranial nerve IX provides taste sensation to the pharynx.
- Cranial nerve X provides taste sensation to the larynx and the hypopharynx.

Points to Ponder

- The main function of the pharynx is to regulate the flow of air to the lungs and the passage of food to the esophagus.
- The eustachian tube on the lateral wall of the nasopharynx helps equalize the pressures in the middle ear with that of the atmosphere.
- The pharynx allows for resonance of sound and improves the quality of speech.
- Mucous from the glands of the pharyngeal wall allows for lubrication of the food bolus.
- The pharynx has a role to play in the defense mechanism through Waldeyer's ring.

Case-Based Questions

1. **A 70-year-old woman presented with a history of difficulty in swallowing and aspiration of fluid while swallowing. She complained that she would cough on taking fluids.**

   a. What are the mechanisms involved in the pharynx that prevent aspiration in normal people?

   b. Name the crania nerves involved in swallowing.

   Answers

   a. During the pharyngeal phase, the position of the tongue blocks the oral cavity. The elevation of the soft palate and uvula blocks the nasopharynx from the oropharynx preventing nasal regurgitation. Then the larynx is elevated by the suprahyoid muscles and the longitudinal pharyngeal muscles. This will allow the epiglottis to close off the laryngeal inlet. Finally, the cricopharyngeal muscles relax to propel food into the esophagus.

   b. The swallowing center is located in the lower pons and medulla oblongata of the brainstem. Swallowing is a complex mechanism involving five cranial nerves. They include the vagus, trigeminal, glossopharyngeal, facial, and hypoglossal nerves.

Frequently Asked Questions

1. What are the divisions of the pharynx?
2. What are the functions of the pharynx?
3. What are the three phases of swallowing?
4. Describe the pharyngeal phase of swallowing.
5. What is Waldeyer's ring and what is its function?

Endnote

Uvula means "little grape" in Latin. It consists of connective tissue, glands, and muscle fibers. The exact function of the uvula is not known, but only humans have an uvula. The possible functions include lubrication of food while swallowing through production of saliva, preventing nasal regurgitation because it seals off the oropharynx from the nasopharynx while swallowing along with the soft palate, and helping form certain sounds during speech especially in the German and French languages. Also, touching it elicits the gag reflex, which is a protective mechanism.

39 History Taking and Examination of the Throat

Deepa R.

The competencies covered in this chapter are as follows:

EN2.6 Demonstrate the correct technique of examining the throat including the use of a tongue depressor.

PE28.11 Perform throat examination using tongue depressor.

History Taking

A detailed and accurate history has to be elicited. This includes:

- **Chief complaints**—documented in chronological order.
- **History of presenting illness**: A detailed description is to be obtained of the presenting complaints with onset, duration, progression, severity, aggravating and relieving factors, and other accompanying or related symptoms.
- **Note**: Lesions of the oral cavity and oropharynx can present with referred otalgia.
- **Past history**, including similar complaints in the past and history of comorbidities such as diabetes mellitus, hypertension, tuberculosis, bronchial asthma, and coronary artery disease.
- **Medical history,** including medications and allergies, prior surgeries, and previous radiation.
  - Postcricoid and posterior pharyngeal wall carcinomas are associated with previous radiation.
  - History of radiation in childhood is associated with increased incidence of thyroid cancer.
- **Personal history**: Patient's personal habits (smoking, alcohol consumption, chewing paan/tobacco):
  - Combined use of tobacco and alcohol increases the risk of oral cavity, oropharyngeal, laryngeal, and hypopharyngeal cancers. Tobacco contains over 30 known carcinogens such as polycyclic aromatic hydrocarbons and nitrosamines. When used synergistically with alcohol there is increased mucosal absorption of these carcinogens due to increased solubility of the carcinogens in alcohol.
  - Paan (betel nut, tobacco, and lime placed in a betel leaf pouch) chewing is strongly associated with oral submucous fibrosis (a premalignant condition) and buccoalveolar cancer.
  - Beedi smoking is associated with cancer of oral commissure, oral tongue, and base of tongue.
  - Chutta (a smokeless tobacco) use is associated with cancer of hard palate and palatine arch.
  - Diet: High intake of fruits and vegetables is associated with decreased risk of head and neck cancer.
  - Poor dental hygiene may be an etiological factor for carcinoma of oral cavity.
  - Lower socioeconomic status and manual occupations are at high risk of developing oral cavity and laryngeal cancer.
  - Social history: Social circumstances of a patient significantly influence management decisions of malignancies.
- **Family history**: Similar illnesses in the family.

◼ Oral Cavity

It starts at the mucocutaneous junction of lips (vermilion border) extending posterosuperiorly to the junction of hard and soft palates, up to anterior pillars laterally and inferiorly the junction of anterior two-thirds and posterior one-third of tongue.

The following structures are included in the oral cavity:

- Lips form the anterior boundary of oral cavity.
- Buccal mucosa lines the inner surface of the cheeks and lips.
- Gums and teeth, gingivae (gums), cover the upper and lower alveolar ridges and the roots of teeth.
- Gingivolabial and gingivobuccal sulci (upper and lower) are grooves formed between the gingivae and the labial mucosa and the gingivae and buccal mucosa, respectively.
- Hard palate forms the roof of oral cavity.
- Anterior two-thirds of tongue (oral tongue) is the mobile portion of the tongue which is included in oral cavity. It has got tip, dorsum, ventral surface, and lateral borders.

- Floor of mouth is the area which lies in between the under surface of the tongue and the lower gingivae. The submandibular ducts, called Wharton's ducts, open on the summit of the raised papillae on either side of the frenulum of tongue with the lingual veins on either side.
- Lateral gutters are spaces on either side of floor of mouth.
- Retromolar trigone comprises of mucosa overlying ascending ramus of the mandible. It is triangular in shape and its base is posterior to the lower last molar and apex is adjacent to maxillary tuberosity.
- Surgeon's graveyard: These are sites in the oral cavity where malignant growths are easily missed:
  - Tonsillo-lingual sulcus.
  - Retromolar trigone.
  - Floor of mouth.

■ Symptomatology

The common complaints of a patient presenting with diseases of oral cavity are discussed in the following.

Pain

It may be localized to a particular area like tooth, tongue, buccal mucosa, floor of mouth, etc. The patient may sometimes present with pain referred to the ipsilateral ear from oral cavity lesion. This is due to referred otalgia via the trigeminal nerve.

Disturbances of Salivation

Dryness of mouth or xerostomia can be due to mouth breathing, postradiation therapy, or salivary gland disease. Excessive salivation is seen secondary to oral ulcers (including malignancy), ill-fitting dentures, sharp edges of broken tooth, poor orodental hygiene, and iodine therapy.

Distortion of Sense of Taste

Sweet taste is appreciated by the taste buds in front, salty and sour taste at the sides, and bitter at the back of tongue:

- The patient can present with diminished sense of taste (*hypogeusia*), absent taste sensation (*ageusia*), or abnormally heightened taste sense (*hypergeusia*), which can be unilateral or bilateral. It can be seen secondary to viral infections (corona virus), certain medications (angiotensin-converting enzyme [ACE] inhibitors, antibiotics, and post chemotherapy), injury to chorda tympani branch of facial nerve, or heavily coated tongue. Cacogeusia indicates sensation of bad taste in the absence of gustatory stimuli.
- *Dysgeusia or parageusia* indicates distorted taste sensation.

Trismus or Difficulty in Opening the Mouth

It is due to conditions in the oral cavity like ulcerative lesions in oral cavity, oral submucous fibrosis, dental abscess, trauma to mandible and maxilla, and malignant tumors of oral cavity with deep infiltration to pterygoid muscles.

Abnormal Appearance/Lesions

The patient can self-examine the oral cavity in the mirror and detect abnormal "growth" (circumvallate papillae), coated tongue, cleft (palate or lip), fistula (oroantral), and *Fordyce spots* or bleeding from oral cavity.

Halitosis or Foul Breath

It could be due to oral cavity conditions like poor oral hygiene, dental caries/abscess, aphthous ulcers, malignancy, etc.

> **Pearls**
> - The five primary taste sensations are sweet, salty, sour, bitter, and umami.
> - Umami is a Japanese word and means "savory taste." It was coined in Japan in 1908. The taste of umami can be picked up through receptors that pick up the taste of glutamates. Food items that have an umami flavor include meat broth, tomatoes, and fish sauce.

Examination

Examine all the structures included in oral cavity by inspection and palpation.

- *Lips*: Examine the upper and lower lips, the outer (cutaneous) and inner (mucosal) surface, and the vermilion border. Look for swellings, growths, vesicles, ulcers, scars, crusts, and unilateral or bilateral clefts (**Figs. 39.1** and **39.2**).
- *Buccal mucosa*: Examine by asking the patient to open the mouth and retracting the cheek using the Lack's tongue depressor (**Fig. 39.3**). Look for any change in color of the buccal mucosa and vestibule:
  - Also look for any ulceration, vesicles (herpes stomatitis, pemphigus vulgaris), white striae/lace-like plaque (lichen planus), blanched appearance with submucosal scarring (oral submucous fibrosis), white patch (leukoplakia), raised red lesion (erythroplakia), erosion (superficial ulcers), creamy white plaque (oral thrush), pigmentation, atrophic changes, and swelling or growth.

Opening of the parotid duct (Stenson's duct) is seen opposite the crown of upper second molar tooth. It will be congested and swollen in viral and bacterial parotitis. Purulent discharge is seen from the duct's orifice on parotid gland massage in suppurative parotitis.

- *Gums and teeth*: Outer surface of gums are examined by retracting cheeks and lips using a tongue depressor

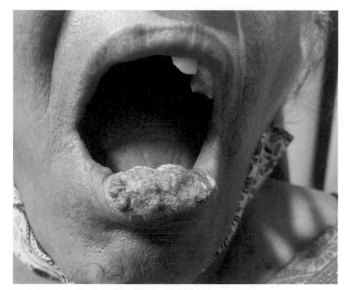

Fig. 39.1 Carcinoma of the lower lip.

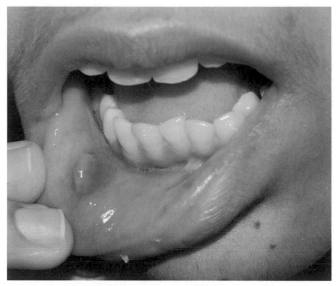

Fig. 39.2 Mucous retention cyst in lower lip.

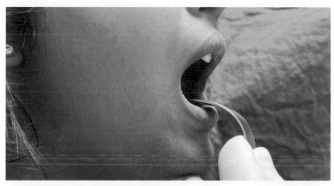

Fig. 39.3 Examination of the oral cavity using Lack's tongue depressor. Note the position of the middle finger to support the chin.

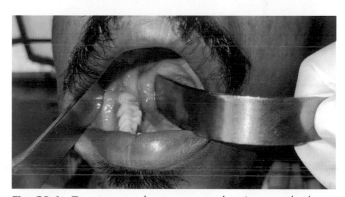

Fig. 39.4 Two tongue depressors used to inspect the lower gingiva.

and inner surface by pushing the tongue away with the tongue depressor (**Fig. 39.4**). The following findings are noted:
- Red and swollen gums—gingivitis.
- Hyperplasia of gums—pregnancy, phenytoin therapy.
- Erosion/ulcers—herpes simplex, pemphigus, aphthous ulcer, drug reaction.
- Membranous lesion—Vincent's angina, candidiasis.
- Growth—benign or malignant tumors.
- Loose teeth—malignancy of maxilla or mandible, periodontitis.
- Caries in teeth—upper (second premolar and first molar): Dentogenic maxillary sinusitis; lower: Ludwig's angina.
- Malocclusion of teeth—seen in fracture of mandible and maxilla, temporomandibular joint abnormalities.
- *Hard palate*: Look for:
  - Cleft palate.
  - High arched palate—mouth breathers.
  - Fistula (oronasal)—trauma, previous surgery, syphilis.

  - Bulge—benign/malignant tumors of palate, nasal cavity, maxilla.
  - Growths/ulcers—benign/malignant tumors.
  - Bony growth in midline—torus palatine.
  - Infections—oral candidiasis or thrush (**Fig. 39.5**).
- *Anterior two-thirds of tongue*:
  Inspection: Examine the tongue in its natural position first; then ask the patient to protrude the tongue and move it in different directions. Examine the tip, dorsum, lateral borders, and under surface. Look for:
  - Large tongue—macroglossia, hemangioma, lymphangioma, cretinism, edema, or abscess.
  - Inability to protrude tongue or ankyloglossia. The causes include congenital (tongue tie), advanced malignancy of tongue (frozen tongue) or floor of mouth malignancy, painful ulcer, abscess.
  - Deviation on protrusion of tongue—paralysis of cranial nerve XII on the side of deviation.
  - Bald tongue—iron deficiency anemia, median rhomboid glossitis, geographical tongue.

- *Palpation*: Palpate the tonsil with a gloved finger:
  - If the consistency of the mass is hard, it can be tonsillolith or malignancy.
  - Pulsations felt in tonsillar fossa could be due to an internal carotid artery aneurysm.
  - An elongated styloid process can be palpated through the tonsillar fossa.
- **Brodsky grading scale:**
  - Grade 1: Enlarged tonsil causing <25% of obstruction.
  - Grade 2: Enlarge tonsil causing 26 to 50% of airway obstruction.
  - Grade 3: Enlarged tonsil causing 51 to 75% airway obstruction.
  - Grade 4: >75% airway obstruction.
- *Anterior and posterior pillars*: Uniformly congested pillars along with tonsils and adjacent pharyngeal mucosa is seen in acute tonsillitis. The presence of a persistent band of congestion of anterior pillars is a feature of chronic tonsillitis. Proliferative or ulcerative growths could be an extension of malignancy from tonsil, base of tongue, soft palate, or retromolar trigone.
- *Soft palate*:
  Look for:
  - Congestion—peritonsillitis.
  - Absence of uvula: Uvulectomy is still performed as a cultural ritual in sub-Saharan African countries like Nigeria by traditional healers with the indigenous belief that it would help to prevent throat and chest infections.
  - Uvula is displaced to opposite side in peritonsillar abscess.
  - Elongated uvula is a normal variant (**Fig. 39.10**).
  - Bifid uvula is a feature of submucous cleft palate; here a V-shaped notch can also be palpated at the junction of hard palate and soft palate in the midline.
  - Ulceration, growth, swelling, and creamy white plaque-like lesion (candidiasis) should be noted.
  - Palatal movements are assessed when the patient says "Aa." In vagal paralysis, there is deviation of uvula and soft palate to the healthy side. When there is unilateral paralysis of pharyngeal wall, it causes

drooping of the pharyngeal wall of the affected side and a "curtain movement" of the pharynx to the opposite side on phonation.

- *Base of tongue and valleculae*: The posterior one-third of tongue is otherwise called base of tongue. It lies between the V-shaped row of circumvallate papillae and the valleculae. Valleculae are two shallow depressions situated between base of tongue and the epiglottis. Base of tongue and valleculae are examined by indirect laryngoscopy and by palpation.
- *Posterior pharyngeal wall*:
  Look for:
  - Presence of lymphoid nodules—granular pharyngitis.
  - Purulent postnasal drip trickling down the posterior pharyngeal wall—sinusitis.
  - Hypertrophy of lateral pharyngeal bands (seen adjacent the posterior pillars)—chronic sinusitis.
  - Thin glazed mucosa with crusting—atrophic pharyngitis.
- *Indirect laryngoscopy* (for base of tongue and vallecula):
  Look for:
  - Color of mucosa—normal/congested.
  - Base of tongue:
    - Prominent veins/varicosities.
    - Ulceration: Tuberculosis, syphilis, malignancy.
    - Solid swelling: Lingual tonsil, lingual thyroid, lymphoma, carcinoma.
    - Cystic swelling: Vallecular cyst, dermoid cyst, thyroglossal cyst.

Palpation of base of tongue: Palpation is mandatory in all cases to diagnose malignancy of base of tongue; a submucosal tumor can be better appreciated by palpation than by inspection. The tumor can spread from the supraglottis directly or via the pre-epiglottic space. The extent of induration is to be carefully noted by palpation preferably under general anesthesia where there will be adequate relaxation of tongue muscles. While palpating oropharyngeal structures, especially in a child, the examiner should invaginate the patient's cheek between his/her teeth with the opposite hand to prevent biting on the examiner's finger (**Video 39.1**).

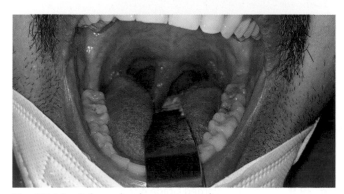

Fig. 39.10 Enlarged, edematous uvula.

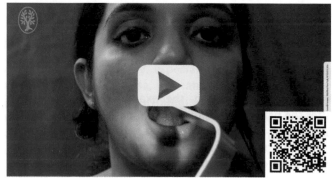

Video 39.1 Examination of throat.

Points to Ponder

- A systematic examination of the throat includes examination of the lips, oral cavity proper, and oropharynx.
- Instruments required include a good light source, one or two tongue depressors, and indirect laryngeal mirror to examine the base of tongue and vallecula.
- After inspection, palpation must always be performed when there is a lesion to determine consistency, tenderness, induration, and whether it bleeds on touch.
- A white patch in the oral cavity should raise suspicion for leukoplakia which is a premalignant condition.
- India has the highest incidence of oral malignancies in the world and all suspicious lesions should be biopsied.

Case-Based Questions

1. A 65-year-old male with history of tobacco chewing and alcohol intake presents to the clinic with a swelling over the right lateral border of the tongue of 3 months duration. It was associated with pain and difficulty in eating and talking. What are the important points in the examination that must be brought to make a provisional diagnosis?

Answer

Since there is a lesion over the right lateral border of the tongue, examination should include inspection and palpation. During inspection, note the site (lateral border of tongue is the commonest site for malignancy of the tongue), size, shape, surface, and margins of the swelling. During palpation, it is important to determine the size of the lesion (for staging purpose), tenderness, whether it bleeds on touch, and the extent of induration. The surface in squamous malignancy of the tongue is usually ulceroproliferative. Lastly, note the tongue movements (to determine fixity of the tongue), and whether there are any metastatic lymph nodes in the neck.

2. A 36-year-old female complains of swelling and pain over the upper part of the neck on the right side (submandibular region) whenever she eats. Examination revealed a firm mass over the right submandibular region thought to be an enlarged submandibular gland. How will you distinguish a submandibular gland enlargement from an enlarged submandibular lymph node clinically, by palpation?

Answer

A bimanual palpation must be carried out to distinguish the two. One finger is place on the floor of the mouth medial to the lower alveolus and the other finger is placed on the neck outside, medial to the margin of the mandible. Both the fingers should be pressed against each other. A submandibular gland is bimanually palpable whereas a lymph node is not.

Frequently Asked Questions

1. What are the common lesions affecting the upper lip?

2. What are the uses of Lack's tongue depressor?

3. How will you visualize the base of tongue and vallecula?

4. What is the importance of palpation of an oral cavity lesion?

5. What is the differential diagnosis for a white patch in the oral cavity?

6. How do you perform a septic squeeze test?

7. How do you do a bimanual palpation of the submandibular salivary gland?

Endnote

There are numerous mucous glands on the floor of the mouth. When their ducts get blocked, they develop into retention cysts which are filled with mucus. If there is extravasation of the mucus from a retention cyst, the term "ranula" is applied, especially in relation to the sublingual gland. The word comes from rana or "frog," because the cyst looks like a "frog's belly." It is a transparent, bluish, fluctuant swelling on the floor of the mouth, and if it passes through the mylohyoid muscle into the neck, it is called a "plunging ranula."

Adenoids, Inflammation of the Nasopharynx, and Adenoidectomy

Udayabhanu H.N.

The competencies covered in this chapter are as follows:

EN4.26 Elicit, document, and present a correct history; demonstrate and describe the clinical features; choose the correct investigations; and describe the principles of management of adenoids.

PE28.1 Discuss the etiopathogenesis, clinical features, and management of nasopharyngitis.

EN4.40 Observe and describe the indications for and steps involved in adenoidectomy.

Introduction

Adenoid tissue is situated at the junction of the roof and the posterior wall of the nasopharynx. Wilhelm Meyer coined the term adenoid (**Fig. 40.1**). It is composed of vertical ridges of lymphoid tissue separated by deep clefts and is covered by ciliated columnar epithelial cells (**Fig. 40.2**). It is the first site of immunological contact for inhaled antigens. Adenoid tissue is present at birth, shows physiological enlargement up to the age of 6 years, then tends to atrophy by puberty, and slowly starts to disappear. It is usually not seen in adults. Adenoid tissue is devoid of a capsule and does not have crypts.

Pearl

When adenoid enlargement is seen in adults, one should rule out lymphoma and acquired immunodeficiency syndrome (AIDS). Adenotonsillar hypertrophy is a common cause for obstructive sleep apnea in children. Adenoid hyperplasia is also seen in some adults with obstructive sleep apnea.

Adenoid Hypertrophy

■ Etiology

Adenoid tissue is subject to physiological enlargement during childhood. There is a tendency for generalized lymphoid hyperplasia (including adenoid tissue) in children. Recurrent attacks of rhinitis, sinusitis, and upper airway allergy may cause chronic adenoid infection and hyperplasia.

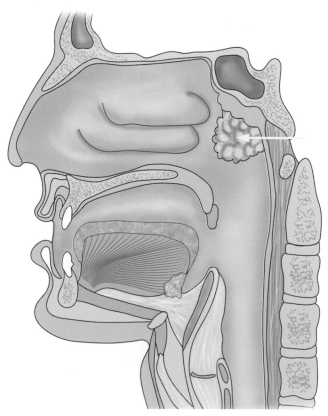

Fig. 40.1 Adenoids is located in the nasopharynx along the superior and posterior walls.

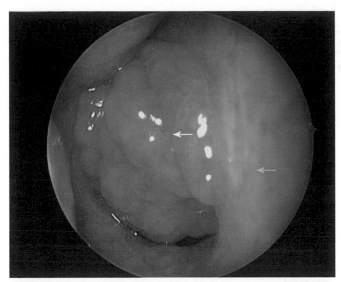

Fig. 40.2 Endoscopic view (right side) of adenoids completely filling the choana. Clefts can be seen (*yellow arrow*). Nasal septum (*blue arrow*).

■ Clinical Features and Assessment

A history with special attention to symptoms of middle ear disease and nasal obstruction should be elicited. The symptoms and signs in adenoid hypertrophy not only depend on the size of the adenoid mass but also the relative space available in the nasopharynx. The enlarged and infected adenoids cause nasal, aural, and obstructive symptoms.

Nasal Symptoms

- Nasal obstruction is the commonest symptom, leading to mouth breathing and noisy breathing (snoring).
- Upper airway obstruction and obstructive sleep apnea.
- Due to obstruction at the choanae, the nasal discharge can be thick and copious. The child has a wet bubbly nose as the discharge tends to flow anteriorly.
- Rhinosinusitis may occur secondary to the choanal obstruction and stasis.
- Inflamed adenoids can cause purulent nasal and postnasal discharge.
- Epistaxis on sneezing or blowing of the nose can occur due to inflamed adenoids and persistent associated rhinitis.
- Rhinolalia clausa, loss of nasal tone of voice, can occur due to obstruction.

Ear Symptoms

- Ear block: Tubal obstruction by enlarged adenoids causes eustachian tube dysfunction affecting middle ear ventilation leading to ear block sensation. The tympanic membrane may be retracted.

- Hearing loss can occur due to eustachian tube dysfunction, which leads to otitis media with effusion (OME). Children may be inattentive or need to be called in a louder voice. Older children may have poor scholastic performance due to conductive hearing loss.
- Inflamed adenoids can lead to recurrent acute otitis media in children.
- Adenoiditis can be a source of infection, causing recurrent ear discharge in chronic otitis media—mucosal type.

General Symptoms

- Olfactory sensitivity is reduced in relation to adenoid size, which accounts for the poor appetite reported in children with adenoid hypertrophy.
- *Failure to thrive*: Nasal obstruction interferes with feeding or suckling in a child. In younger children, respiration and feeding cannot take place simultaneously.
- Lack of concentration (aprosexia).
- Pulmonary hypertension and cor pulmonale.

Adenoid Facies

Chronic nasal obstruction and mouth breathing leads to the characteristic facial appearance called *adenoid facies*. The child will have the following characteristics:
- Elongated face with dull expression.
- Loss of the nasolabial fold.
- Open mouth with prominent and crowded upper teeth.
- Hitched-up upper lip.
- Pinched nose appearance due to disuse atrophy of the alae nasi.
- Hard palate in these children is highly arched as the molding action of the tongue on the palate is lost.
- Dull look.
- Hypoplasia of the maxilla.

Assessment of the external nose should be made before anterior rhinoscopy. Skin crease in the supratip region may indicate frequent nose rubbing from symptoms of rhinitis. The nasal airway patency may be assessed with a Lack metallic tongue depressor.

Posterior rhinoscopy is difficult to perform in children. In some older children, nasal endoscopy can be done under topical anesthesia (**Fig. 40.3**).

■ Diagnosis

A detailed nasal examination should be followed by a nasal endoscopy, either rigid nasal endoscopy or flexible nasopharyngoscope, to examine the nasopharynx. Lateral soft-tissue X-ray of the neck (for nasopharynx) in children unable to tolerate nasal endoscopy will reveal the size of adenoids and also the extent of nasopharyngeal airspace compromise (**Fig. 40.4**). The upper respiratory allergy should be excluded.

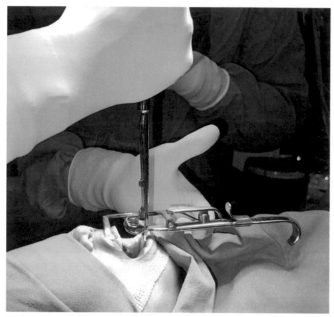

Fig. 40.6 Adenoid curette introduced into the nasopharynx.

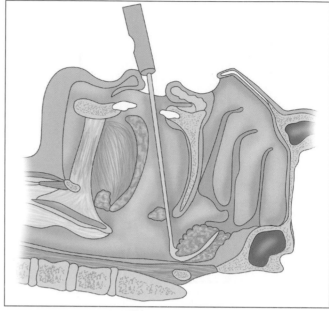

Fig. 40.7 Adenoidectomy by curettage.

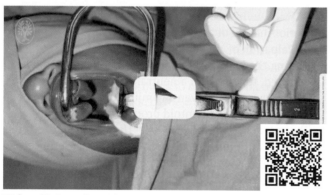

Video 40.1 Adenoidectomy.

the palate for better visualization. The adenoid mass can be removed with a microdebrider or by coblation or by using curettage under visualization. Endoscopes also help achieve hemostasis with cautery under vision (**Video 40.1**).

The advantages of endoscopic adenoidectomy are the following:

- It provides direct visualization.
- It prevents injury to the eustachian tube opening.
- It allows precise removal of the adenoid mass.
- Techniques employing direct vision have the advantage of reduced blood loss.
- It allows for use of additional instrumentation like microdebriders and coblators (**Figs. 40.8, 40.9, 40.10, and 40.11**).

■ Complications

- Bleeding (primary, reactionary, and secondary hemorrhage).

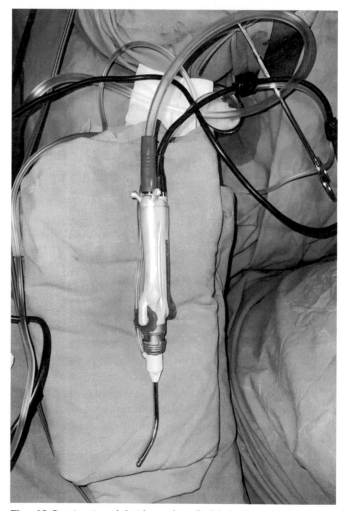

Fig. 40.8 A microdebrider, a handheld device with blades at the tip that can cut and suck out the tissue and blood.

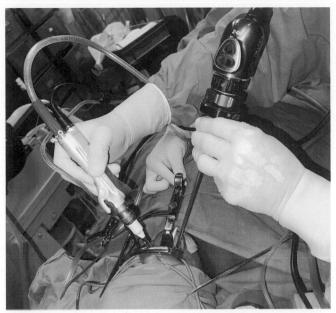

Fig. 40.9 Microdebrider-assisted adenoidectomy. Approach through the oral cavity. A microdebrider in the right hand and an endoscope in the left hand.

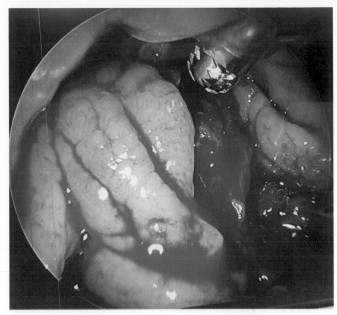

Fig. 40.10 Adenoidectomy using a microdebrider.

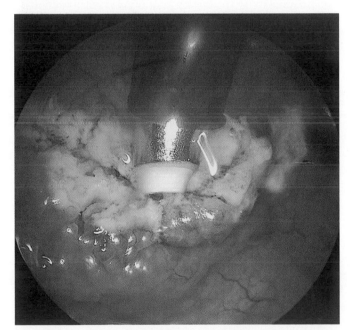

Fig. 40.11 Adenoidectomy using a coblator. Radiofrequency energy is used to break up sodium chloride into ions, which results in tissue destruction at temperatures of 60°C.

- Dental trauma and trauma to the lips, tongue, and palate.
- Airway obstruction due to aspiration of retained swab or nasopharyngeal blood clot (referred to as Coroner's clot).
- Infection.
- Cervical spine injury (particularly in syndromic children).

- Velopharyngeal insufficiency.
- Regrowth of the adenoid.

> **Pearl**
>
> Grisel's syndrome is a nontraumatic subluxation of the atlantoaxial joint. This can occur following adenoidectomy, especially in the presence of inflammation, which causes laxity of the ligament.

Inflammation of the Nasopharynx

■ Thornwaldt's Disease (Pharyngeal Bursitis)

It is an infection of the pharyngeal bursa, which is a median recess representing attachment of the notochord to the endoderm of the primitive pharynx. The pharyngeal bursa is located in the midline of the posterior wall of the nasopharynx in the adenoid mass. It presents as persistent postnasal discharge with crusting in the nasopharynx and nasal obstruction due to swelling. Eustachian tube obstruction leading to serous otitis media can occur. Other symptoms are occipital headache, sore throat, and fever.

Nasal endoscopic examination would reveal a cystic, fluctuant swelling in the posterior wall of the nasopharynx. There may be crust formation in the nasopharynx due to dried discharge. The infection can be managed conservatively. Marsupialization of the cystic swelling is the treatment of choice.

■ Acute Nasopharyngitis

Acute infection of the nasopharynx may be isolated or can be a part of a generalized upper respiratory infection caused by a virus (influenza, parainfluenza, rhinovirus, or adenovirus) or bacteria (*Streptococcus Pneumococcus* or *Haemophilus influenzae*). Rhinovirus is the most common and contagious of all these. The spread is mostly through air droplets or by touching objects contaminated by virus or bacteria and then touching the eyes, nose, or mouth.

Clinical Features

Dryness, irritation, and burning sensation above the soft palate are usually the first symptoms as experienced with the common cold. This is followed by pain and discomfort localized to the back of the nose with some difficulty in swallowing. Nasal stuffiness, nasal discharge, sneezing, postnasal drip, sore throat, cough, watery or itchy eyes, headache, body ache, and lethargy are the accompanying symptoms. In severe infection, there may be pyrexia and enlarged cervical lymph nodes. Examination of the nasopharynx reveals congested and swollen mucosa often covered with exudate.

A nasopharyngeal swab will help in the diagnosis of diseases like in Covid-19 and swine flu.

Treatment

It is mainly symptomatic. In children, there is an associated adenoiditis leading to nasal obstruction, which will require topical nasal decongestants. Depending on the severity, symptomatic cases can be treated with anti-inflammatory and analgesic drugs. Antibiotics are started for secondary bacterial infection. Saline nasal douches are helpful in clearing the discharge and crusts.

■ Chronic Nasopharyngitis

It is associated with a chronic infection of the nose, paranasal sinuses, and/or pharynx. It is commonly seen in chronic smokers, due to excess intake of alcohol, and in those exposed to dust and fumes.

Clinical Features

Thick postnasal discharge with crusting and irritation at the back of the nose is the most common complaint. The patient has a constant desire to clear the nose by hawking or inspiratory snorting.

Treatment

Chronic infection of the nose, paranasal sinuses, and oropharynx should be treated. Excessive smoking and drinking should be avoided. Preventive measures should be taken to avoid dust and fumes. Nasal douches with normal saline will help clear the exudates and crusting.

Points to Ponder

- Adenoid hypertrophy are a common disease of childhood and is due to enlargement of the lymphatic tissue in the nasopharynx.
- Adenoid enlargement is seen in children around 5 to 6 years of age, typically schoolgoing children.
- Adenoid facies can occur in children with severe nasal obstruction.
- Adenoidectomy or surgical removal of the adenoids is the treatment of choice when there is nasal obstruction.
- Adenoidectomy can be combined with tonsillectomy.
- One of the commonest complications of adenoidectomy is hemorrhage.
- Hemorrhage can be classified as primary, reactionary, or secondary.

Case-Based Questions

1. **An 8-year-old boy was brought to the ear, nose, and throat (ENT) outpatient clinic with a history of mouth breathing and snoring of 2 years' duration. He had disturbed sleep. The teacher in his school reported that he was inattentive and was not doing well in his studies.**

   a. What is the possible diagnosis?

   b. What are investigations that can be done to confirm the diagnosis?

   c. What is the treatment?

Answers

a. Adenoid hypertrophy with OME.

b. Lateral soft-tissue X-ray of the neck and diagnostic nasal endoscopy for adenoid hypertrophy. Pure tone audiogram (conductive hearing loss) and impedance audiometry ("B"-type tympanogram in OME) should be carried out to exclude OME.

c. Adenoidectomy. Myringotomy with grommet insertion should be done if there is associated OME.

2. A 4-year-old girl underwent adenoidectomy under general anesthesia. Postoperatively, after 2 hours, she developed choking spells and breathing difficulty, which were managed by assessing the laryngotracheal airway using bronchoscopy in the operating room. On postoperative day 2, she was noted to have a hypernasal voice.

   a. Why did she have airway obstruction that required bronchoscopy?

   b. What is the type of voice she developed on postoperative day 2?

   c. What is the etiology of this type of voice?

Answers

   a. She may have aspirated blood clots or swabs.

   b. Rhinolalia aperta.

   c. Velopharyngeal insufficiency. This may be due to pain and usually recovers. Occasionally, it may be due to a prior undetected submucous cleft palate that gets manifested following the adenoidectomy.

Frequently Asked Questions

1. What are the ear diseases associated with adenoids?

2. Describe the clinical features associated with adenoid facies.

3. How will you go about investigating suspected adenoids in children?

4. What are the indications for adenoidectomy?

5. What are the different methods of adenoidectomy?

6. Enumerate the complications of adenoidectomy.

Endnote

Hans Wilhelm Meyer, in 1868, was the first person to point out the relationship between adenoids and ear disease. Adenoidectomy soon became popular for a variety of conditions like otitis media, problems related to speech, cognitive problems, and obstructive sleep apnea. Techniques of removal of adenoids included use of bare fingernails, curette, knife, and electrocautery. From the 1930s to the 1960s, radiation therapy was widely used to cure adenoids, instead of surgery. Around 2.5 million children and adults were subjected to radiation during this period because radiation caused a rapid melting of lymphoid tissue. The side effect of this radiation was increased risk of cancer, and this form of therapy fell into disrepute.

41 Acute and Chronic Pharyngitis

Mahesh Santhraya G.

The competencies covered in this chapter are as follows:

PE28.2 Discuss the etiopathogenesis of pharyngotonsillitis.

PE28.3 Discuss the clinical features and management of pharyngotonsillitis.

Introduction

Sore throat is a common presentation to a general practitioner and in an ENT clinic. Pharyngitis refers to the inflammation of the pharynx and/or tonsils, that is, generalized or localized. The term "pharyngotonsillitis" is sometimes used for generalized inflammation of the posterior pharyngeal wall and the tonsillar region.

The oropharyngeal mucosa is exposed to inhaled substances, either directly or through the nose and nasopharynx, and to ingested substances. Infection and irritation are the prime causes of inflammation. Pharyngitis may be a primary disease, or part of an upper respiratory tract infection. The pharynx can be affected anteriorly from the oral cavity, superiorly from the secretions from the sinuses, and inferiorly from the aerodigestive tract.

Causes of Pharyngitis

■ Infections

Acute Pharyngitis

- Viral: Rhinovirus, corona virus, adenovirus, parainfluenza, influenza A & B, Coxsackie virus, herpes simplex 1 & 2, Epstein–Barr virus, cytomegalovirus, and human immunodeficiency virus (HIV).
- Bacterial: Group A beta-hemolytic *streptococcus* (GABHS), *Haemophilus influenzae*, *Moraxella catarrhalis*, *Mycoplasma pneumoniae*, *Corynebacterium diphtheriae*.
- Fungal: *Candida*.
- Protozoal: *Toxoplasma gondii*.

Chronic Pharyngitis

- *Nonspecific types*: Hypertrophic, granular, and atrophic.
- *Specific*: Tuberculosis, syphilis, scleroma, and leprosy.

■ Noninfectious/Contributing Factors

- Gastroesophageal reflux disease (GERD).
- Rhinosinusitis (postnasal drip).
- Upper respiratory allergy.
- Atmospheric (dry air, dusty surroundings, and pollution).
- Smoking.
- Radiotherapy.
- Poor dental hygiene.
- Caustic injury.
- Post endotracheal intubation.
- Toxins.

Pearl

In persistent sore throat, especially in the older age group, one should rule out malignancy. Conversely, in oropharyngeal malignancy, there will be some amount of surrounding inflammation, which will contribute to pain.

Acute Pharyngitis

It is a common inflammation that is often a part of an upper respiratory tract infection.

■ Etiology

Majority of the cases of pharyngitis are viral in origin. The common viruses include rhinovirus, influenza A & B, adenovirus, coxsackie, coronavirus, and parainfluenza. Other viruses that can affect the pharynx are herpes simplex, Epstein–Barr virus, HIV, and cytomegalovirus (**Table 41.1**).

A bacterial infection tends to be more severe and may develop secondary to a viral infection. The most common bacteria that affects the pharynx is GABHS.

Environmental pollutants, allergens, and chemical exposures may also cause acute pharyngitis.

Pharyngitis may be a symptom of locoregional conditions like peritonsillar abscess, retropharyngeal abscess, and epiglottitis. Other less common causes of pharyngitis include allergies, trauma, reflux, and certain toxins.

Pearl

Spread of the viral infection can be through airborne droplets, skin-to-skin contact, saliva, or from contaminated surface.

Viral pharyngitis, in addition to sore throat, may have other features like sneezing, nasal discharge, fever, cough,

Table 41.1 Common viruses causing pharyngitis

Virus	Associated disease	Pharyngitis	Features
Rhinovirus	Common cold	With nasal discharge, sneezing	Most common viral infection; rarely, bronchiolitis and pneumonia can occur in infants
Coronavirus	Common cold	Common	Two types, i.e., SARS-CoV and MERS-CoV cause severe respiratory symptoms. Others cause mild to moderate symptoms
Adenovirus	Pharyngoconjunctival fever and acute respiratory disease	With nasal congestion/discharge, conjunctivitis, and cough	Common in military recruits and boarding schools
Herpes simplex virus type 1	Gingivostomatitis	Vesicular and ulcerative	Along cranial nerves V, IX, and X
Herpes simplex virus type 2		Severe ulcerative pharyngitis	Orogenital contact
Parainfluenza virus	Common cold and croup	With cough, breathing difficulty/wheezing	Upper and lower respiratory tract infection
Coxsackievirus A (or by enterovirus 30, 71) Coxsackie A10	Herpangina Acute lymphonodular pharyngitis	With high fever, headache and neck pain With mild fever, dysphagia	Grayish papulovesicular lesions White-yellow nodules
Coxsackie A16 (or by enterovirus)	Hand, foot, and mouth disease	With malaise/fatigue	Oral/oropharyngeal vesicles; vesicular lesions over the hand and feet
Influenza A and B viruses	Influenza/flu	With myalgia, dry cough, nasal congestion, and breathing difficulty	Can be severe with lower respiratory symptoms; flu season
Respiratory syncytial virus	Bronchiolitis and croup	Not common; mainly nasal congestion and lower respiratory symptoms	Pneumonia can occur in children
Epstein–Barr virus	Infectious mononucleosis	With odynophagia, cervical lymphadenopathy and enlarged tonsils	Grayish white membrane; hepatosplenomegaly
Cytomegalovirus	Mononucleosis like syndrome	Mild sore throat	Symptoms are similar to infectious mononucleosis but in an older age group; thrombocytopenia
Human immunodeficiency virus	Primary HIV infection		High-risk groups

Note: Viruses are the most common cause of pharyngitis.

The uvula may be elongated and edematous (especially in snorers).

Features of inciting factors may be noted, for example, postnasal drip, signs of GERD, and lower respiratory disease.

Diagnosis

- The diagnosis is mainly by history and physical examination.
- Throat swab for culture and sensitivity when a persistent infection is suspected.
- Other conditions like malignancy should be ruled out.
- Diagnostic nasal endoscopy can be done to look out for sinonasal disease, (rhinosinusitis and nasal obstruction/ mouth breathing). A CT scan of the nose and paranasal sinuses is done when chronic rhinosinusitis is suspected.
- Rigid telescopy of laryngopharynx is performed to look for features of reflux and to rule out malignancy.

Complete blood count, thyroid function tests, serum immunoglobulin E (IgE) levels, and other special tests to rule out various causes of pharyngitis may be required in persistent cases.

Treatment

- Treat the inciting disease, for example, allergic rhinitis (with steroid nasal spray).
- Chronic rhinosinusitis with nasal douches and steroid nasal spray, ± antibiotics.
- GERD with proton pump inhibitors.
- Avoid the inciting factors, whether it is inhaled, ingested, or environmental.
- Antibiotics when the throat swab is positive, indicating a persisting infection. A broad-spectrum antibiotic like amoxycillin with clavulanic acid can be tried.
- Adequate hydration.
- Warm saline gargles.
- Avoid smoking and alcohol consumption.
- Lifestyle changes will help reduce stress and avoid mouth breathing.

Tonsillar Keratosis

This condition is characterized by the appearance of a single or multiple, white cheesy projections from the crypts of the tonsillar surface. If it occurs from the pharyngeal wall, it is known as "keratosis pharyngis." It usually affects young adults. It is a benign condition.

The patient is usually asymptomatic and pick up this lesion incidentally while examining the throat in the mirror. In mild cases, there may be irritation of the throat or halitosis. On examination, there will be white horny plugs over the surface of the tonsil. There are no signs of

inflammation. This will distinguish it from acute follicular tonsillitis (**Fig. 41.3**).

If it is asymptomatic, no treatment is required, only reassurance. Antiseptic gargles will help. If patient is still symptomatic, tonsillectomy may be done.

Chronic-Specific Pharyngitis

Tuberculosis

It is caused by *Mycobacterium tuberculosis* organism, rarely by atypical mycobacteria. In adults, it is usually secondary to pulmonary tuberculosis or miliary tuberculosis. It can occur in individuals with HIV. In children, there may be focus on the tonsil or adenoids, which can be asymptomatic.

Syphilis

It is caused by *Treponema pallidum* and is due to sexual contact. It can mimic other conditions and is also known as the "great pretender." Syphilis can present in the congenital or acquired forms, which include primary, secondary, and tertiary syphilis.

Primary syphilis, in which the lesion is called the chancre, can occur in the tonsil as papule that forms a painless ulcer with indurated margins. There will be painless, cervical lymphadenopathy.

Secondary syphilis presents with fever, headache, malaise, generalized lymphadenopathy, sore throat, and mucocutaneous rash. There may be "snail-track" ulcers over the pharynx with congested mucosa. The ulcer will have a grayish-white membrane.

Tertiary syphilis presents with a gumma (painless, granulomatous, and necrotic lesion), involving the posterior pharyngeal wall, tonsil, palate, and larynx.

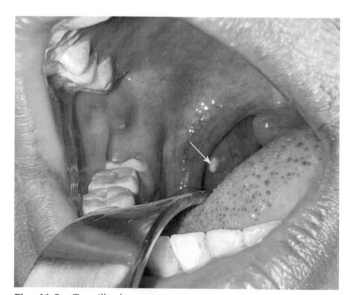

Fig. 41.3 Tonsillar keratosis.

Leprosy

The involvement of the pharynx is due to spread from the nose. Commonly it is the lepromatous leprosy that can affect the pharynx. It presents as ulcers that heal by fibrosis.

Scleroma

It occurs secondary to nasal involvement. It presents as a granulomatous lesion that subsequently undergoes scarring.

Case-Based Questions

1. A 19-year-old man presented with a 2-day history of fever, nasal discharge, sore throat, and cough. The patient also had conjunctivitis. On examination, the posterior pharyngeal wall was congested. There were no palpable cervical lymph nodes.

a. What is the diagnosis?
b. What is the possible organism?
c. What is the treatment?

Answers
a. Acute pharyngitis, which is part of an acute viral upper respiratory tract infection.
b. Adenovirus since the patient has conjunctivitis.
c. Symptomatic treatment with NSAIDs, adequate hydration, and oral antihistamine with decongestant can be given for nasal symptoms.

2. A 46-year-old man presented with an 8-month history of persistent sore throat. He works in a factory and is a chronic smoker. He also gives a history of occasional retrosternal burning sensation. He had a history of discomfort duration phonation. On examination, the posterior pharyngeal wall was congested and thickened. Rigid telescopic examination of the laryngopharynx did not show any lesion. The diagnostic nasal endoscopy did not show any significant sinonasal pathology.

a. What is the possible diagnosis?
b. What are the factors causing the condition?
c. What is the treatment?

Answers
a. Chronic simple pharyngitis.
b. Work environment, smoking, and GERD.
c. Quitting smoking, treatment of the GERD, precautions at work environment (use of mask), warm saline gargles, and adequate hydration.

3. A 43-year-old housewife presented with a 7-month history of sore throat. She also complained of bilateral nasal obstruction, hawking, and occasional mouth breathing and cough. There was no history suggestive of GERD. On examination, the posterior pharyngeal wall was granular and congested. There was mucopurulent postnasal drip noted on the posterior pharyngeal wall.

a. What is the diagnosis?
b. What are the investigations required to be done?
c. What is the treatment?

Answers
a. Chronic hypertrophic/granular pharyngitis which has occurred secondary to a sinonasal etiology.
b. Diagnostic nasal endoscopy and CT scan of the paranasal nasal sinuses.
c. Treatment of the sinonasal cause. Saline nasal douches, antibiotics, and steroid nasal spray are the initial line of treatment. Septoplasty with or without turbinoplasty and endoscopic sinus surgery can be considered depending on the symptoms and CT scan findings.

Frequently Asked Questions

1. What are the common causes for acute pharyngitis?
2. What are the predisposing factors for oropharyngeal candidiasis?
3. What is the etiology for chronic nonspecific pharyngitis?
4. What are the clinical types of chronic nonspecific pharyngitis?
5. What is tonsillar keratosis?

Endnote *Clergyman's sore throat or CST was defined as chronic inflammation of the pharynx due to habitual overuse or misuse of voice. It has been classified as a form of chronic pharyngitis. It is also known as dysphonia clericorum. Old texts regarding this disease opine that this not only affects clergymen but also lawyers, senators, and professional singers.*

42 Acute and Chronic Tonsillitis

Yogeesha B.S., Venkatesha B.K., and Nagaraj Maradi

The competencies covered in this chapter are as follows:

AN36.1 Describe the (1) morphology, relations, blood supply, and applied anatomy of palatine tonsil and (2) composition of soft palate.

EN4.39 Elicit, document, and present a correct history; demonstrate and describe the clinical features; choose the correct investigations; and describe the principles of management of squamosal type of acute and chronic tonsillitis.

PE28.2 Discuss the etio-pathogenesis of pharyngotonsillitis.

PE28.3 Discuss the clinical features and management of pharyngotonsillitis.

EN4.40 Observe and describe the indications for and steps involved in a tonsillectomy.

Anatomy of Tonsils

The subepithelial lymphoid tissue situated in the oropharynx between the anterior and posterior pillars on either side is referred to as the palatine tonsil (**Fig. 42.1**). They are a part of mucosa-associated lymphoid tissue (MALT) known as Waldeyer's ring. They are prone to recurrent infections as they provide protection to the respiratory and alimentary tracts from bacterial invasion.

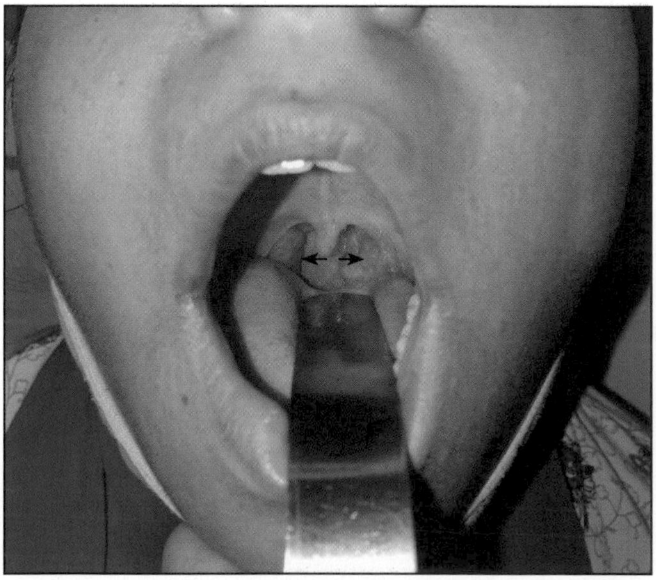

The palatoglossal and palatopharyngeal folds along with the tonsillolingual sulcus (lateral part of the base of tongue) form the *tonsillar fossa*. The fold of mucous membrane connecting the superior parts of the palatoglossal and palatopharyngeal folds is called *plica semilunaris*. The fold of mucous membrane connecting the palatoglossal and palatopharyngeal folds at the lower pole of the tonsil is called *plica triangularis*.

The tonsil is lined by stratified squamous epithelium. There are mucosal invaginations into the substance of tonsil on its medial surface which form 12 to 15 tonsillar crypts. *Crypta magna* (**Fig. 42.2**) is the largest and is situated at the upper part of the tonsil. Crypta magna is a remnant of the second pharyngeal pouch.

The tonsils are partially encapsulated and has a fibrous capsule on the lateral surface which loosely attaches to

Fig. 42.1 Tonsils shown with *black arrowheads*.

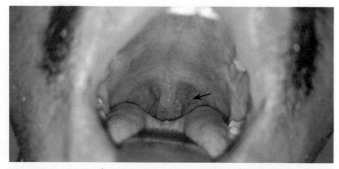

Fig. 42.2 Note the crypta magna on the left side indicated in the clinical photograph with a *black arrow*.

the tonsillar bed. There is loose areolar tissue between the tonsil capsule and its bed which forms the peritonsillar space.

■ Relations of Tonsil

- Anteriorly, it is bounded by palatoglossus which forms anterior pillar.
- Posteriorly, it is bounded by palatopharyngeus which forms posterior pillar.
- The oropharyngeal lumen is located medially.
- Laterally, it is bounded by the structures on the tonsillar bed (**Fig. 42.3**).
- The soft palate lies superiorly.
- The lateral part of tongue base, that is, the tonsillo-lingual sulcus, is located inferiorly.

■ Tonsillar Bed

It is formed by loose areolar tissue, pharyngobasilar fascia, superior constrictor muscle, and buccopharyngeal fascia. From within outwards, tonsillar bed consists of the pharyngobasilar fascia, superior constrictor muscle in posterosuperior two-third, and styloglossus muscle (in anteroinferior one-third) accompanied by the glossopharyngeal nerve.

Relations of Tonsillar Bed

- Arteries:
    - Facial artery and its ascending palatine branch.
    - Ascending pharyngeal artery.
    - Internal carotid artery (lies about 25 mm behind and lateral to the tonsil).
- Styloid process (if enlarged).
- Submandibular salivary gland.
- Medial pterygoid muscle.
- Angle of mandible.

■ Blood Supply of Tonsil

The arterial supply is mainly from the tonsillar branch of the facial artery. In addition, the branches of the arteries mentioned below also supply the tonsils (**Fig. 42.4**):

- Ascending pharyngeal artery, a branch of the external carotid artery.
- Descending palatine artery, a branch of the internal maxillary artery.
- Dorsalis linguae artery, a branch of the lingual artery.
- Ascending palatine artery, a branch of the facial artery.

■ Venous Supply

The veins emerge on the lateral surface and lower pole of the tonsil. The *paratonsillar vein* exits from the lateral surface to pierce the superior constrictor muscle, and ends in the common facial vein and pharyngeal plexus of veins.

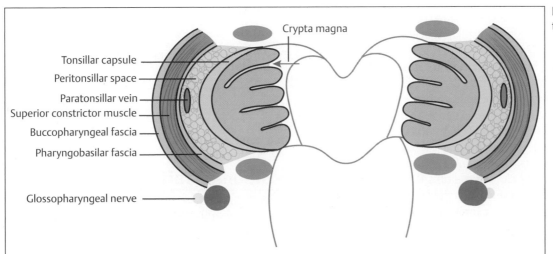

Fig. 42.3 Lateral relations of the tonsil.

Crypta magna

Tonsillar capsule
Peritonsillar space
Paratonsillar vein
Superior constrictor muscle
Buccopharyngeal fascia
Pharyngobasilar fascia

Glossopharyngeal nerve

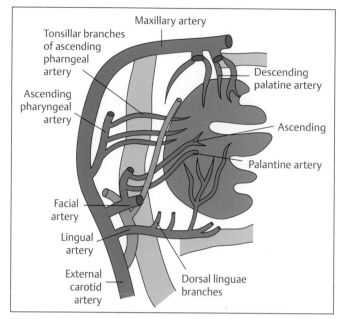

Fig. 42.4 Blood supply of the tonsil.

■ Lymphatic Drainage

The palatine tonsils are peculiar in that there are no afferent lymphatics. The efferent lymphatics exit from the lateral surface and drain into the jugulodigastric group of deep cervical nodes.

■ Applied Anatomy of Tonsils

- Crypts increase the surface area of tonsil.
- Peritonsillar abscess (quinsy) occurs due to the collection of pus in the peritonsillar space secondary to chronic tonsillitis. Drainage of the pus is done at the most prominent site which is felt as a soft area.
- Jugulodigastric lymph node, also known as the tonsillar node, is usually palpable in tonsillitis.
- Although the tonsils produce IgA to improve immunity, tonsillitis can be a septic foci in the body, especially when recurrent. This necessitates surgical removal.
- During tonsillectomy, the peritonsillar space is used as the plane for dissection.
- In tonsillectomy, the tonsil requires to be separated from the tonsillar bed along with its capsule.
- The fatty tissue around the carotid sheath protects the internal carotid artery, which is 2.5 cm lateral to the tonsillar bed, and is therefore not injured in tonsillectomy.
- Although in most surgeries preserving the clots helps prevent hemorrhage, this rule doesn't apply to the tonsils and uterus. The blood clots in the tonsillar fossa are removed as they prevent the contraction of surrounding muscles, thereby preventing the retraction of vessel walls. Removing the clots thus prevents postoperative hemorrhage.

Table 42.1 Contrasting features between adenoid and tonsil

Adenoid	Tonsil
Ciliated columnar epithelium	Nonkeratinizing squamous epithelium
No capsule	Partially encapsulated
Has furrows	Has crypts
Peak growth: 6 years	Peak growth: 8 years
Growth stops: 12 years	Growth stops: 15 years
Disappears: 20 years	Partial regression: 18 years

Table 42.2 Contrasting features between tonsil and lymph node

Tonsil	Lymph node
Subepithelial in position	Connective tissue
Hemicapsule	Fully encapsulated
Efferent lymphatics only	Afferent and efferent lymphatics
Crypts present	Crypts absent
Cortex or medulla absent	Cortex or medulla present
Growth curve present	Growth curve absent

- Ligature of the tonsillar arteries, especially inferior tonsillar artery, is important during tonsillectomy.
- The paratonsillar vein may be injured during tonsillectomy leading to profuse hemorrhage.
- Referred otalgia due to diseases of the tonsils (peritonsillar abscess, post tonsillectomy, or malignancy) can occur due to common nerve supply (cranial nerve IX).

Differences between Adenoid and Tonsil

Table 42.1 shows differences between adenoid and tonsil.

Differences between Tonsil and Lymph Node

Differences between tonsil and lymph node are described in **Table 42.2.**

Composition of Soft Palate

Soft palate is the movable posterior one-third part of palate. It is suspended from posterior border of hard palate, and it has no bony skeleton. It is composed of five muscles, namely, tensor veli palatini, levator veli palatini, palatoglossus, palatopharyngeus, and musculus uvulae (**Fig. 42.5**).

The tensor veli palatini is supplied by mandibular division of trigeminal nerve. All the other muscles of the soft palate are supplied by the vagus nerve through pharyngeal plexus.

Soft palate helps in closing off the nasal passages posteriorly during the oropharyngeal phase of swallowing.

> ### Pearl
>
> Bifid uvula indicates incomplete closure of soft palate with the Passavant's ridge. To compensate the deficiency of the muscle, the adenoid hypertrophies to seal the nasopharyngeal aperture. Hence, in these cases, adenoidectomy is contraindicated, and if done it leads to velopharyngeal insufficiency. Similarly, in submucosal cleft also, adenoidectomy is contraindicated. Clinically, it can be identified by digital palpation of the posterior edge of hard palate. Normally, there is spine in the midline to which soft palate muscles attach. In submucosal cleft, there is a notch, a V-shaped deficit in the midline of hard palate.

Acute Tonsillitis

Acute infections of the palatine tonsils predominantly occur in school-going children, but any age group may be affected (**Fig. 42.6a–c**). Peak incidence is between 5 and 6 years of age.

■ Etiology

It commonly occurs following viral upper respiratory tract infection. It can also occur as a primary infection of the tonsil. *Group A beta-haemolytic Streptococcus (GABHS),* *Staphylococcus, Hemophilus influenzae,* and *Pneumococcus* are the common bacterial pathogens. Among these, infection by GABHS (*Streptococcus pyogenes*) is important because this can be precursor of two serious conditions, namely, *acute rheumatic fever* and *poststreptococcal glomerulonephritis.* Rarely, anaerobes like bacteroides and fusobacterium can present with foul-smelling pus.

■ Pathology

The process of inflammation originates within the tonsil. There is hyperemia and edema, and the lymphoid follicles are converted into small micro-abscesses which drain into the crypts.

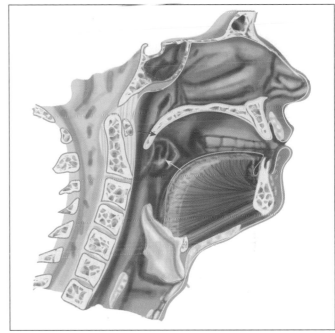

Fig. 42.5 Soft palate—sagittal section (*red arrow*). Note its relation to the palatine tonsils inferiorly (*yellow arrow*).

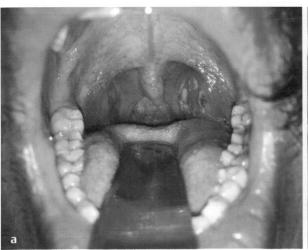 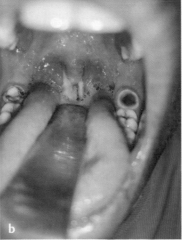 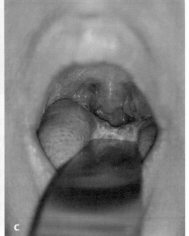

Fig. 42.6 **(a)** Acute follicular tonsillitis. **(b)** Acute membranous tonsillitis. **(c)** Acute parenchymatous tonsillitis.

The course of the disease may be self-limiting, lasting for 8 to 10 days but the infection (GABHS) is contagious during and even after 1 week after the symptoms subside, and there is possibility of developing sequelae or complications. Antibiotics are initiated without waiting for the culture report to avoid the complications and reduce the contagious period. Penicillins are the drug of choice. Amoxycillin (30–50 mg/kg body weight/day) in three divided doses with beta lactamase inhibitors like clavulanic acid is preferred. If the patient is allergic to penicillin, then azithromycin (10 mg/kg/day orally; once a day for 3 to 5 days), clindamycin (20–30 mg/kg/day orally; every 8 hours), or cephalosporins are preferred. Antibiotics reduce the duration and severity of symptoms and prevent the sequelae or complications.

Tonsillectomy is done for recurrent episodes (more than six episodes in 1 year, more than five episodes per year in 2 consecutive years, or more than three episodes per year in 3 consecutive years) and in GABHS carrier state.

> **Pearl**
>
> Coryza has a similar presentation of sore throat and fever but with additional features of nasal symptoms like rhinorrhea. The treatment does not necessitate antibiotic use, unless there is secondary infection.

Complications

- Chronic tonsillitis.
- Peritonsillitis (**Fig. 42.12**).
- Peritonsillar abscess (quinsy).
- Parapharyngeal abscess.
- Acute otitis media.
- Acute glomerulonephritis—presentation is with generalized edema, hypertension, and bradycardia/tachycardia.
- Rheumatic fever—the involvement of the mitral and tricuspid valves leads to relapsing fever and stenosis or incompetence of the valves.
- Sepsis.
- Suppurative lymphadenitis.
- Septic arthritis—can lead to osteitis, arthrodesis, and reduced joint movements.

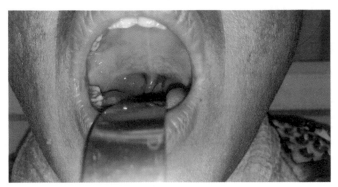

Fig. 42.12 Picture showing right peritonsillitis.

- Scarlet fever:
  - From trunk to extremities (except palms and soles), there is generalized, nonpruritic, erythematous, macular rash.
  - Strawberry tongue (bright, red, painful tongue due to desquamation of papilla).
  - Circumoral pallor may occur and last for 6 to 9 days.
- Pediatric autoimmune neuropsychiatric disorders associated with streptococcal infection (PANDAS). This is an obsessive-compulsive disorder along with tics. The symptoms go into remission after some weeks but may recur after the next infection.

Differential Diagnosis for Membrane over the Tonsils

Table 42.5 lists differential diagnosis for membrane over the tonsils.

Infectious Mononucleosis (Glandular Fever)

It is caused by Epstein-Barr virus and transmitted by close contact. It can also involve the spleen, liver, and central nervous system.

Clinical Features

The incubation period can be up to 6 weeks. The symptoms vary from mild to severe. The presentation is with fatigue, malaise, and sore throat. There will be enlargement of the cervical lymph nodes (Waldeyer's ring). The tonsils will be enlarged with an overlying grayish membrane which can be easily removed. The enlarged tonsils can cause noisy breathing and airway obstruction. There may be petechiae on the palate.

In addition, there may be a maculopapular skin rash, splenomegaly, hepatomegaly, and cranial neuropathies. There may be edema of the upper eye eyelid.

Investigations

A peripheral smear done will show abnormal lymphocytes. Paul-Bunnell test or monospot test will show heterophile antibodies. Serology tests to detect IgM-specific antibodies to viral capsid antigen is the gold standard. The liver function tests may be abnormal.

Treatment

Mainly supportive treatment is given for the symptoms. Antibiotics are given only if there is secondary infection. Ampicillin is avoided as a rash can develop. Intravenous steroids are given for enlarged tonsils causing airway

Table 42.5 Membrane over the tonsils—differential diagnosis (**Figs. 42.13, 42.14,** and **42.15**)

Lesions producing tonsillar membrane	Characteristics of the lesion
Acute membranous tonsillitis (Fig. 42.13)	• Membrane limited to tonsils; easily removed • High grade fever • Enlarged tender jugulodigastric nodes
Agranulocytosis	• Ulcerative necrotic lesions, fever • Total leukocyte count: 50–2,000/mm³ • Neutrophils: 5% or less
Diphtheria (Fig. 42.14)	• *Corynebacterium diphtheria* • Low grade fever • Child looks ill • Dirty, gray, tenacious membrane extends beyond tonsils to soft palate, posterior pharyngeal wall, and larynx, which bleeds on removal • Cervical lymph nodes are enlarged (bull-neck appearance) • Albert's stain—cuneiform pattern of bacilli • Exotoxin-mediated myocarditis, neurological complications • Treated with anti-diphtheric serum, penicillins/erythromycin
Leukemia	• Acute lymphoblastic leukemia more common in children • Total leukocyte count >100,000/cumm • Progressive anemia • Bone marrow examination—blast cells seen
Aphthous ulcers	• Solitary/multiple painful ulcers with erythematous base • Severe odynophagia • Total counts are normal
Malignancy	• Ulcer with indurated base • Bleeds on touch • Referred otalgia • Hard palpable cervical lymph node
Traumatic ulcer	• Accidental • Healing by formation of a membrane which appears within 24 h
Vincent's angina	• Fusiform bacilli and spirochetes • Mild fever, throat discomfort • Membrane usually on one tonsil • Pseudomembrane can be easily removed to reveal an irregular ulcer
Infectious mononucleosis (Fig. 42.15)	• Epstein-Barr virus • Fever, sore throat, enlarged tonsils with exudate • Lethargy, enlarged posterior triangle neck nodes • Splenomegaly • Increased total lymphocyte count, >10% atypical • Monospot or Paul-Bunnell test • Serological tests are more sensitive (VCA, EBNA) • Symptomatic treatment

Abbreviations: EBNA, Epstein-Barr nuclear antigen; VCA, viral capsid antigen.

compromise. The patient is counseled regarding rest and to avoid contact sports.

Chronic Tonsillitis

■ Etiopathology

Chronic inflammatory changes in the tonsil are the result of recurrent acute infections treated inadequately. The tonsils are denuded of the epithelium. Micro-abscesses occur in the lymphoid follicles due to the recurrent infection. The fibrous tissue and adjacent inflammatory cells (mainly lymphocytes) seal off the micro-abscesses. There is decreased production of IgA antibodies in response to antigenic stimulation.

Persistent or recurrent infection of the nose and paranasal sinuses with resultant postnasal discharge can be a source of infection to the tonsils.

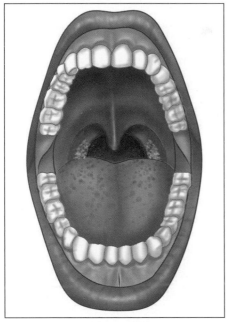

Fig. 42.13 Acute membranous tonsillitis.

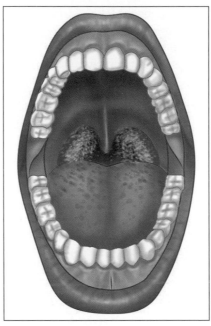

Fig. 42.14 Diphtheria.

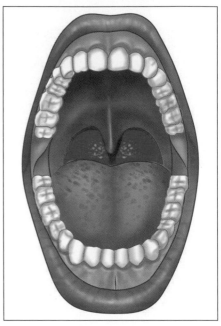

Fig. 42.15 Infectious mononucleosis.

■ Types

- *Chronic follicular*: Crypts are filled with cheesy material, which can be expressed by applying pressure on the anterior pillar (*Irwin Moore sign*).
- *Chronic parenchymatous*: Tonsils may be markedly enlarged causing difficulty in swallowing, snoring, and sleep apnea in children.
- *Chronic fibrotic*: Tonsils are small but infected.

■ Clinical Features

Symptoms

The patient presents with discomfort in the throat, recurrent episodes of sore throat, unpleasant taste (*cacogeusia and dysgeusia*), and foul smell from mouth (*halitosis*). There may be difficulty in swallowing or breathing, and a change in voice. The attacks may be associated with fever and throat discomfort. It may affect the scholastic performance of the child because of the loss of school days. In some children, along with difficulty in swallowing there may be failure to thrive. Breathing difficulty mainly manifests as obstructive sleep apnea and may need further evaluation. Halitosis is due to the secondary bacterial infection of the oral cavity and the resultant poor oral hygiene.

Signs

The tonsils may be enlarged (parenchymatous) or small (fibrotic). The three cardinal signs of chronic tonsillitis are (**Fig. 42.16**):
- Hyperemia of the anterior pillars.

- Enlarged, nontender jugulodigastric (tonsillar) nodes.
- Positive Irwin Moore sign or septic squeeze test. For the Irwin Moore sign, two tongue depressors are used; one is used to depress the anterior part of the tongue and the other tongue depressor is used to gently press on the anterior pillar. The tonsillar crypts are observed for exudation of yellowish, cheesy material.

The diagnosis is mainly clinical with the classical history of recurrent attacks of sore throat, and the cardinal signs as described earlier.

■ Treatment

- Antibiotics are mainly helpful during acute exacerbations of chronic tonsillitis. Penicillins are the drug of choice. Amoxycillin (30–50 mg/kg body weight/day) in three divided doses with a beta lactamase inhibitor like clavulanic acid is preferred. A throat swab should be taken prior to starting antibiotics.
- A source of infection if present in the nose or paranasal sinuses should be treated. Povidone iodine (2%) mouth wash and gargle help in maintaining good oral hygiene by controlling the oral and oropharyngeal bacterial flora.
- The surgical management is *tonsillectomy* for patients who continue to have recurrent episodes or persistent sore throat or halitosis.

■ Complications

- Peritonsillar abscess.
- Parapharyngeal abscess.
- Intratonsillar abscess.

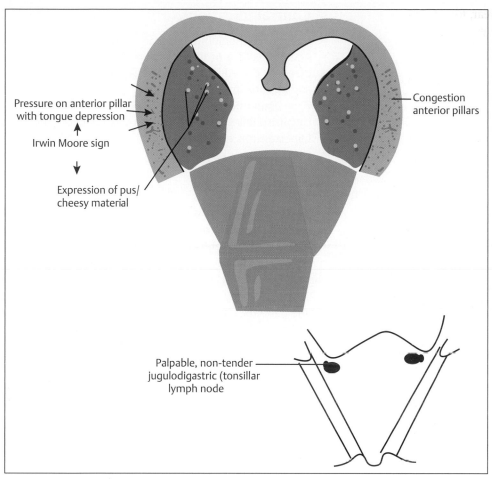

Fig. 42.16 Signs of chronic tonsillitis.

- Tonsillar cyst.
- Tonsillolith.
- Rheumatic fever.
- Acute nephritis.

■ Differential Diagnosis of a White Patch on the Tonsil

- Infection:
  - Viral—herpes simplex, Epstein-Barr (infectious mononucleosis).
  - Bacterial:
    ○ Acute—GABHS, corynebacterium, Vincent's angina.
    ○ Chronic—tuberculosis, syphilis.
  - Fungal—candida.
- Traumatic—acid or alkali ingestion, iatrogenic trauma, foreign body.
- Systemic—agranulocytosis, aplastic anemia, leukemia.
- Tumors—benign, malignant.
- Miscellaneous—tonsillolith, tonsillar cyst, keratosis pharyngis, aphthous ulcer, leukoplakia.
- HIV-related infections, hairy leukoplakia, tumors.

■ Investigations

These should be done based on the clinical presentation. Blood tests like a complete blood count, peripheral smear, and monospot test. A throat swab can be taken for culture and sensitivity. Serological tests are done to detect virus and syphilis infection. Albert's stain is done if diphtheria is suspected. Bone marrow studies may be required for certain systemic diseases. When the diagnosis is in doubt, a biopsy is taken.

Tonsillectomy

It is the procedure done for removal of both tonsils. The commonest technique used is the dissection and snare method.

■ Indications

Absolute

- Chronic or recurrent tonsillitis:
  - Seven or more episodes in 1 year.

- Five or more episodes in a year, for 2 years.
- Three or more episodes in a year, for 3 years.
- Peritonsillar abscess in children after 4 to 6 weeks and after second attack in adults. Abscess (hot) tonsillectomy is done in the presence of the abscess and interval tonsillectomy is done 4 to 6 weeks after the infection subsides.
- Tonsillitis causing febrile seizures.
- Cardiac valvular disease associated with recurrent streptococcal tonsillitis.
- Tonsillar hypertrophy causing obstructive sleep apnea, sleep disturbances, snoring, feeding problems, speech problems.
- Malignancy is suspected when there is asymmetric or unilateral tonsillar hypertrophy.

Pearl

Paradise criteria are used for deciding candidates for tonsillectomy in children with chronic or recurrent tonsillitis. It states that the child should have:

- Seven or more episodes in 1 year.
- Five or more episodes in a year, for 2 years.
- Three or more episodes in a year, for 3 years.
- Two or more weeks of lost school in a year.

Relative

- Tonsillolithiasis.
- Tonsillitis with lymph node abscess.
- Chronic tonsillitis with persistent sore throat and/or halitosis.
- Diphtheria carriers unresponsive to antibiotics.
- Streptococcal carriers in a family with rheumatic fever and acute nephritis patients.
- Chronic tonsillitis with bad taste or halitosis.
- Failure to thrive; enlarged tonsils with swallowing difficulties.
- Obstructive tonsils in infectious mononucleosis not responding to medical therapy.

As Part of Other Procedures

- Styloid process removal in patients with stylalgia or Eagle's syndrome.
- Palatopharyngoplasty for obstructive sleep apnea syndrome.
- Glossopharyngeal neurectomy in patients diagnosed with glossopharyngeal neuralgia.
- Removal of tonsils to identify the inner end of branchial fistula of second arch.
- Removal of tonsils to reroute the submandibular duct in a drooling child.

Contraindications

- Anemia: Hemoglobin less than 10 gram%.
- Acute tonsillitis or upper respiratory tract infection.
- Bleeding disorders like leukemia, hemophilia, purpura, and aplastic anemia.
- Polio epidemic.
- Uncontrolled systemic diseases like diabetes mellitus, hypertension, and asthma.
- During menses or pregnancy.

Preoperative Assessment

The patient should be evaluated for history of easy bruising or family history of coagulation disorders. Coagulation studies is done in relevant cases. In patients with obstructive sleep apnea syndrome, a polysomnography, X-ray chest, and electrocardiography (ECG) are required along with a cardiology consultation. In velocardiofacial syndrome patients, angiography will help to rule out medially placed carotid artery.

Procedure

Preoperative Measures

- The patient is not allowed to take anything orally for 8 hours before planned surgery time and intravenous fluids are started.
- Intravenous antibiotic is given half an hour before incision. Ceftriaxone, 30 mg/kg/day in two divided doses, is preferred.

Anesthesia

- The procedure is usually done under general anesthesia with endotracheal intubation. In adults a nasotracheal intubation may be done. In cooperative adults, local anesthesia can be used, although this is seldom carried out.

Position

The patient is put in Rose's position—supine position with pillow under the shoulders and head stabilized using rubber ring. This allows for extension of neck and head.

Tonsillectomy Surgical Instruments (Fig. 42.17)

From top to bottom and from left to right:
- Eve's tonsillar snare.
- Waugh's tenaculum forceps.
- St. Claire Thompson adenoid curette with cage.
- Draffin's bipods.
- Yankauer's suction tip.

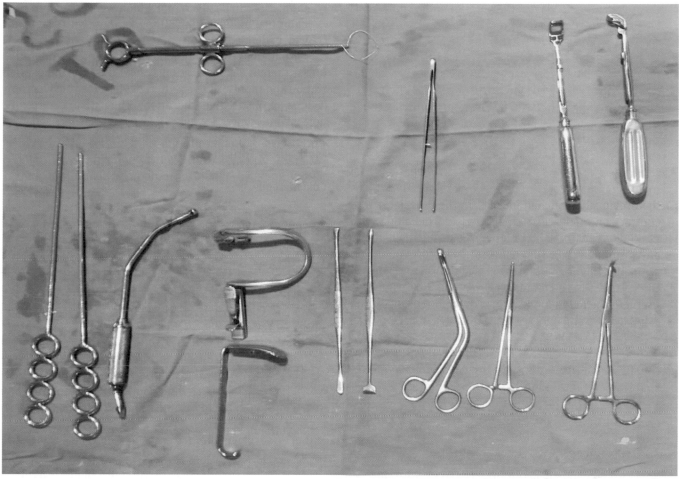

Fig. 42.17 Tonsillectomy instruments. The above image includes adenoid curette used for adenoidectomy.

- Boyle Davis mouth gag.
- Gwynne-Evan's tonsillar dissector.
- Mollison's anterior pillar retractor.
- Dennis Brown tonsil holding forceps.
- Burkitt first artery forceps.
- Negus second artery forceps.

Operative Steps: Dissection and Snare Method (Fig. 42.18)

- After the patient is put in Rose's position, a Davis Boyle's mouth gag with tongue blade is used to open the mouth and retract the tongue. A Doughty's tongue blade may be used when there is an orotracheal tube.
- The tonsil is grasped at the upper pole, using the Dennis Browne's tonsil holding forceps, and gently pulled medially.
- An incision is made in the mucosa of the anterior pillar at the upper pole at its junction with the tonsil, using Waugh's tenaculum forceps or a No. 15 surgical blade.
- Using Gwynne-Evan's dissector (or Mollison anterior pillar retractor with tonsillar dissector), the tonsil with its capsule is separated from the loose areolar tissue on

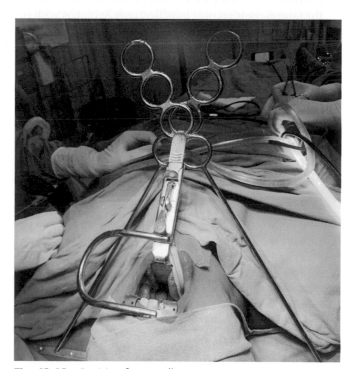

Fig. 42.18 Position for tonsillectomy.

Case-Based Questions

1. A 6-year-old boy was brought by the mother to the hospital with complaints of frequent sore throat associated with fever. The last episode was 2 weeks back. A local doctor diagnosed this as tonsillitis and advised surgery.

   a. What are the cardinal signs of chronic tonsillitis?

   b. Is it advisable to operate on this patient immediately, 2 weeks after the last episode of fever and sore throat?

   c. What are the complications of tonsillectomy?

   Answers

   a. The cardinal signs of chronic tonsillitis include congested anterior pillars, enlarged but nontender jugulodigastric lymph nodes, and positive Irwin Moore sign.

   b. During an acute infection, tonsillectomy is contraindicated due to the risk of bleeding from inflamed tissues and spread of infection through the tissue planes. Ideally it should be performed 6 to 8 weeks after the last infection.

   c. Immediate complications include hemorrhage, trauma to surrounding structures, and aspiration of blood.

2. A 7-year-old girl presents with history acute throat pain and fever. She finds it painful to swallow food. On examination, the tonsils are enlarged and congested (Grade 3), with a white membrane over the medial surface of the tonsil on both sides. Palpation of the neck revealed tender lymph nodes. She is febrile.

   a. What is the diagnosis?

   b. What is the differential diagnosis for a white membrane over the tonsil?

   c. How will you treat this girl?

   Answers

   a. Acute membranous tonsillitis.

   b. In addition to acute membranous tonsillitis, they include diphtheria, leukemia, and agranulocytosis and infectious mononucleosis.

   c. She can be treated with antibiotics such as a combination of amoxycillin with clavulanic acid. Paracetamol can be given for the pain and fever, and povidone-iodine mouth gargle can be advised. This is an antiseptic agent.

Frequently Asked Questions

1. What are the differences between adenoids and tonsils?

2. What is the blood supply of the tonsil?

3. What are the symptoms of acute tonsillitis in a child?

4. What are the signs of acute tonsillitis?

5. How will you grade tonsillar enlargement?

6. What are the absolute indications for tonsillectomy?

7. What are the complications of tonsillectomy?

Endnote

Tonsillectomy was first described in medical literature by Cornelio Celsus in the first century BC. His description involved dissection of the tonsillar bed and application of a mixture of milk and vinegar for hemostasis. Without anesthesia, this was a difficult procedure. This surgery was performed mainly by general surgeons till the end of the 19th century when ENT surgeons started performing this procedure. With better illumination with the advent of the mouth gag, tongue depressors, better positioning with the head suspended as described by Killian, and the use of ligatures for bleeding, tonsillectomy became a relatively safe surgery.

43 Tumors of Oral Cavity

Vijendra Shenoy S. and Sreenivas Kamath K.

The competencies covered in this chapter are as follows:

DE4.1 Discuss the prevalence of oral cancer and enumerate the common types of cancer that can affect tissues of the oral cavity.

SU20.1 Describe etiopathogenesis of oral cancer and symptoms and signs of pharyngeal cancer. Enumerate the appropriate investigations and discuss the principles of treatment.

DE4.2 Discuss the role of etiological factors in the formation of precancerous/cancerous lesions.

DE4.3 Identify potential precancerous/cancerous lesions.

EN2.11 Describe and identify by clinical examination malignant and premalignant ENT diseases.

Brief Anatomy

The oral cavity extends anteroposteriorly from the vermilion border of lips to the oropharyngeal isthmus. It is bounded laterally by the buccal mucosa, superiorly by the hard palate, and inferiorly by the floor of mouth (**Fig. 43.1**).

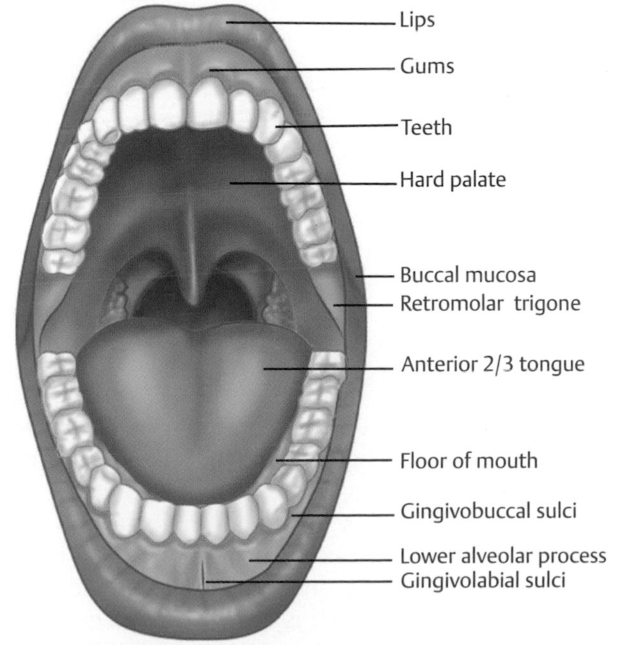
Lips
Gums
Teeth
Hard palate
Buccal mucosa
Retromolar trigone
Anterior 2/3 tongue
Floor of mouth
Gingivobuccal sulci
Lower alveolar process
Gingivolabial sulci

Fig. 43.1 Anatomy of the oral cavity.

The lining epithelium is nonkeratinized stratified squamous cell lining, except the occlusal line over the buccal mucosa may get keratinized. This is supported by fibrous connective tissue and submucosal fibroadipose tissue. The minor salivary glands, nerves, and capillaries are present in the submucosa. The lymphatics are outlined in **Table 43.1** and **Fig. 43.2.**

Classification of Oral Cavity Tumors

Oral cavity tumors can be classified as:

- Benign tumors.
- Premalignant lesions and conditions.
- Malignant tumors.

Benign Tumors

There is a wide variety of benign tumors in the oral cavity but most of them are rare and they are classified by the tissue of origin.

Classification of benign tumors:

- *Epithelial tumors*:
  - Papillomas.
- *Salivary gland tumors*:
  - Pleomorphic adenoma.
- *Soft tissue tumors*:
  - Lymphangioma.
  - Hemangioma (**Fig. 43.3**).

Table 43.1 Lymphatic drainage of the oral cavity

Subsite	Lymphatic drainage
Lips	Submental (Ia), submandibular (Ib), preparotid (upper lips) and level II
Buccal mucosa, alveolar ridge	Ia, Ib, II, III
Hard palate	II, III, retropharyngeal group
Tongue	Ia, Ib, II, III, IV (midline lesion could have bilateral spread)
Floor of mouth	Ia, Ib, II, III (lesions could have bilateral spread)

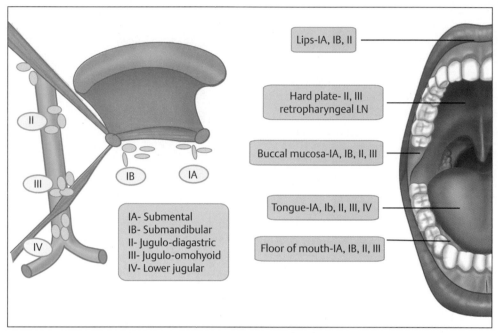

Lips-IA, IB, II

Hard plate- II, III retropharyngeal LN

Buccal mucosa-IA, IB, II, III

Tongue-IA, Ib, II, III, IV

Floor of mouth-IA, IB, II, III

IA- Submental
IB- Submandibular
II- Jugulo-diagastric
III- Jugulo-omohyoid
IV- Lower jugular

Fig. 43.2 Pictorial representation of lymphatic drainage. A, keratin pearls; B, keratinocyte with high N/C ratio.

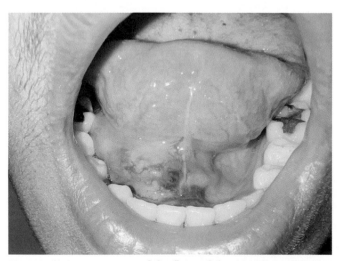

Fig. 43.3 Hemangioma of the floor of the mouth.

- Neurofibroma.
- Lipoma.
- *Benign odontogenic tumors and cysts*:
  - Osteoma.
  - Ossifying fibroma.

- *Benign conditions*:
  - Candidiasis (thrush).
  - Aphthous ulcers (canker sores).
  - Recurrent herpes labialis (cold sores).
  - Erythema migrans (geographic tongue).
  - Hairy tongue.
  - Lichen planus.
  - Frictional hyperkeratosis.
  - Mucocele, for example, ranula.

■ Premalignant Lesions and Premalignant Conditions of the Oral Cavity

Premalignant lesion is a single isolated area on the oral mucosa with morphologically altered tissue in which cancer is most likely to occur.

Premalignant condition of the oral mucosa is a more generalized mucosal disease which can lead to formation of a morphologically and genetically altered tissue (premalignant lesion), which is at high risk of malignant transformation. Due to their genetic damage, these lesions have distinguished phenotypic appearance that are easily noted during clinical examination. Early treatment of these conditions and/or regular follow-up can help avoid malignant transformation or help in early detection and management of the malignancy (**Table 43.2**).

Leukoplakia

The definition of leukoplakia is: "a white plaque with a growing debatable oral cancer risk after excluding other known diseases and disorders that do not increase the risk" (WHO Consensus, 2007).

It can also be defined as a white patch or plaque, not less than 5 mm in diameter, that cannot be removed or scraped off by rubbing and cannot be classified as any other diagnosable disease. There is a 4 to 6% chance of malignant transformation.

Epidemiology

It represents 85% of oral premalignant lesions more commonly seen in Southeast Asian countries. The incidence in India varies from 0.2 to 5.2%. The peak incidence is at 40 to 70 years of age. The male to female ratio is 2:1. The main risk factors are tobacco smoking (global) and betel nut chewing (Asian).

Clinical Features (Figs. 43.4 and 43.5)

It is diffuse or multiple and can affect any site. There are two clinical variants:
- *Homogenous.*
- *Nonhomogenous.*

The homogenous leukoplakia is superficial and flat, with a uniform white appearance and clear margins.

The nonhomogenous leukoplakia carries a higher risk of malignant transformation and has three variants, namely:
- Speckled.
- Nodular/granular.
- Verrucous/verruciform.

The speckled form presents as islands of red patches.

The nodular type appears as a small, whitish, rounded, polyp-like growth.

The verrucous form has elevated proliferative surface and is often misdiagnosed as verrucous carcinoma.

The high-risk factors for malignant transformation are:
- Female sex.

- Longer duration of disease.
- Diffuse lesion.
- Nonhomogenous type.
- Site at floor of mouth and ventrolateral part of tongue.
- Lesion larger than 2 cm.
- Rapid progression in size.
- Coinfection with human papilloma virus (HPV) or candidiasis.

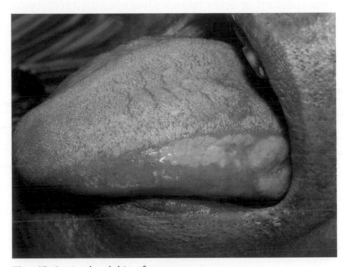

Fig. 43.4 Leukoplakia of tongue.

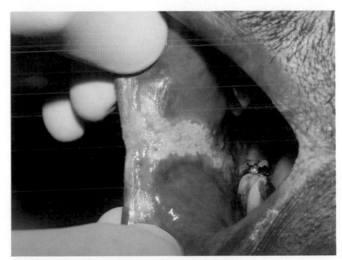

Fig. 43.5 Leukoplakia of buccal mucosa.

Table 43.2 Differential diagnosis of premalignant lesions and conditions

Definitive (premalignant lesion)	Probable (premalignant condition)	Doubtful
Leukoplakia	Syphilitic glossitis	Discoid lupus erythematosus
Erythroplakia	Sideropenic dysphagia	Dyskeratosis congenita
Oral submucosal fibrosis	Oral lichen planus	Smokeless tobacco keratosis
Proliferative verrucous leukoplakia (PVL)	Chronic hyperplastic candidiasis Actinic keratosis (lip only)	

Microscopy

Leukoplakia is a clinical diagnosis. On histopathology, the presence or absence of epithelial dysplasia is noted. Epithelial dysplasia and surface hyperkeratosis are the hallmarks of leukoplakia.

Management

Other causes should be ruled out by biopsy, which is the gold standard, or other methods like cytology/brush cytology, chemiluminescence, and tissue autofluorescence (**Box 43.1**).

Preventive treatment involves cessation of habits (smoking, alcohol, tobacco chewing). Public information and health care program to be conducted for awareness.

Conservative treatment is often preferred as many lesions may disappear spontaneously. Vitamin A, retinoids, beta carotene, lycopene, and local bleomycin have been advocated with varying success.

Surgical management involves complete excision with or without laser (KTP-532 laser, CO_2 laser, or Nd:YAG laser).

Erythroplakia

It is defined as a fiery, red patch which cannot be characterized clinically or pathologically as any other definable condition.

Epidemiology

It is a rare entity accounting for <1% of oral premalignant lesions. It is seen in the 45 to 55 years age group and more commonly in males. The risk factors are:
- Tobacco chewing.
- Smoking.
- Alcohol consumption.
- Human papilloma virus 16.
- Genomic instability is thought to play a role in pathogenesis (p53).

The risk of malignant transformation is 14 to 50%.

Clinical Features

It presents as a well-defined, smooth, reddish, velvety lesion, which is soft on palpation without any induration. It is reddish in appearance due to thinning of the surface epithelium, resulting in close proximity of vascular lamina propria to the surface.

Buccal mucosa, soft palate, and floor of mouth are the most commonly affected areas.

The clinical variants are:
- Homogenous erythroplakia.
- Erythroplakia interspersed with patches of leukoplakia (erythro-leukoplakia).
- Granular or speckled erythroplakia (speckled leukoplakia).

Microscopy

It can range from epithelial dysplasia to carcinoma. There are two variants, namely, neoplastic and inflammatory.

The differential diagnosis for erythroplakia is given in **Table 43.3**.

Management

It is the same as for leukoplakia (see above). In addition, chemoprevention by p-53 targeted drugs such as ONYX-015, thalidomide, epidermal growth factor receptor (EGFR) inhibitors, and vitamin E have been tried without much reported benefit.

Oral Submucosal Fibrosis (OSMF)

Synonyms: Diffuse oral submucosal fibrosis, idiopathic palatal fibrosis, sclerosing stomatitis.

Epidemiology

In 2002, around 5 million cases were reported in India. The prevalence in India is 1.3% (more common in North India), and is predominantly seen in Southeast Asian countries. The male to female ratio is 1:1. The 20 to 40 years age group is more commonly involved. The rate of transformation to malignancy is around 1 to 15%.

Table 43.3 Differential diagnosis for erythroplakia

Infective pathology	Inflammatory causes
- Bacterial—tuberculosis - Fungal—Erythematous oral candidiasis, general candida erythema, histoplasmosis	- Pemphigoid - Pemphigus - SLE - Lichen planus
Other differential diagnosis: Hemangiomas, Kaposi sarcoma, oral purpura, amelanotic melanoma	

Abbreviation: SLE, systemic lupus erythematosus.

Box 43.1 Differential diagnosis of leukoplakia		
Candidiasis	Discoid lupus erythematosus	Frictional lesion
Hairy leukoplakia	Leukoedema	Lichen planus
Papilloma-like diseases	Tobacco-induced lesions	White sponge nevus

Risk factors are areca nut chewing, local irritants (spicy food), nutritional deficiency, and autoimmune pathology.

Etiopathogenesis

Areca nut plays an important role in OSMF. This is one of the constituents of "paan" which is chewed in India. The main alkaloid found to be the culprit is *arecoline*. Other compounds are alkaloids, polyphenols, and trace elements. Long-term exposure to areca nut causes fibroblast to produce excessive collagen. Tannins and catechin stabilize the collagen and thereby reduce the synthesis of collagenase. Fibroblasts produce stable collagen and excess collagen. Collagen cross linking is increased due to upregulation of lysyl oxidase. There is reduced collagen phagocytosis. In addition, there is deficiency of micronutrients and vitamins. The mucosa lacks elasticity, collagen becomes avascular, and there may be skeletal muscle atrophy.

Clinical Features

The early symptoms are burning sensation in oral cavity, especially with intake of spicy food and associated dryness of mouth.

The late symptoms are:
- Stiffening of the mucosa leading to *trismus* (restricted mouth opening).
- Difficulty in swallowing, whistling, or blowing a candle.
- Due to palatal fibrosis, there could be rhinolalia aperta (increased airflow through the nose).

On examination in early stages, there may be blisters, vesicles, ulcer, and/or recurrent stomatitis.

In later stages, the mucosa will appear blanched and whitish due to fibrosis. Fibrotic bands may be seen and palpable with the buccal mucosa and lower lip initially affected. There will be restricted mouth opening (**Fig. 43.6**).

The grading depends on the number of fingers the patient can accommodate between the upper and lower alveolus (mild—three fingers; moderate—two fingers; severe—less than one finger). Hooked up uvula or bud-like uvula is noted. There may be impaired tongue movement (**Flowchart 43.1**).

Laboratory findings show anemia, raised erythrocyte sedimentation rate (ESR), and eosinophilia.

Histopathology shows epithelial atrophy, juxta epithelial inflammation, and excessive collagen in lamina propria and submucosa. Sometimes hyperkeratosis, parakeratosis, and acanthosis may also be seen.

Imaging by orthopantomogram shows elongation of coronoid process due to prolonged trismus.

Management

The aim is symptomatic relief, prevention of disease progression, and reduction of possible malignant transformation. The patient should be counseled regarding the condition and the possible long-term outcome.

The initial supportive measures are mainly preventive, that is, discontinuation of tobacco chewing, smoking, alcohol consumption, and public health awareness program. Nutritional supplementation with multivitamins, iron, and micronutrients. Physiotherapy by massage therapy, muscle stretch exercise (using ice cream stick exercise), and ultrasound therapy.

Medical Treatment

It is given to alleviate burning sensation, increase mouth opening, and reduce fibrosis. Steroids reduce the synthesis of inflammatory markers and increase the apoptosis of inflammatory cells. It relieves the symptoms but fail to reduce the fibrotic tissue deposition. Hence, there is a high relapse rate when steroid is used as a single modality. It can be used by (1) topical, (2) systemic, and (3) intralesional routes. The steroids commonly used are short acting

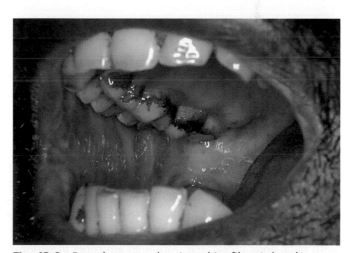

Fig. 43.6 Buccal mucosa showing white fibrotic bands.

Stage 1	Stage 2	Stage 3	Stage 4
- Stomatitis - Burning sensation - no fibres present	- Palpable fibrous bands (more on soft palate) - Mouth opening 26–35 mm.	- Blanched mucosa - Tongue involved - Mouth opening 6–25 mm	- Fibrosis of lips - Mouth opening 0–5 mm

Flowchart 43.1 Flowchart of pathophysiology.

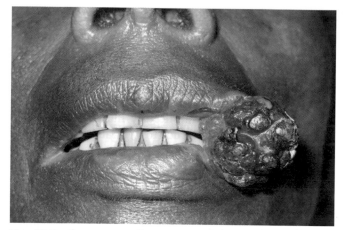

Fig. 43.7 Squamous cell carcinoma of the lip.

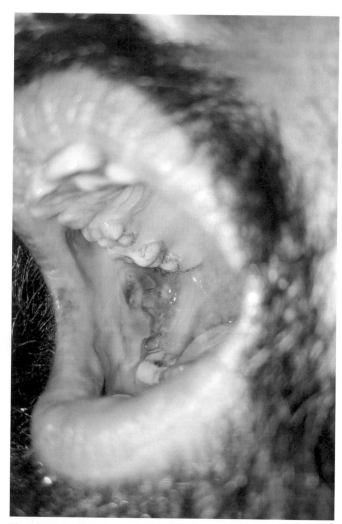

Fig. 43.8 Malignancy of the right buccal mucosa.

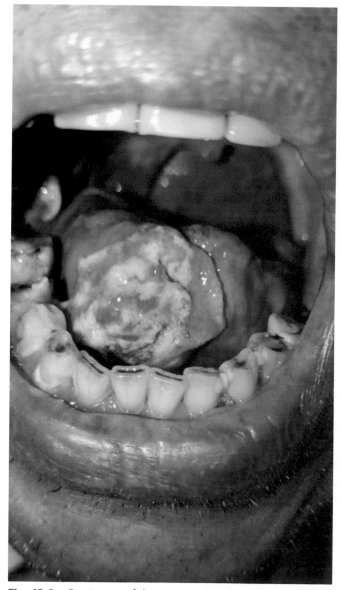

Fig. 43.9 Carcinoma of the anterior two-thirds of the tongue.

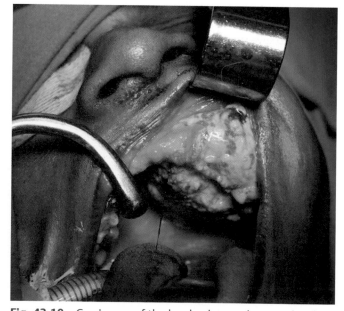

Fig. 43.10 Carcinoma of the hard palate and upper alveolus.

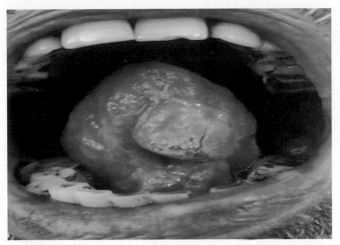

Fig. 43.11 Carcinoma involving the ventral surface of tongue and floor of mouth.

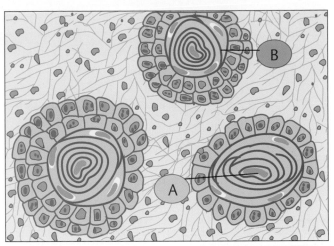

Fig. 43.12 Schematic diagram of histopathological finding in squamous cell carcinoma (SCC). A, keratin pearls; B, squamous cell with high nuclear/cytoplasmic (N/C) ratio.

Investigations

Screening of early suspicious areas can be performed by brush cytology, tissue reflectance system, or narrow emission tissue fluorescence.

Toluidine blue, which stains dark blue with malignant tissue, has been used for screening of suspicious lesions.

A biopsy is taken from the ulcer edge along with the adjoining normal-appearing mucosa. The central areas of the tumor tissue will lack blood supply leading to necrosis; hence, the tissue sample may not be representative for histopathological diagnosis.

The histology of SCC can range from well-differentiated SCC to poorly differentiated SCC (Broder's classification) (**Fig. 43.12**).

A fine-needle aspiration cytology (FNAC) of the neck mass can be done to evaluate neck metastasis but it is not necessary when the primary has been confirmed and the node is in the draining area. An ultrasound of the neck is useful for evaluation of neck metastasis.

Imaging by a contrast-enhanced computed tomography (CECT) will show contrast enhancement in malignant tumors and neck metastasis. Bone involvement is better picked up with a CECT.

Magnetic resonance imaging (MRI) with gadolinium contrast is better for soft tissue assessment especially for the depth of invasion in the tongue. Perineural and bone marrow invasions are better noted on MRI. A computed tomography (CT) scan of the thorax is done to rule out lung metastasis. In advanced lesions, a positron emission tomography–computed tomography (PET-CT) scan can be done to rule out distant metastasis. It is also done when a recurrence (local or regional) or a second primary is suspected.

Staging

The AJCC 8th edition TNM (tumor, node, metastasis) staging is given in **Table 43.5.**

Dental assessment and treatment for caries teeth are done prior to definitive treatment by radiotherapy to avoid osteoradionecrosis.

Treatment of Oral SCC

There are three modalities of treatment for SCC of the oral cavity:
- Surgery.
- Radiotherapy.
- Chemotherapy.

Most cases involve surgery as the mainstay of treatment as can be seen in **Table 43.6**.

Surgery can be followed by adjuvant radiotherapy and chemotherapy unless they are early lesions in which case only a single modality of treatment is required.

Surgery

While planning for surgical resection of oral cavity malignancy one has to understand the functions that may be compromised, that is, swallowing, articulation (speech), and taste. Accordingly, reconstruction is done to:
- Fill the defect.
- Give bulk.
- Reduce cosmetic deformity.
- Allow for postoperative rehabilitation.

For upper alveolar lesions, after resection a dental obturator can be used to fill the gap and allow for mastication.

Table 43.5 TNM staging of oral cavity tumors

T category	T criteria
Tx	Primary tumor cannot be assessed
Tis	Carcinoma in situ
T1	Tumor < 2 cm, < 5 mm DOI, DOI is depth of invasion and not tumor thickness
T2	Tumor < 2 cm, DOI > 5 mm and < 1 0 mm or tumor > 2 cm but < 4 cm, and < 10 mm DOI
T3	Tumor > 4 cm or any tumor > 10 mm DOI
T4	Moderately advanced or very advanced local disease
T4a	Moderately advanced local disease (lip); tumor invades through cortical bone or involves the inferior alveolar nerve, floor of mouth, or skin of face (i.e., chin or nose) (oral cavity); tumor invades adjacent structures only (e.g., through cortical bone of the mandible or maxilla, or involves the maxillary sinus or skin of the face). Note: Superficial erosion of bone/tooth socket (alone) by a gingival primary is not sufficient to classify a tumor as T4
T4b	Very advanced local disease Tumor invades masticator space, pterygoid plates, or skull base and/or encases the internal carotid artery

N category	Clinical N criteria
Nx	Regional lymph nodes cannot be assessed
N0	No regional lymph node metastasis
N1	Metastasis in a single ipsilateral lymph node, 3 cm or smaller in greatest dimension ENE(−)
N2	Metastasis in a single ipsilateral node larger than 3 cm but not larger than 6 cm in greatest dimension and ENE(−); or metastases in multiple ipsilateral lymph nodes, none larger than 6 cm in greatest dimension and ENE(−); or in bilateral or contralateral lymph nodes, none larger than 6 cm in greatest dimension, and ENE(−)
N2a	Metastasis in a single ipsilateral node larger than 3 cm but not larger than 6 cm in greatest dimension, and ENE(−)
N2b	Metastasis in multiple ipsilateral nodes, none larger than 6 cm in greatest dimension, and ENE(−)
N2c	Metastasis in bilateral or contralateral lymph nodes, none larger than 6 cm in greatest dimension, and ENE(−)
N3	Metastasis in a lymph node larger than 6 cm in greatest dimension and ENE(−); or metastasis in any node(s) and clinically overt ENE(+)
N3a	Metastasis in a lymph node larger than 6 cm in greatest dimension and ENE(−)
N3b	Metastasis in any node(s) and clinically overt ENE(+)

M category	M criteria
M0	No metastasis
M1	Distant metastasis

Stage	T stage	N stage	M stage
I	T1	N0	M0
II	T2	N0	M0
III	T3	N0	M0
III	T1, 2, 3	N1	M0
IVA	T4a	N0, N1	M0
IVA	T1-4a	N2	M0
IVB	Any T	N3	M0
IVB	T4b	Any N	M0
IVC	Any T	Any N	M1

Abbreviations: DOI, depth of invasion; ENE, extranodal extension.

Prosthetic teeth can be incorporated in a reconstructed mandible. Postoperative swallowing therapy would be useful in the rehabilitation.

Management of mandible: Subperiosteal excision, i.e., stripping of periosteum in the vicinity of the tumor, is done in cases of confirmed noninvolvement of cortical bone of mandible. Marginal mandibulectomy is removal of part of mandible involved, leaving behind minimum of 1 cm bone along the inferior margin of mandible. It is done in cases of confirmed periosteum involvement and tumor adjacent to periosteum.

Reverse marginal mandibulectomy is when the inferior part of the mandible is removed for clearance while removing a submandibular metastatic lymph node.

Segmental mandibulectomy is removal of a segment of mandible with 1 cm margins. Hemimandibulectomy is removal of mandible from symphysis menti to condylar process (**Fig. 43.13**).

Neck management for extent of clearance of neck nodes can be planned based on the N staging. For N0, a selective neck dissection (levels 1–3, which is also known as supra-omo-hyoid neck dissection or SOND) is performed.

Level 4 may be included for tongue lesions.

For N+ status, a comprehensive neck dissection has to be done. Comprehensive neck dissection is further classified into:
- Modified radical neck dissection (**Fig. 43.14**).
- Radical neck dissection.
- Extended radical neck dissection.

Radiation Therapy

It can be given as a definitive treatment for early-stage lesions or as adjuvant therapy.

There are two modes of administration of radiotherapy to oral cavity lesions, namely:
- Brachytherapy.
- Teletherapy: Teletherapy is more commonly used. A total dose of 66 to 70 Grays (Gy) over 33 to 35 fractions is administered. (Each fraction is 200 cGy given 5 days in a week.)

Chemotherapy

It is a nonsurgical modality of treatment of oral cancer, and it can be administered as the sole neoadjuvant or as palliative treatment or as an adjuvant to surgical treatment with or without radiotherapy.

Table 43.6 Treatment for malignant tumors of the various subsites of the oral cavity

Carcinoma of lip	Carcinoma of buccal mucosa
• Best outcomes • Wide surgical excision with adequate reconstruction when needed • Reconstruction options: – Local advancement flaps – Pedicled flaps – Free flaps	**Mandible not involved:** • Wide excision with reconstruction • Reconstruction options: – Primary closure – Split-thickness skin/collagen graft – Local advancement flap – Pedicled flap – Free flap **Mandible involved:** • Marginal mandibulectomy • Segmental mandibulectomy • Hemimandibulectomy
Anterior two-third of tongue	**RMT**
• Wide excision with primary closure • Hemiglossectomy with reconstruction • Total glossectomy with reconstruction: – Local advancement flap – Pedicled flaps – Free flaps • Mandible managed if involved as mentioned above	• Wide excision/block resection with or without reconstruction
	Hard palate
	• Wide excision with or without reconstruction
	Floor of mouth
	• Wide excision with reconstruction

Abbreviation: RMT, retromolar trigone.

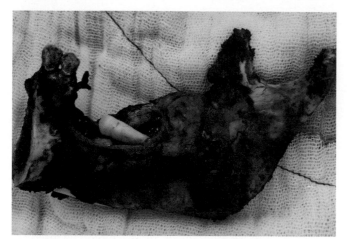

Fig. 43.13 Hemimandibulectomy specimen.

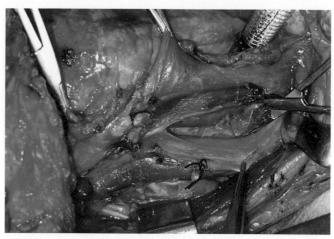

Fig. 43.14 Modified radical neck dissection.

Chemotherapy is a part of adjuvant treatment, after surgery, in the following conditions:
- In advanced lesions.
- Where there are positive surgical margins.
- Perineural invasion.
- Perivascular invasion.
- Extra-nodal extension.
- N2 or above nodal status.

Based on which phase of treatment chemotherapy is given, it can be classified into:
- Neoadjuvant chemotherapy (prior to definitive treatment).
- Concurrent (along with definitive treatment, i.e., combined with radiation therapy).
- Adjuvant therapy (after the definitive treatment).

Points to Ponder

- In leukoplakia, the risk of malignancy depends on the sex, site, type, progression, and association with HPV or candidiasis.
- Oral submucous fibrosis is a relatively common premalignant condition in the Indian subcontinent. It is often due to chewing betel quid or areca nut.
- Chronic smoking and alcohol intake increase the risk of oral cancer. Field cancerization can occur leading to synchronous or metachronous cancers.
- SCC is the commonest malignancy of the oral cavity.
- Early-stage oral cancers can be treated by surgery or radiotherapy.
- Advanced stage oral cancers require surgery followed by postoperative radiotherapy with or without chemotherapy.
- When treating cancer of the oral cavity one should keep in mind its effects on the functions of the oral cavity.

Case-Based Questions

1. **A 52-year-old male presented with a 2 × 1 cm ulceroproliferative growth in the left lateral border of the tongue. Biopsy taken from the lesion was suggestive of moderately differentiated squamous cell carcinoma. There were no palpable cervical lymph nodes. He is a chronic smoker.**

   a. What are the radiological investigations required?

   b. What is the stage of the tumor?

   c. What is the treatment?

   Answers
   a. Ultrasound of the neck to assess for cervical lymph node metastasis. Contrast-enhanced computed tomography (CT) scan or magnetic resonance imaging (MRI) of neck to assess the primary and for cervical lymph node metastasis.

   CT scan of thorax to assess for lung metastasis, second primary in the lung, and for prior lung disease.

   b. Clinically, T1N0Mx, Stage I.

   c. Partial glossectomy (wide local excision), with supraomohyoid (levels I, II, and III) or extended supraomohyoid neck dissection (levels I, II, III, and IV). If the patient does not want surgery or is medically unfit for surgery, radiotherapy is given.

2. **A 33-year-old male patient presented with an ulceroproliferative lesion in the right-side buccal mucosa. It was 5 × 3 cm and was encroaching the lower alveolus. The rest of the oral mucosa appeared blanched and whitish. There were palpable right level Ib and IIa cervical lymph nodes. There was history of betel quid**

chewing for 15 years. The patient had burning sensation of the mouth for 4 years associated with trismus.

a. What are the radiological investigations required?

b. How would you confirm the diagnosis?

c. What was the initial condition the patient had prior to developing this malignancy?

d. What is the treatment?

Answers

a. Contrast-enhanced computed tomography (CT) scan of the neck (puffed cheek during the scan) to assess the primary including mandibular involvement and to look for metastatic cervical lymph nodes. CT scan of the thorax to assess for lung/rib metastasis and for a second primary.

b. Biopsy from the margin of the lesion for histopathological examination.

c. Oral submucous fibrosis.

d. Wide excision of buccal mucosa with segmental or hemi-mandibulectomy (depending on the extent of mandibular involvement), modified radical neck dissection of the right side, and reconstruction of the defect. As it is in an advanced stage, postoperative radiotherapy will be required with or without chemotherapy.

Frequently Asked Questions

1. What is leukoplakia and erythroplakia?

2. Enumerate the premalignant lesions of the oral cavity.

3. What is oral submucous fibrosis?

4. What is the surgical management of oral submucous fibrosis when there is trismus?

5. What are the etiological factors for oral cavity cancer?

6. What is the differential diagnosis for a white patch on the buccal mucosa?

Endnote

Oral submucous fibrosis is a debilitating, chronic condition which is caused by inflammation of the submucosa of the oral cavity. It results in stiffening of the tissues and trismus. It was first reported by Schwartz in 1952 when he came across this condition among five Indian women and he termed it "atrophia idiopathica mucosae oris." It was Joshi, in 1953, who coined the term "oral submucous fibrosis," and it was widespread in the Indian subcontinent. But this condition was known from the time of Sushruta (600 BC), who coined the term "Vidari" for this condition.

44 Tumors of the Nasopharynx

Anil Kumar R. and B. Vishwanath

The competencies covered in this chapter are as follows:

EN4.32 Describe the clinical features, investigations, and principles of management of nasopharyngeal angiofibroma.

EN4.35 Describe the clinical features, investigations, and principles of management of tumors of the nasopharynx.

Introduction

Nasopharyngeal tumors are rare. Due to the site, which is posterior to the nasal cavity and above the soft palate, visualization of these tumors is difficult. The early symptoms may be missed and are therefore detected when they are in an advanced stage.

The tumors of the nasopharynx can be divided into benign and malignant lesions. Benign lesions or tumors of the nasopharynx can be classified based on their tissue of origin:

- *Developmental* lesions or tumors include Thornwaldt's cyst, teratoma, hairy polyp, branchial cyst, Rathke's cyst, and hamartoma.
- *Epithelial* tumors include papilloma and adenoid mucous retention cyst.
- *Mesenchymal* tumors are juvenile nasopharyngeal angiofibroma (JNA), craniopharyngioma, choanal polyp, hemangioma, and paraganglioma.
- *Salivary gland*: The most common salivary gland tumor is pleomorphic adenoma.

Adenoid hypertrophy and adenoiditis are the commonest diseases of the nasopharynx. Among the tumors of the nasopharynx, JNA (benign) and nasopharyngeal carcinoma (malignant) are relatively common.

Juvenile Nasopharyngeal Angiofibroma

It is a rare, benign, locally aggressive fibrovascular tumor of the nasopharynx seen exclusively in adolescent males. It comprises less than 1% of the head and neck tumors.

■ Etiopathology

Various theories have been proposed for the formation of a JNA like vascular malformation and hamartoma. It may be a vascular remnant from incomplete regression of the first pharyngeal arch artery. Androgen receptors, progesterone receptors, and estrogen receptors have been identified, which explains the hormonal influence. It has been associated with familial adenomatous polyposis.

The tumor is not capsulated, having vascular and fibrous stromal tissue. The irregular shaped vessels, which are embedded in a fibrous stroma, have an endothelial lining with a poorly developed myoid-type cells but no true muscular coat, and lack elastic fibers. This causes profuse bleeding as it cannot contract.

■ Spread

The site of origin has been noted to be the basisphenoid adjacent to the sphenopalatine foramen at the junction of the orbital and sphenoidal processes of the palatine bone, and the body of the sphenoid.

The common spread is through the sphenopalatine foramen to the pterygopalatine fossa (PPF). From the PPF, it can spread to the middle cranial fossa via the foramen rotundum or the vidian canal. It can also spread to the orbit via the inferior orbital fissure, and from the orbit it can spread to the cavernous sinus and the parasellar region via the superior orbital fissure. From the PPF, it can spread to the infratemporal fossa. From the nasopharynx, it can spread via the sphenoid sinus to the cavernous sinus and the sella. Through the nasal cavity, it involves the ethmoid sinus and the cribriform plate, and can spread to the anterior cranial fossa.

■ Clinical Features

Nasal obstruction and epistaxis are the common presenting symptoms. The nasal bleed is typically *unprovoked, painless*, and *profuse*. Other symptoms are based on the extension of the tumor:

- Orbit (proptosis, reduced vision, and diplopia).
- Infratemporal fossa (cheek swelling and trismus).
- Nasopharynx (conductive hearing loss).
- Intracranial (headache).

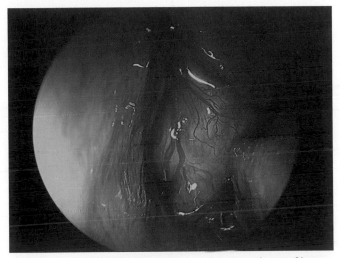

Fig. 44.1 Endoscopic view of a nasopharyngeal angiofibroma (JNA) tumor in the nasopharynx with prominent vessels.

■ Investigations

- Diagnostic nasal endoscopy will show a well-defined, lobulated pinkish mass that may have prominent vessels on its surface (**Fig. 44.1**) in the posterior part of the nasal cavity and the nasopharynx.
- A contrast-enhanced computed tomography (CT) scan or magnetic resonance imaging (MRI) will help delineate the enhancing lesion and its extent including orbital and intracranial involvement, relation to the internal carotid artery, and a possible alternate diagnosis. Spread to the PPF will show a widening of the sphenopalatine foramen (**Fig. 44.2**). The *Holman–Miller (antral) sign* is the anterior bowing of the posterior wall of the maxillary sinus due to the expanding JNA (**Fig. 44.3**).
- Digital subtraction angiography (DSA) will show a highly enhancing mass (**Fig. 44.4**). It will help in assessing the blood supply, whether it is from the external carotid artery or the internal carotid artery or both or from a contralateral vessel to the tumor. In addition, a selective embolization can be done to block the blood supply, that is, the internal maxillary artery and the ascending pharyngeal artery, within 48 hours of the scheduled surgery.
- A biopsy is discouraged as profuse bleeding can occur unless the diagnosis is in doubt in which case the biopsy is taken in the controlled setting of an operating room.

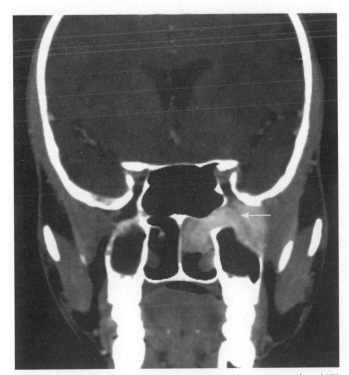

Fig. 44.2 Contrast-enhanced computed tomography (CT) scan (coronal cut) showing widening of the sphenopalatine foramen with tumor extension to pterygopalatine fossa.

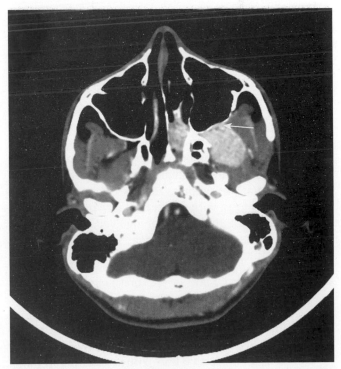

Fig. 44.3 Computed tomography (CT) scan, axial view showing bowing of the posterior wall of the maxillary sinus: Holman–Miller sign.

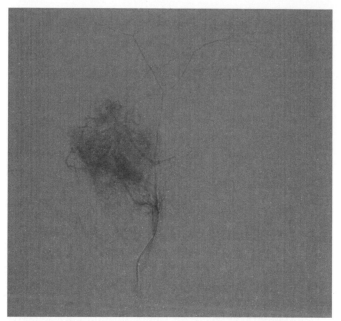

Fig. 44.4 Digital subtraction angiography showing the tumor blush. The feeding vessel is from the maxillary artery.

Pearl

JNA is a clinical and radiological diagnosis. Probing or biopsy should not be done as it can cause profuse bleeding.

■ Staging

Staging is required for counseling, treatment planning, predicting outcomes, and reporting.

- *Staging by Andrews et al (1989):*
  - **Stage I:** The tumor is limited to the nasopharynx and the nasal cavity. There is negligible bone destruction.
  - **Stage II:** The tumor invades the PPF, or the maxillary, ethmoid, or sphenoid sinus with bone destruction.
  - **Stage IIIa:** The tumor invades the infratemporal fossa or orbit with no intracranial extension.
  - **Stage IIIb:** The tumor invades the infratemporal fossa or orbit with intracranial extradural extension.
  - **Stage IVa:** The tumor invades the cavernous sinus and pituitary fossa with intracranial intradural extension, but the optic chiasma is not involved.
  - **Stage IVb:** The tumor invades the cavernous sinus and pituitary fossa with intracranial intradural extension and optic chiasma invasion.

■ Treatment

- The aim of treatment is to remove the tumor with minimal blood loss and morbidity. The bleeding can be minimized by preoperative DSA with embolization. Direct tumor embolization can be done using cyanoacrylate glue or onyx. Internal maxillary artery ligation or carotid control (temporary clamp on the ipsilateral external carotid artery), prior to resecting the tumor, will also facilitate removal with minimal bleeding.
- Flutamide, a nonsteroidal androgen receptor blocker, can be given prior to surgery for 6 weeks. It causes volume reduction and reduced vascularity in larger tumors.
- The removal of JNA can be done by an endoscopic endonasal approach or an open approach. The endoscopic approach, with improved instrumentation and expertise, is the preferred technique.
- The various open approaches that can be used to facilitate removal of the tumor include a midfacial degloving approach, lateral rhinotomy/maxillary swing, transpalatal, Le Forte I, and anterior subcranial approach. Combined approaches can be used for intracranial extensions.
- Recurrence can be as high as 35%.

Other Benign Tumors

Hairy polyp/dermoid comprises ectoderm and mesodermal tissue. It can be associated with other anomalies like cleft palate, external ear deformities, choanal atresia, and left carotid artery atresia. It may be asymptomatic or present as a polypoid mass causing respiratory and feeding problems.

Teratoma comprises all three germinal layers. It presents as a lobular, solid cystic lesion. It is often seen protruding into the oropharynx. Serum alpha fetoprotein levels are raised in immature teratomas. Complete excision is the treatment.

Hamartoma is an excess or haphazard growth of local differentiated tissue, which can be epithelial, mesenchymal, or mixed. It appears as polypoidal mass. These do not infiltrate the surrounding tissues.

Craniopharyngioma arise from epithelial remnants of Rathke's pouch (from which the anterior pituitary gland develops).

Thornwaldt's cyst presents in the midline, deep to the pharyngobasilar fascia. When infected, it can cause postnasal drip, nasal block, neck or occipital pain, and middle ear effusion. Treatment is by marsupialization.

Malignant Tumors of the Nasopharynx

The majority (80–99%) of nasopharyngeal malignancies arise from the lining epithelium, and histologically are variants of squamous cell carcinomas.

Malignant lesions of the nasopharynx are classified based on tissue of origin as the following:

- *Epithelial*: Keratinizing and nonkeratinizing carcinoma.
- *Embryonal*: Chordoma.
- *Lymphoid*: Lymphoma.
- *Mesodermal*: Rhabdomyosarcoma, hemangiopericytoma, and plasmacytoma.
- *Salivary*: Adenoid cystic carcinoma and mucoepidermoid carcinoma.
- *Metastasis* from the breast, renal cell, hepatocellular, and bronchogenic carcinomas.

Nasopharyngeal Carcinoma

Nasopharyngeal carcinomas (NPCs) are epithelial tumors that originate from the nasopharyngeal mucosa. The common site of involvement is the posterolateral part of the nasopharynx, that is, *the fossa of Rosenmuller.*

■ Epidemiology

The incidence and geographic distribution of NPC vary with respect to multiple factors like genetic susceptibility, environment, diet, and personal habits. NPC is endemic to Southeast Asia (Hong Kong and Singapore), southern China, North Africa, and Alaska where there is a high incidence. It constitutes 0.41% of all cancers in India. The male-to-female ratio is 3:1.

■ Etiology

Various factors have been associated with NPC:

- Environmental factors include nitrosamines from dry salted fish and vegetables, and smoke from burning incense sticks and hard wood.
- Epstein–Barr virus (EBV) is associated with the non-keratinizing form of NPC. The immunoglobulin A (IgA) of two antigens, that is, viral capsid antigen (VCA) and early antigen (EA), can be detected by immunofluorescence.
- Tobacco use and alcohol may increase the risk although a clear association has not been proven.
- Genetic susceptibility: There is high risk among Chinese in Southern China and southeast Asia. There is higher incidence in family/siblings among Chinese. Certain human leukocyte antigens (HLA) are more prevalent in NPC. Deletions of some chromosomes and inactivation of *p16* have also been noted.
- Occupational: Exposure to nickel, chromium, radioactive metal, and inhalation of chemical fumes and formaldehyde can cause NPC.
- Chinese herbal medicine and nutritional deficiencies (vitamins) have also been implicated.
- Patients with dermatomyositis have a 10% risk of developing NPC.

■ Pathology

According to the World Health Organization (WHO) classification, NPCs are of three histologic types:

- Keratinizing squamous cell carcinoma (WHO 1)
- Nonkeratinizing carcinoma: differentiated (WHO 2a) and undifferentiated (WHO 2b).
- Basaloid squamous cell carcinomas are a rare variety.

■ Clinical Features

The symptoms are based on the spread to surrounding structures (like the bone of skull base and the parapharyngeal space) and through the foramina (lacerum, ovale, and rotundum), and metastasis.

- Males between 30 and 60 years are affected. Younger individuals may also be affected in endemic areas.
- *Nasal symptoms* include nasal obstruction and nasal/postnasal discharge (blood-stained) epistaxis, blood-stained saliva; hyponasal speech due to mass in nasopharynx.
- *Aural symptoms*: Conductive hearing loss due to serous otitis media may be the presenting symptom. It could also present with ear block and tinnitus.
- *Orbital symptoms* are diplopia (**Fig. 44.5**) and ophthalmoplegia (third, fourth, and sixth cranial nerves), proptosis (orbital extension), and blindness (second cranial nerve).
- *Neurological symptoms* are facial pain (fifth cranial nerve) and jugular foramen syndrome when the 9th, 10th, and 11th cranial nerves are involved, which may be due to the pressure of lymph nodes on the nerves. Horner's syndrome may be present. Commonly the 5th, 6th, 9th, 10th, and 12th cranial nerves can be involved.
- *Headache*: Skull base erosion and secondary sinusitis.

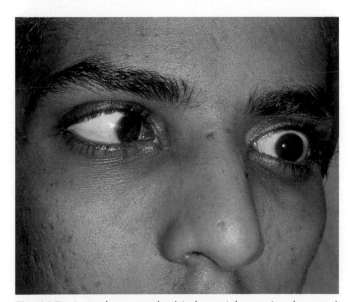

Fig. 44.5 Lateral rectus palsy (sixth cranial nerve involvement) in nasopharyngeal carcinoma, left side.

- *Trotter's triad* (sinus of Morgagni syndrome) is ipsilateral conductive deafness/serous otitis media (due to eustachian tube dysfunction), facial pain/neuralgia (due to involvement of the mandibular division of the trigeminal nerve in the region of the foramen ovale), and palatal asymmetry (due to infiltration of the levator veli palatini muscle).
- *Neck swellings* may be the presenting symptom due to metastatic cervical lymph nodes, which may be unilateral or bilateral. The retropharyngeal group of lymph nodes are the first to be involved. The second echelon of lymph nodes are levels II and V. Lymph node metastasis occurs in 60% of the cases. Level III may also be involved.
- Other symptoms like neck pain, trismus, or weight loss may be present.
- The lesion in the nasopharynx may be exophytic, ulcerative, or infiltrative (submucosal; **Fig. 44.6**).
- Distant metastasis can occur to the bone, lung, liver, brain, and retroperitoneal lymph nodes.

■ Diagnosis

- Diagnostic nasal endoscopy and biopsy are done to assess and confirm the diagnosis. Immunohistochemistry can be done to rule out lymphoma.
- IgA antibodies to VCA and immunoglobulin G (IgG) antibodies to EA to assess for EBV can be performed.
- Fine-needle aspiration cytology of the metastatic lymph node can be performed.
- Contrast-enhanced CT scan delineates the primary growth, erosion of the skull base (**Fig. 44.7**) and clivus, and parapharyngeal, retropharyngeal, and intracranial

extensions. Metastatic cervical nodes can also be appreciated.
- MRI is done for intracranial extension and soft-tissue extension.
- CT scan of the thorax can be done to assess for secondaries or second primary in the lung. Ultrasound of the abdomen is done to rule out liver secondaries.
- Positron emission tomography (PET) CT scan will delineate the primary, metastatic lymph nodes and secondaries. It is also useful for follow-up assessment.
- Pure tone audiometry: A baseline audiogram is done to diagnose serous otitis media, and also prior to starting chemotherapy because it can cause ototoxicity.

TNM Classification (American Joint Committee on Cancer)

According to the American Joint Committee on Cancer (AJCC), 8th edition, staging is done based on clinical and radiological findings.

- **T staging:**
  - T1: Nasopharynx, oropharynx, or nasal cavity without parapharyngeal extension.
  - T2: Parapharyngeal extension and adjacent soft-tissue involvement (medial pterygoid, lateral pterygoid, and prevertebral muscles).
  - T3: Bony structures (skull base and cervical vertebra) and/or paranasal sinuses.
  - T4: Intracranial extension, cranial nerve, hypopharynx, orbit, and extensive soft-tissue involvement (beyond the lateral surface of the lateral pterygoid muscle and the parotid gland).

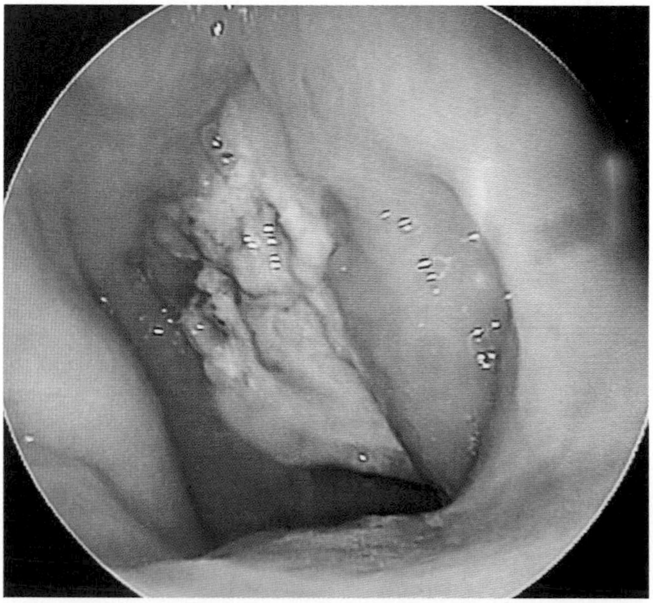

Fig. 44.6 Endoscopic view of the left nasopharynx showing white-colored slough covering the tumor over the left fossa of Rosenmuller.

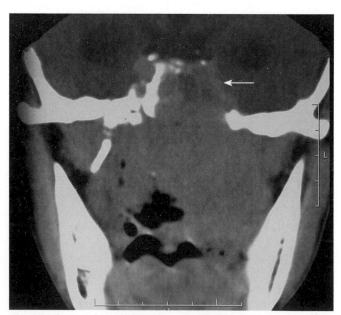

Fig. 44.7 Contrast-enhanced computed tomography (CT) scan (coronal cut) showing tumor invasion of the skull base and the sphenoid sinus.

- **N staging:**
  - N0: No regional lymph node involvement.
  - N1: Retropharyngeal (regardless of laterality); cervical unilateral <6 cm, and above the caudal border of the cricoid cartilage.
  - N2: Cervical, bilateral <6 cm, and above the caudal border of the cricoid cartilage.
  - N3: >6 cm, and/or below the caudal border of the cricoid cartilage.
- **M staging:**
  - MX: Distant metastasis cannot be assessed.
  - M0: No metastasis.
  - M1: Distant metastasis is present.
  - Stage I: T1, N0, and M0.
    Stage II: T2, N0–N1, and M0; T1, N1, and M0.
  - Stage III: T3, N0–N2, and M0; T1–T2, N2, and M0.
  - Stage IVa: T4, N1–N2, and M0.
  - Stage IVb: any T, N3, and M0.
  - Stage IVc: any T, any N, and M1.

■ Treatment

- **Radiotherapy:** It is the mainstay of treatment for NPC (Stages I and II). A total dose of 6,000 to 7,000 cGy (200 cGy per day, 5 days a week over 6–7 weeks), covering the primary tumor and the cervical lymph node region, is administered. NPC is usually radiosensitive. Intensity-modulated radiotherapy (IMRT) has the advantage of better outcomes with less complications and morbidity.
- **Chemotherapy:** It is given along with radiotherapy as neoadjuvant or concurrent, in locoregionally advanced stages (Stages III and IV). Cisplatin and 5-fluorouracil are commonly used. Palliative chemotherapy is sometimes given in advanced disease with distant metastasis.
- **Recurrent and residual disease:** Re-radiation is possible only after 2 to 3 years due to its local tissue reaction, and toxicity to the surrounding structures including the cervical spine; radiation-induced myelitis can occur.

For cervical nodes, a radical neck dissection can be done. For local disease, a nasopharyngectomy can be done via an endoscopic, transpalatal, robotic, or maxillary swing approach.
- Molecular-targeted therapy with bevacizumab has been tried for radiorecurrent/residual disease, and distant metastatic disease.

Other Malignant Tumors

They are rare and include the following:
- **Lymphomas:** Non-Hodgkin's (B-cell type) is more common than Hodgkin's.
- **Rhabdomyosarcomas:** These are embryonal type. These tumors occur rarely, and are more common in children.
- **Plasmacytoma:** It may be solitary or part of a generalized multiple myeloma.
- **Chordoma:** It arises from the remnant of the notochord; it is locally aggressive.
- **Adenoid cystic carcinoma:** It usually arises from minor salivary glands.

Points to Ponder

- Tumors of the nasopharynx are uncommon.
- Angiofibroma is the most common benign tumor of the nasopharynx seen in adolescent males. It is commonly treated by endoscopic resection.
- Nasopharyngeal tumors present with symptoms including nasal obstruction, epistaxis, and otological symptoms.
- NPC is the most common malignant tumor of the nasopharynx.
- NPC is commonly treated by radiotherapy or chemoradiation, depending on the stage of the disease.

Case-Based Questions

1. **A 16-year-old adolescent boy presented with a 4-month history of left-sided, recurrent, profuse, unprovoked epistaxis. On diagnostic nasal endoscopy, there was a reddish-purple mass with prominent vessels on its surface occupying the posterior part of the left nasal cavity. Contrast-enhanced CT scan showed a highly enhancing mass extending to the PPF.**

   a. What would be the most likely diagnosis?

   b. What is the Holman–Miller sign?

   c. What approach would be best suited for removal of this mass?

   d. What is the role of DSA?

Answers
a. JNA.
b. Anterior bowing of the posterior wall of the maxillary sinus due to extension of the tumor into the PPF.
c. Endoscopic (transnasal) approach.
d. DSA will confirm the vascular nature of the tumor, delineate the feeding vessels, and allow for guided embolization of the feeding vessels through the external carotid artery system.

2. **A 48-year-old Chinese male presented with a 3-month history of bilateral upper neck swelling. He had right-**

sided ear block sensation for the last 2 months. Diagnostic nasal endoscopy showed an exophytic lesion in the right posterolateral part of the nasopharynx adjacent to the eustachian tube (torus tubarius).

a. What is the most likely diagnosis?
b. How would you confirm the diagnosis?
c. What is Trotter's triad?
d. What is the role of various imaging modalities?
e. What is the treatment?

Answers

a. NPC.

b. Biopsy from the lesion. IgA of VCA and EA for detection of Epstein–Barr virus. Immunohistochemistry is also done.

c. Trotter's triad is unilateral conductive hearing loss, facial pain, and palatal asymmetry.

d. Contrast-enhanced CT scan or MRI to assess the primary tumor and regional lymph nodes, and CT scan of thorax for the second primary or secondaries in the lung. Perform an ultrasound of the abdomen to rule out liver metastasis. PET CT scan can be done for assessment of the primary and metastatic disease and for follow-up.

e. As it is in an advanced stage, chemotherapy with radiotherapy is the treatment of choice.

Frequently Asked Questions

1. What is the commonest site for malignancy of the nasopharynx?

2. Describe the etiological factors of carcinoma of the nasopharynx.

3. How will you manage a patient with malignancy of the nasopharynx?

4. What is the etiology of juvenile nasopharyngeal angiofibroma?

5. What radiological investigations will help establish a diagnosis of juvenile nasopharyngeal angiofibroma?

6. What is the Holman–Miller sign?

Endnote

The highest rate of NPC is in Hong Kong and Southern China. Besides the genetic susceptibility of the Chinese population, one other factor considered for the development of NPC is eating salt-cured fish and meat. The meat is coated with dry salt or the food items are immersed in a salt solution. The incidence of NPC is highest in areas where salt-cured food items are eaten, proving the etiological link.

45 Tumors of the Oropharynx

Vijendra Shenoy S. and Sweekritha N. Bhat

The competency covered in this chapter is as follows:

SU20.1 Describe the etiopathogenesis, symptoms, and signs of oropharyngeal cancer. Enumerate the appropriate investigations and discuss the principles of its treatment.

Introduction

The oropharynx is an important structure at the crossroads of the nasopharynx, oral cavity, and laryngeal and hypopharyngeal regions (**Fig. 45.1**). It performs the role of a respiratory and alimentary conduit and has an important part in normal swallowing and speech.

■ Benign Tumors

About 10% of all oropharyngeal tumors are benign.
The benign tumors/lesions can be congenital or acquired.
The congenital lesions include the following:
- Vascular malformations.
- Lingual thyroid.
- Dermoid cysts.

Acquired lesions include the following:
- Inflammatory lesions like abscesses.
- Neoplastic lesions like hemangiomas or pleomorphic adenomas.
- Mucous cysts.
- Papillomas.

Lingual Thyroid

The base of the tongue is a common location for an ectopic thyroid tissue. Around 90% of all ectopic thyroid tissue are located in this region, because the thyroid fails to descent into the neck during development. It is located in the midline and is usually asymptomatic, but it can be associated with hypothyroidism. If the patient is symptomatic, they will complain of a lump in the throat, dysphagia, and breathing difficulty. Treatment includes thyroid replacement therapy, which may reduce the size of the lingual thyroid and the symptoms. But in euthyroid individuals with enlarged ectopic thyroid, treatment is surgical excision.

The routes of excision include transoral, transhyoid, and transcervical by a lateral pharyngotomy approach.

Vallecular Cyst

These are benign cystic lesions arising from the vallecula or the lingual surface of the epiglottis (**Fig. 45.2**). The vallecula has numerous mucous glands and their ducts get blocked due to trauma or inflammation leading to the development of mucous retention cysts or vallecular cysts. The cysts are usually small and the patient is asymptomatic. These are detected incidentally during clinical examination or during imaging. Gradually, the cyst can attain a large size resulting in symptoms like breathing difficulty, stridor, dysphagia, and hot potato voice. Treatment is surgery. Surgery includes deroofing, marsupialization, and excision with laser.

Papilloma of the Oropharynx

Squamous papillomas are benign, exophytic, warty growths protruding from the surface, squamous, epithelium of the oropharynx (**Fig. 45.3**). It is thought to be caused by the human papilloma virus (HPV). It is asymptomatic and appears as a pedunculated, sessile, or verrucous lesion. Common sites include the tonsil and the base of the tongue. Large papillomas can cause symptoms like dysphagia, globus sensation, dry cough, and throat irritation. Treatment is surgical excision.

■ Malignancy of the Oropharynx

The oropharynx accounts for about 10 to 12% of all head and neck cancers. Squamous cell carcinoma is the most common malignancy. Based on the other tissues in the oropharynx, minor salivary gland malignancy and lymphoma can also occur. Sarcomas are rare. The various subsites of the oropharynx are depicted in **Fig. 45.4**.

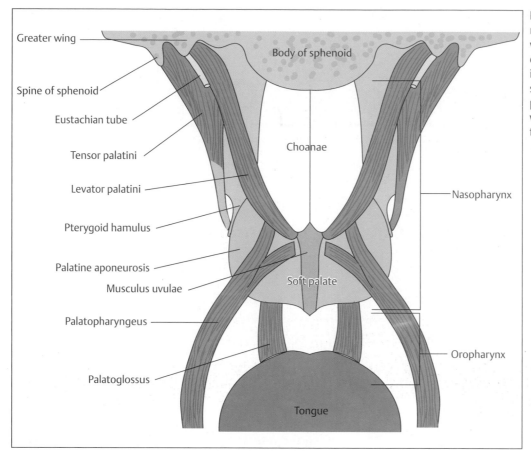

Greater wing
Spine of sphenoid
Eustachian tube
Tensor palatini
Levator palatini
Pterygoid hamulus
Palatine aponeurosis
Musculus uvulae
Palatopharyngeus
Palatoglossus

Body of sphenoid
Choanae
Soft palate
Tongue
Nasopharynx
Oropharynx

Fig. 45.1 Diagram of the nasopharynx and oropharynx when viewed from posteriorly". Nasopharynx can be indicated with a "}" from the sphenoid spine to the soft palate and the Oropharynx with a "}" from the soft palate to the tongue.

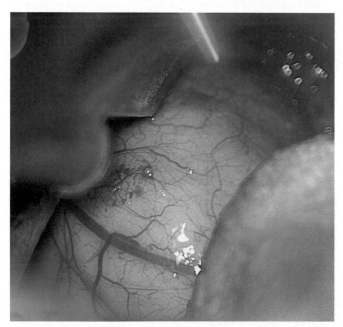

Fig. 45.2 Large vallecular cyst in an adult.

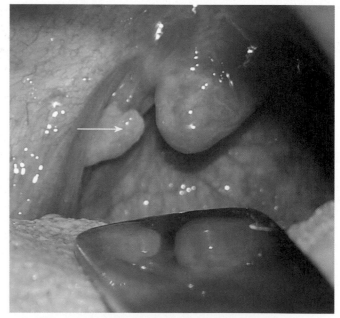

Fig. 45.3 Squamous papilloma of the right tonsil.

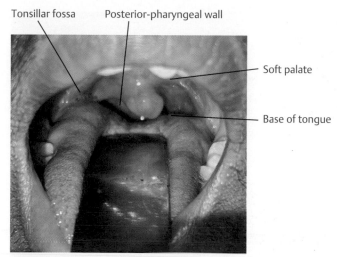

Fig. 45.4 Picture depicting the various subsites of the oropharynx.

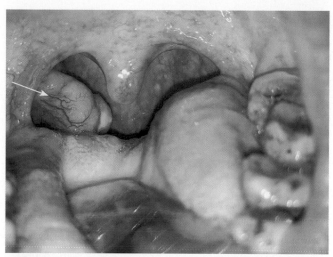

Fig. 45.5 Growth over the right tonsil.

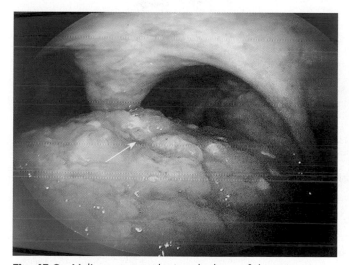

Fig. 45.6 Malignant growth over the base of the tongue.

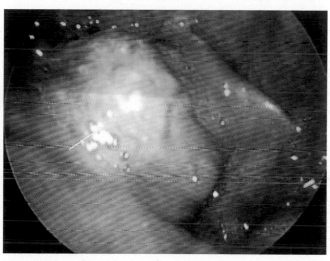

Fig. 45.7 Malignant growth in the vallecula pushing the epiglottis posteriorly.

■ Sites of Malignancy in the Oropharynx and Incidence

- *Laterally*: Tonsillar region (tonsil, anterior pillar, and posterior pillar)—60% (**Fig. 45.5**).
- *Anteriorly*: Base of the tongue, vallecula, and the lingual surface of the epiglottis—25% (**Figs. 45.6** and **45.7**).
- *Superiorly*: Soft palate—10% (**Fig. 45.8**).
- *Posteriorly*: Posterior pharyngeal wall—5% (**Fig. 45.9**).

■ Etiology

- Tobacco and alcohol act synergistically.
- Betel quid.

- HPV 16 & 18 genotypes (refer to **Table 45.1** for the contrasting features between HPV and non-HPV tumors).
- Dietary deficiency of carotenes, vitamin A, and riboflavin.
- Others: leather industry products, poor oral hygiene, etc.

Pearl

The incidence of oropharyngeal cancers has been increasing over the last 20 years. The HPV has been implicated as the etiology for this steady rise in cases. An HPV infection increases the risk of developing oropharyngeal carcinoma by 32 times, whereas smoking increases the risk by 3 times and alcohol by 2.5 times.

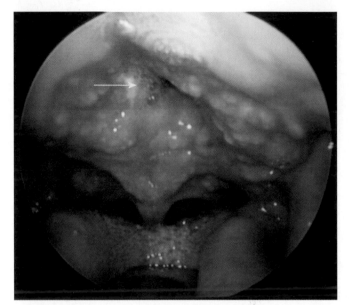

Fig. 45.8 Malignant growth over the soft palate.

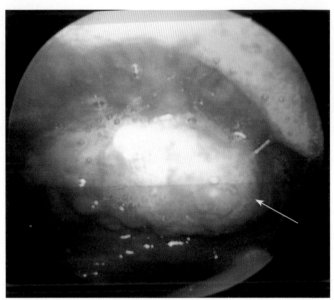

Fig. 45.9 Malignant growth over the posterior pharyngeal wall.

Table 45.1 Differences between HPV and non-HPV tumors of the oropharynx

Characteristics	Non-HPV	HPV +
Age	5–7 decades	4–5 decades (younger)
Sex	Males	Females
Cause	Tobacco and alcohol	HPV 16 (orogenital sex)
Socioeconomic status	Poor	Higher
Sites	No specific site	Base tongue and tonsil
Differentiation	Well to moderate	Poorly differentiated
Dysplastic epithelium	Prior dysplasia +	No dysplasia
Immunohistochemistry	p16 lost	p16 intact
Locoregional recurrence	High	Low
Prognosis	Variable	Better

Abbreviation: HPV, human papilloma virus.

■ Clinical Presentation

The clinical presentation of the tumor depends on the site (**Fig. 45.2**).

Initial Disease

- It is asymptomatic in the early stage.
- It shows nonspecific symptoms like soreness/fullness/globus/foreign body sensation, etc.
- There may be painless cervical lymphadenopathy.

Advanced Disease

- Foul odor from the mouth.
- Dysphagia/odynophagia (fixity of deep muscles of the base of the tongue).
- Unexplained deep pharyngeal pain.
- Difficulty in speech (mass effect or involvement of the soft palate and fixity of the tongue).
- Bleeding.
- Otalgia (referred pain due to involvement of cranial nerves IX and X).

- Trismus (pterygoid muscle involvement).
- Spread to the adjoining areas can occur, that is, oral cavity, larynx, hypopharynx, and nasopharynx.

Neck Nodes

- In all, 15 to 75% have cervical lymphadenopathy, commonly at levels II, III, and IV.
- Presentation may be as a cervical carcinoma with unknown primary (metastasis of unknown origin).
- High incidence of cervical metastasis is due to rich lymphatics.
- Midline and paramedian tumors in the oropharynx have bilateral lymphatic spread.

Distant Metastasis

- About 5 to 10% at presentation.
- Sites: Lungs > bone > liver.

■ Evaluation

Physical Examination

- Assess the size, location, and appearance of the lesion, and mouth opening.
- Check the mobility of the tongue.
- Assess the induration/depth of invasion by digital palpation.
- Check the palpation of the neck for cervical lymphadenopathy.

Endoscopy

- Fiberoptic laryngoscopy to evaluate for the posterior extent of the lesion and the upper aerodigestive tract for any second primary lesions.
- Peroral panendoscopy to assess the lesion and look for a second primary.
- Nasal endoscopy to look for nasopharyngeal extension in case of soft palate and posterior pharyngeal lesions.

Radiological Evaluation

- Contrast-enhanced computed tomography (CT) scan of the neck: Look for primary and nodal disease, bony invasion, and destruction of the following: skull base/pterygoid plates/mandible.
- CT of the thorax is done to rule out distant metastasis or a second primary in the lung.
- Magnetic resonance imaging (MRI): This offers better soft-tissue delineation, base of the tongue invasion and extension to the parapharyngeal space, involvement of the pterygoid musculature, masticator space, and skull base, and to detect perineural invasion.

- Ultrasound (US) of the neck is done to look for nonpalpable nodal disease.
- US-guided fine-needle aspiration cytology (FNAC) can be done from a suspected node.
- Positron emission tomography CT (PET-CT) can be done to assess the primary, regional nodes, and distant metastasis, especially in advanced disease, and posttreatment assessment for recurrence.

Examination under Anesthesia

- Biopsy from the primary tumor; histopathological examination should include immunohistochemistry (p16) and for the presence of HPV deoxyribonucleic acid (DNA).
- It is done to determine the extent of the tumor and operability, if surgery is feasible.

American Joint Committee on Cancer Classification and Staging (8th Edition) of Oropharyngeal Tumors

The TNM (tumor, node, and metastasis) staging for oropharyngeal tumors depends on whether it is mediated by HPV or not. Therefore, there are two sets of classification:
- HPV-mediated oropharyngeal cancer.
- Non-HPV-mediated oropharyngeal cancer.

■ TNM Classification for HPV-Mediated Oropharyngeal Cancer

The TNM classification for HPV-mediated oropharyngeal cancer is presented in **Table 45.2**.

Staging for HPV-Associated Oropharyngeal Cancer

Staging for HPV-associated oropharyngeal cancer is presented in **Table 45.3**.

■ TNM Classification for Non-HPV-Mediated Oropharyngeal Cancer

The TNM classification for non-HPV-mediated oropharyngeal cancer is presented in **Table 45.4**.

Staging for HPV-Negative Oropharyngeal Cancer

Staging for HPV-negative oropharyngeal cancer is presented in **Table 45.5**.

Table 45.2 TNM classification for human papilloma virus (HPV) mediated oropharyngeal cancer

T Category[3]	Criteria
T0	No primary tumor identified
T1	Tumor size ≤ 2 cm in greatest dimension
T2	Tumor size > 2 cm but ≤ 4 cm in greatest dimension
T3	Tumor size > 4 cm in greatest dimension or extension to lingual surface of epiglottis
T4	Moderately advanced tumor invading larynx, extrinsic tongue muscles, medial pterygoid, hard palate, or mandible or beyond

Clinical N Category	Criteria
Nx	Regional nodes cannot be assessed
N0	No regional nodal metastasis
N1	Metastasis to one or more ipsilateral nodes, ≤ 6 cm
N2	Metastasis to contralateral or bilateral lymph nodes, ≤ 6 cm
N3	Metastasis in any cervical lymph node > 6 cm

Pathologic N Category	Criteria
Nx	Regional nodes cannot be assessed
pN0	No regional nodal metastasis identified
pN1	Metastasis to 4 or fewer lymph nodes
pN2	Metastasis to 5 or fewer lymph nodes

M Category	Criteria
M0	Absence of distant metastasis
M1	Presence of distant metastasis

Table 45.3 Staging for human papilloma virus (HPV) associated oropharyngeal cancer

T Category	N Category	M Category	Stage Group
T0, T1, or T2	N0 or N1	M0	I
T0, T1, or T2	N2	M0	II
T3	N0, N1, or N2	M0	II
T0, T1, T2, T3, or T4	N3	M0	III
T4	N0, N1, N2, or N3	M0	III
Any	Any N	M1	IV

Management

Most oropharyngeal carcinomas are treated depending on the stage of the tumor.

- Stages I and II:
  - The primary treatment is surgery or radiotherapy, but surgery is not preferred in most centers because of the difficulties in reconstruction in these subsites, and the associated morbidity.
- Stages III and IV:
  - Concurrent chemotherapy and radiation is the standard of care for the locally advanced disease.

The general principles of treatment are described in **Table 45.6**.

■ Surgical Approaches

- Transoral: Small lesions can be resected with the following:
  - Cautery.
  - CO_2 or KTP laser.
  - Transoral robotic surgery (TORS).
- Open approaches:
  - Mandibulotomy or mandibular swing approach.

Table 45.4   TNM classification for non-HPV-mediated oropharyngeal cancer

T category[3]	Criteria
Tx	Primary tumor cannot be assessed
Tis	Carcinoma in situ
T1	Tumor size > 2 cm in greatest dimension
T2	Tumor size > 2 cm but ≤ 4 cm in greatest dimension
T3	Tumor size > 4 cm in greatest dimension or extension to lingual surface of epiglottis
T4	Moderately advanced or very advanced tumor
T4a	Moderately advanced tumor invading larynx, extrinsic tongue muscles, medial pterygoid, hard palate, or mandible
T4b	Very advanced tumor invading lateral pterygoid muscle, pterygoid plate, lateral nasopharynx, or skull base or encasement of the carotid artery
Clinical N category	**Criteria**
Nx	Regional nodes cannot be assessed
N0	No regional nodal metastasis
N1	Metastasis to single ipsilateral node, ≤ 3 cm and ENE-negative
N2	Metastasis in a single ipsilateral lymph node > 3 cm but ≤ 6 cm in greatest dimension and ENE-negative or metastases in multiple ipsilateral lymph nodes, ≤ 6 cm in greatest dimension and ENE-negative or metastases in bilateral or contralateral lymph nodes, ≤ 6 cm in greatest dimension and ENE-negative
N2a	Metastasis in a single ipsilateral lymph node > 3 cm but < 6 cm in greatest dimension and ENE-negative
N2b	Metastasis in single ipsilateral lymph node ≤ 6 cm in greatest dimension and ENE-negative
N2c	Metastases in bilateral or contralateral lymph nodes, ≤ 6 cm in greatest dimension and ENE-negative
N3	Metastasis in lymph node > 6 cm in greatest dimension and ENE-negative or metastasis in any lymph node(s) and clinically overt ENE-positive
N3a	Metastasis in a lymph node > 6 cm in greatest dimension and ENE-negative
N3b	Metastasis in any lymph node(s) and clinically overt ENE-positive
Pathologic N category	**Criteria**
Nx	Regional nodes cannot be assessed
N0	No regional nodal metastasis
N1	Metastasis to single ipsilateral node, ≤ 3 cm and ENE-negative
N2	Metastasis to single ipsilateral node, ≤ 3 cm and ENE-positive or metastasis in a single ipsilateral lymph node, > 3 cm but ≤ 6 cm in greatest dimension and ENE-negative or metastases in multiple ipsilateral lymph nodes, < 6 cm in greatest dimension and ENE-negative or metastases in bilateral or contralateral lymph nodes, ≤ 6 cm in greatest dimension and ENE-negative
N2a	Metastasis to single ipsilateral node, ≤ 3 cm and ENE-positive or metastasis in a single ipsilateral lymph node > 3 cm but ≤ 6 cm in greatest dimension and ENE-negative
N2b	Metastases in multiple ipsilateral lymph nodes, ≤ 6 cm in greatest dimension and ENE-negative
N2c	Metastases in bilateral or contralateral lymph nodes, ≤ 6 cm in greatest dimension and ENE-negative
N3	Metastasis in a lymph node > 6 cm in greatest dimension and ENE-negative or metastasis in a single ipsilateral lymph node > 3 cm in greatest dimension and ENE-positive or metastases in multiple ipsilateral, contralateral, or bilateral lymph nodes, with any ENE-positive
N3a	Metastasis in a lymph node > 6 cm in greatest dimension and ENE-negative
N3b	Metastasis in a single ipsilateral lymph node > 3 cm in greatest dimension and ENE-positive or metastasis in multiple ipsilateral, contralateral, or bilateral lymph node with any ENE-positive or a single contralateral node < 3 cm and ENE-positive
M category	Criteria
M0	Absence of distant metastasis
M1	Presence of distant metastasis

Table 45.5 Staging for human papilloma virus (HPV) negative oropharyngeal cancer

T Category	N Category	M Category	Stage Group
Tis	N0	M0	0
T1	N0	M0	I
T2	N0	M0	II
T3	N0	M0	III
T1, T2, T3	N1	M0	III
T4a	N0, N1	M0	IVA
T1, T2, T3, T4a	N2	M0	IVA
Any T	N3	M0	IVB
T4b	Any N	M0	IVB
Any T	Any N	M1	IVC

Abbreviation: HPV, human papilloma virus.

Table 45.6 General principles of treatment for oropharyngeal carcinomas

Definitive radiotherapy	Concurrent chemotherapy with radiotherapy	Surgery	Palliative
Early T1/T2 disease without nodal metastasis	Early disease with cervical metastasis or in advanced stage	Residual disease In selective advanced cases along with adjuvant therapy	Distant metastasis Locally or regionally advanced or recurrent disease

- Midline vallecular (pharyngotomy) approach with pull-through.
- Composite resection with mandibulectomy.
- Neck dissection is done with the primary surgery.
- Salvage neck dissection is done for residual lymph node disease (post radiotherapy residual nodes).

Radiotherapy

- Curative dose: 66–70 Gy, that is, 2.0 Gy/fraction over 6 to 7 weeks.

Palliative

- Chemotherapy or radiotherapy.
- For swallowing, a nasogastric tube or feeding gastrostomy (percutaneous endoscopic gastrostomy) may be used in the presence of dysphagia and/or aspiration.

- Tracheostomy may be performed in case of stridor and/or aspiration.
- Pain management.

Points to Ponder

- Benign tumors of the oropharynx are rare.
- Squamous cell carcinoma is the most common malignant tumor.
- The commonest site of involvement is the tonsillar region.
- HPV is an important etiological agent for oropharyngeal tumors, and the worldwide incidence is increasing because of the rise in HPV infection.
- The TNM classification for oropharyngeal tumors depends on whether it is mediated by HPV or not. Therefore, there are two sets of classification, HPV mediated and non-HPV-mediated tumors.

Case-Based Questions

1. **A 57-year-old man, chronic smoker, presented with a history of right-sided throat pain with referred otalgia. On examination of the throat, there was an ulceroproliferative growth involving the right tonsil extending to the anterior pillar. There was a 2 × 1 cm hard right level II cervical lymph node.**

   a. What is the most likely diagnosis?

   b. What are the investigations required to assess the condition and confirm the diagnosis?

   c. What is the treatment?

   Answers

   a. Malignancy of the right tonsil.

   b. Investigations include biopsy from the tonsil, rigid telescopy of the oropharynx and hypopharynx to determine the extent of the tumor, and a contrast-enhanced CT scan to map the disease in the oropharynx (primary), neck (regional nodes), and thorax (distant metastasis).

   c. For advanced stage tumors, T3 or T4 with neck nodes, organ preserving concurrent chemoradiation is administered.

2. **A 45-year-old man noticed a swelling in the back of the throat. He was seen in the ear, nose, and throat (ENT) Department where they noticed a small ulceroproliferative growth, 1.5 cm in diameter, over the soft palate on the right side, 1 cm lateral to the base of the uvula. There were no neck nodes or signs of metastasis.**

   a. What is the probable diagnosis?

   b. What is the clinical TNM staging of this tumor?

   c. What relevant investigations should be performed?

   d. What is the treatment?

   Answers

   a. When an ulceroproliferative lesion is encountered, in an oropharyngeal subsite like the soft palate, a malignant tumor like squamous cell carcinoma must be kept in mind. In the soft palate, 80% of the malignancies are squamous cell carcinomas.

   b. T1 N0 M0. The size of the tumor is less than 2 cm, and there were no neck nodes or distant metastasis.

   c. A contrast-enhanced CT scan of the head and neck will help in determining the extent of the disease and allow an accurate staging of the tumor, including the sites of metastatic nodes if any. A metastatic workup by CT thorax and ultrasound abdomen is done for distant metastasis.

   A biopsy can be easily obtained from this site in the outpatient department under local anesthesia. The biopsy should be carried out from the edge of the tumor, rather than the necrotic center.

   d. When the tumor is small, either T1 or T2, involving the soft palate, the treatment is either surgery or radiotherapy. Because of the difficulties in reconstruction of the soft palate, if the patient undergoes surgery, radiation is the recommended treatment in T1, T2, and T3 lesions.

Frequently Asked Questions

1. What are the oropharyngeal subsites?

2. What are the etiological factors for oropharyngeal tumors?

3. What is the role of HPV in oropharyngeal malignancy?

4. What is the treatment for early oropharyngeal malignancy?

5. How will you manage advanced tumors of the oropharynx?

Endnote

Vallecula means depression. The vallecula in the oropharynx consists of a mucosa-lined depression, posterior to the base of the tongue on either side of the median glossoepiglottic folds. The function of the vallecula is to trap or collect saliva during sleep. Trapping of the saliva prevents the swallowing reflex from being activated constantly during sleep. It is also an important landmark during intubation of a patient for anesthesia for surgery. The tip of a Macintosh laryngoscope is inserted deep into the vallecula so that the epiglottis is lifted up, allowing good visualization of the laryngeal inlet and vocal cords.

46 Tumors of the Hypopharynx

Vijendra Shenoy S. and Sanchit Bajpai

The competency covered in this chapter is as follows:

EN4.46 Describe the clinical features, investigations, and principles of management of malignancy of the hypopharynx.

Introduction

The pharynx is divided into the nasopharynx, oropharynx, and hypopharynx (**Fig. 46.1**). The hypopharynx has three regions (**Figs. 46.2** and **46.3**):

- Pyriform fossa.
- Postcricoid region.
- Posterior pharyngeal wall.

Hypopharyngeal cancers arise from the mucosa of one of the three anatomical subsites of the hypopharynx. It is characterized by advanced disease at presentation mainly because of its abundant lymphatic drainage, and its anatomic diversity, which allows tumors to grow silently for a substantial period of time before symptoms occur. Hypopharyngeal cancers have an unfavorable prognosis among all cancers due to their aggressive behavior at the site involved. The quality of life is affected as it compromises swallowing, voice, and airway. Around 95% of hypopharyngeal malignancies are squamous cell carcinomas.

Epidemiology

It comprises 3 to 5% of all head and neck cancers. It is more common in men than in women with a peak incidence in

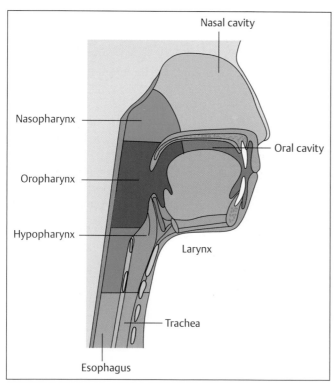

Fig. 46.1 Divisions of the pharynx.

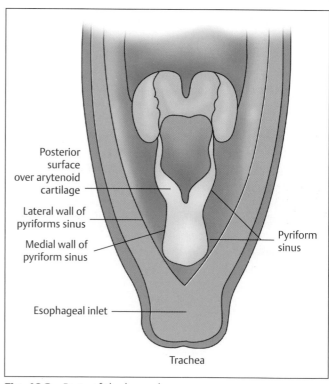

Fig. 46.2 Parts of the hypopharynx.

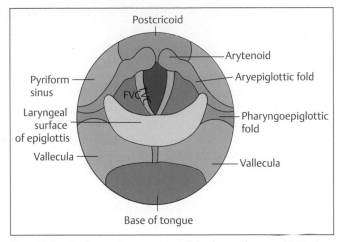

Fig. 46.3 Endoscopic anatomy of the hypopharynx (TVC, true vocal cords; FVC, false vocal cords).

the sixth and seventh decades of life. The most common site of origin of hypopharyngeal cancer is the pyriform sinus (66–75%), posterior pharyngeal wall (15–20%), and postcricoid area (5–15%).

Etiology

- Tobacco use and chronic alcohol intake have a synergistic effect.
- Poor nutrition and vitamin deficiency can exacerbate hypopharyngeal cancer.
- There is an association with poor socioeconomic status.
- Plummer–Vinson syndrome, a premalignant condition in middle-aged females with iron deficiency anemia and postcricoid web, is associated with the development of hypopharyngeal carcinoma.
- Genetic factors:
  - There is an association between tobacco use and p53 mutations.
  - The loss of heterozygosity at 9p and abnormalities in chromosome 11 has been reported.
  - Mutations in the p21 gene have also been identified.
- Human papilloma virus (HPV) is a contributing factor to carcinogenesis in head and neck squamous cell carcinomas, but the role in hypopharyngeal cancer is not clear.
- Occupational exposures mainly asbestos, wood smoke, and welding fumes increase the risk of cancer.

Patterns of Spread in Hypopharyngeal Cancers

The submucosal spread is more extensive than the appearance on the surface. There is a high incidence of lymph node metastasis.

Table 46.1 Patterns of spread in hypopharyngeal cancers

Area involved	Pattern of spread
Pyriform sinus involvement	Laterally: Through the thyroid cartilage (ossified cartilage more prone to invasion) Extralaryngeal structures Medially: Laryngeal inlet Anteromedially: Paraglottic space Posteriorly: Posterior pharyngeal wall and postcricoid region
Posterior pharyngeal wall	Fairly larger in size due to its location Anteriorly: Laryngeal inlet Posteriorly: Prevertebral muscles/fascia Inferiorly: Postcricoid area and cervical esophagus
Postcricoid area	Spreads circumferentially causing obstruction to swallowing Anteriorly: Larynx Posteriorly: Prevertebral fascia Laterally: Pyriform fossae Inferiorly: Esophagus

In pyriform sinus malignancy, lymph node metastasis is 60 to 75% (highest incidence). This spread is usually to levels II and III. From the postcricoid region, lymph node metastasis occurs to levels VI and VII (**Table 46.1**).

Distant metastasis at the time of clinical diagnosis is 17%. Approximately half of the recurrences have distant metastatic disease. The most common sites for distant metastases are the lung, liver, bones, and brain.

Clinical Features

■ Symptoms

- Early hypopharyngeal cancers show symptoms of mild, nonspecific sore throat or vague discomfort on swallowing.
- Predominant symptoms are those related to the locoregional disease spread.
- Sore throat: Typically, pain is unilateral and well localized.
- Odynophagia.
- Dysphagia more to solids than liquids. It progresses to absolute dysphagia.
- Weight loss.
- A lump or mass in the neck: In 50% of patients, it may be the first sign. This lump is due to lymph node metastasis.
- Hoarseness indicates either involvement of the recurrent laryngeal nerve, which runs deep to the anterior wall of the pyriform sinus, or direct invasion of the larynx.
- Coughing on swallowing liquids may indicate aspiration.
- Breathing difficulty/stridor.
- Otalgia (referred pain).

Pearl

Lesions on the medial wall tend to present earlier than lateral wall lesions due to their proximity to the larynx resulting in airway symptoms.

Signs

- Widening of thyroid cartilage.
- Anterolateral infiltration can present as a thyroid swelling and can be misdiagnosed as goiter.
- Loss of laryngeal crepitus (*Bocca's sign* and *Trotter's sign*).
- Fullness in the thyrohyoid membrane.
- Palpable neck nodes.
- Look for sign of dehydration and hyponatremia.

On Indirect Laryngoscopy or Rigid Telescopy of the Larynx

- It can present in the following ways: as an infiltrative mass, ulceroproliferative lesion, ulcer, or a mucosal fullness or bulge (**Figs. 46.4** and **46.5**).
- Pooling of secretions in pyriform fossa—*Jackson's sign*.
- Restricted mobility of vocal cords or fixed vocal cords is indicative of laryngeal involvement.
- Edematous arytenoids.

Investigations

- Laboratory investigations:
  - Complete blood count to rule out anemia and leucocytosis.
  - Serum electrolytes for electrolyte imbalance.
  - Liver function tests to test the protein, bilirubin, and liver enzyme levels.
  - Renal function tests.
- *Contrast-enhanced computed tomography (CECT) scan*: It is used to assess the extent and spread of tumor. It is useful for assessing laryngeal cartilage involvement, extralaryngeal or extrapharyngeal spread, paraglottic space spread, spread to the retropharyngeal space, and for clinically occult metastatic lymphadenopathy.
- *Magnetic resonance imaging (MRI) scan*: It is a better radiological assessment of soft-tissue involvement, prevertebral fascia involvement, and perineural invasion.
- *Endoscopy*: Direct laryngoscopy, hypopharyngoscopy, and esophagoscopy ± bronchoscopy can be conducted to assess the lesion and look for skip lesion and a second primary.
- *Biopsy* is done during the endoscopy to confirm the diagnosis.
- *Fine-needle aspiration cytology (FNAC) of the neck mass* should be done to evaluate for neck metastasis.
- *Barium esophagogram* should be done to delineate the filling defect, map the extent of disease, and look for synchronous lesions in the esophagus.
- *Flexible transnasal esophagoscopy* can be done as an initial assessment.
- *Chest X-ray* can be done to look for secondaries in lungs, second primary in the lung, aspiration pneumonia, superior mediastinal lymph nodes, and other pathologies like chronic obstructive pulmonary disease (COPD) and tuberculosis. A CT scan of the thorax is preferred.
- *Ultrasonography (USG) of the abdomen* can be done to rule out abdominal secondaries (liver).
- *X-ray of the neck* (anteroposterior and lateral views) can be done to note the shift of the trachea, airway

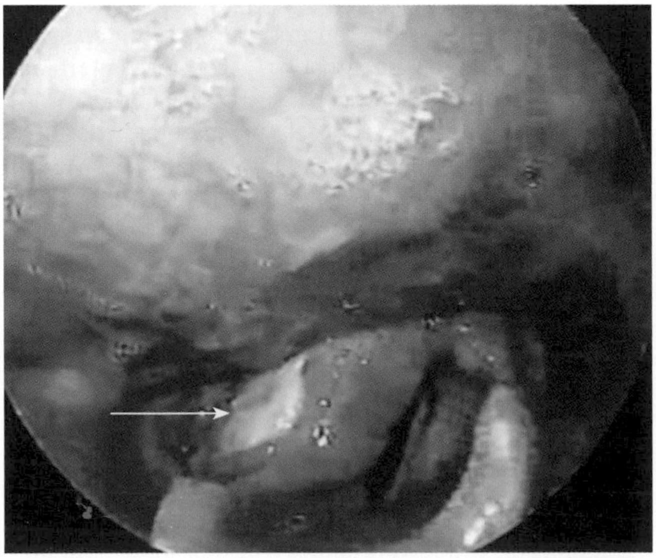

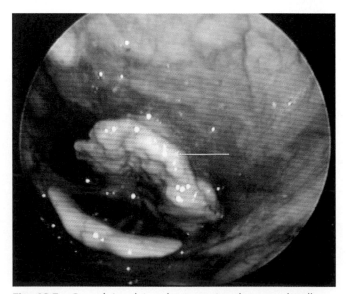

Fig. 46.4 Video laryngoscopic image showing growth in the right pyriform fossa (medial wall).

Fig. 46.5 Growth involving the posterior pharyngeal wall.

compromise/patency of the airway, and to rule out cervical spine pathology before direct laryngoscopy. This will be noted better on a CT scan.

- *Bone scan* can be done to rule out bone metastasis.
- *Positron emission tomography (PET) scan* is helpful in staging and in ruling out distant metastasis in advanced and recurrent cases.

Staging in Hypopharyngeal Cancers

TNM (tumor, node, and metastasis) staging of the hypopharyngeal cancers according to the American Joint Committee on Cancer (AJCC), 8th edition, is described in **Tables 46.2, 46.3, 46.4**, and **46.5**.

Management of Hypopharyngeal Cancers

Hypopharyngeal cancers are difficult to treat due to the following reasons:
- Biologically more aggressive than cancers of the larynx.
- Submucosal spread.
- Invasion of the laryngeal framework.
- High incidence of lymph node metastasis.
- Silent and asymptomatic in early stages with late presentation.

Treatment options of hypopharyngeal cancers depend on the following factors:
- Location of the lesion.
- T stage.

Table 46.2 T staging of hypopharyngeal tumor

Stage	Criteria
Tx	Primary tumor cannot be assessed
T0	No evidence of primary tumor
Tis	Carcinoma in situ
T1	Tumor limited to one subsite of the hypopharynx and or 2 cm or less in greatest dimension
T2	Tumor invades more than one subsite of the hypopharynx or an adjacent site, or measures more than 2 cm but 4 cm or less in greatest dimension without fixation of the hemilarynx
T3	Tumor measures more than 4 cm in greatest dimension or with fixation of the hemilarynx
T4a	Tumor invades the thyroid/cricoid cartilage, hyoid bone, thyroid gland, esophagus or central compartment soft tissue, which includes the prelaryngeal strap muscles and subcutaneous fat
T4b	Tumor invades the prevertebral fascia, encases the carotid artery, or involves the mediastinal structures

Table 46.3 N staging of hypopharyngeal tumor

N Category	N Criteria
NX	Regional lymph nodes cannot be assessed
N0	No regional lymph node metastasis
N1	Metastasis in a single ipsilateral lymph node, 3 cm or smaller in greatest dimension and ENE-negative
N2	Metastasis in a single ipsilateral lymph node larger than 3 cm but not larger than 6 cm in greatest dimension and ENE-negative; or metastases in multiple ipsilateral lymph nodes, none larger than 6 cm in greatest dimension and ENE-negative; or metastasis in bilateral or contralateral lymph nodes, none larger than 6 cm in greatest dimension and ENE-negative
N2a	Metastasis in a single ipsilateral lymph node larger than 3 cm but not larger than 6 cm in greatest dimension and ENE-negative
N2b	Metastasis in multiple ipsilateral lymph nodes, none larger than 6 cm in greatest dimension and ENE-negative
N2b	Metastasis in bilateral or contralateral lymph nodes. none larger than 6 cm in greatest dimension and ENE-negative
N3	Metastasis in a lymph node larger than 6 cm in greatest dimension and ENE-negative; or metastasis in any lymph node(s) and clinically overt ENE-positive
N3a	Metastasis in a lymph node larger than 6 cm in greatest dimension and ENE-negative
N3b	Metastasis in any node(s) and clinically overt ENE-positive

Abbreviation: ENE, extranodal extension.

Table 46.4 M staging of hypopharyngeal tumor

Stage	Criteria
MX	Distant metastasis cannot be assessed
M0	No distant metastasis
M1	Distant metastasis

Table 46.5 Staging of tumor according to TNM

Group	T	N	M
0	Tis	N0	M0
I	T1	N0	M0
II	T2	N0	M0
III	T3	N0	M0
	T1, T2, T3	N1	M0
IVA	T1, T2, T3	N2	M0
	T4a	N0, N1, N2	M0
IVB	T4b	Any N	M0
	Any T	N3	M0
IVC	Any T	Any N	M1

Abbreviation: TNM, tumor, node, and metastasis.

- N stage.
- M stage.
- Performance status of the patient.
- Facilities and expertise available.
- Patient preference.
- Associated comorbidities.

The *treatment options* are the following:
- Surgery.
- Radiotherapy.
- Chemotherapy.
- Targeted therapy.
- Combined modality of treatment.

■ Early Hypopharyngeal Cancers

Stages I and II (T1/T2, N0): A single modality of treatment, either surgery or radiotherapy is advised. Both modalities were found to be equally effective.

Advantages of Radiation Therapy

- Probability of functional morbidity or cosmetic defects is reduced.
- Risk of a major postoperative complication is avoided.
- Elective neck radiotherapy can be included with little added morbidity.
- Surgical salvage of radiotherapy failure is supposed to have better outcome than the radiotherapy for salvage of a surgical failure.

Surgery

- External approach:
  - Extended supraglottic partial laryngopharyngectomy.
  - Supracricoid hemilaryngopharyngectomy (SCHLP).
- Transoral approach:
  - Transoral laser microsurgery.
  - Transoral robotic surgery.
  - Transoral videoendoscopic surgery.

Management Options of Neck Nodes

- With a T1N0 neck, a regular follow-up with an USG every 2 months during the first 2 years.
- Selective (levels II–IV)/bilateral neck dissection: Selective neck dissection can be done at the time of resection of the primary due to high incidence of occult metastasis.

■ Advanced Hypopharyngeal Cancers

(Stage III/IV) T1–T2, N1–N3/T3–T4, N0–N+. Combined modality of treatment is preferred.

The following are the options, which can be selected in managing advanced tumors:
- Radiotherapy with altered fractionation schedules.
- Radiotherapy with chemotherapy.
- Radiotherapy with biological therapy.
- Neoadjuvant chemotherapy followed by surgery.
- Surgery followed by radiotherapy/chemotherapy and radiotherapy.

Role of Surgery

- *Indications*:
  - Good general condition.
  - Compromised laryngeal function (aspiration).
  - Laryngeal framework is involved.
  - Recurrence after radiotherapy (±chemotherapy) may require a salvage surgery.
- *Contraindications*:
  - Poor performance status.
  - Disease extension—root of the neck:
    ○ encasing the carotid.
    ○ involving the oropharynx.
    ○ prevertebral involvement.
  - Distant metastasis.

Surgical Options (Based on the Extent of the Disease)

- Near-total laryngectomy with partial pharyngectomy.
- Total laryngectomy with partial pharyngectomy.
- Total laryngectomy with total pharyngectomy.
- Total laryngopharyngoesophagectomy with gastric pull-up (**Fig. 46.6**).
- Neck nodes:
  - Comprehensive bilateral neck dissection (levels II–V) is cleared as nodal metastasis is high in advanced tumors.

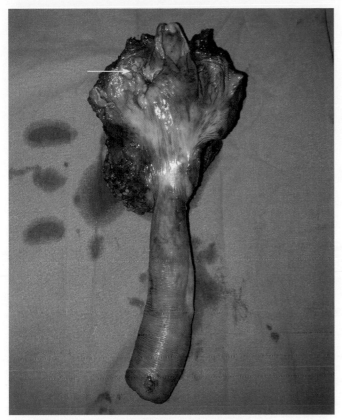

Fig. 46.6 Total laryngopharyngoesophagectomy specimen with tumor seen in the right pyriform fossa.

■ Indications for Adjuvant (Radiation ± Chemotherapy) Treatment after Surgery

- T3/T4 disease.
- Close margins.

- Positive margins.
- Perineural invasion.
- Lymphovascular spread.
- Invasion of the cartilage, bone, and soft tissues.
- Multiple nodal involvement.
- Extracapsular spread (in the lymph node).

■ Follow-Up in Hypopharyngeal Malignancy

Due to the high recurrence rates, regular follow-up is required.
- First 2 years: Every 2 months.
- Third year: Once in 4 months.
- Fourth year: Once in 6 months.
- Greater than 5 years: Once a year.

Points to Ponder

- Hypopharyngeal cancers are rare tumors and usually arise from the pyriform fossa.
- Pyriform fossa tumors can affect both the food passage and the airway.
- The Plummer–Vinson syndrome is a premalignant condition for the development of hypopharyngeal malignancy.
- Metastatic nodes are common because of the rich lymphatic supply in this area.
- Postcricoid tumors will result in loss of laryngeal crepitus or Trotter's sign.
- Relevant investigations include a rigid endoscopic examination to find out the upper extent and lower extent of the tumor and also to take a biopsy.
- Treatment options depend upon the TNM staging of the tumor.

Case-Based Questions

1. **A 42-year-old female patient presented with a 3-year history of dysphagia. She was treated twice before for her dysphagia, which improved after blood transfusion. She has pallor and glossitis. Indirect laryngoscopy showed pooling of saliva in the pyriform fossae and edematous arytenoids with left vocal cord fixity. Bocca's sign was positive.**

   a. What is the possible diagnosis?
   b. What was the initial condition and what are its features?
   c. How would you confirm the diagnosis?
   d. How would you have treated the initial condition?

   Answers
   a. Postcricoid malignancy of the hypopharynx.

   b. Plummer–Vinson/Paterson–Kelly–Brown syndrome. The features are anemia, glossitis, angular cheilitis, koilonychia, and esophageal or cricopharyngeal web.

   c. Hypopharyngoscopy and biopsy.

   d. Esophagoscopy and dilatation of the web, and correction of anemia.

2. **A 53-year-old man, a chronic smoker and alcoholic, presented with a 6-month history of progressive dysphagia. At present, he is not able to swallow liquids and has cough on swallowing with mild breathing difficulty. Indirect laryngoscopy showed an ulceroproliferative growth involving the right pyriform fossa medial and lateral wall, with fullness of the right ventricular band and fixity of the right vocal cord. There was spillover of saliva into the larynx.**

a. What is the most probable diagnosis?

b. What is absolute dysphagia?

c. What are the laboratory and radiological investigations required?

d. How would you confirm the diagnosis?

Answers

a. Malignancy of the hypopharynx (right pyriform fossa).

b. Dysphagia to solids and liquids.

c. The laboratory investigations required are complete blood count, serum electrolytes, and liver function tests. The required radiological investigations are CECT of the neck and thorax.

d. Hypopharyngoscopy and direct laryngoscopy to determine the upper and lower extent and biopsy for obtaining a tissue diagnosis.

Frequently Asked Questions

1. What is the type of malignancy commonly seen in the hypopharynx?

2. What are the subsites of the hypopharynx?

3. Describe the clinical features of a patient with pyriform fossa malignancy.

4. What is Bocca's sign/Trotter's sign?

5. What are the relevant investigations done for a patient with hypopharyngeal malignancy?

6. What are the treatment options for early malignancy of the hypopharynx?

Endnote

In advanced hypopharyngeal malignancy, the esophagus (along with the laryngopharynx) was removed earlier via a thoracotomy. Since this led to higher chest complications, it was modified to a downward eversion stripping technique of the esophagus, using a vein stripper. The whole laryngopharyngoesophagectomy specimen can be removed in toto by the upward eversion stripping technique, a technique initially described by Rajan et al. Esophageal stripping is also done as an emergency procedure in acute necrosis of the esophagus by a concentrated caustic solution.

47 Miscellaneous Conditions of the Pharynx

Ashish Chandra Agarwal and Kailesh Pujary

The competencies covered in this chapter are as follows:

EN2.13 Identify, resuscitate, and manage ear, nose, and throat (ENT) emergencies in a simulated environment including removal of foreign bodies in the ear, nose, throat, and upper respiratory tract.

EN3.4 Observe and describe the indications for and steps involved in the removal of foreign bodies from the ear, nose, and throat.

Foreign Bodies in the Throat

■ Introduction

Foreign bodies in the throat are commonly encountered in the ear, nose, and throat (ENT) practice. The propensity to get lodged and the subsequent manifestations depend on the physical and chemical characteristic of the foreign body. The tonsil is a common site for lodgment of foreign bodies like fish bone. Early identification and removal of the foreign body is the mainstay of treatment and prevents the development of complications.

■ Etiology

The following individuals are at risk:
- Pediatric age group.
- Adults having psychiatric issues or in a state of altered sensorium (e.g., alcohol intoxication).
- Individuals having organic pathologies in the esophagus like tumors and postcorrosive or radiation strictures, which prevent the passage of the foreign body.

Foreign bodies are classified into the following types:
- *Organic* foreign bodies, which include seeds, nuts, and fish or chicken bones.
- *Nonorganic* foreign bodies, which include sharp objects (needles/pins), blunt objects (small toys, coins), and corrosives (battery).

The common *sites of lodgment* in the pharynx from superior to inferior include the following:
- Tonsillar crypts.
- Tonsillolingual sulcus.
- Base of the tongue (**Fig. 47.1**).
- Vallecula.

- Pyriform sinus (**Fig. 47.2**).
- Cricopharynx—at the cricopharyngeal sphincter.

■ Clinical Features

Symptoms

It depends on the site of lodgment. The common symptoms are foreign body sensation in the throat and throat pain. There may be difficulty in swallowing and drooling of saliva. Breathing difficulty and neck swelling may be seen

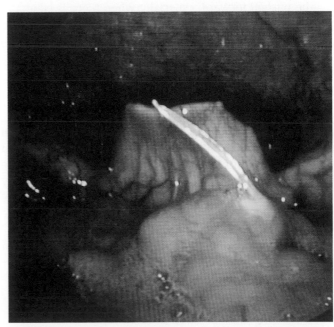

Fig. 47.1 Fishbone embedded in the base of the tongue. Epiglottis can be seen posterior to it.

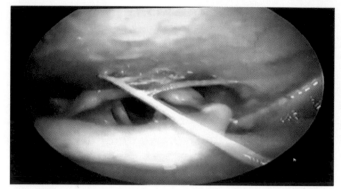

Fig. 47.2 Fishbone being removed from the pyriform fossa.

in long-standing cases where localized inflammation or abscess formation has started. The patient may complain of referred pain to the ipsilateral ear due to secondary infection in the throat.

Signs

- On examination, a foreign body of the pharynx is usually visible. It may be lodged on the medial surface of the tonsil, which can then be visualized by depressing the tongue. Foreign bodies in the base of the tongue, vallecula, or pyriform fossa can be seen on indirect laryngoscopy or rigid telescopy.
- Pooling of secretions in the vallecula or pyriform fossa may be noted. Slough formation and edema can occur at the site of lodgment.
- On examination of the neck, the larynx may be found to be pushed forward, especially when there is edema of the hypopharynx or retropharyngeal abscess. Laryngeal crepitus is painful or absent. In long-standing foreign bodies, there may be a neck swelling due to abscess formation.

■ Investigations

A plain x-ray of the neck in the anteroposterior and lateral views will reveal a radio-opaque foreign body. Prevertebral widening with or without air–fluid level will be visible in cases of long-standing cricopharyngeal foreign body (**Fig. 47.3**). Rarely, a computed tomography (CT) scan may be required especially when the foreign body is not visible or lodged in the deeper tissues (e.g., within the tonsil).

A rigid-angled telescopy or a flexible nasopharyngeal laryngoscopy may help in the assessment, if clinical examination has not been helpful.

■ Treatment

- A foreign body lodged in the tonsillar crypt or tonsillo-lingual sulcus can be removed with the help of forceps.

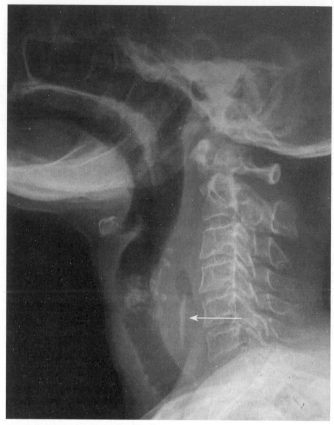

Fig. 47.3 Bone lodged at the cricopharyngeal sphincter (C6 vertebra).

- Curved forceps or upturned forceps can be used to remove the foreign body from the base of the tongue, valleculae, or pyriform sinus while simultaneously doing an indirect laryngoscopy examination or rigid telescopy.
- A direct laryngoscopy or a rigid hypopharyngoscopy under general anesthesia needs to be done to remove a foreign body from the cricopharynx.
- Incision and drainage are performed in cases of abscess formation.
- Medications in the form of antibiotics, analgesics, and anti-inflammatory agents are required if there is superadded infection. If the foreign body is lodged within the tonsil and not visible (but seen on CT scan), an ipsilateral tonsillectomy can be carried out.

■ Complications

- Aspiration of the foreign body can occur if the patient attempts to swallow or the foreign body slips from the forceps during removal.
- Abscess formation at the site of lodgment or in the deep neck spaces can occur in long-standing foreign bodies.
- Tracheoesophageal fistula and stricture formation in the pharynx are rare complications.

Obstructive Sleep Apnea

■ Introduction

Apnea is the cessation of breathing for more than 10 seconds in an adult.

In children, it is defined as cessation of breathing for 20 seconds or more. It is less than 20 seconds if it is accompanied by bradycardia or cyanosis.

Sleep apnea can be of three types:
- Obstructive sleep apnea (OSA).
- Central apnea.
- Mixed.

Obstructive sleep apnea syndrome (OSAS) is part of the spectrum of obstructive hypoventilation, which includes snoring, upper airway resistance syndrome, obstructive hypopnea syndrome, and OSA. OSAS is when there are more than five obstructive episodes per hour. In some patients, there can be coexisting central apnea.

■ Etiopathogenesis

OSAS is more commonly seen in obese individuals. In children, it is commonly seen with adenotonsillar hypertrophy with or without craniofacial anomalies including Down's syndrome.

During sleep, the individual has snoring and multiple cycles of apnea associated with decreased partial pressure of oxygen and increased carbon dioxide, which increases the respiratory drive, leading to arousal. More than 30 such episodes over 6 hours of sleep is considered significant.

There may be a partial obstruction in the nose, nasopharynx, and oropharynx. During sleep, the pharyngeal muscle tone reduces and the tongue also falls back. This increases the obstruction. Due to the venturi effect during attempted inspiration, the oropharyngeal mucosa (especially when there is loose, redundant mucosa) collapses inward. The vibration of the mucosa contributes to the noisy breathing. There is poor airflow but marked effort in breathing (**Fig. 47.4**).

■ Clinical Features

Symptoms

Snoring is the commonest symptom. It is an inspiratory, low-pitched, noisy breathing during sleep.

In the Michelson snoring scale:
- 0: No snoring.
- 1: Occasional soft snoring.
- 2: Daily soft snoring.
- 3: Persistent loud snoring.
- 4: Persistent terrible snoring.
- 5: "Heroic" snoring.

Other nocturnal symptoms are sweating, nocturia, reflux, and dry mouth. There will be witnessed apneic episodes. In children, there will be restlessness, nocturnal enuresis, and bruxism.

The daytime symptoms include excessive daytime sleepiness, behavioral problems, and headache. This is due to reduced partial pressure of oxygen and fragmented sleep. Children, in addition, may have mouth breathing, swallowing problems, and poor scholastic performance.

■ Signs

On examination:
- There may be a bulky or long, soft palate and uvula.
- There may be redundant oropharyngeal mucosa (snorer's throat).

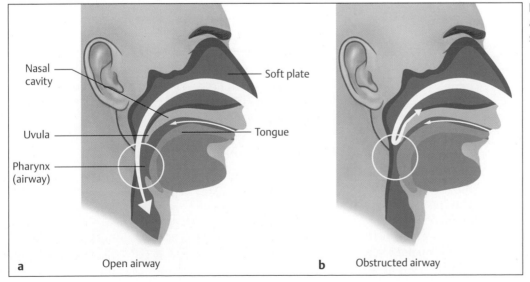

Fig. 47.4 **(a)** Normal airway and **(b)** airway in obstructive sleep apnea.

Nasal cavity

Soft plate

Uvula

Tongue

Pharynx (airway)

a — Open airway

b — Obstructed airway

- There may be maxillary hypoplasia, retrognathia, or other craniofacial abnormalities.
- The neck may be short with a large circumference (short fat neck).
- The examination should include the face, neck, nose, oral cavity, oropharynx, and laryngopharynx for the possible levels of obstruction, which may be multilevel.

The person may have social and workplace-related problems like marital disharmony, poor work performance, accidents at home or at work or while driving, cognitive problems, and behavioral problems. Additional morbidity includes cardiac arrhythmias, myocardial infarction, stroke, decreased libido and impotence, and insulin resistance.

Pearl

Heroic snoring is snoring that is loud enough to be heard by another individual in the next room through a closed door.

Investigations

- A complete blood count, thyroid function tests (hypothyroidism may present with snoring), and blood sugar levels.
- Lateral view of the neck X-ray may be done for adenoid hypertrophy in children.
- A dynamic magnetic resonance imaging (MRI) done during sleep may show the sites of obstruction.
- A flexible nasopharyngoscopy will help assess the nose, soft palate during Muller's maneuver, laryngopharynx, and base of the tongue.
- Polysomnography is a comprehensive test that involves recording of the following events and electrical activity during sleep (**Fig. 47.5**):
  – Electroencephalogram (EEG).
  – Electrocardiogram (ECG).
  – Electro-oculography (EOG).
  – Electromyogram (EMG).
  – Snoring intensity.
  – Chest and abdominal movements.
  – Oxygen saturation.
  – Heart rate.
  – Body position.
  – Esophageal pressure.

This battery of tests is the gold standard for assessment of OSA before and after treatment. Polysomnography helps document and assess the severity of sleep apnea, evaluates pre- and posttreatment status (i.e., following weight reduction, use of continuous positive airway pressure [CPAP], and surgery), and is helpful in the titration of CPAP.

- Drug-induced sleep endoscopy (DISE), using dexmedetomidine (midazolam, halothane, or propofol can also be used), induces a sleeplike condition and a transnasal flexible endoscope is used to assess the upper airway to look for obstruction. It is done preferably in the operating room with a standby for any emergency airway management. This would help document the sites contributing to obstruction.

Treatment

Conservative

Weight reduction through diet and exercise; control of habits like smoking and alcohol intake; avoiding sedatives; sleeping in the lateral position; treating medical problems like hypothyroidism; and use of oral appliances (to keep the tongue from falling back or the lower jaw forward) all play a role in reducing the symptoms of OSAS.

The commonest method used to treat OSAS is *CPAP*. Using a mask or nasal prongs, air with pressure helps keep the pharyngeal tissues apart, which improves the airway. The pressure can be titrated during polysomnography and can also be changed for inspiration and expiration, that is, bi-level positive airway pressure (*BiPap*).

Obesity can also be treated by centrally or peripherally acting appetite suppressants. In severe and moderate obesities with severe medical conditions, bariatric surgery, (laparoscopic, adjustable, silicone, gastric banding) can be done.

Surgical Treatment

It depends on the site of the obstruction, which can be multiple.

In children, it is mainly adenotonsillectomy. Other procedures done are for craniofacial anomalies, choanal atresia, glossoptosis, and congenital cysts.

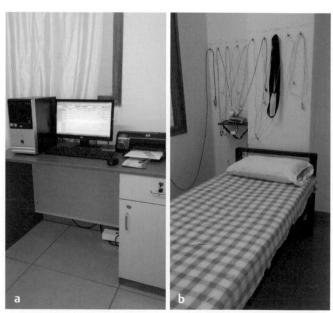

Fig. 47.5 (a, b) Modified sleep laboratory for polysomnography. (This image is provided courtesy of Dr. Aswini Kumar Mohapatra.)

In adults, nasal surgeries like septoplasty, turbinate reduction, and nasal valve surgery are done to improve the nasal airway, which may also facilitate better use of CPAP. Palatal surgeries like uvulopalatopharyngoplasty are aimed at increasing the oropharyngeal space especially the retropalatal space. Tongue base reduction procedures like partial midline glossectomy or radiofrequency reduction are aimed at increasing the retrolingual space. Maxillary and mandibular advancement procedures are aimed at increasing the retropalatal and retrolingual space, respectively. The implantable hypoglossal nerve stimulator prevents the tongue from falling back. In multilevel obstruction, a combination of procedures can be done although sometimes it is done in two sittings. In severe obesity with OSAS and other comorbidities, the treatment of choice would be a tracheostomy, which bypasses the upper airway obstruction.

Zenker's Diverticulum (Pulsion Diverticulum)

■ Introduction

Pharyngeal diverticulum or pouch is a herniation of the mucosa and submucosa through a weakness in the muscular wall. It can occur at various sites in the pharynx. It commonly occurs at Killian's dehiscence, which is between the oblique fibers of the thyropharyngeus and the horizontal fibers of cricopharyngeus. It is commonly seen after the sixth decade and the male-to-female ratio is 2:1 (**Figs. 47.6** and **47.7**).

■ Etlopathogenesis

Various theories have been put forward for the formation of the pouch. It occurs at a site of anatomical weakness. Cricopharyngeal spasm does not allow the free passage of bolus and this can put pressure at a site of weakness. It is due to incoordination of muscles with poor propulsion of food from pharynx, along with early cricopharyngeal closure. Since this occurs in the older age group, reduced muscle tone and loss of tissue elasticity may contribute. With the progression of the pouch size, a septum forms between the pouch and the esophagus and the food goes preferably toward the pouch as it becomes in line with the pharynx above it. In a long-standing pouch, malignancy can occur.

■ Clinical Features

Symptoms

The symptoms vary in severity at presentation and are gradually progressive. There is a sticking sensation on swallowing (globus), which requires a second swallow.

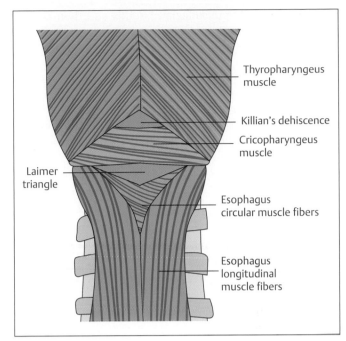

Fig. 47.6 Zenker's diverticulum usually presents through the muscular dehiscence between the fibers of the thyropharyngeus and cricopharyngeus muscles. Both are parts of the inferior constrictor muscle.

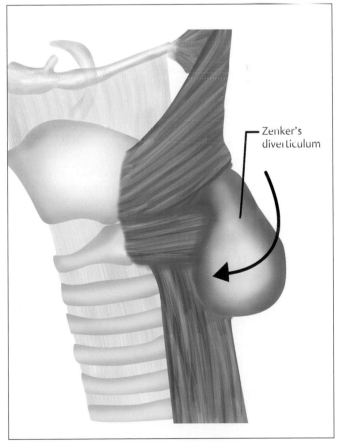

Fig. 47.7 Zenker's diverticulum protruding between the muscle fibers.

This progresses to dysphagia to solids and then absolute dysphagia. Regurgitation of meals can occur while lying down. This can predispose to hoarseness, cough, and aspiration.

Signs

On palpation, there may be a gurgling feel on the left side of the neck (Boyce's sign). Indirect laryngoscopy or rigid telescopy may show pooling of saliva.

■ Investigations

- Using functional endoscopic evaluation of swallowing, the "rising tide sign" may be seen. This occurs when liquids with dye are swallowed and may be seen to rise back up after initial ingestion.
- Barium swallow will show the pouch with its approximate size.

■ Treatment

- Conservative treatment with botulinum toxin injection (percutaneous or endoscopic) can be done in the early stages in patients who are not fit for surgery or refuse surgery.
- Open surgical procedures (via an external incision) include cricopharyngeal myotomy, excision of the pouch and myotomy, and inversion of the pouch and myotomy.
- Endoscopic procedures include cricopharyngeal myotomy (with laser or cautery), removal of the septum between the pouch and the esophagus by cutting and

sealing with stapler, and division of the septum with laser or cautery. Endoscopic stapler diverticulotomy is the preferred procedure. The aim is to remove the septum between the pouch and the esophagus with cricopharyngeal myotomy to allow for free passage of food, preferentially into the esophagus.

Points to Ponder

- Early identification of a foreign body in the pharynx and its prompt removal is the mainstay of management.
- Examination with the help of an angled telescope helps rule out a foreign body in hidden areas like tonsillar crypts, vallecula, and tonsillolingual sulcus.
- Self-manipulation by the patient should be discouraged as the foreign body in the pharynx can get lodged deeper.
- OSAS is a part of a spectrum of disease called obstructive hypoventilation and snoring is one component of it.
- OSA has social and medical consequences. These include marital discord and pulmonary hypertension.
- Polysomnography is the gold standard for the diagnosis of OSAS.
- Zenker's diverticulum is due to a gap between the thyropharyngeus and the cricopharyngeus.
- The main symptoms of this diverticulum are dysphagia and regurgitation of food.
- Endoscopic diverticulotomy is the preferred surgical procedure.

Case-Based Questions

1. **A 45-year-old man presented to the outpatient clinic with difficulty in swallowing of 1-day duration. He gives history of ingestion of chicken the previous day.**

   a. What is the commonest site for lodgment of a chicken bone?

   b. How will you manage this patient?

   Answers

   a. The commonest site is the cricopharynx, which is the site of the upper esophageal sphincter. This is usually closed and if there is a failure of relaxation during swallowing or if the foreign body is big, it will get lodged at this site, which is on the opposite side of the C6 vertebra.

   b. Lateral view of a plain X-ray of the neck will reveal the radiopaque shadow of the bone at the C6 level. This can then be removed during hypopharyngoscopy.

2. **A 55-year-old, obese man came with complaints of feeling tired and exhausted all day. He often falls asleep at his workplace, and his wife complains of snoring at night.**

   a. What is the diagnosis?

   b. How will you manage this condition?

   Answers

   a. Obesity with symptoms of excessive daytime sleepiness, feeling of tiredness, and snoring all point to OSAS.

   b. The gold standard test to diagnose this condition is polysomnography. Treatment should be in a graded manner. Weight loss through dieting and exercise should be advised. If that is not successful, CPAP or BiPap should be tried. This drives the air into the respiratory passageway to keep it patent. If this is also unsuccessful, surgery at the level of the obstruction should be carried out like uvulopalatopharyngoplasty.

Frequently Asked Questions

1. What are the common sites of lodgment of foreign bodies in the pharynx?

2. How do you classify foreign bodies?

3. How will you remove a foreign body stuck at the cricopharyngeal sphincter?

4. What is apnea?

5. How do you classify sleep apnea?

6. What is DISE and how is it useful in OSA?

7. What is the gold standard investigation in OSAS?

8. What is Zenker's diverticulum?

9. What radiological investigation will help confirm the diagnosis of a pharyngeal pouch?

10. What is the rising tide sign?

Endnote

Chevalier Jackson (1865–1958) is regarded by some as the father of endoscopy. He invented hollow tubes with illumination at one end, called bronchoscopes and esophagoscopes, to peer into the body. In the process, he was able to remove a considerable number of foreign bodies from the pharynx, esophagus, and bronchus. He extracted 2,374 swallowed or inhaled foreign bodies during a span of 75 years, and they are now exhibited in the Mütter Museum in Philadelphia in the United States.

48 Anatomy of the Larynx

Suresh Pillai and Prerit Rao

The competencies covered in this chapter are as follows:

EN1.1 Describe the anatomy and physiology of the ear, nose, throat, and head and neck.

AN38.1 Describe the morphology, and identify structure of the wall, nerve supply, blood supply and actions of the intrinsic and extrinsic muscles of the larynx.

Introduction

The larynx is called the gateway between the esophagus and the trachea. It plays a crucial role in the protection of the lower airway from aspiration. This is achieved with the help of various muscles, joints, and ligaments present in the larynx. Hence, it is important to have a basic understanding of the anatomy of these structures.

Embryology

During the fourth week of life, the respiratory tract develops as an outgrowth from the primitive gut termed the tracheobronchial groove. The tracheoesophageal septum separating the larynx from the esophagus forms in the fourth week. The laryngeal lumen temporarily closes between the 7th and 10th week, following which recanalization occurs. The larynx itself develops in two parts:
- The supraglottis arises from the buccopharyngeal bud.

- The glottis and the subglottis arise from the tracheobronchial bud.

The laryngeal innervation is by the superior and recurrent laryngeal nerves and these are derivatives of the fourth and sixth branchial arches, respectively.

Pearl

The embryological development of the larynx may help limit spread of malignancy from one subsite to the other in the early stages of the disease.

Anatomy

The larynx is a fibrocartilaginous framework formed by various cartilages, ligaments, membranes, and muscles.

■ Laryngeal Cartilages

These are *paired* and *unpaired cartilages* (**Flowchart 48.1**).

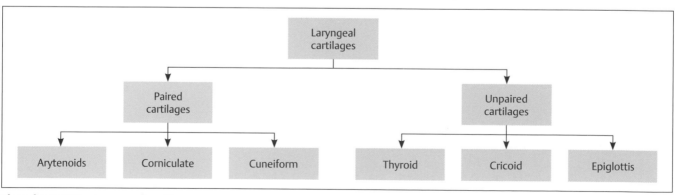

Flowchart 48.1   Laryngeal cartilages.

■ Thyroid Cartilage

It is a *V*-shaped cartilage (shieldlike) formed by two quadrilateral laminae. These laminae are more prominent in males and form an angle of around 90 degrees, which forms a prominence called Adam's apple. The angle between the laminae in females is 120 degrees.

From the posterior border of the thyroid cartilage arise the superior and inferior cornua. The superior cornua articulate with the hyoid bone by the lateral thyrohyoid ligaments, whereas the inferior cornua articulate with the cricoid cartilage, thereby forming the cricothyroid joint (**Fig. 48.1**).

■ Cricoid Cartilage

It is a signet ring-shaped cartilage, which has a narrow anterior lamina and a broader posterior lamina (**Fig. 48.2**).

■ Epiglottis

It is a leaf-shaped, elastic cartilage found in the upper part of the larynx in the anterior wall. It has a broad upper free part and a lower part attached to the angle between the two thyroid cartilage laminae. This attachment is known as the petiole or the thyroepiglottic ligament. The hyoepiglottic ligament attaches the hyoid bone to the epiglottis.

The epiglottis has two surfaces, the lingual surface, and the laryngeal surface. It can be divided into the suprahyoid and infrahyoid parts.

■ Arytenoid Cartilages

These are paired cartilages situated at the upper border of the cricoid cartilage. These are pyramidal in shape. The apex of the cartilage articulates with the corniculate cartilage. The base of the cartilage is concave, and it articulates

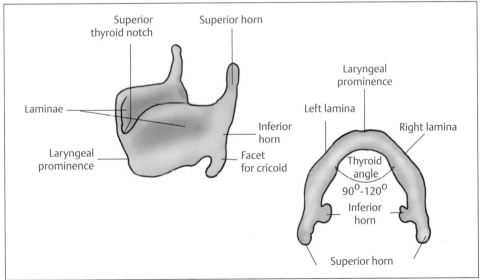

Fig. 48.1 The various parts of the thyroid cartilage.

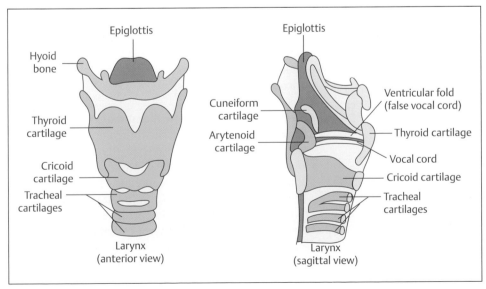

Fig. 48.2 The laryngeal framework, anterior view, and sagittal view.

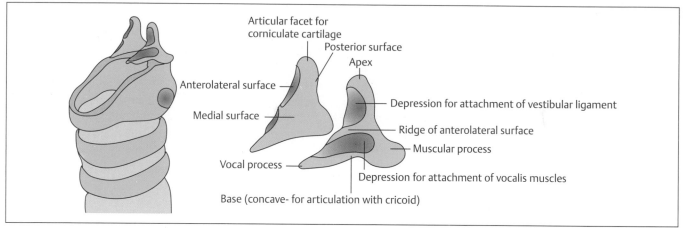

Fig. 48.3 Parts of the arytenoid cartilage and the position in relation to the cricoid.

with the upper border of the cricoid lamina. At the base, anteriorly is the vocal process and posterolaterally the muscular process (**Fig. 48.3**).

■ Corniculate Cartilages

These are also called Santorini's cartilage. These are horn-shaped and articulate with the apex of the arytenoid cartilage in the posterior part of the aryepiglottic fold (**Fig. 48.4**).

■ Cuneiform Cartilages

These are small wedge-shaped, paired cartilages present in the aryepiglottic fold ventral to the corniculate cartilage (**Fig. 48.4**).

Pearl

The infrahyoid epiglottis has fenestrations through which malignancy can spread to the preepiglottic space and vallecula.

■ Laryngeal Joints

Cricothyroid joint: It is a synovial joint between the thyroid cartilage (inferior cornu) and the cricoid cartilage. It allows rotatory movements in the horizontal plane and gliding movements.

Cricoarytenoid joint: It is a synovial joint between the base of the arytenoid and the upper border of the cricoid. It facilitates rotatory movements in the vertical plane, and gliding movements, which are responsible for adduction and abduction of the vocal cords.

■ Laryngeal Ligaments and Membranes

Laryngeal ligaments and membranes are the following (**Fig. 48.5**):
• Extrinsic:
  – Thyrohyoid membrane is pierced in the lateral aspect by the superior laryngeal nerve and artery along with

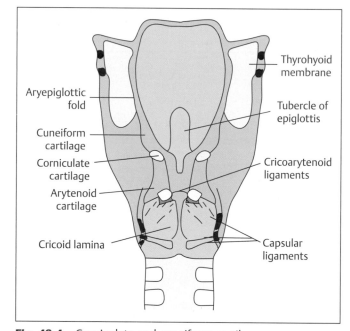

Fig. 48.4 Corniculate and cuneiform cartilages.

the lymphatics from the supraglottis to the deep cervical nodes.
  – Hyoepiglottic ligament.
  – Cricotracheal ligaments.
• Intrinsic:
  – Formed by the fibroelastic membrane.
  – The quadrangular membrane is the upper part, which extends from the arytenoids to the epiglottis. The lower free border forms the ventricular folds, and the upper border forms the aryepiglottic folds.
  – The conus elasticus runs from its attachment to the inner surface of the cricoid cartilage superiorly and medially. Between the thyroid cartilage and arytenoid cartilage, it is thickened to form a part of the vocal cord between the epithelium and the muscle layers, that is, the vocal ligament. The cricothyroid

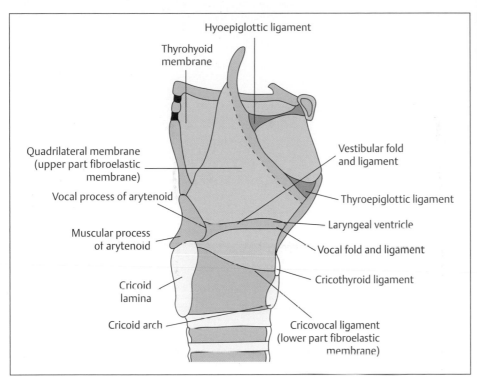

Fig. 48.5 Ligaments of the larynx showing the quadrilateral (quadrangular membrane) and the cricovocal ligament (conus elasticus).

Table 48.1 Intrinsic muscles of the larynx

Name of the muscle	Origin	Insertion
Cricothyroid	Lower border and lateral surface of the cricoid	Inferior cornu and lower border of the thyroid cartilage
Posterior cricoarytenoid	Posterior surface of the lamina of the cricoid	Muscular process of the arytenoid
Lateral cricoarytenoid	Lateral part of the upper border of the cricoid	Muscular process of the arytenoid
Transverse arytenoid	Posterior surface of one arytenoid	Posterior surface of the opposite arytenoid
Oblique arytenoid	Muscular process of the arytenoid	Apex of the opposite arytenoid
Thyroarytenoid (vocalis and thyroepiglottic)	Thyroid angle and adjacent cricothyroid ligament	Anterolateral surface of the arytenoid cartilage

membrane extends upward and medially from the anterosuperior part of the cricoid cartilage to the anteroinferior part of the thyroid cartilage, forming a thick anterior part, which is known as the cricothyroid ligament.

> **Pearl**
>
> The cricothyroid membrane is the site for the emergency procedure, cricothyroidotomy, and for transconioscopy.

■ Muscles of the Larynx

The muscles that attach within the laryngeal cartilages are known as intrinsic muscles. The extrinsic muscles join the laryngeal framework to the adjacent structures and aid in the movement of the larynx. The extrinsic muscles are strap muscles and pharyngeal muscles, which help in the elevation and depression of the larynx. The intrinsic muscles move the cartilages relative to each other, which helps in altering the position, length, and tension of the vocal cords. These are described in **Table 48.1** and illustrated in **Figs. 48.6, 48.7,** and **48.8.** Their actions are outlined in **Flowchart 48.2.**

> **Pearl**
>
> The interarytenoid muscles (transverse and oblique) are supplied by the recurrent laryngeal nerve of both sides. In unilateral recurrent laryngeal nerve palsy, there will be some movement of the arytenoid on the affected side due to this bilateral innervation.

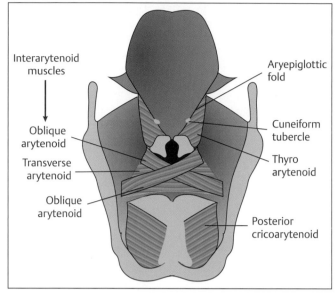

Fig. 48.6   Posterior view of the intrinsic muscles of the larynx.

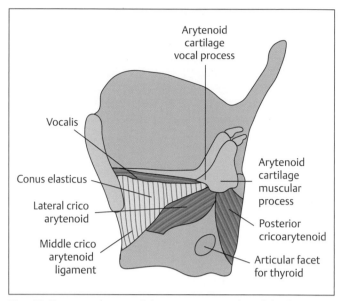

Fig. 48.7   Lateral view of the intrinsic muscles of the larynx.

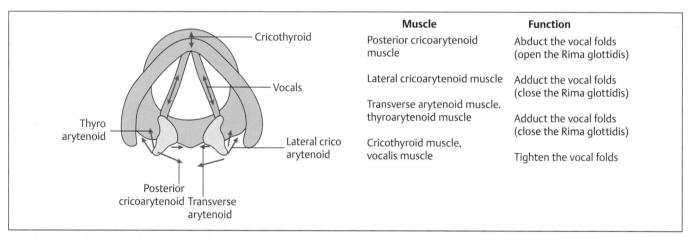

Muscle	Function
Posterior cricoarytenoid muscle	Abduct the vocal folds (open the Rima glottidis)
Lateral cricoarytenoid muscle	Adduct the vocal folds (close the Rima glottidis)
Transverse arytenoid muscle. thyroarytenoid muscle	Adduct the vocal folds (close the Rima glottidis)
Cricothyroid muscle, vocalis muscle	Tighten the vocal folds

Fig. 48.8   Action of the intrinsic muscles.

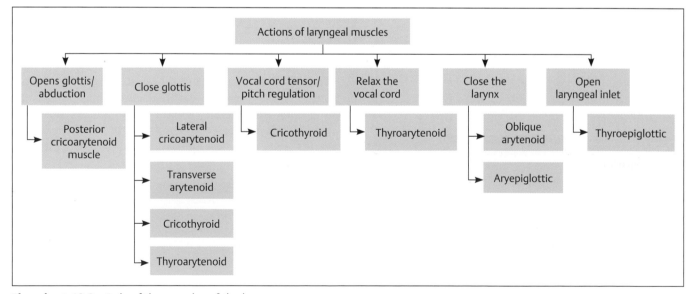

Flowchart 48.2   Role of the muscles of the larynx.

■ Laryngeal Inlet and Cavity

The laryngeal inlet known as the vestibule is oblique, positioned backward and upward, and opens into the laryngopharynx. The inlet boundaries are as follows:

- Anterior: The tip of the epiglottis.
- Posterior: The apex of the arytenoids and the interarytenoid region.
- Lateral: The superior aspect of the aryepiglottic folds.

The larynx is divided into three parts as depicted in **Flowchart 48.3**.

The cavity of the larynx extends from the laryngeal inlet to the lower border of the cricoid cartilage. Inside the laryngeal cavity, on each side, are the upper and lower folds. The upper fold is called the ventricular fold or false vocal fold, and the lower fold is known as the vocal fold (vocal cord). The space between the vestibular folds is the rima vestibule, and the space between the vocal cords is the rima glottidis.

The supraglottis comprises the laryngeal surface of the epiglottis, aryepiglottic folds, arytenoids, ventricular folds, and ventricle. The ventricle of the larynx is a narrow space and extends anteriorly as the saccule of the larynx between the vestibular folds and the thyroid lamina. It contains mucous glands, which provide lubrication to the larynx.

The glottis comprises the vocal cords, anterior commissure, and posterior commissure. The vocal cords are attached anteriorly to the middle of the thyroid cartilage by Broyles' ligament. At the site of attachment, there is no inner perichondrium. Posteriorly, it is attached to the vocal process of the arytenoid. The vocal cord has five layers: the lining epithelium, the superficial lamina propria (Reinke's space), the intermediate lamina propria, the deep lamina propria (vocal ligament), and the vocalis muscle (**Fig. 48.9**). The epithelium is stratified squamous epithelium devoid of mucous glands. The length of the vocal cord is 15 to 23 mm in males and 13 to 17.5 mm in females. This accounts for the difference in pitch of the male and female voices.

The subglottis starts just below the level of the vocal cords and extends up to the lower border of the cricoid cartilage.

> ### Pearl
>
> The subglottis is formed by the cricoid cartilage, which is the only complete ring in the laryngotracheobronchial airway. Hence, this subsite is prone to stenosis, and mild edema can cause stridor especially in children.

■ Mucous Membrane of the Larynx

The anterior surface and the upper half of the laryngeal surface of the epiglottis, upper parts of the aryepiglottic folds, and the vocal folds are lined by the stratified squamous epithelium. The rest of the laryngeal mucous membrane

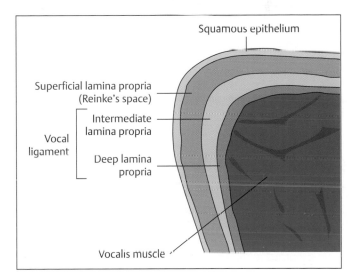

Fig. 48.9 Diagram showing the five layers of the vocal cord.

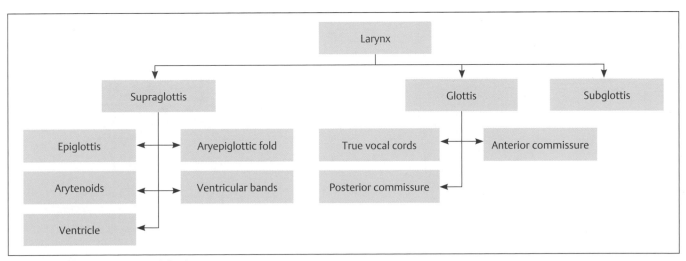

Flowchart 48.3 Divisions of the larynx.

is composed of columnar ciliated epithelium interspersed with goblet cells.

All the parts of the mucous membrane are loosely attached to the cartilages except over the vocal ligaments and posterior (laryngeal) surface of the epiglottis, where it is thin and firmly adherent. The mucous glands are absent over the vocal cords but numerous over the anterior surface of the epiglottis, around the cuneiform cartilage, and in the vestibular folds.

■ Preepiglottic Space of Boyer

Boundaries

The boundaries of the preepiglottic space are the following (**Fig. 48.10**):
- Anteriorly: The thyroid cartilage and thyrohyoid membrane.
- Posteriorly: The anterior surface of the epiglottis and thyroepiglottic ligament.
- Superiorly: The hyoid bone, hyoepiglottic ligament, and vallecula.
- Laterally: Continuous with the paraglottic space.

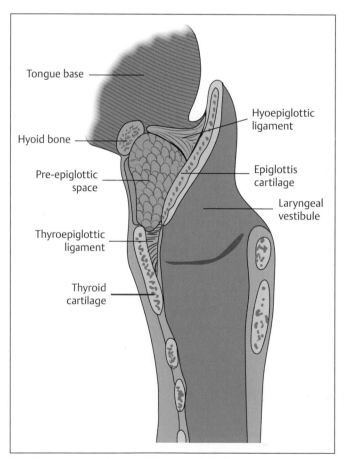

Fig. 48.10 Boundaries of the preepiglottic space.

> **Pearl**
>
> Malignancy from the supraglottis can spread to the preepiglottic space because of multiple fenestrations in the infrahyoid epiglottis. Spread can also occur via the paraglottic space. It contains fat, which makes it relatively resistant to radiotherapy.

■ Paraglottic Space of Tucker

Boundaries (**Fig. 48.11**):
- Medially: Quadrangular membrane, laryngeal ventricle, and conus elasticus.
- Laterally: Thyroid cartilage, mucosa of the medial wall of the pyriform fossa.
- Inferolaterally: Cricothyroid membrane.
- Anteriorly: Continuous with the preepiglottic space.

> **Pearl**
>
> The involvement of the paraglottic space by malignancy leads to impaired cord mobility or fixity. Tumor spread through the paraglottic space from the supraglottis can involve the glottis, subglottis, and thyroid cartilage.

■ Reinke's Space

It is a potential space present in the vocal cords between the epithelium and the vocal ligament containing cells, special fibers, and extracellular matrix with lymphatics (**Fig. 48.8**). It plays an important role in the vibration of vocal cords. It can potentially act as a barrier, preventing the early spread of cancer.

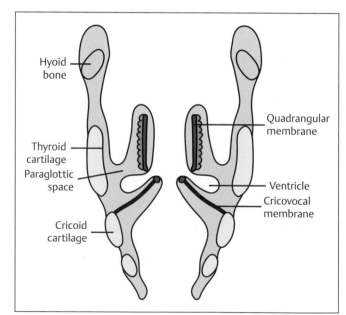

Fig. 48.11 Diagram showing the boundaries of the paraglottic space.

Table 48.2 Outline of the blood supply of the larynx

	Above the vocal cords	**Below the vocal cords**
Arterial supply	Superior laryngeal artery, a branch of the superior thyroid artery	Inferior laryngeal artery, branch of the inferior thyroid artery
Venous drainage	Superior laryngeal vein drains into the superior thyroid vein	Inferior laryngeal vein drains into the inferior thyroid vein

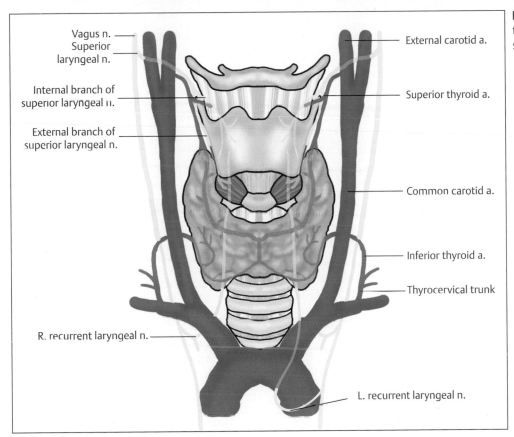

Fig. 48.12 Diagram showing the blood supply and nerve supply of the larynx.

Relations of the Larynx

- Anterior: Skin and deep cervical fascia.
- Posterior: Prevertebral fascia and muscles and body of C3–C6 vertebrae.
- Lateral: Carotid sheath, infrahyoid muscles, sternocleidomastoid muscle, and thyroid gland.

Blood Supply of the Larynx

The blood supply of the larynx is described in **Table 48.2**.

Nerve Supply of the Larynx

The nerve supply of the larynx is illustrated in **Fig. 48.12**.

■ Motor Supply

The cricothyroid muscle is the only intrinsic laryngeal muscle supplied by the external branch of the superior laryngeal nerve. The other intrinsic laryngeal muscles are supplied by the recurrent laryngeal nerve.

■ Sensory Supply

The sensation in the larynx from the supraglottis to the level of vocal cords is carried by the internal branch of the superior laryngeal nerve. The sensation below the level of vocal cords is by the recurrent laryngeal nerve.

Pearl

The region of the thyrohyoid membrane adjacent to the greater cornu of the hyoid bone, where the superior laryngeal vessels and nerve pierce to enter the larynx, is the site where the superior laryngeal nerve block can be given via an external approach.

Table 48.3 Differences between an adult larynx and an infant larynx

	Adult larynx	Infant larynx
Situation	C3–C6 vertebral level	C2–C3 vertebral level
Position	Behind the base of tongue at a lower level	More superior and anterior; obligate nasal breathers
Size	4–5 cm in length and width	One-third the adult size
Epiglottis	Leaf shaped	Longer, tubular, and narrower
Laryngeal inlet	Tubular	Conical/funnel shaped
Vocal cords	Horizontal	Shorter and concave
Arytenoids and aryepiglottic folds	Proportionate	More prominent with a large vocal process in comparison to the vocal cord
Cartilages	Firm	Soft
Subglottis	10 mm	4 mm
1 mm of circumferential subglottic edema	30% reduction in the subglottic airway	60–75% reduction in the subglottic airway

Lymphatic Drainage

Lymphatics from the supraglottic region drain along the superior thyroid vessels, pass through the thyrohyoid membrane to the deep cervical lymph nodes (levels II–IV).

Lymphatics in the vocal cords are sparse, which account for the lower incidence of lymph node metastasis in glottic malignancy.

Lymphatics from below the vocal cord region (subglottis) drain predominantly into the pretracheal, paratracheal, prelaryngeal (Delphian node), and superior mediastinal lymph nodes.

Pearl

The supraglottis is rich in lymphatics. Malignancy of the supraglottis has a high incidence of lymph node metastasis, which can be bilateral.

Differences between an Adult and an Infant Larynx

Differences between adult and infant larynxes are presented in **Table 48.3**.

Pearl

The higher position of the larynx in infants allows for the suck–swallow–breathe sequence during feeds.

Points to Ponder

- The larynx is made of cartilages supported by membranes.
- The supraglottis, glottis, and subglottis are the three subsites of the larynx.
- The superior laryngeal nerve (internal branch) provides sensation above the glottis, and the recurrent laryngeal nerve supplies sensation below the glottis.
- The recurrent laryngeal nerve supplies all the intrinsic muscles of the larynx except the cricothyroid muscle, which is supplied by the external branch of the superior laryngeal nerve.
- The size of the larynx, shape of the laryngeal inlet, laxity of mucosa, and soft cartilages in infants and young children make them more prone for early airway compromise with minimal edema.

Case-Based Question

1. **A 56-year-old chronic smoker presented to the ear, nose, and throat (ENT) clinic with a 3-year history of change in voice. He had a low-pitched, hoarse voice. Indirect laryngoscopy showed bilateral, edematous, mobile, and congested vocal cords, with a slightly translucent appearance. He also gives history of overuse of voice.**

   a. What is the diagnosis?

   b. What is the etiopathology of this condition?

   c. How will you treat this condition?

   Answers

   a. Reinke's edema.

   b. Reinke's space is a potential space on the vocal cords between the outer squamous epithelium and the intermediate lamina propria. This space, the superficial laminal propria, normally contains a gelatinous fluid, but due to constant irritation, like cigarette smoking, excessive fluid can accumulate leading to swollen vocal cords.

   c. Treatment consists of cessation of smoking, voice therapy, and treatment of gastric reflux. If medical treatment does not improve the condition, surgery must be performed through the microflap technique in order to reduce the edematous, redundant mucosa.

Frequently Asked Questions

1. What are the parts of the larynx?

2. What are the muscles of the larynx and their actions?

3. What is the nerve supply of the larynx?

4. Enumerate the cartilages of the larynx.

5. Describe the anatomical boundaries of the preepiglottic space.

6. What is Reinke's space? What is its clinical importance?

7. What is the conus elasticus? Describe its attachments.

Endnote

Giovanni Domenico Santorini (1681–1737) was an Italian anatomist and lived in the city of Venice. He was a meticulous and outstanding anatomist who dissected out complex structure of the human body like the accessory pancreatic ducts of Santorini. His ENT contributions include the fissures of Santorini, the supreme or Santorini's turbinate, and the risorius or smiling muscle of facial expression called the muscle of Santorini. In the larynx, the corniculate cartilage is named after him, Santorini's cartilage. The cuneiform and corniculate cartilages are thought to strengthen the aryepiglottic folds.

49 Physiology of the Larynx

Suresh Pillai and Prerit Rao

The competency covered in this chapter is as follows:
EN1.1 Describe the anatomy and physiology of the ear, nose, throat, and head and neck.

Introduction

The larynx is in a unique position in the aerodigestive tract. It is nestled between the pyriform fossae on either side and is also the portal of entry toward the lower respiratory tract. The position and structure of the larynx, with regard to the cartilages, muscles, and membranes, along with the neural network and neuromuscular control, are responsible for the physiological functions of the larynx. Abnormalities in any of these can affect the laryngeal and lower airway in terms of respiration, aspiration, swallowing, and phonation. The glottis opens during respiration and closes during swallowing.

Functions of the Larynx

The functions of the larynx are the following:
- Protection of the lower respiratory tract.
- Respiration.
- Phonation.
- Increasing intrathoracic pressure.

■ Larynx in Protection of the Lower Respiratory Tract

The lower airway, the tracheobronchial tree, is further protected during the pharyngeal phase of deglutition from ingested and inhaled materials at the larynx by the following mechanisms:
- The upward and anterior movement of the larynx.
- The three-tier mechanism of valvular closure.
- Cough.

In addition, there are mechanoreceptors and chemoreceptors, which, along with the central nervous system (supratentorial and brainstem), play an important role in the action of the larynx during the pharyngeal phase of deglutition.

The upward and anterior movement of the larynx occurs due to the following:
- Mylohyoid action causing laryngeal elevation.
- Stylopharyngeus action causing laryngeal tilting.

This enlarges the pharynx, creates a vacuum in the hypopharynx and larynx, and opens up the cricopharynx sphincter for the bolus of food to move downward.

The Three-Tier Mechanism

The epiglottis passively moves to cover the laryngeal inlet, which helps divert food toward the pyriform fossae (**Flowchart 49.1**). It also slows down the movement of fluids to allow time for the vocal cords to adduct and the larynx to elevate.

Pearl

Mechanical or neural pathologies affecting the larynx can compromise these protective mechanisms during swallowing leading to aspiration.

Cough

It occurs due to an increased inspiratory effort with exaggerated abduction of the vocal cords (preparatory inspiratory phase) followed by the tight closure of the vocal cords (compressive phase). Subsequently there is increased intrapulmonary and subglottic pressure, which leads to an abrupt opening of the vocal cords. This releases air at high velocity.

It can occur by involuntary stimulation of the network of afferent sensory innervation (the internal branch of

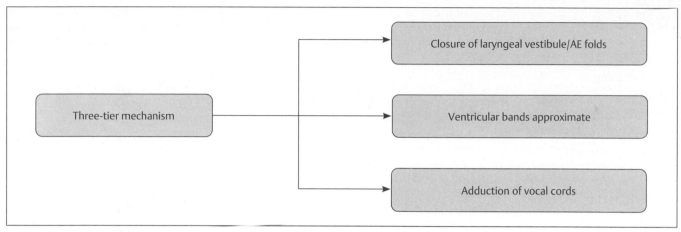

Flowchart 49.1   A three-tier mechanism of protection of the lower respiratory tract by the larynx.

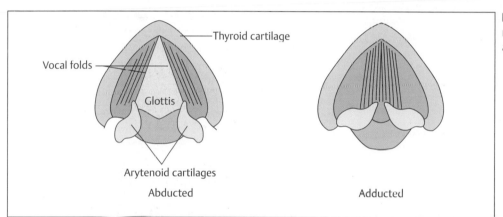

Fig. 49.1   Diagram showing the movements of the vocal cords, abduction, and adduction.

the superior laryngeal nerve) or it can be voluntary. This is important for expulsion of material that has wrongly entered the airway.

> ### Pearl
> Coughing can occur even in bilateral laryngeal paralysis due to the passive closure of the ventricular bands, which is sufficient for effective cough.

■ Larynx in Respiration

- In the resting state, abduction of the cords is by the action of the posterior cricoarytenoid muscle and it maintains the laryngeal patency during inspiration (**Fig. 49.1**).
- Adduction of the cords is by the adductors and passive relaxation of the posterior cricoarytenoid resulting in a small amount of positive end-expiratory pressure, which slows the exhalation rate. This helps in preventing collapse of distal bronchi.
- The larynx regulates airflow to and from the lungs. Inspiratory collapse of the laryngeal airway during respiration is prevented by the cricoid cartilage.

> ### Pearl
> The pathological exaggeration of the protective glottal closure through adduction, even after stopping the stimulus, leads to laryngospasm. This is forceful and prolonged. It can occur due to laryngeal instrumentation, foreign body in the airway, and laryngopharyngeal reflux.

■ Larynx in Phonation

The human voice is a complex sound that emanates from the vocal cords and, when articulated by the structures above, results in speech. This is important for communication.

The role of the larynx in voice production is facilitated by the change in shape and movement of the vocal cords. The shape of the vocal cords is due to its five layers.

- The epithelial lining and superficial lamina propria form the *cover*.
- The intermediate and deep layers form the *transition zone*.
- The vocalis muscle forms the *body* of the vocal cord.

The movements occur due to the action of the intrinsic muscles of the larynx and they include the following:
- Abduction.
- Adduction.
- Lengthening.
- Mass.
- Stiffness.
- Tension of the vocal cords.

The vocal cords vibrate when air starts escaping, causing vibratory tones. These tones are then converted into speech with the help of articulators and resonators.

The resonators are present in the chest, pharynx, nose, and paranasal sinus, whereas the articulators are present in the oral cavity.

Pearl

Rhythmic opening and closing occur due to vibration of the "cover" of the vocal cord resulting in pulses of air perceived as sound. Injury of the transition zone due to surgery or trauma leads to scarring. Vocal cord tension and regulation of resistance to airflow is affected when the "body" of the vocal cord is involved.

There are various theories that have been described in the literature regarding the mechanism of phonation. The most accepted one is the myoelastic aerodynamic theory.

The *myoelastic aerodynamic theory* of phonation states that when the vocal cords are completely adducted, escape of air is prevented, leading to a positive pressure air column. This air column or subglottic pressure, when sufficient, pushes the vocal cords apart. This is responsible for the vibration of the vocal cords, which results in vibratory tones. These tones are further amplified by the resonators. The articulators give the characteristic speech.

The prerequisites of normal phonation are as follows:
- Adequate respiratory support.
- Adequate glottic closure.
- Intact mucosal cover of vocal cords.
- Adequate control of the vocal fold length and tension.

If any of the above four factors are not met, then phonation is affected. For example, if a patient has abductor palsy due to a cerebrovascular accident, there will not be adequate glottic closure, which will result in voice change as the chief complaint.

Each cycle consists of the following:
- Subglottic pressure from below pushing up against a closed glottis.
- Added pressure from the lungs leads to opening of the inferior part of the vocal cords.
- This opening travels upward like an "air bubble" toward the superior surface of the vocal cord like a traveling wave (**Fig. 49.2**).
- As the superior surface opens, pressurized air escapes as a jet (opening phase of the vibratory cycle).
- The wave on the superior surface propagates laterally during which the inferior part moves medially due to reduced subglottic pressure.
- Closure of the vocal cords occurs from inferior to superior (closing phase of the vibratory cycle).
- Repetition of the cycle.

Pearl

The pitch of the voice depends on the frequency of the vocal cord vibration, which is related to length. Loudness of voice depends on the subglottic pressure and amplitude of vibration of the vocal cords. Subglottic pressure depends on the pressure generated from the lungs and the extent of closure of the glottis.

■ Larynx in Increasing Intrathoracic Pressure

Laryngeal closure with increase in intrathoracic pressure, via a Valsalva maneuver, is important for activities like coughing, straining, lifting, and pushing.

Pearl

Laryngeal stimulation can initiate cardiovascular reflexes leading to bradycardia, cardiac arrhythmias, and cardiac arrest. This can even occur during intubation.

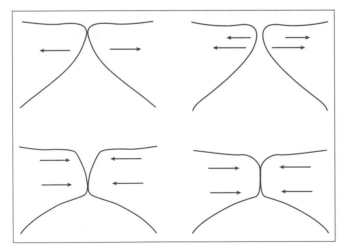

Fig. 49.2 Vocal cord movements from an inferior surface to a superior surface, during phonation as subglottic pressure builds up and the cords are pushed apart.

Points to Ponder

- Diseases of the larynx can affect the lower airway (aspiration, collapse of the distal bronchiole, and airway obstruction).
- The three-tier mechanism at the larynx and the cough reflex are important for protecting the lower airway.
- Diseases of the lower airway can affect the production of voice due to the inadequate intrapulmonary pressure, which in turn results in inadequate subglottic pressure.
- Voice production occurs due to rhythmic repetitive cycles of vibration of the "cover" over the "body" of the vocal cords.

Case-Based Question

1. **A 65-year-old woman was brought to the ear, nose, and throat (ENT) clinic on a wheelchair, with a history of breathy voice and cough on taking food. She had given a history of a cerebrovascular accident (CVA), previously. On examination, both vocal cords were in an abducted position with a large phonatory gap.**

   a. What is the reason for the breathy voice?

   b. What is the reason for the cough?

Answers

a. Since both the vocal cords are in the abducted position, due to the neurological pathology, there is no subglottic pressure build to generate sound against the adducted vocal cords.

b. One of the protective functions of the lungs is lost due to the inability of the vocal cords to adduct and abduct. Also, the neurological lesion may have affected the sensation of the larynx, leading to aspiration.

Frequently Asked Questions

1. Enumerate the functions of the larynx.
2. How does the larynx protect the lower airway?
3. What are the prerequisites for normal phonation?
4. Explain the physiology of sound production.
5. Describe the muscles involved in abduction and adduction.

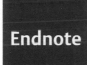

Endnote

Minoru Hirano (1932–2017) was one of the prominent figures of laryngology of the 20th century. He knew that the larynx was capable of producing an astonishing variety of sounds in term of pitch, quality, and intensity, and he wanted to know how professional singers can produce these sounds. In 1974, he published the Cover Body theory of vocal cord vibration, where he divided the vocal cords, biomechanically, into the cover and the body. He said that the epithelium and the superficial lamina propria moved as a single unit and called it the cover, whereas the body consisted of the vocal ligament and the thyroarytenoid muscle. So according to his theory, the vocal cords function as a double-structured vibrator, the cover and the body.

50 History Taking and Examination of the Larynx

Sathappan Subramanian

> **The competencies covered in this chapter are as follows:**
>
> EN2.1 Elicit, document, and present an appropriate history in a patient presenting with an ear, nose, and throat (ENT) complaint.
>
> EN4.42 Elicit, document, and present a correct history; demonstrate and describe the clinical features; choose the correct investigations; and describe the principles of management of hoarseness of voice.

History-Taking Skills

- Enquire about the chief complaints from the patient and the duration. The common symptoms include the following:
  - Change in voice.
  - Pain on swallowing.
  - Difficulty in swallowing.
  - Breathing difficulty.
  - Cough.
  - Swelling in the neck.
- History of present illness (HOPI): The chief complaints have to be explored in detail with reference to the type, duration, onset, progression, associated symptoms, and aggravating and relieving factors.
- Other relevant history related to laryngeal symptoms should include the following:
  - Change in voice or hoarseness of voice. This can occur due to laryngeal lesions or vocal cord palsy.

The type of voice such as harsh, breathy, and muffled should be noted. Note whether there are any voice breaks, delayed phonatory onset, diplophonia, or inability to use a high pitch. Also consider that in boys, voice changes occur during puberty (puberphonia). Also evaluate whether there is any diurnal variation. Chronic laryngitis is worse in the morning, while in myasthenia gravis, the voice deteriorates by evening.

  - Voice abuse (shouting/talking loudly), overuse (talks for a long duration without frequent breaks), or misuse (altering ones voice like in mimicry) can all contribute to voice change.
  - Cough with phlegm can occur in tuberculous laryngitis or chronic obstructive pulmonary disease. Chronic cough can cause a contact ulcer or granuloma.
  - Frequent clearing of throat or hawking.
  - Difficulty in swallowing or dysphagia. It can occur due to malignancy.
  - Painful swallowing or odynophagia. It can occur in acute laryngitis, tuberculous laryngitis, and advanced malignancy.
  - Cough on swallowing or aspiration.
  - Difficulty in breathing or stridor seen in laryngomalacia, carcinoma of the larynx, granulomas, edema, stenosis, and inflammatory disorders. Note if there is any improvement with change in position. In laryngomalacia, the stridor reduces in the prone position, whereas in acute epiglottitis, the patient is more comfortable in the sitting-up and forward positions, also known as the tripod sign.
  - Sore throat (laryngitis and pharyngitis).
  - Swellings in the neck (thyroid, cervical lymph nodes, and laryngocele).
  - Foreign body sensation in the throat (laryngopharyngeal reflux).
  - Referred ear pain (carcinoma larynx and laryngitis).
  - History suggestive of gastroesophageal reflux disease.
  - History of sinonasal infection and upper respiratory allergy.
  - Neurological history.
  - Endocrine history: menopause and thyroid.
- Past medical history:
  - Is there diabetes mellitus, hypertension, bronchial asthma, and exposure to tuberculosis?
  - Prior history of radiotherapy to the neck.
- Past surgical history:
  - Enquire about previous surgical history in the neck, throat, or thorax, especially thyroid surgery and neck dissection.
  - Prior history of intubation or endoscopy.

- Drug history:
  - Thyroid hormone replacement therapy or nonsteroidal anti-inflammatory drugs (NSAIDs).
  - Use of inhalers.
- Personal history:
  - Occupation (teacher, salesperson, and singer).
  - Smoking.
  - Drinking alcohol.
  - Food habits.
- Family history:
  - Tuberculosis.

Examination of the Larynx

The examination of the external framework of the larynx is done along with the examination of the neck. Specific examination related to the larynx is mentioned below.

- External laryngeal framework examination in the neck. Look for the following:
  - Swelling or fullness in the thyrohyoid or cricothyroid membrane, which can occur in benign conditions like laryngocele and in extralaryngeal spread of malignancy.
  - Redness of skin.
  - Fistula or sinus.
  - Discharge.
  - Splaying of the thyroid cartilage with tenderness, which signifies malignancy.
  - Laryngeal crepitus: This is performed by moving the laryngeal cartilage from side to side against the cervical vertebra with a gentle posterior pressure. A crackling sound or grating sensation is produced. This is called Muir's crackle. This is normal. It is absent in postcricoid carcinoma, retropharyngeal abscess, and laryngeal trauma. It is also referred to as positive *Bocca's sign.*
- *Indirect laryngoscopy* is a standard method of examining the base of the tongue, larynx, and hypopharynx using a mirror. It allows for visualizing the anatomical structures, mucosal color and integrity, and vocal cord mobility. The patient is seated in front of the examiner at a slightly higher level such that the eyes of the examiner are at the level of the patient's mouth (**Fig. 50.1**). The examiner can use a head mirror with a light source or a headlight. The patient with a straight back should lean forward at the hips along with lifting of the chest and chin ("sniffing" position). This makes the base of the tongue more anterior to the larynx allowing for better visualization. A laryngeal or dental mirror (**Fig. 50.2**) is warmed or dipped in antifog solution. The patient is asked to protrude the tongue, which is grasped with a gauze sponge by the examiner using the left hand. The index finger of the left hand is used to elevate the upper lip. The mirror is introduced into the mouth, after dipping in a soap solution, and placed against the soft palate (**Fig. 50.3**). It is angled in various directions to visualize the structures. The larynx and vocal cords should be examined while the patient says "EEE" and also during respiration (**Fig. 50.4** and **50.5**).

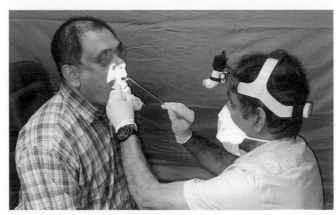

Fig. 50.1 The position of the patient and examiner during laryngeal examination.

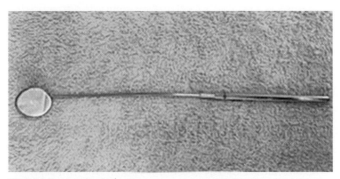

Fig. 50.2 Laryngeal mirror.

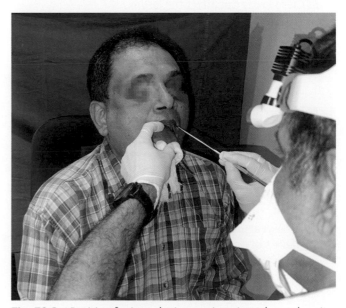

Fig. 50.3 Position for introducing a mirror into the oral cavity.

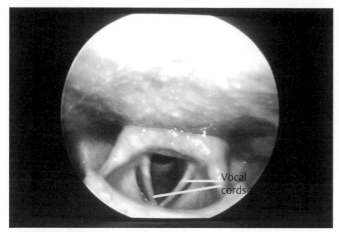

Fig. 50.4 View of vocal cords during indirect laryngoscopy.

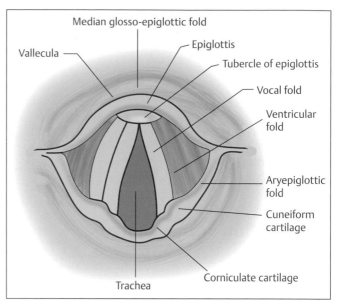

Fig. 50.5 Diagrammatic representation of the structures seen during laryngeal examination.

- Rigid or flexible laryngoscopy is currently more frequently used as the visualization of the structures is better. When used with a camera, the videolaryngoscopy can be used to counsel the patient, and also for teaching purposes.
- Voice assessment during history-taking and examination is valuable in getting an indication toward the type and quality of voice. A more formal assessment is done by the speech pathologist using parameters like the GRBAS (grade, roughness, breathiness, asthenia, and strain) scale.
- The neck is observed for contraction or tightness of the cervical muscles during phonation, which is mainly seen in muscle tension dysphonia.
- Examination of the neck for other swellings including lymph nodes and goiter.
- Examination of the nose and paranasal sinuses, oral cavity, oropharynx, and chest is required as pathologies in these areas can affect the larynx.
- Palpation of the base of the tongue and vallecula is necessary in laryngeal and hypopharyngeal malignancy.

Here induration may be felt when there is spread to the pre-epiglottic space or vallecula. This is better felt if the patient is under general anesthesia (for the biopsy of the primary lesion) as the muscles will be relaxed and the changes can be better felt.

Points to Ponder

- The commonest complaint with regard to laryngeal disease is change in voice.
- Enquire about gastroesophageal reflux disease in hoarseness of voice.
- Positive Bocca's sign means absence of laryngeal crepitus.
- Flexible laryngoscopy is more useful when assessing the larynx in children and infants.

Case-Based Question

1. **A 35-year-old primary school teacher presents with a 6-month history of change in voice. There is history of voice breaks and delayed phonatory onset. He is not a smoker and does not consume alcohol. There is no history of an upper respiratory tract infection.**

   a. What is the most likely diagnosis?
   b. What will be the expected findings on laryngoscopy?
   c. A 60-year-old man, who is a smoker, came with complaints of hoarseness of voice. How will you examine his larynx?

Answers
a. Vocal cord nodules (Singer's nodule).
b. Both the vocal cords will be mobile, but nodules will be noted at the junction of the anterior one-third and posterior two-thirds of the vocal cords.
c. With the patient seated in front, the examiner uses a light source and a laryngeal mirror. The mirror is dipped in savlon or a soap solution so that it does not mist when it is introduced into the oral cavity. Gag reflex is prevented by avoiding touching the posterior pharyngeal wall. The mirror is rotated so that the entire larynx is visualized, and the patient is made to phonate to see the vocal cord movements.

Frequently Asked Questions

1. What are the common symptoms associated with laryngeal disorders?

2. What are the steps involved in indirect laryngoscopy?

3. What is laryngeal crepitus?

4. In which condition is the voice worse in the morning?

Endnote

Manuel Patricio Garcia (son of a famous Spanish tenor) was a music composer, singer, and teacher. He is credited to have first used a dentist's mirror to view his own larynx. This was done by reflecting the sunlight behind him, onto a mirror he placed in front so that the light would be reflected into his mouth. He then introduced another warmed mirror into the back of his throat. He used both the mirrors simultaneously to see the structure and movement of the vocal cords. His paper on Physiological observations on the human voice was presented at the Royal society of London in 1855. For his contribution, he is considered the father of laryngology.

Investigations for Laryngeal Disease and Evaluation of Hoarseness of Voice

51

Sathappan Subramanian

The competencies covered in this chapter are as follows:

EN3.3 Observe and describe the indications for and steps involved in the performance of rigid/flexible laryngoscopy.

EN4.42 Elicit, document, and present a correct history; demonstrate and describe the clinical features; choose the correct investigations; and describe the principles of management of hoarseness of voice.

Introduction

The purpose of any investigation in medical practice is to make a possible diagnosis, to know the extent of disease, to plan appropriate treatment, to know the prognosis, and for documentation during medicolegal proceedings. Voice is an important component of communication. Disorders of voice are quite common, with change in voice being the most common symptom. According to Aronson, "a voice disorder exists when there is a difference in the voice quality, pitch, loudness or flexibility from the voices of others of similar age, sex, and cultural group."

Definitions for Different Types of Altered Voice

Dysphonia/hoarseness is an abnormal quality of voice.
Breathy voice is due to incomplete closure at the glottic level during phonation, giving it an "airy" quality. The voice is weak. It is seen in unilateral vocal cord palsy and vocal cord atrophy.

Muffled voice is when the voice appears as if it is wrapped or covered. It is also known as "hot potato voice." It is seen in oropharyngeal space occupying tumors, quinsy, and some supraglottic tumors.

Strained voice is tightness of the neck or throat during attempted phonation. It is usually seen in muscle tension dysphonia or spasmodic dysphonia.

Functional aphonia is the inability to produce voice in the absence of an organic pathology.

Puberphonia is the persistence of a high-pitched voice in males, after puberty.

Voice abuse is using a loud voice either suddenly or frequently.

Voice misuse is the alteration of the pitch or quality of voice, for example, in mimicry.

Voice overuse is when the voice is used for long durations without sufficient breaks.

Causes of Hoarseness

■ Organic Voice Disorders

- Congenital: Glottic web.
- Inflammatory: Acute laryngitis and chronic laryngitis including granulomatous conditions like tuberculosis.
- Neurological conditions: Vocal cord paralysis or paresis, myasthenia gravis, Parkinson's disease, amyotrophic lateral sclerosis, and spasmodic dysphonia.

- Neoplasms.
- Benign: Papilloma/papillomatosis.
- Malignant: Squamous cell carcinoma.
- Miscellaneous: Vocal cord atrophy, keratosis, amyloidosis, and leukoplakia.

■ Nonorganic/Behavioral Voice Disorders

- Habitual: Nodules, polyp, cyst, Reinke's edema, and contact ulcer/granuloma.
- Psychogenic: Muscle tension dysphonia and functional aphonia.

The investigations for diseases of the larynx are preceded by a focused and relevant history, and examination, which includes laryngoscopy. History taking and examination of the larynx are described in Chapter 50.

Investigation of Laryngeal Disorders

The evaluation of laryngeal disorders should include the following:
- Laryngeal videoendoscopy/rigid telescopy of larynx.
- Flexible laryngoscopy.
- Hematological investigations.
- Imaging studies.
- Biopsy.
- Voice assessment using software like VAGMI is useful in documenting the type of voice and analyzing the progress during and after treatment. Voice handicap index (VHI), a quality-of-life score, is useful for the purpose of documentation.
- Additional evaluation modalities:
  - Videostroboscopy.
  - High-speed kymography.
  - High-speed digital imaging.
  - Laryngeal electromyography.
  - Narrowband imaging (NBI).

The larynx and hypopharynx can be examined by a laryngeal mirror, a 90-degree rigid laryngeal telescope, a flexible nasopharyngolaryngoscope, or a direct laryngoscope. Each of these has advantages and disadvantages.

Few decades ago, use of the *laryngeal mirror* was the standard practice for examining the larynx, hypopharynx, and base of the tongue. The mirror needs to be warmed to avoid fogging. An overhanging epiglottis may block the view of the vocal cords. The advent of good-quality endoscopes has largely replaced its use in many centers.

■ Rigid-Angled Laryngeal Telescopes

A 90-degree rigid endoscopy is commonly used to examine the larynx and its adjacent structures (**Fig. 51.1**). It is slightly expensive, but the resolution (high definition) of images is good and can be recorded. During the procedure, the patient is asked to protrude the tongue, which is grasped by the examiner using a gauze. The patient breathes normally through the mouth. The rigid endoscope is introduced from the side of the mouth (commonly near the right oral commissure) and then directed medially toward the posterior pharyngeal wall. If it is passed from the midline, the bulk of the tongue may manipulate the endoscope and make viewing difficult. The patient is asked to say "EEE," which makes the soft palate move upward and backward, and also makes the base of the tongue move inferiorly, which allows for better manipulation and visualization of the larynx and hypopharynx. To negate the gag reflex, a 10% xylocaine spray is used (**Fig 51.2**).

■ Flexible Nasopharyngolaryngoscopy

The flexible nasopharyngolaryngoscopy (FNPLS; **Fig. 51.3**), which is made up of a bundle of fiberoptic rods, is another method used to examine the larynx and hypopharynx. Even though it is expensive, it is comfortable when compared to a rigid telescope, and can be used in both children and adults. In addition, since the tongue is not held by the

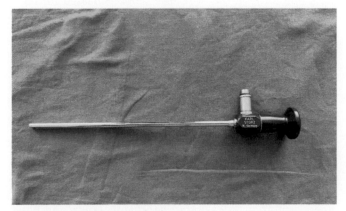

Fig. 51.1 Rigid laryngeal telescope.

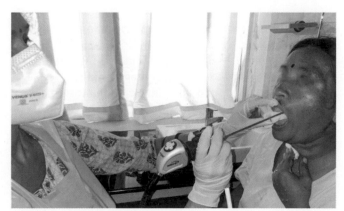

Fig. 51.2 Rigid laryngoscopy in progress.

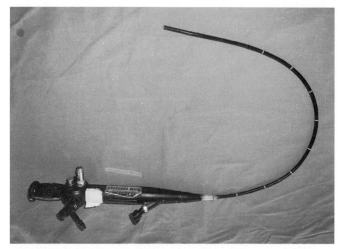

Fig. 51.3 Flexible nasopharyngolaryngoscope.

examiner, visualization of the structures is in an anatomic position, and the vocal cord movement is more dynamic. The nasopharyngolaryngoscope may have a channel with it, which can be used to do suction and take biopsy at the same time with minimal discomfort. Therapeutic procedures may be done when the scope has a channel for instrumentation (**Fig. 51.4a** and **b**).

Indications

- Diagnostic:
  - Evaluation of pediatric and adult stridor.
  - Evaluation of lesions in the nose, nasopharynx, oropharynx, larynx, and hypopharynx.
  - Evaluation of voice disorders.
  - Evaluation of neurological conditions of the larynx.
  - Fiberoptic endoscopic evaluation of swallowing.
  - Biopsy.
- Therapeutic:
  - Assessment of correction during medialization thyroplasty.
  - Confirm the site for injection of botulinum toxin in spasmodic dysphonia.
  - Confirm the site and the correction of injection laryngoplasty (vocal cord augmentation).
  - Assist in mucosal injections (cidofovir in papillomatosis and steroids in contact granuloma).
  - It can be used with laser for papillomatosis, contact granuloma, and glottic web.
  - Removal of vocal cord polyp.
  - Removal of small foreign body.

Anesthesia

Topical decongestant with an anesthetic agent can be placed in the nasal cavities. The oropharynx can be sprayed with 10% topical xylocaine. The laryngeal inlet may also be anesthetized by a topical agent.

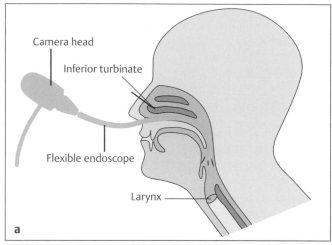

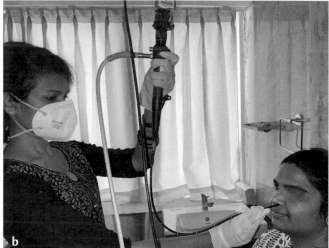

Fig. 51.4 **(a)** Flexible nasolaryngoscopy to visualize the larynx. **(b)** Flexible nasopharyngoscopy in progress.

Procedure

The outer surface of the scope toward the tip is prepared with KY or Xylocaine jelly for smooth introduction of the scope through the nose. The scope is passed through the nasal cavity along the floor (between the inferior turbinate and septum; it may also be passed between the middle and inferior turbinates) till it reaches the postnasal space. The tip of the scope is turned downward. During that time, the patient is asked to breathe through the nose to open the nasopharyngeal isthmus, to advance the scope. Once the scope reaches the oropharynx, there will be a clear view of the base of the tongue, epiglottis, larynx, and hypopharynx. The patient is asked to protrude the tongue for visualization of the vallecula. The patient is asked to puff the cheeks with closed lips to distend the pyriform fossae. The structure and mobility of vocal cords are also assessed during quiet respiration, speaking voice, singing voice, and phonation during various maneuvers. The pyriform fossa of the hypopharynx is also visualized during phonation.

■ Hematological investigations

Investigation	Reasons
Complete blood count	To rule out acute or chronic infection
C-reactive protein	To rule out acute infection
ESR	Increased chronic infections
Thyroid function test (TSH, T3, T4)	To rule out hyper-/hypothyroid diseases

Abbreviations: ESR, erythrocyte sedimentation rate; TSH, thyroid-stimulating hormone.

■ Imaging studies

Investigation	Justification
Neck X-ray	Foreign body, retropharyngeal abscess, and laryngotracheal stenosis
Chest X-ray	To rule out pulmonary tuberculosis and sarcoidosis
Scan of the neck/larynx	Extension of lesion or mass; laryngotracheal stenosis
MRI of the neck/larynx	Soft-tissue extension of lesion/mass in the neck/larynx
PET scan	Early detection of carcinoma; screening for metastasis or second primary cancer, in advanced malignancy, and for recurrent malignancy

Abbreviations: CT, computed tomography; MRI, magnetic resonance imaging; PET, positron emission tomography.

For the larynx, a high-resolution CT scan with 1-mm cuts with or without contrast is preferred. It is useful in laryngeal trauma, recurrent granuloma, ventricular band fullness, immobile cords, tumors, and laryngeal stenosis.

■ Biopsy

Histopathological examination is necessary before formulating any treatment. Biopsy is essential to confirm the neoplastic diseases and to grade the tumors. It is also useful in diagnosing or confirming benign conditions of the larynx including tuberculosis, papillomatosis, etc. The biopsy can be taken by visualizing through a rigid telescope, a flexible endoscope, a direct laryngoscope, or by microlaryngoscopy.

■ Videostroboscopy

Principle

Talbot's law states that the retention of an image on the retina is 200 milliseconds after exposure. Using this principle, when rapid flashes of light are projected on a quasiperiodic vibratory (cyclically moving) source like the oscillating vocal cords, the recorded images can be made slower or frozen. These can be reproduced in sequence, giving the illusion of continuous images. It can be done with the help of a rigid or a flexible endoscope.

Parameters Assessed

- Symmetry of vibration of the two cords.
- Periodicity of vibration (length of glottal cycle).
- Phase closure (percentage of time the cord edges are open or closed).
- Amplitude of vibration (lateral movement of cords).
- Glottic configuration (vocal cord closure pattern).
- Mucosal wave (movement of the superficial layers with air movement).

Uses

- Detailed visual analysis of vocal cord vibration.
- Hoarseness with relatively normal structure and mobility.
- Documentation of vocal cord function prior to treatment.
- Evaluation of outcomes of treatment.
- Planning surgery especially in unilateral vocal cord palsy.

Examples

- Posterior gap is common in females.
- Anterior or spindle-shaped gap is seen in scars, atrophy, and sulcus.
- Hourglass shape is seen in nodules, cyst, and polyp.
- Incomplete closure is seen in vocal cord palsy.
- Amplitude of vibration is reduced in glottal incompetence and increased stiffness, and the amplitude is increased in palsy.

■ High-Speed Videokymography

Principle

The vocal cord movements at adduction and abduction during phonation are rapid, that is, around 100 times per second. The velocity of vibration is also high, that is, approximately 1 m per second. These movements are captured by a continuous light (in contrast to stroboscopy, which is flashes of light) using high-speed imaging. Here the full movement including intracycle images is captured. But in kymography, the images are captured in a single horizontal line.

■ High-Speed Digital Imaging

Principle

A high-speed camera captures real-time images at a minimal rate of 2,000 to 10,000 frames per second. The full length of the vocal cord and pattern of vibration are recorded regardless of phonatory duration or severity of dysphonia. These are played back in slow motion. Using computer-based programs, the large amount of data captured can be processed to reduce the viewing time. The denervation, reinnervation potential, and recruitment patterns are assessed.

Uses

It gives a better assessment of vocal fold vibratory function. Even different singing styles can be studied.

■ Laryngeal Electromyography

Principle

The action potentials of the muscles of the larynx are recorded during voluntary and involuntary contraction. The right and left cricothyroid muscles (for the corresponding superior laryngeal nerve) and the right and left thyroarytenoid muscles (for the corresponding recurrent laryngeal nerve) are mainly assessed.

Uses

- To differentiate paresis from palsy.
- Mechanical fixation from ankylosis and dislocation (cricoarytenoid joint).
- Denervation and myopathy from neuropathy.
- It is also useful while assessing the site of injection and the response in the treatment for botulinum toxin in spasmodic dysphonia.

■ Narrowband Imaging

Principle

It is endoscopy with optical interference filters. The differential absorption characteristics for tissues and blood vessels are utilized. White light is filtered into specific light wavelengths: blue (400–430 nm) and green (515–555 nm). Switch to either wavelengths can be done. On endoscopy, using this technique, the intraepithelial papillary capillary loops are enhanced. Changes in these microvascular characteristics in relation to the mucosa are classified (Ni classification) to potential benign, preneoplastic, and malignant possibilities.

Uses

It can be used for detecting early malignancy and preneoplastic lesions. Biopsy can be taken from suspicious areas based on NBI findings.

Management of Hoarseness

■ Medical

Treatment of the underlying condition like laryngitis. Treatment of factors that affect the larynx like sinonasal infection, upper respiratory allergy, and gastroesophageal reflux disease.

■ Voice Therapy

- It may start with voice rest.
- It can be the main treatment for disorders like vocal nodules, and is also used in the postoperative period to enhance/maintain prior voice quality.
- Appropriate use of voice and phonation exercises.
- Professional voice users are trained in the use of voice.
- Appropriate use of pitch, volume, and rate of speech.
- Singing voice therapy is individualized to restore and maximize singing quality of the voice especially after an injury or phonomicrosurgery.
- Vocal hygiene: These are the steps taken to keep the vocal cord healthy and include the following:
  - Increased intake of fluids to prevent dehydration.
  - Avoiding alcohol.
  - Avoiding repeated clearing of throat.
  - Avoiding smoking.
  - Normal conversational use of voice instead of whispering or shouting.
  - Avoiding spicy food and environmental pollution.

■ Behavioral Therapy

- Reduce musculoskeletal tension.
- Breathing exercises that help improve breath support for voice.
- Reduce stress factors that cause strain to voice.

■ Invasive Procedures

- Botulinum injection: It is used in spasmodic dysphonia and nonhealing contact granuloma.
- Injection laryngoplasty: It is used for augmentation of vocal cord for vocal cord paralysis.
- Phonomicrosurgery: It is used for benign lesions and tumors, and in early glottic malignancy. It is also useful for assessment of the vocal cords and taking biopsy.
  - Excision biopsy for benign lesions.
  - Cordectomy for malignant lesions in carcinoma of the vocal cord.
- Laryngeal framework surgery is commonest is medialization thyroplasty done for unilateral vocal cord palsy.

Points to Ponder

- Dysphonia or hoarseness of voice is an important symptom pointing to laryngeal disease. The colloquial term "hoarseness" is retained because it is a term patients understand.
- Laryngeal examination must be carried out if dysphonia fails to improve even 3 weeks after treatment so that the underlying pathology is not missed.
- There is a wide range of instruments and equipment available to look into the larynx including rigid and flexible laryngoscopes.
- Flexible laryngoscopy is more comfortable for the patient and the indications are divided into diagnostic and therapeutic.
- Vocal hygiene is an important component of the medical management of voice disorders.

Case-Based Question

1. **A 45-year-old woman underwent hemithyroidectomy following which she developed hoarseness of voice. She was referred to the ear, nose, and throat (ENT) department for further management since the hoarseness was not improving.**

   a. What is the likely cause of hoarseness of voice?

   b. What relevant investigations should be carried out?

   c. What is the management of this condition?

Answers

a. Following thyroidectomy, if there is immediate hoarseness of voice, the most likely etiology is injury to the recurrent laryngeal nerve, which can paralyze the vocal cord.

b. A rigid-angled laryngeal telescope is sufficient to visualize the vocal cords in adult patients. However, if the patient is uncomfortable or uncooperative, an FNPLS can be used.

c. Hoarseness, in this condition, persists because of a paralyzed vocal cord. Injection laryngoplasty can be tried to push the vocal cord medially and improve the voice. Another option is laryngeal framework surgery in the form of medialization thyroplasty.

Frequently Asked Questions

1. What are the different types of altered voice?
2. What are the causes of hoarseness of voice?
3. List the indications for flexible laryngoscopy.
4. Describe the steps involved in flexible laryngoscopy.
5. How will you medically manage a patient with hoarseness of voice?
6. What is stroboscopy?

Endnote

The capturing of a series of images in rapid succession followed by creating an optical illusion of apparent motion is the principle used in the making of motion pictures. This principle is made use of in stroboscopy to observe and study vocal cord vibration. Stroboscopy uses flashes of light that pass through a laryngoscopy, either rigid or flexible. The flashes of light allow for a slow motion picture of vocal cord movements much like the disco lights in a night club.

52 Acute and Chronic Inflammation of the Larynx

Jaspal Singh Sahota and Kamlesh Dubey

The competencies covered in this chapter are as follows:

EN4.43 Describe the clinical features, investigations, and principles of management of acute and chronic laryngitis.

AN38.2 Describe the anatomical aspects of laryngitis.

PE28.6 Discuss the etio-pathogenesis, clinical features, and management of acute laryngo-tracheo-bronchitis.

PE28.5 Discuss the etio-pathogenesis, clinical features, and management of epiglottitis.

Introduction

The larynx, cradled behind the base of tongue and between the pyriform fossae, is exposed to inhaled and ingested substances. It can be involved from an extension of disease of the upper respiratory tract (nose, nasopharynx, and oropharynx) or secondary to lower respiratory conditions.

Classification

- *Acute*:
  - Acute laryngitis.
  - Acute epiglottitis/supraglottitis.
  - Acute laryngotracheobronchitis.
  - Diphtheria.
- *Chronic (specific)*:
  - *Bacterial*:
    - ○ Tuberculous.
    - ○ Scleroma.
    - ○ Syphilitic.
    - ○ Leprosy.
    - ○ Actinomycosis.
  - *Fungal*:
    - ○ Candidiasis.
    - ○ Histoplasmosis.
    - ○ Cryptococcosis.
    - ○ Blastomycosis.
- *Nonspecific (noninfective)*:
  - Wegener's granulomatosis.
  - Amyloidosis.
  - Sarcoidosis.
  - Relapsing polychondritis.
  - Angioedema.

- *Other noninfective conditions* which can cause or predispose to *inflammation of the larynx* include:
  - Vocal abuse.
  - Laryngopharyngeal reflux (LPR).
  - Reinke's edema.
  - Iatrogenic (radiotherapy, intubation, endoscopy).
  - Upper respiratory allergy.
  - Trauma: External (blunt or penetrating injury) and internal (chemicals and corrosive, iatrogenic).
  - Environmental pollution and/or smoke.
  - Chronic rhinosinusitis with postnasal drip.

Pearl

Chronic cough referred to an otolaryngologist is mainly to assess sinonasal infection, upper respiratory allergy, or LPR or gastroesophageal reflux disease (GERD) as possible causes. An intrinsic lesion in the laryngotracheal airway and an extrinsic swelling like a thyroid nodule pressing on the trachea can also present with cough.

Acute Laryngitis

Acute laryngitis is an acute inflammation of the larynx. The condition starts abruptly and lasts less than 3 weeks.

■ Etiology

- It is usually a part of a viral upper respiratory tract infection commonly caused by adenovirus, rhinovirus, parainfluenza, or respiratory syncytial virus. Later there can be secondary bacterial infection with *Streptococcus pneumoniae* or *Hemophilus influenzae*.

- It can also be the result of vocal misuse or exposure to chemical agents during inhalation. It can also be caused by allergy and reflux disease (GERD).

■ Symptoms and Signs

- Fever, malaise, sore throat, painful swallowing, and hoarseness are the common symptoms.
- Other symptoms include dry cough and frequent throat clearing.
- Indirect laryngoscopy or rigid telescopy will show congestion of the larynx (red color), with or without edema (**Fig. 52.1**).
- Sticky secretions may also be seen between the vocal cords or in the interarytenoid region.

■ Treatment

- The symptoms resolve spontaneously in 5 to 14 days.
- Symptomatic treatment is with analgesics and antipyretics. Antibiotics are reserved for secondary bacterial infection.
- Voice rest. Complete voice rest is ideal, but it may be difficult for the patient to follow. Whispering is to be avoided as it increases the strain on the vocal cords.
- Steam inhalation will keep the upper airway moist and help to clear the secretion and exudate.
- Cessation of smoking.
- Persistent symptoms will require re-evaluation of the larynx by rigid or flexible endoscopy.

Acute Laryngotracheobronchitis (Croup)

This is a viral upper respiratory tract infection commonly seen in children. It mainly affects the larynx and trachea, but it can also extend to the bronchus. It is also known as croup because of the characteristic barking cough seen in these patients.

■ Etiology

The viruses causing this infection are spread during coughing and sneezing as well as by hand contamination through fomites and then subsequently touching the eyes, nose, or mouth.

- Inflammatory changes to the subglottis secondary to viral and bacterial infections may often present as stridor and cough.
- Parainfluenza virus types 1, 2, and 3 account for 75 to 80% of all croup cases. Influenza A and B, adenovirus, respiratory syncytial virus, rhinovirus, and enterovirus have also been associated with causing laryngeal and cervical tracheal edema.
- It is usually seen in children in the age group of 6 months to 3 years.

■ Clinical Features

- Common presenting symptoms include rhinorrhea, dysphonia progressing to aphonia, fever, and "seal bark" cough. Low grade fever may be present. The symptoms are worse at night.
- Stridor may be present.
- Viral subglottic edema is usually self-limiting and will resolve within 5 days.
- The edema (exudate rich in neutrophils) extends from the subglottis to the bronchi.

■ Management

- A plain film radiograph (X-ray of neck in anteroposterior [AP] view) reveals a *steeple sign* (or wine bottle sign). This is pathognomonic of croup (**Fig. 52.2**).
- Supportive care with analgesics, antipyretics, systemic corticosteroids, nebulized adrenaline, humidification, and supplemental oxygen in majority of croup cases is paramount.
- Endotracheal intubation or tracheostomy may be required in some cases.

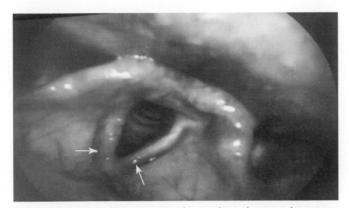

Fig. 52.1 Acute laryngitis. Both vocal cords are edematous and congested.

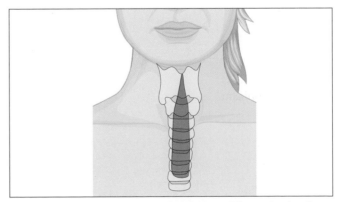

Fig. 52.2 Diagrammatic representation of "steeple sign."

- Laryngoscopy is rarely indicated in the acute or subacute phases of the illness.
- Recurrent cases of croup should prompt more detailed ENT investigation. This may be indicative of underlying subglottic stenosis that makes the child more susceptible to airway compromise with minimal subglottic edema with a more difficult recovery. These patients will likely need hospitalization, supplemental oxygen, and possible intubation during the disease course.
- Gastroesophageal reflux has been associated with subglottic stenosis and may leave the child more susceptible to recurrent croup.
- Airway endoscopy should be considered in the workup of patients with recurrent croup in order to identify a subglottic pathology such as stenosis or hemangioma.

> ### Pearl
> Steeple sign is produced by edema of the subglottis and upper trachea due to inflammation. This results in narrowing or tapering of the upper trachea. On an AP view of X-ray of the neck, the narrowed part resembles a church steeple.

Acute Epiglottitis or Supraglottic Laryngitis

This is an acute inflammation of the supraglottic region of the larynx which includes epiglottis, vallecula, arytenoids, and aryepiglottic folds. The resulting edema can result in obstruction of the airway.

■ Etiology

- It is seen in children in the 2 to 4 years age group and is caused by the bacteria *Hemophilus influenza* type B (HIB). The incidence has reduced nowadays due to HIB vaccine. Post HIB vaccination other organisms like group A *Streptococcus pneumoniae*, *Staphylococcus aureus*, *Klebsiella pneumoniae*, and β hemolytic streptococci can cause this infection.
- In adults it is seen in immunocompromised individuals including those with uncontrolled diabetes.

■ Clinical Features

- There is a sudden onset of symptoms. Fever, sore throat, drooling of saliva, and odynophagia are the presenting symptoms. This can rapidly lead to stridor.
- On examination, a cherry-red appearance of the epiglottis due to inflammation and edema will be seen. Abscess can form especially in adults with epiglottitis. Do not use a tongue depressor for examination as it can precipitate stridor.
- The child will sit up, leaning forwards with hands on the sides for support. This is known as the tripod position (**Fig. 52.3**). On leaning back, the airway may get compromised due to the enlarged epiglottis, occluding the laryngeal inlet.
- There will be tachycardia and tachypnoea with accessory muscles of respiration acting and tracheal tug. The child is restless with a toxic appearance. Cough will be absent.

■ Management

- X-ray of neck in lateral view will show a prominent epiglottis (*thumb sign*) and narrow or absent pre-epiglottic air shadow known as the *vallecula sign* (**Fig. 52.4**).
- Admit the child in the intensive care unit (ICU) and start on adrenaline nebulization which may help reduce the edema. Starting an intravenous line should be done in a controlled setting as agitation of the child can also aggravate the airway compromise.
- Intravenous antibiotics (third-generation cephalosporins, chloramphenicol) are started.

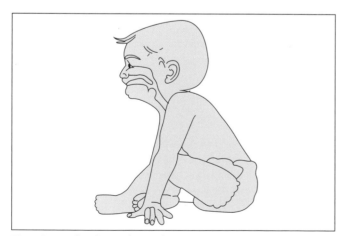

Fig. 52.3 The classical tripod position seen in acute epiglottitis in children.

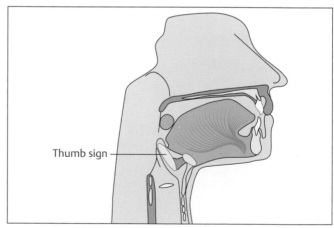

Fig. 52.4 Lateral view of oropharynx showing thumb sign.

- Swab may be taken from the epiglottis in a controlled setting of an ICU or operating room after securing the airway. The blood is sent for culture and sensitivity test.
- Tracheostomy is sometimes required to secure the airway.

■ Differential Diagnosis

Croup, airway foreign body, anaphylaxis, retropharyngeal abscess, peritonsillar abscess, trauma, airway burns, or ingestion of corrosives.

Chronic Laryngitis

Laryngitis or inflammation of the larynx that lasts longer than 3 weeks is known as chronic laryngitis. The disease process involves the mucosa and submucosa. The chronic inflammation can be due to infectious or noninfectious causes.

The infectious variety of chronic laryngitis can be further classified into *nonspecific* and *specific* chronic laryngitis. In the latter there is a definite etiology like tuberculosis or syphilis.

Chronic nonspecific laryngitis can further be classified into *chronic hyperemic laryngitis* in which there is a diffuse inflammation of the larynx and *chronic hypertrophic* or *hyperplastic laryngitis* which can be diffuse or localized like vocal cord polyp and Reinke's edema (**Flowchart 52.1**).

Examples of noninfectious causes of chronic laryngitis include allergy, smoking, voice abuse, and LPR.

Chronic Nonspecific Laryngitis

This is a common condition presenting with dysphonia or hoarseness of voice. The severity of dysphonia depends on the etiology. It can vary from mild to severe hoarseness of voice ultimately leading to aphonia or absence of voice.

■ Etiology

- Incompletely treated or unresolved acute laryngitis.
- Focus of chronic infection at other sites like chronic sinusitis, chronic tonsillitis, dental caries, and lung infection.
- Vocal abuse or vocal misuse.
- Smoking.
- Environmental factors like exposure to dust and chemical fumes.
- Chronic cough and constant clearing of throat.
- LPR.

■ Clinical Features

Symptoms

- Hoarseness of voice.
- Voice fatigue.
- Discomfort in throat.
- Persistent throat clearing.
- Halitosis.
- Globus pharyngeus like symptoms.

Signs

- There is diffuse hyperemia of the larynx.
- Vocal cords are congested and edematous.
- Thick secretions may be seen over the vocal cord.

■ Investigations

- Investigations include flexible fiberoptic laryngoscopy.
- In most of the cases, diagnosis can be made from the history and the clinical examination.
- In cases of long-standing duration, biopsy should be considered to rule out other conditions like candidiasis, tuberculosis, or malignancy.

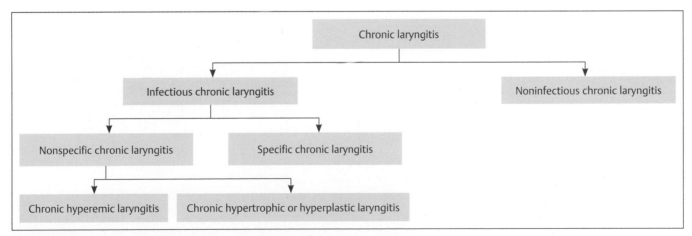

Flowchart 52.1 Flowchart depicting the classification of chronic laryngitis.

■ Treatment

- Treatment of chronic infections of the sinuses, tonsils, teeth, and lungs if present.
- Cessation of smoking.
- Speech therapy if there is voice abuse or voice misuse.
- Treatment of LPR and GERD with proton pump inhibitors like pantoprazole.

The causes and features of acute and chronic laryngitis are outlined in **Table 52.1**.

Laryngeal Diphtheria

It is usually secondary to spread of infection from the oropharynx. Treatment is with antitoxin and antibiotics (penicillin or macrolides). Intubation or tracheostomy may be required to secure the airway.

Laryngeal Tuberculosis

■ Etiology

Tuberculosis of the larynx is caused by *Mycobacterium tuberculosis* and is usually secondary to pulmonary tuberculosis. Primary laryngeal involvement is rare. It spreads from a pulmonary site and reaches the larynx through the blood or through sputum. Atypical mycobacteria (like *Mycobacterium avium* complex, *Mycobacterium fortuitum*, and *Mycobacterium malmoense*) can involve the larynx especially in immunocompromised individuals.

Table 52.1 Causes and features of acute and chronic laryngitis

Etiology	Acute laryngitis	Chronic laryngitis
Infections:		
Viral (most common infectious causes)	Parainfluenza, influenza, RSV, rhinovirus, coronavirus, adenovirus, chickenpox, measles	HPV-associated with RRP, EBV
Bacterial	*Streptococcus pneumoniae, Hemophilus influenzae, Moraxella catarrhalis* (most common bacteria in order), *Bordetella pertussis* (whooping cough)	*Staphylococcus aureus* (methicillin sensitive and resistant variants), *Pseudomonas aeruginosa*, other enterobacteria (*Klebsiella, Escherichia coli*), *Serratia marcescens*; chronic granulomatous diseases (tuberculosis, leprosy, rhinoscleroma)
Fungal	Mostly secondary to antibiotics and steroid inhaler use; common fungus isolated are *Candida albicans*, Cryptococcus, *Histoplasma capsulatum*, Blastomyces, and Coccidioides; seen in both immunocompromised and immunocompetent patients	Candidiasis, aspergillosis, cryptococcosis, blastomycosis, histoplasmosis; also seen in patients with history of diabetes, immunodeficiency status, and immunosuppressive medication (long-term steroids, chemotherapeutic drugs)
Allergy	Both acute and chronic inflammation	Chronic cases with recurrent acute inflammation presentations
LPR diseases	Both acute and chronic inflammation	A major cause for chronic laryngitis
Voice abuse/overuse	Both acute and chronic inflammation	When associated with LPR, greater risk for vocal nodules and contact ulcer or granuloma
Pollution	Both acute and chronic inflammation	Wide prevalence with environmental pollution
Lifestyle habits	Both acute and chronic inflammation	Smoking, alcohol use
Chronic rhinosinusitis		PND causes chronic inflammation of pharynx as well as larynx
Autoimmune disorders		Wegener's granulomatosis (polyangiitis granulomatosis) Rheumatoid arthritis SLE Relapsing polyangiitis Amyloidosis
Trauma	Intubation, endoscopy procedures, surgeries in lower respiratory tract	Pollutants, smoke, LPR-induced injuries, RT

Abbreviations: EBV, Epstein-Barr virus; HPV, human papillomavirus; LPR, laryngopharyngeal reflux; PND, postnasal dip; RRP, respiratory recurrent papillomatosis; RSV, respiratory syncytial virus; RT, radiotherapy; SLE, systemic lupus erythematosus.

■ Pathology

The tubercle bacilli present in the sputum reaches the larynx when it is expectorated. It generally tends to affect the posterior part of the larynx with infiltration of the submucosa of the interarytenoid region, ventricular bands, vocal cords, and epiglottis. There is initial exudation of the subepithelial space followed by round cell infiltration. The submucosal tubercles undergo caseation and ulceration, eventually healing by fibrosis.

■ Clinical Features

The symptoms in addition to pulmonary symptoms are odynophagia, dysphagia, painful phonation, change in voice, and vocal fatigue.

The signs are as follows (**Figs. 52.5** and **52.6**):
- Monochorditis (unilateral vocal cord congestion).
- Mouse-nibbled appearance (ulcerations on the vocal cord).
- Nodular lesions.
- Involvement of posterior glottis and interarytenoid region due to coughed up sputum stagnating in this region.
- Reduced vocal cord mobility due to myositis, or nerve or cricoarytenoid joint involvement.
- Turban epiglottis in the later stages due to pseudoedema secondary to lymphatic obstruction.
- Tuberculosis can mimic other diseases including malignancy.

■ Management

- Investigations include chest X-ray, sputum acid-fast bacilli (AFB), and culture and biopsy from the laryngeal lesions.
- Antitubercular treatment.

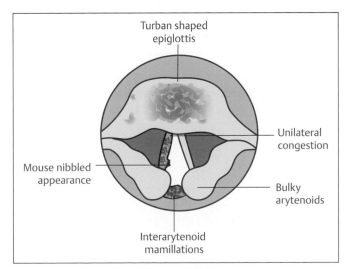

Fig. 52.5 Tuberculous lesions of the larynx.

Laryngeal Leprosy

- It is caused by *Mycobacterium leprae* (Hansen's bacilli). Laryngeal involvement is rare.
- It usually involves the supraglottis with painless edema, congestion, and a nodular appearance. The voice may be muffled.
- Ulceration and fibrosis of the larynx may lead to stenosis.
- Diagnosis is by biopsy from the lesion.
- Treatment is with diaminodiphenyl sulphone (dapsone), rifampicin, or clofazimine. It is administered until subsequent biopsies are negative.

Laryngeal Syphilis

This is caused by *Treponema pallidum*. It is a rare condition and is associated with secondary or tertiary syphilis.
- In the secondary stage there are maculopapular lesions with erythema.
- In the tertiary stage, the lesions present as nodular lesions with ulceration which later lead to perichondritis and scarring and fibrosis.

Pearl

Perichondritis of the laryngeal cartilages can occur due to radiotherapy, infections like tuberculosis and syphilis, trauma, or following fracture of the cartilage and advanced malignancy.

Scleroma of Larynx

- The causative organism is *Klebsiella rhinoscleromatis*. It usually involves the nose.
- In the larynx, the subglottis may be involved leading to fibrosis and stridor.

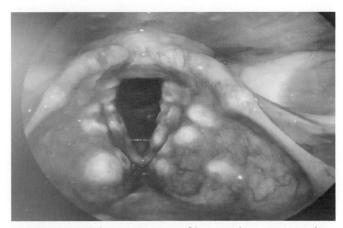

Fig. 52.6 Nodular appearance of laryngeal mucosa in tuberculous laryngitis.

- Treatment is with tetracycline. Tracheostomy may be required to secure the airway.

Laryngeal Actinomycosis

- It is caused by *Actinomycosis bovis* or *Actinomycosis israelii* and affects devitalized tissue.
- There will be edema and congestion of the larynx. An abscess can develop which is followed by a discharging sinus.
- Histopathology shows sulfur granules of actinomyces.
- Treatment is with penicillin or tetracycline.

Laryngeal Candidiasis

■ Etiology

- Prolonged use of systemic or inhaled steroids.
- Reduced immunity due to uncontrolled diabetes, acquired immunodeficiency syndrome (AIDS), chemotherapy, and chronic alcoholism.
- After radiotherapy to the head and neck region laryngopharynx.

■ Presentation

- Sore throat, odynophagia, change in voice.
- Whitish patches can be seen over the supraglottis with mucosal erythema (**Fig. 52.7**).

■ Treatment

- Treat the underlying cause.
- Oral nystatin suspension for local application. Systemic treatment with antifungals like fluconazole.

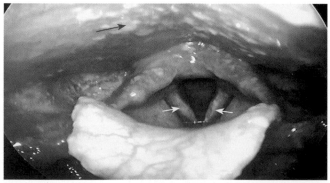

Fig. 52.7 White patches seen over the vocal cords (*yellow arrows*) and posterior pharyngeal wall (*red arrow*) in laryngeal candidiasis.

Granulomatosis with Polyangiitis (GPA) (Wegener's Granulomatosis)

- It is a rare, multisystem disorder of unknown etiology.
- It is characterized by necrotizing granulomatous inflammation of small and medium sized vessels leading to vasculitis.
- It can present with subglottic stenosis and airway obstruction.
- Diagnosis is based on antineutrophilic cytoplasmic antibodies (cANCA) or anti-proteinase3 tests, and histopathological examination of the lesion.
- Treatment is with steroids and cyclophosphamide.

Laryngeal Amyloidosis

- Amyloidosis is a disturbance in metabolism leading to extracellular eosinophilic proteinaceous filament deposits.
- Congo red stain shows apple green birefringence under polarized light microscopy.
- It can be hereditary or acquired, systemic or localized.
- The common symptom in laryngeal amyloidosis is hoarseness.
- Laryngeal examination shows ventricular band fullness and polypoid or nodular lesions. The lesions can be diffuse or localized.
- Localized laryngeal amyloidosis can be resected.
- Systemic involvement leads to renal or cardiac failure.

Points to Ponder

- Viral laryngotracheobronchitis is the most common emergency inflammatory laryngitis condition in young children of the 6 months to 3 years age group.
- Acute laryngitis is inflammation of the larynx of less than 3 weeks in duration.
- Chronic laryngitis is inflammation of the larynx of more than 3 weeks duration.
- The commonest organism causing croup is Parainfluenza virus types 1, 2, and 3.
- *Hemophilus influenzae* is the commonest cause for acute epiglottitis.
- Tripod position and thumb sign are seen in acute epiglottitis.
- Monochorditis and turban epiglottis are features of tuberculosis of the larynx.
- LPR disorder, pollution, smoking, and voice abuse are becoming common factors associated with chronic laryngitis in adults.

Case-Based Questions

1. **A 1-year-old male child was brought to the emergency department with a history of low grade fever, cough, and change in the quality of voice. An X-ray of the neck was done, and it showed narrowing of the subglottis and upper trachea.**

a. What is the most probable diagnosis?

b. What are the common causative organisms?

c. What is the typical X-ray finding in this condition?

d. What is the treatment?

Answers

a. Croup or acute laryngotracheobronchitis.

b. Parainfluenza virus types 1, 2, and 3. Other viruses implicated are influenza A and B, adenovirus, respiratory syncytial virus, rhinovirus, and enterovirus.

c. Steeple sign.

d. Supportive treatment with analgesics, antipyretics, intravenous corticosteroids, nebulized adrenaline, humidified air, and supplemental oxygen.

2. **A 3-year-old female child presented with fever, throat pain, pain on swallowing, and breathing difficulty. The child was sitting up and leaning forwards. X-ray of neck in lateral view showed a prominent soft tissue shadow of the epiglottis.**

a. What is the most probable diagnosis?

b. What is the common organism responsible?

c. What is the sign on the X-ray and the name of the position adopted by the child?

d. What is the treatment?

Answers

a. Acute epiglottitis.

b. *Hemophilus influenza* type B.

c. Thumb sign; tripod position.

d. Intravenous antibiotics (third-generation cephalosporins), intravenous fluids, and nebulized adrenaline. Tracheostomy may be required to secure the airway.

3. **A 37-year-old male presented with chronic cough and evening rise of temperature. There is a recent history of change in voice. Rigid telescopy showed congestion of the left vocal cord with thickening in the interarytenoid region.**

a. What is the most probable diagnosis?

b. What are the investigations required for diagnosis?

c. What are the other features of laryngeal involvement of this disease?

d. What is the treatment?

Answers

a. Pulmonary tuberculosis with secondary laryngeal tuberculosis.

b. Chest X-ray, sputum for acid-fast bacilli (AFB) staining and culture; biopsy may be done to confirm laryngeal involvement.

c. Monochorditis (unilateral vocal cord congestion), mouse-nibbled appearance (ulcerations on the vocal cord), nodular lesions, involvement of posterior glottis and interarytenoid region due to coughed up sputum stagnating this region, reduced vocal cord mobility due to myositis, or nerve or cricoarytenoid joint involvement, turban epiglottis in the later stages due to pseudoedema secondary to lymphatic obstruction. This can mimic other diseases including malignancy.

d. Antitubercular treatment.

Frequently Asked Questions

1. What is the etiology of acute laryngitis?

2. What is croup? How will you manage this condition?

3. What is tripod position? Why does the child adopt this posture?

4. What are the laryngeal features of tuberculosis of the larynx?

5. What is the etiology of chronic nonspecific laryngitis?

6. What is thumb's sign? In which condition is this seen?

Endnote

GERD has been implicated in laryngitis since the 1960s. There are two theories stated as to the pathophysiology of laryngitis due to GERD. One theory states that there is direct injury to the tissues of the larynx due to the pepsin and acid content of gastric secretions. The second theory states that the acid content in the lower esophagus stimulates the vagus resulting in bronchospasm, cough, and chronic throat clearing. These two mechanisms may bring about changes in the larynx leading to chronic laryngitis. The association of GERD and laryngitis is known as acid laryngitis.

53 Vocal Cord Paralysis

Udayabhanu H.N.

Introduction

Vocal cord paralysis or vocal fold paralysis (VFP) is due to a reduced or absent movement of one or both vocal folds. A neural or neurological cause is the main etiological factor for a vocal cord paralysis, and it is rarely due to neuromuscular junction disorders. The morbidity due to the paralysis can adversely affect the patient's quality of life.

Vocal cord paralysis can be unilateral or bilateral. It may involve the recurrent laryngeal nerve (RLN) or superior laryngeal nerve (SLN), or both. The glottic airway, phonation, protection of lower airway, and swallowing can get affected depending on whether one or both cords are involved. Males are more commonly affected than females (8:1).

The symptoms depend on whether it is a unilateral or bilateral cord palsy. The other associated symptoms, based on the etiology, include:
- Referred otalgia.
- Cough.
- Hemoptysis.
- Neck lumps.

Unilateral and bilateral cord paralysis symptoms vary due to the functional movement of the cords. Abduction is required for respiration, while adduction is necessary for phonation and prevention of aspiration. There will also be an inability to obtain a positive subglottic pressure which is important for straining (Valsalva maneuver) and phonation.

The subspeciality of laryngology has brought in better diagnostic tools, clinical assessment, and treatment options in the management of unilateral vocal cord palsy.

Pearl

VFP can be a sign of an underlying disease in the neck or thorax and investigations should include these two regions.

Definitions

Vocal cord paralysis is complete absence of movement (immobility) of the vocal cord.

Vocal cord paresis is a condition where there are weak or varying degrees of movement (impaired mobility) of the vocal cord.

Laryngeal Innervation

Phonation is initiated by *Area 4* in the Sylvian fissure of the cerebrum. The vagal nuclei are thus bilaterally innervated. The nucleus of the vagus nerve is in the brainstem (medulla), that is, nucleus ambiguus. It passes through the jugular foramen and travels below in the carotid sheath. Three branches are given off in the neck (**Fig. 53.1**):
- Pharyngeal branch.
- Superior laryngeal nerve.
- Recurrent laryngeal nerve.

The SLN divides into two branches:
- Internal laryngeal nerve.
- External laryngeal nerve.

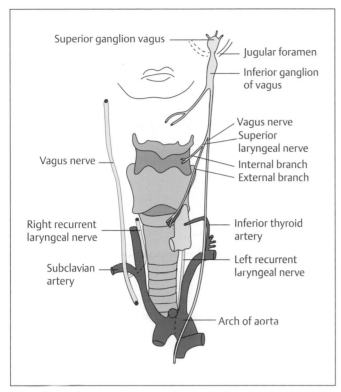

Fig. 53.1 The vagus nerve and its branches.

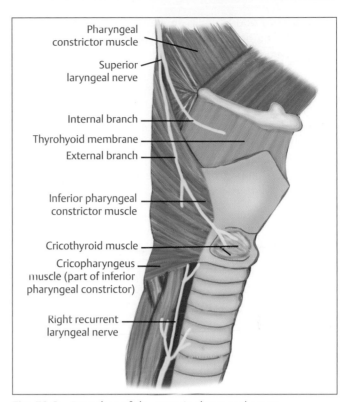

Fig. 53.2 Branches of the superior laryngeal nerve.

The *internal branch of the SLN* is a sensory branch providing sensation to the supraglottis which is above the level of the vocal cords. The *external branch of the SLN* is a motor branch innervating the cricothyroid muscle (**Fig. 53.2**).

The origin of the RLN from the vagus is in the superior mediastinum. On the left side the vagus descends posteromedial to the aortic arch, loops around it through the aorticopulmonary window. On the right side, it descends posterior to the subclavian artery, loops around it to ascend upwards into the neck. As it courses upwards it is situated in or adjacent to the tracheoesophageal groove. It enters the larynx posterior to the cricothyroid joint. The RLN supplies all the muscles of the larynx except for the cricothyroid muscle (**Fig. 53.3**).

The RLN supplies the unpaired interarytenoid muscle; therefore, it receives bilateral innervation. This allows adduction of the vocal cord during ipsilateral RLN paralysis. The cricothyroid muscle is a tensor of the vocal cord and does not adduct or abduct the cords.

The final position of the vocal cord is not static and results from a number of forces such as the degree of muscle atrophy, the degree of reinnervation, and the extent of synkinesis (mass movement).

Muscles Acting on the Vocal Cord

The intrinsic muscles of larynx are those which act on the vocal cord and laryngeal inlet.

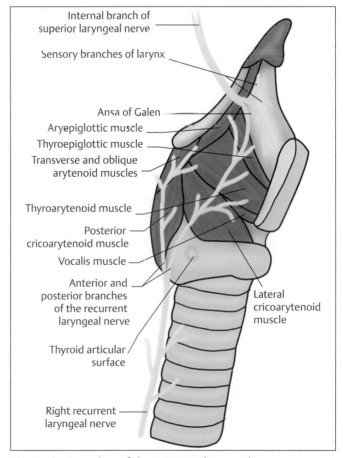

Fig. 53.3 Branches of the recurrent laryngeal nerve.

Vocal cord adduction is movement of the vocal cords toward the midline. This is carried out by adductor muscles which include:

- Lateral cricoarytenoid.
- Interarytenoid (transverse arytenoid).
- Thyroarytenoid (external part).

Vocal cord abduction (movement of vocal cords away from the midline) is carried out by the sole abductor which is the posterior cricoarytenoid muscle. The cricothyroid and vocalis (internal part of thyroarytenoid) help in tensing or lengthening of the vocal cord and are called tensors.

Pathophysiology

Palsy or paresis of the vocal cord in most cases is due to neural involvement which can affect the motor and sensory nerves. Pathology in the brain and cricoarytenoid joint fixity or dislocation can also affect vocal cord mobility.

The left RLN has a longer course and is more prone to chronic demyelination neuropathy. Injury to the RLN can also cause demyelination, and the rate of recovery depends on the severity of the injury. When Wallerian degeneration occurs due to a severe injury, recovery will depend on the number of viable fibers and the gap between the cut ends of the nerve. The human RLN has a strong tendency for reinnervation. Reinnervation seems to be the rule. Due to this tendency for reinnervation, the position of the vocal cord varies with time and there will be a gradual improvement in the voice. This improvement is also due to the compensatory action by the contralateral vocal cord.

For the vocal cords to vibrate, or for alternate opening and closing, two antagonistic forces are required to work, out of phase with each other, on the vocal cords. The opening force derives from subglottal pressure, whereas the closing force stems from elastic recoil and the Bernoulli effect.

Pearl

One should be able to differentiate between fixity and paralysis of the vocal cord as the pathological processes involved are usually different.

Causes of Vocal Cord Paralysis

The causes of vocal cord paralysis in general are:

- Malignant diseases like bronchial carcinoma, esophageal carcinoma, and thyroid carcinoma.
- Surgical trauma like thyroid surgery, congenital heart surgery, cervical spine surgery, and skull base surgery.
- Nonsurgical trauma like road traffic accident, violence (blunt or penetrating injury to neck or chest), and excessive cuff pressure of endotracheal tube.

- Idiopathic (possibly viral neuritis).
- Central neurological causes like cerebrovascular accidents and multiple sclerosis.
- Inflammatory causes like pulmonary tuberculosis and neck abscess.
- Neuromuscular disorders like myasthenia gravis and Eaton-Lambert syndrome.
- Miscellaneous causes like collagen diseases.

■ Anatomical Basis of Laryngeal Paralysis

Laryngeal paralysis may be unilateral or bilateral and may involve (1) RLN, (2) SLN, or (3) both recurrent and SLNs (combined or complete paralysis).

The causes for laryngeal paralysis could be at the following levels:

The cause may be central or peripheral, congenital, or acquired.

Central causes may be supranuclear, nuclear, or infranuclear (based on the nucleus ambiguus—upper and lower motor neurons synapse here):

- *Supranuclear*: Supranuclear lesions of the cortex leading to isolated paralysis of the vocal cord are extremely rare. It may be due to massive, diffuse bilateral lesions in the brain.
- *Nuclear*: There is involvement of nucleus ambiguus in the medulla. The causes are vascular, neoplastic, motor neurone disease, polio, and syringobulbia. Nuclear lesions have an associated paralysis of other cranial nerves and neural pathways (**Table 53.1**).
- *Infranuclear*:

Table 53.1 Causes of combined paralysis, both recurrent and superior laryngeal nerves

Location of lesion*	Etiology for paralysis
Intracranial	Posterior fossa lesions
	Tubercular meningitis
	Cerebrovascular accidents
	Arnold-Chiari malformation
	Meningomyelocele
	Hydrocephalus
Skull base	Fractures
	Nasopharyngeal carcinoma
	Skull base paraganglioma
	Surgical procedures
Neck	Penetrating/surgical trauma
	Parapharyngeal tumors/abscess
	Metastatic nodes
	Lymphomas

*The lesions are high vagal lesions and those involving nucleus ambiguus.

– *High vagal lesions*: Vagus nerve may be involved in the skull base areas, at the level of jugular foramen or parapharyngeal space.
– *Low vagal nerve or RLN* injury.

It is idiopathic in about 12 to 22% of cases. The cause remains obscure.

■ Anatomical Basis of Recurrent Laryngeal Nerve Paralysis

Recurrent Laryngeal Nerve

The RLN provides motor nerve to all of the intrinsic laryngeal muscles, except cricothyroid, and sensory nerve to the mucosa at and below the level of the vocal cords. The right RLN arises from the vagus at the level of subclavian artery, hooks around it, and then ascends (initially at an angle) between the trachea and esophagus, parallel to the tracheo-esophageal groove.

The left RLN arises from vagus in the mediastinum at the level of arch of aorta, loops around it, and then ascends into the neck in the tracheo-esophageal groove. The left recurrent has a longer course than right and is more prone to paralysis. The ratio of injury is 4:1 in comparison to right side.

The important relations of the RLN in the neck and thorax are outlined in **Table 53.2**. Lesions in these structures can cause paralysis.

The various etiologies for recurrent laryngeal paralysis are mentioned in **Table 53.3**.

Pearl

Although left vocal cord palsy is more common, during thyroidectomy the right RLN is more likely to be injured as it is placed away from the tracheo-esophageal groove.

Pearl

A *non-RLN* arises directly from the vagus and enters the larynx. It may be seen on the right side especially when there is an aberrant right subclavian artery. It occurs in 1% of cases. The nerve may be more prone to injury during thyroid surgery if the surgeon is not aware of this condition.

Systemic disease leading to vocal cord paralysis include the following:
- Diabetes mellitus.
- Rheumatoid arthritis.
- Collagen vascular diseases.
- Viral infections.

Table 53.2 Important relations of the recurrent laryngeal nerve

Right side	Left side
Right subclavian artery	Aortic arch
Apex of right upper lobe of lung	Esophagus
Supraclavicular lymph nodes	Left mainstem bronchus
	Mediastinal lymph nodes
	Left atrium

Table 53.3 Etiology of recurrent laryngeal nerve paralysis

Unilateral—right or left side	Left side	Bilateral
Congenital conditions	*Mediastinum*:	Congenital
Postsurgical trauma: Post thyroid/parathyroid surgery, tracheostomy, esophageal and lung surgery for carcinoma, partial laryngectomy, neck dissection, removal of pharyngeal pouch, anterior approaches for cervical spine fusion	• Bronchogenic carcinoma • Pulmonary tuberculosis • Aneurysm of aorta • Mediastinal mass **(Fig. 53.4)** • Mediastinal lymphadenopathy **(Fig. 53.5)**	Post thyroid/parathyroid surgery Malignancy of thyroid or cervical esophagus
Nonsurgical neck trauma, including birth trauma, i.e., use of forceps, blunt or penetrating injury, cuff of endotracheal tube	• Ortner's syndrome (enlarged left atria) • Intrathoracic surgery—patent ductus arteriosus, tracheo-esophageal repair, cardiac/pulmonary surgery	Cervical lymphadenopathy Guillain-Barre syndrome
Malignant disease: Malignancy of thyroid, cervical esophagus, nasopharynx, larynx	• Sarcoidosis • Syphilitic aortitis	Idiopathic
Cervical lymphadenopathy: Metastatic, tuberculosis, lymphoma		
Inflammatory causes: Pulmonary tuberculosis, parapharyngeal abscess; viral neuritis due to influenza or infectious mononucleosis viruses		
Aneurysm of subclavian artery		
Neurological diseases: Cerebrovascular accident, multiple sclerosis, amyotrophic lateral sclerosis, syringomyelia and Parkinsonism, Guillain-Barre syndrome		
Idiopathic		

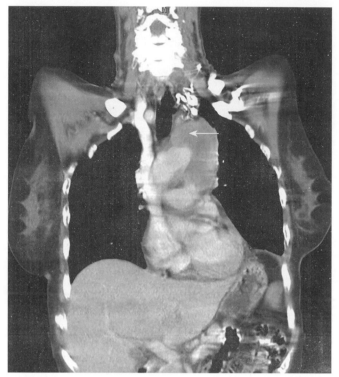

Fig. 53.4 Mediastinal mass causing left recurrent laryngeal nerve palsy.

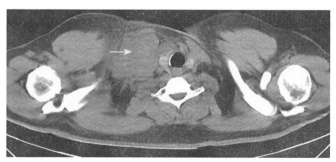

Fig. 53.5 Mediastinal lymphoma leading to right recurrent laryngeal nerve palsy.

- Gout.
- Polyarteritis nodosa.
- Toxic neuritis (lead, zinc, alcohol).
- Granulomatosis with polyangiitis (Wegener's granulomatosis).
- Relapsing polychondritis.
- Drug toxicity (vincristine, organophosphates).
- Radiation to the head and neck region.

■ Causes for SLN Palsy

- Surgical procedures like thyroidectomy, neck dissection, carotid endarterectomy, cricopharyngeal myotomy, supraglottic laryngectomy, and anterior approach to cervical spine.

- Laryngopharyngeal and thyroid malignancy.
- Neuritis.

Unilateral Vocal Cord Paralysis

Lesion or injury at the level of the RLN is the common cause for unilateral vocal cord paralysis. Lesions at the brainstem and along the path of the vagus nerve can also cause unilateral vocal cord palsy.

■ Etiology

The causes for unilateral vocal cord palsy are varied (**Table 53.3**). Iatrogenic surgical traumas, as in during thyroidectomy, esophagectomy, and anterior approach to the cervical spine, are some of the common etiological factors.

■ History

In addition to the onset, duration, and severity, a history of trauma, surgery, systemic illnesses, and recent infections should be documented. Associated symptoms of cough, aspiration (cough on swallowing), dysphagia, odynophagia, and breathing difficulty should be elicited.

Voice Quality

- Patients with unilateral vocal cord palsy may go undetected with minor change in voice without any other symptoms.
- Change in voice is the main symptom. The voice will be *breathy or weak* voice due to imperfect closure of the glottis. The muscle tone and the position of the vocal cord defines the quality of the voice.
- "Paralytic falsetto," a high-pitched voice, that occurs due to contraction of the ipsilateral cricothyroid muscle as a compensatory mechanism, may be present.
- There will be vocal fatigue and an inability to lift, pull, or push objects.

Dysphagia with aspiration can occur when there is vagus nerve involvement at a higher level. The pharyngeal constrictors are affected, and there is loss of sensation in the larynx.

Shortness of breath can occur due to incomplete glottic closure with air leak during phonation.

Pearl

The pharyngeal branch of the vagus, through its innervation, plays an important role in the elevation of the larynx and in regulating the upper esophageal sphincter pressure which is important for swallowing and for protecting the lower airway.

■ Clinical Examination

Larynx

- Flexible fiberoptic laryngoscopy is done to assess the mobility of the vocal cords. Rigid endoscopy and indirect laryngoscopy involve grasping the tongue which can affect the movements of the larynx or vocal cords.
  - When the patient says "eee" the vocal cords adduct. In vocal cord palsy, the position of the affected vocal cord may be median, paramedian, or cadaveric, depending on the nerves involved. Reinnervation and synkinesis can later affect the vocal cord position (**Fig. 53.6**).
  - Falling forward/anteriorly of the arytenoid on the affected side can occur due to total denervation or incomplete reinnervation of the thyroarytenoid muscle.

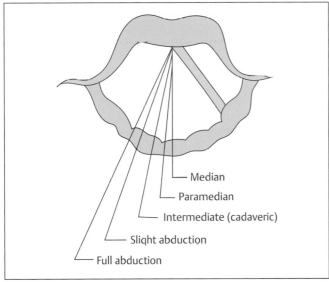

- Median
- Paramedian
- Intermediate (cadaveric)
- Slight abduction
- Full abduction

Fig. 53.6 Various positions of the vocal cord during paralysis.

- Maximal phonation time (MPT) gives the degree of air leak (glottic incompetence). The patient is asked to take a deep breath and say "eee" for as long as possible. In a normal individual, MPT is 25 seconds. But with a paralyzed vocal cord, the duration can be reduced to 5 to 10 seconds depending on the degree of glottic air leak.
- Manual compression test: It involves compression of the thyroid alae medially during phonation using the thumb, index, and middle fingers at the level of the vocal cord to assess any changes in voice. The test should be repeated with varying forces at various sites. If significant improvement in voice is noted with the procedure, the patient could have good prognosis following surgery.

Sometimes it is important to distinguish between a paralyzed vocal cord from one which does not move due to fixity of the cricoarytenoid joint. Fixity prevents the arytenoid from rotating. The main differences between the two are outlined in **Table 53.4**.

In *unilateral RLN palsy*, the vocal cord will be in the paramedian position. There may be a slightly breathy voice. On examination, the vocal cord will be in the paramedian position which leads to a small phonatory gap. Compensation by the opposite vocal cord will occur. Later, mainly the singing voice will be affected (**Figs. 53.7** and **53.8**).

In *unilateral SLN palsy*, due to paralysis of cricothyroid, there may be diplophonia, inability to change the pitch (not able to achieve a high pitch), especially for singers, monotony of voice, and vocal fatigue. Due to anesthesia of larynx above the level of vocal folds, there may be paroxysmal coughing, frequent clearing of the throat, and foreign body sensation.

In *unilateral combined palsy*, there will be severe breathiness of the voice. There will be aspiration. The cough will be ineffective. On examination, the vocal cord will be in the intermediate position and the opposite cord will not be able to compensate. There may be pooling of saliva in the pyriform fossa.

Table 53.4 Difference between vocal cord paralysis and cricoarytenoid joint fixation on endoscopy

Characteristic feature	Vocal cord paralysis	Cricoarytenoid joint fixation
Bowing of vocal cord	Present	Absent
Floppy vocal cord	Present	Absent
Position of cord	Higher	Normal
Tilt of larynx	To paralyzed side	Absent
Flicker of movement on phonation	Present	Absent
Pyriform fossa	Shallow	Normal
Position of cord	Depends on type of palsy	Any position
Arytenoid position	Falls forwards	No movement
Arytenoid mobility on palpation (endoscopy)	Mobile	Fixed

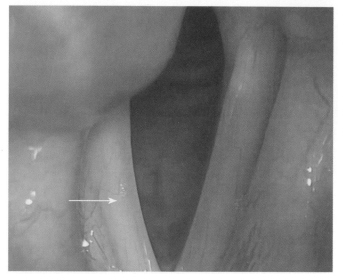

Fig. 53.7 Right vocal cord paralysis (*yellow arrow*). Left vocal cord in full abduction.

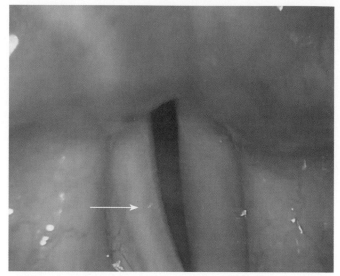

Fig. 53.8 Right vocal cord paralyzed (*yellow arrow*), with left vocal cord in full adduction while phonating. Note the space between the two vocal cords.

Pearl

Patients with high vagal lesions above the level of the pharyngeal nerve will present with nasal regurgitation and dysphagia in addition to change in voice and aspiration.

Neck

Examination for cervical lymphadenopathy, thyroid gland swelling/solitary nodule, and other neck masses should be done.

■ Cranial Nerves Examination

The function of the cranial nerves, especially IX, X, XI, and XII, should be examined to assess for generalized neuropathy. If the vagus is affected at a higher level, the soft palate will move toward the uninvolved side. The gag reflex should also be noted.

Pearl

Wagner and Grossman theory states that in unilateral RLN paralysis, the vocal fold is in the paramedian position. The adduction action of the cricothyroid pulls the paralyzed cord toward the midline. The vocal fold paralyzed in the intermediate position is due to paralysis of the SLNs and the RLNs.

■ Investigations

- Endoscopy of larynx with rigid or flexible scopes and stroboscopy are useful for assessing the movement of the vocal cords, and to look for any local pathology.

- Laryngeal electromyography can be prognostic when done in the 6 months of the palsy, as it provides information on the integrity of laryngeal innervation.
- Voice recording for the purpose of acoustic analysis and aerodynamic measurements are other useful tests.
- Preoperative evaluation includes a variety of subjective and objective voice parameters such as maximum phonation time, amplitude perturbation (shimmer), and pitch perturbation (jitter).
- Imaging studies are done when there is no known traumatic cause for the vocal cord palsy. A computed tomography (CT) scan with contrast or magnetic resonance imaging (MRI) of the neck (including skull base) and thorax is done to identify the presence of any lesion. When there is palatal paralysis and vocal cord paralysis, MRI should include the brainstem. MRI of the brain may be required for posterior fossa lesions.
- Esophagoscopy or barium swallow can be done if there is history of dysphagia.

Features of unilateral RLN palsy on flexible endoscopy:
- Immobile cord in the paramedian position.
- Falling forwards of the arytenoid.
- Bowing of the affected cord.
- Affected cord at a lower level when compared to the normal cord (during phonation).
- The ventricle may appear prominent/roomy.
- Compensation by the opposite cord (by shortening to allow the vocal processes to be opposite each other) helps close most of the glottis chink, except posteriorly.
- The ipsilateral pyriform fossa may appear shallow.

Features of unilateral SLN palsy on flexible endoscopy:
  – Askewed position of glottis.
  – Shortening of cord with loss of tension or bowing.
  – Cord may be at a lower level.
  – Wavy, asymmetrical cord seen during phonation at high pitch.
  – Posterior commissure points toward the paralyzed side.

■ Treatment

Four treatment options can be considered in unilateral vocal cord paralysis:

* *Observation* with regular follow-up for 6 to 9 months to assess for recovery or compensation.
* *Treat the cause* when feasible. Steroids may be helpful especially in idiopathic cases and in suspected viral etiology.
* *Voice therapy* or vocal cord strengthening exercises. Swallowing therapy especially in combined palsy.
* *Surgery*: Although the aim is to improve the voice, in combined palsy, the more important indication is to protect the lower airway and prevent aspiration.
    – Temporary: Medialization laryngoplasty, i.e., augmentation of the vocal fold with a filler substance like gelfoam, fat, collagen derivatives, or teflon. This can be done under local anesthesia transcutaneously with fiberoptic endoscopy guidance, or under general anesthesia using an operating microscope.
    – Permanent:
      o *Medialization thyroplasty*: This type I thyroplasty can be done using silastic, titanium, or Gore-Tex. It is done early in patients with aspiration. The silastic and titanium can be removed to reverse the procedure.
      o *Arytenoid adduction* procedure can be done along with medialization thyroplasty for better posterior glottic chink closure.
      o *Reinnervation* procedures, like end-to-end anastomosis, hypoglossal-to-RLN anastomosis, and ansa hypoglossi-to-RLN anastomosis, may help obtain neural continuity.
      o *Cricopharyngeal myotomy* may help facilitate swallowing and reduce aspiration in combined palsy.

The period of 6 to 9 months is recommended before any permanent surgical intervention; the exception being the presence of aspiration which requires early intervention.

Bilateral Vocal Cord Paralysis

■ Etiology

Bilateral vocal cord paralysis occurs in about 6% of cases. The common cause for bilateral vocal cord paralysis is thyroidectomy. Malignancy of the laryngopharynx, esophagus, and thyroid, thyroiditis, viral infection, trauma to the larynx (whiplash, post intubation), neurological conditions, and idiopathic causes are other etiological factors. The neurological causes include stroke, encephalitis, syringobulbia, progressive bulbar palsy, multiple sclerosis, and Arnold-Chiari malformation in children.

■ Clinical Presentation

Bilateral RLN (abductor) palsy has a dramatic presentation with mild to severe stridor or breathing difficulty on exertion. The presentation can be early or can present in the following days or weeks after the incident. The glottic airway varies from 1 to 3 mm. The voice will be good. There may be a history of a surgery like thyroidectomy. Rheumatoid arthritis and prior intubation history should be sought (**Fig. 53.9**).

Bilateral SLN palsy is not common and is usually part of a combined palsy. There will be some aspiration. A high pitch of voice cannot be achieved. On examination, the epiglottis will overhang the laryngeal inlet obscuring the view of the anterior glottis.

Bilateral combined palsy presents with severe breathiness to aphonia. There will be severe aspiration due to an incompetent larynx. On examination, both the cords will be in the intermediate position or cadaveric position.

> **Pearl**
>
> A voice which is normal in the morning and tires as the day goes on occurs in unilateral abductor paralysis. Stridor occurs in bilateral abductor paralysis whereas aspiration implies bilateral adductor paralysis.

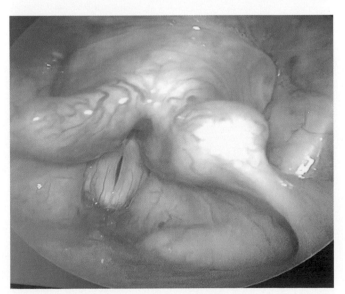

Fig. 53.9 Bilateral vocal cord palsy. Note the reduced airway between the vocal cords. This patient will be in stridor.

■ Clinical Examination

In addition to examination of the larynx and neck, a neurological examination (including examination of the cranial nerves) should be done.

■ Investigations

- When there is a history of surgical trauma, other investigations to evaluate for the cause is not necessary.
- MRI of the brain would be useful in children to rule out hydrocephalus and Arnold-Chiari malformation.
- Laryngoscopy (flexible) is done to assess the mobility of the vocal cords. A rigid, direct laryngoscopy done under anesthesia without an endotracheal tube can help in assessing cricoarytenoid joint fixation and interarytenoid scarring.

■ Treatment

For Bilateral Abductor Palsy

The aim is to achieve a safe and stable airway, preserve the voice quality, and allow for safe swallowing without aspiration.

Immediate Airway Management

Secure the airway by endotracheal intubation. If bilateral vocal cord paralysis still persists a tracheostomy is done.

Reversible/Temporary Procedures

- *Tracheostomy* is the commonest emergency procedure that is done to secure the airway. The patient should be assessed over a period of 6 to 12 months for spontaneous recovery.
- *Suture lateralization* involves using a nonabsorbable suture from the skin of the neck to around vocal process and then back out from the neck where it is secured over a button externally with adequate pressure to pull the posterior part of the ipsilateral cord laterally.
- *Botox injection* into the thyroarytenoid–lateral cricoarytenoid muscle complex may help in improving the airway for 2 to 4 months.

Permanent Procedures

- *Posterior transverse cordotomy or cordectomy,* using laser or coblation, is done in front of the vocal process to create posterior glottis space which improves airway but does not significantly affect the voice (**Figs. 53.10** and **53.11**).
- *Arytenoidectomy* is done either alone or with other procedures like cordotomy. There is a risk of aspiration after the procedure.
- *Arytenoidopexy* uses suture to displace the arytenoid and cord laterally.
- *Laryngeal pacing* involves placing an implant under the skin which gives electrical stimulation to the posterior cricoarytenoid muscle during inspiration. The inspiration is detected by an electrode placed on the diaphragm.

For Bilateral Combined Palsy

The aim of the treatment is to protect the lower airway.

The various positions of the vocal cord and the symptoms experienced by the patient in different types of palsies are summarized in **Tables 53.5** and **53.6.**

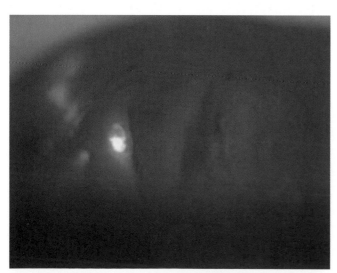

Fig. 53.10 The white spot on the posterior part of the right vocal cord indicates the position of the beam of the carbon dioxide laser during laser cordotomy. This cuts and vaporizes the vocal cord in order to create space for breathing in bilateral vocal cord paralysis.

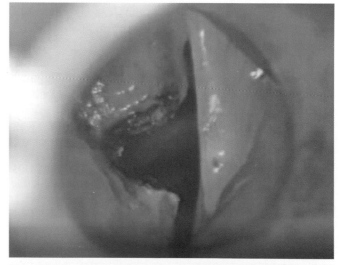

Fig. 53.11 Laser cordotomy performed. Note the space obtained after the posterior part of the right vocal cord has been vaporized.

Table 53.5 Characteristic feature of various types of palsies

Characteristic feature	Unilateral RLN palsy	Bilateral RLN palsy	Unilateral SLN palsy	Bilateral SLN palsy
Position of cords	Paramedian	Midline	Apparent shortening with asymmetric length	Apparent shortening
Voice	Breathy/normal	Normal/strained due to stridor	Diplophonia; cannot achieve high pitch	Loss of vocal range
Airway	Adequate	Compromised	Adequate	Adequate
Aspiration	Absent	Absent	Possible	High risk
Treatment	Medialization	Lateralization		

Abbreviations: RLN, recurrent laryngeal nerve; SLN, superior laryngeal nerve.

Table 53.6 Characteristics of combined nerve palsies

Characteristic feature	Unilateral combined palsy	Bilateral combined palsy
Position of cords	Intermediate on affected side	Intermediate or cadaveric position on both sides
Voice	Severe breathiness	Aphonia
Airway	Persistently open at glottic level; no compensation from opposite cord	Persistently open at glottic level; incompetent larynx
Aspiration	Present	Severe
Treatment	Medialization of cord +/− cricopharyngeal myotomy; voice and swallowing therapy	Protection of lower airway

> **Pearl**
>
> Involvement of the external branch of SLN will lead to inability to change the pitch of the voice, especially high pitch, and affects singers.

Specific Neurological Conditions Affecting the Vocal Cords

■ Wallenberg Syndrome or Lateral Medullary Syndrome

It is the infarct of the lateral medulla due to occlusion of the posterior inferior cerebellar artery. In addition to dysphagia, dysarthria, impaired pain, and temperature sensation in the ipsilateral face and contralateral trunk and extremities, there will be unilateral vocal cord paralysis.

■ Myasthenia Gravis

Due to reduced availability of acetylcholine at the myoneural junction, there will be weakness during sustained muscular effort. There will be a breathy voice with reduced loudness. The symptoms worsen with sustained speaking.

There may be associated hypernasality with nasal regurgitation, dysphagia, and articulation defects.

The various multiple cranial nerve syndromes involving the vagus nerve are outlined in **Table 53.7**.

> **Pearl**
>
> Functional aphonia is the inability to phonate which usually occurs after a specific event. On flexible endoscopy, the cords do not adduct during phonation but do so when the patient is asked to cough. Previously called hysterical aphonia.

■ Laryngeal Framework Surgery or Thyroplasty

Laryngeal framework surgery can change the position, shape, and tension of the vocal cord. From the functional view point this type of surgery may be classified into four categories:

- *Thyroplasty type I* for medialization of the vocal cords (**Fig. 53.12**).
- *Thyroplasty type II* for lateralization of the vocal cords.
- *Thyroplasty type III* for relaxation of the vocal cords.
- *Thyroplasty type IV* for lengthening or tensing of the vocal cords.

Table 53.7 Vagus nerve involvement in syndromes

Syndrome	Site of disease	Nerves involved
Collet-Sicard	Posterior cranial fossa	IX, X, XI, XII
Hughlings-Jackson	Posterior cranial fossa	X, XI, XII
Vernet	Jugular foramen	IX, X, XI
Tapia	Parapharyngeal space	X, XII
Villaret	Parapharyngeal space	IX, X, XI, sympathetic chain
Klinkert	Superior mediastinum	X (RLN), phrenic
Pancoast	Apex of lung	X, sympathetic chain, phrenic
Garcin	Skull base	Usually, 7 or more cranial nerves; can involve all 12 cranial nerves

Abbreviation: RLN, recurrent laryngeal nerve.

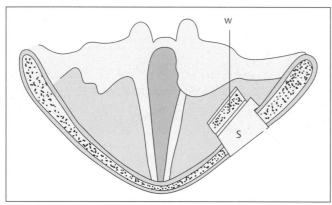

Fig. 53.12 Diagram depicting type 1 thyroplasty. A block of silastic, wedge shaped (*yellow arrow*), is inserted into the left thyroid cartilage pushing the left vocal cord medially in left recurrent laryngeal nerve palsy.

Points to Ponder

- Unilateral SLN palsy is not common.
- In bilateral RLN (abductor) palsy, the vocal cords are in median position. Voice may be good but the glottic airway is compromised, and there will be stridor, especially on exertion, which requires early intervention.
- In bilateral SLN palsy, there is loss of supraglottic sensation leading to aspiration.
- In unilateral combined palsy, the voice is breathy and there is aspiration. Early surgical intervention is done to protect the lower airway.
- In bilateral combined palsy, the vocal cords are in intermediate position leading to complete aphonia and severe aspiration.

Case-Based Questions

1. **A 42-year-old woman had undergone a hemithyroidectomy. Postoperatively, there was a change in voice. There was no aspiration.**

   a. What would be the position of the cord if the recurrent laryngeal nerve was involved?

   b. What would be the position of the cord if the recurrent and superior laryngeal nerves were involved?

   c. What would be the treatment of choice if the change in voice was mild?

   d. What would be the treatment of choice if there was a breathy voice with aspiration?

   Answers

   a. In paramedian position.

   b. In intermediate position or cadaveric position.

   c. Wait and watch with regular follow-up. Compensation by the opposite cord will usually occur. If paralysis is persistent, a medialization thyroplasty can be performed after 6 to 9 months.

   d. Medialization thyroplasty with or without cricopharyngeal myotomy needs to be done early to protect the lower airway.

2. **A 4-month-old infant was brought to the emergency ward with noisy breathing. A flexible endoscopy done in the operating room showed bilateral abductor palsy.**

   a. What further investigation will be required?

   b. What is the position of the vocal cord?

   c. In a 36-year-old woman after total thyroidectomy, with a similar presentation, what would be the treatment options?

Answers

a. A magnetic resonance imaging (MRI) of the brain is required to rule out Arnold-Chiari malformation or hydrocephalus.

b. The cords will be in the median position. Mild edema will precipitate stridor.

c. Wait and watch. If there is stridor, tracheostomy is done. Later, in order to improve the posterior airway, a laser posterior cordotomy, arytenoidectomy, or suture lateralization can be performed.

Frequently Asked Questions

1. What are the causes of unilateral recurrent laryngeal nerve palsy?

2. How does bilateral abductor palsy present?

3. What is the emergency management of bilateral abductor palsy?

4. What is the aim of treatment of unilateral combined palsy?

5. What are the various positions of the vocal cord in lesions of the recurrent laryngeal nerve and superior laryngeal nerve?

Endnote

Vagus means "wandering" in Latin. The vagus nerve is the wandering nerve. It wanders from the head, into the neck and thorax, and enters the abdomen.

Sushruta in Sushruta Samhita (6th century BC) documented what is considered the first reference to the "control of voice in relation to the wind-pipe." Galen (2nd century AD) described a nerve from the brain that courses down toward the heart and winds around in a reversed course toward the larynx. He named it "reversivi."

Frank Lahey (1938) popularized the dissection of the recurrent laryngeal nerve in surgery of the thyroid gland.

54 Benign Lesions of the Vocal Cord

K.P. Basavaraju and Kartik Herkal

The competency covered in this chapter is as follows:

EN4.44 Describe the clinical features, investigations, and principles of management of benign lesions of the vocal cord.

Introduction

Benign lesions of the vocal cord are very common. These can occur in all age groups, and in both genders. In the majority of cases, vocal abuse will be the main cause. Other etiological factors include viral infection, smoking, laryngopharyngeal reflux (LPR), and laryngeal trauma. The majority of these lesions can be diagnosed by indirect laryngoscopy, fiberoptic laryngoscopy, and stroboscopy. Most of these lesions can be treated by conservative management or by a procedure called microlaryngoscopy (MLS).

Benign lesions are usually classified into non-neoplastic and neoplastic lesions.

Classification

The non-neoplastic lesions are more common and include the following:
- Vocal cord nodules.
- Vocal cord polyp.
- Vocal cord cyst.
- Reinke's edema.
- Sulcus vocalis/vocal cord scars.
- Vocal cord granuloma and contact ulcer.
- Leukoplakia/keratosis of the vocal cord.
- Saccular cyst of the larynx.
- Laryngocele.

Benign neoplastic lesions are rare. These include the following:
- Squamous papilloma:
  - Recurrent respiratory papillomatosis (RRP) or juvenile papilloma.
  - Adult solitary papilloma.
- Hemangioma of the larynx.

Benign Non-Neoplastic Lesions

■ Vocal Nodules

Introduction

Vocal nodules are commonly seen in those who abuse their voice or speak for a long time. This lesion develops as a response to voice trauma. Hence, these lesions are also called singer's nodules, teacher's nodules, preacher's nodules, or screamer's nodules.

Etiology

Vocal nodules are more frequently seen in females and children. Voice abuse, overuse, or misuse is the main reason for occurrence of vocal nodules.
- Vocal abuse refers to a behavior that results in vocal cord trauma, such as talking loudly and shouting and screaming. It can also be due to excessive coughing and constant clearing of the throat.
- Vocal overuse refers to talking for prolonged periods.
- Vocal misuse is due to the use of inappropriate pitch such as in singing and mimicry.
- It will also be seen in individuals with cleft palate as they require an increased effort at phonation due to velopharyngeal insufficiency.

Pathology

Vocal nodules are always symmetrical, occurring on both cords, at the junction of the anterior and middle third of the vocal cords. Vocal abuse causes trauma due to forced voice production resulting in edema and submucosal hemorrhage at the point of maximum vibration. Later, fibrosis and hyalinization occur to form vocal nodules.

Clinical Features

The patient presents with a change in voice, mainly hoarseness and voice breaks. Singers will have a loss of range of voice with an inability to sing high notes. The voice tires easily and after prolonged phonation, pain in the neck may occur. On indirect laryngoscopy, bilateral, symmetrical, pinhead-sized (<3 mm), white nodules are seen typically at the junction of the anterior and middle one-third of the vocal cord on the free edge (**Fig. 54.1a, b**).

Investigations

Fiberoptic laryngoscopy is done to confirm the diagnosis. Stroboscopy shows hourglass closure of the glottis with normal mucosal wave.

Treatment

Early nodules resolve with conservative treatment. This includes voice rest for 4 to 6 weeks and voice therapy. Avoidance of vocal abuse, overuse, and misuse is essential. Acid reflux may contribute to this condition, so the use of antireflux medications like proton pump inhibitors may be required. Examples of proton pump inhibitors include omeprazole and pantoprazole.

A minimally invasive option for persistent nodules is intralesional injection of corticosteroids, either triamcinolone or methyl prednisolone. When these measures fail, microlaryngoscopy and excision can be done. It would be prudent to remove the nodule from one side and if required from the other side at a second sitting to avoid adhesions. Postoperative voice therapy and vocal hygiene are required to prevent recurrence. Children with vocal nodules and their parents need to be counseled as the voice can be a learned behavior that will require modifications and behavioral changes to avoid recurrence.

■ Vocal Cord Polyp

Introduction

A vocal polyp is a sessile (**Fig. 54.2a**) or pedunculated lesion (**Fig. 54.2b**), usually unilateral, greater than 3 mm, seen on the free edge of the vocal cord, midmembranous part.

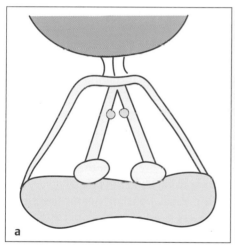
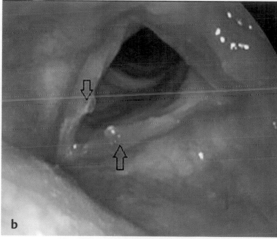

Fig. 54.1 **(a)** Diagrammatic representation of vocal nodules. **(b)** Microlaryngoscopic (MLS) picture of vocal nodules.

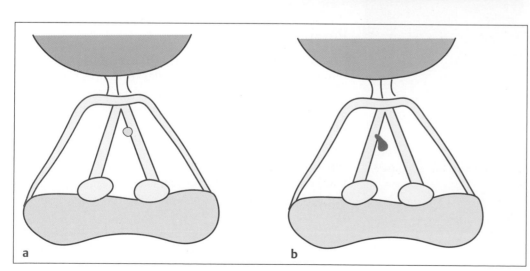

Fig. 54.2 **(a)** Vocal cord polyp sessile. **(b)** Vocal cord polyp pedunculated.

Etiology

It is seen more in adult males between the age of 30 and 50 years. Polyp occurs due to phonotrauma or vocal abuse. It can follow a shouting or yelling episode, especially when the vocal cords are inflamed. Working in a noisy environment and smoking are contributing factors.

Pathology

A vocal cord polyp is usually unilateral, but in 20% of cases, it may be bilateral. Polyps are usually sessile, translucent, and arising close to the anterior commissure. The size varies from a few millimeters to a centimeter. Persistent hyperkinetic phonation leads to recurrent trauma to the vocal cord causing vascular engorgement and microhemorrhages followed by edema with the formation of a polyp. It usually involves the superficial lamina propria.

Cigarette smoking can cause injury to the vocal cord by disrupting the basement membrane of the blood vessels. This leads to microhemorrhage and exudation leading to polyp formation.

Clinical Features

- Symptoms include a persistent hoarseness of voice and diplophonia. Diplophonia is the production of a voice with two tones. A large, pedunculated polyp can cause stridor or intermittent choking attacks.
- On examination by indirect laryngoscopy or rigid telescopy, a single, sessile, or pedunculated mass on the free edge of the vocal cord is seen, which is reddish in color. It moves with respiration, when pedunculated (**Fig. 54.3**).

Investigation

Fiberoptic laryngoscopy helps confirm the diagnosis. Contact changes on the opposite vocal cord can be noted.

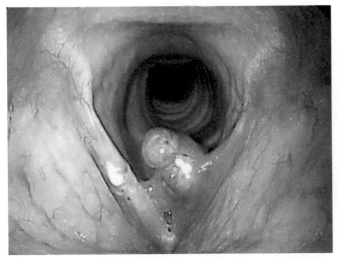

Fig. 54.3 Left vocal cord polyp.

Treatment

Conservative treatment includes voice therapy, but most polyps will require surgical removal under general anesthesia.

A vocal cord polyp is excised through an MLS procedure. This can be done using laser or laryngeal scissors. The excised specimen should be sent for histopathology. The patient is advised to undergo voice therapy following surgery.

■ Vocal Cord Cyst

Introduction

Two types of vocal cord cysts are described:
- Mucous retention cyst.
- Epidermoid or keratin cyst.

Etiopathogenesis

The development of a mucous retention cyst is due to obstruction of the glandular duct. Inflammation and phonotrauma are presumed causes for this obstruction of the glandular duct.

Two theories are proposed for the formation of an epidermoid cyst:
- Acquired.
- Congenital.

The acquired theory proposes microtrauma to vocal cord causing inclusion of small fragment of epithelial tissue, which would grow inward.

Clinical Features

Patients with intracordal cyst present with symptoms of dysphonia. These are unilateral in 90% of cases.

On examination, the most constant feature is slight enlargement of one vocal cord. Stroboscopic examination shows diminished mucosal wave at the site of cyst (**Fig. 54.4**).

Treatment

The lesion is excised by MLS using the microflap technique. In the microflap technique, a flap of mucosa is incised over the cyst and retracted, the cyst is removed, and the flap is replaced. This prevents mucosal loss during surgery and results in less scarring, which can affect the voice. Postoperative voice therapy is advised.

■ Reinke's Edema

Introduction

These lesions are also known as bilateral diffuse polyposis or polypoid corditis. Reinke's edema is a condition that

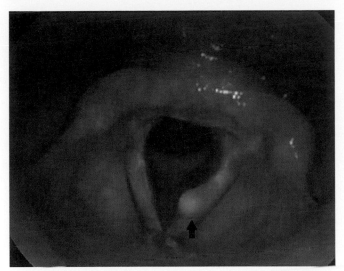

Fig. 54.4 Left vocal cord epidermoid cyst.

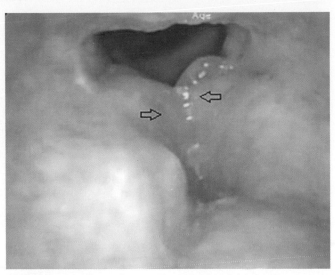

Fig. 54.5 Reinke's edema.

involves deposition of gelatinous material in the subepithelial layer of the entire vocal cord.

Etiopathogenesis

Patients with Reinke's edema often have a *triad* of causative factors:

- Chronic smoking.
- LPR.
- Vocal abuse.

Structurally, the vocal cord has five layers:

- Outermost squamous epithelium.
- Superficial lamina propria or *Reinke's space* filled with gelatinous material.
- Intermediate lamina propria.
- Deep lamina propria.
- Vocalis muscle.

The intermediate lamina propria and the deep lamina propria together form the vocal ligament.

In Reinke's edema, there is an accumulation of gelatinous material in the superficial lamina propria. This occurs throughout the length of the vocal cord.

Clinical Features

The patient presents with a low-pitched hoarse and harsh voice. In females, the voice will have a masculine quality. In advanced stage, there can be stridor due to narrowing of the air space between the vocal cords.

On examination by indirect laryngoscopy (or rigid telescopy), both vocal cords are pale and diffusely polypoidal in appearance, especially on the superior surface with reduction in the glottic space (**Fig. 54.5**).

Investigation

Fiberoptic laryngoscopy is done to assess the lesion. In the initial stages, stroboscopy will show decreased mucosal wave as the pliability of vocal cord is affected, but in the later stage mucosal wave is severely dampened. Thyroid function tests should be done to rule out hypothyroidism.

Treatment

Treatment should be directed to checking the primary causes including cessation of smoking, correcting LPR, and voice therapy.

Surgical treatment includes MLS in which an incision on the superior surface of the vocal cord is given and the polypoidal material is suctioned or dissected out. The excess mucosa is resected and re-approximation of the cut margins is carried out.

> **Pearl**
>
> *LPR* is similar to another condition called gastroesophageal reflux disease (GERD). LPR is due to the reflux of acid content from the stomach through lax esophageal sphincters, upper and lower, into the pharynx and larynx. Around 10% of patients coming to the ear, nose, and throat (ENT) clinic complain of symptoms related to LPR. These include hoarseness of voice, chronic cough, dysphagia, globus sensation, and constant clearing of the throat.

■ Sulcus Vocalis

Sulcus vocalis is a longitudinal groove on the medial edge of the membranous part of the vocal cord.

Etiology

It results from the spontaneous rupture of an epidermoid cyst on the free edge of the vocal cord, followed by adhesion of the epithelium to the underlying vocal ligament. This leads to a deep linear furrow on the free edge of the vocal cord, which results in restriction of vibration and closure during phonation.

Clinical Features

Patients present with an increased pitch, breathy harsh voice, diplophonia, voice fatigue, and foreign body sensation in the throat.

On indirect laryngoscopy and fiberoptic laryngoscopy, there is deep linear furrow on the free edge of the vocal fold with mucosal irregularities. On phonation, there is an oval- or spindle-shaped phonatory gap (**Fig. 54.6**).

Treatment

Voice therapy is the initial line of management. Antireflux therapy is then started. Release of adhesion and sulcus through microlaryngoscopy using laser or cold steel microinstruments can be carried out. Fat implantation into the sulcus may help improve the voice. A slicing mucosal technique or resection of the mucosa of the sulcus to release the tension lines of the vocal cord has been carried out with some success.

■ Contact Ulcer and Vocal Cord Granuloma

Introduction

Vocal cord granulomas typically occur in the posterior portion of the vocal cord over the vocal process of the arytenoid.

Etiology

Vocal cord granuloma is caused by trauma like vocal abuse, intubation, and surgical trauma. Frequent throat clearing and chronic cough can also lead to a contact ulcer and granuloma. Gastroesophageal reflux is a contributing factor.

There is loss of epithelium with exposure of the cartilage over the vocal process leading to perichondritis, which later forms a nonspecific reparative granuloma. During phonation, due to the trauma caused by vocal cord movements, the opposite cord develops an ulcer, known as a contact ulcer.

Clinical Features

Patients present with a husky voice along with repeated clearing of the throat and pain in the throat that worsens on phonation.

On indirect laryngoscopy or rigid telescopy, a sessile or polypoidal reddish mass is seen in the posterior part of the vocal cord and on the vocal process of the arytenoid, and on the opposite cord, there may be a corresponding indenting ulcer (**Fig. 54.7**).

Treatment

Management consists of antireflux therapy for long duration with proton pump inhibitors and voice therapy.

To temporarily reduce movement of the vocal cords (and allow healing), botulinum toxin can be injected into the lateral cricoarytenoid muscle or the thyroarytenoid muscle.

Surgical management should be considered only if medical treatment fails. Excision of the granuloma is carried out by microlaryngoscopy with cold steel instruments or by laser. The specimen is sent for histopathological

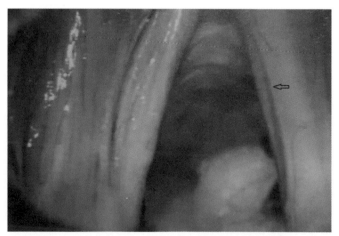

Fig. 54.6 Sulcus vocalis.

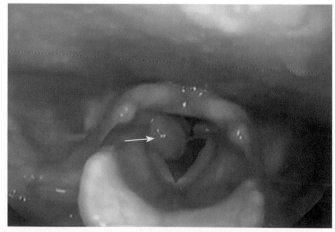

Fig. 54.7 Intubation granuloma of the right posterior vocal cord.

examination to rule out other granulomatous conditions like tuberculosis.

Local injection of corticosteroids or application of mitomycin C may prevent recurrences.

■ Leukoplakia or Keratosis of the Vocal Cord

Introduction

These are premalignant lesions of the vocal cord presenting as a white patch over the vocal cord.

Etiology

Leukoplakia or keratosis of the vocal cord is caused by chronic laryngeal irritation caused by chronic smoking, LPR, inhalational injury, and vocal abuse.

Pathogenesis

Chronic irritation of the vocal cord epithelium leads to epithelial hyperplasia and dyskeratosis forming white warty growth over the vocal cord, impairing cord mobility.

Clinical Features

Symptoms include hoarseness of voice and discomfort during phonation. Indirect laryngoscopy or rigid telescopy of the larynx shows a white warty lesion over the vocal cord involving one or both cords. It may also be an incidental finding picked up in an asymptomatic patient during routine examination of the larynx (**Fig. 54.8**).

Treatment

Using microlaryngoscopy, stripping of the epithelium over the vocal cord is done after injecting saline into the subepithelial space and the tissue is sent for histopathologic examination to rule out carcinoma in situ. Postoperatively, cessation of smoking, antireflux medication, and voice therapy are advised to prevent recurrences.

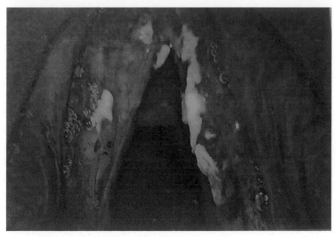

Fig. 54.8 Leukoplakia of both vocal cords.

■ Saccular Cyst

Introduction

The saccule is present in the anterior part of the laryngeal ventricle. It stores mucous secretions of the underlying glands, which are released by the contraction of the adjacent muscles. A saccular cyst is a fluid-filled cystic lesion arising in the saccule of the larynx.

Etiopathogenesis

Obstruction of the laryngeal ventricle leading to the retention of secretion and a cystic swelling. A *laryngopyocele* is an infected saccular cyst. These are classified by size and location into the following:

- *Lateral saccular cysts* extend posterosuperiorly into the false cord and aryepiglottic fold, presenting in the neck through the thyrohyoid membrane.
- *Anterior saccular cysts* are present in the anterior part and extend medially and posteriorly to protrude from the anterior laryngeal ventricle. These usually overhang the anterior glottis obstructing the view of the vocal cords.

Clinical Features

Infants with congenital saccular cyst present with a weak cry, cough, stridor, and cyanosis. In adults, signs and symptoms depend on the size and type of the saccular cyst. Symptoms are caused by the mass effect. If the lesion is small, it may be asymptomatic. A large cyst presents with dysphonia or hoarseness of voice. Indirect laryngoscopy or direct laryngoscopy will reveal the lesion as a fullness in the ventricular band or a fullness in the vallecula.

Investigations

Anteroposterior (AP) and lateral X-ray of the soft tissue of the neck or computed tomography (CT) scan of the neck aids in the diagnosis.

Treatment

Treatment is via endoscopic marsupialization of the cyst or CO_2 laser vaporization. Lateral cysts are approached via a thyrotomy or laryngofissure approach.

■ Laryngocele

Introduction

It is an air-filled, dilated saccule. There are three types:
- *Internal laryngocele*, which extends into the ventricular band and the aryepiglottic fold.
- *External laryngocele*, which pierces the thyrohyoid membrane, extending into the neck in the form of a neck

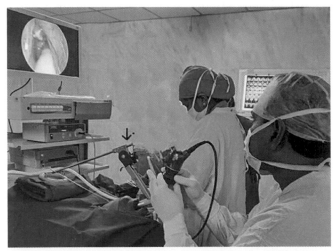

Fig. 54.11 Phonomicrosurgery setup in the operation theater.

known as suspension microlaryngoscopy. This allows both hands to be free for handling instruments.

- Various methods are used for removal of vocal cord lesions, including the following:
  - These include cold steel instruments like cup forceps, micro-scissors, and micro-knife.
  - Lasers like CO_2 laser and potassium-titanyl-phosphate (KTP) laser.
  - Microdebrider and laryngeal shaver.
  - Coblator or by using microcautery.

- Advantages of PMS is good visualization of lesions using adequate illumination and magnification by microscope or telescope with camera.
- Laryngoscope is fixed with a suspension stand, so both hands are free to do precise surgery.
- Photographs of the lesions can be taken.
- Different tools can be utilized through the laryngoscope to treat the vocal cord lesion precisely.

Points to Ponder

- Benign vocal cord lesions are common and most present with change in voice and, if large enough, cause airway obstruction.
- These lesions are generally classified into non-neoplastic and neoplastic lesions. Among the non-neoplastic lesions, vocal nodules and vocal polyps are commonly encountered.
- Vocal abuse, vocal overuse, and vocal misuse are the primary etiological factors in the development of vocal nodules.
- Leukoplakia, found in smokers and in those with LPR, is a premalignant condition and must be evaluated as early as possible.
- RRP is an HPV-induced lesion, both the juvenile and adult types. Both require surgical excision, the juvenile type to prevent airway obstruction and the adult type to rule out malignancy.

Case-Based Questions

1. **A 40-year-old schoolteacher presented with a 4-month history of voice fatigue and hoarseness of voice. The local doctor prescribed antibiotics assuming it to be laryngitis, but the symptoms persisted. In the ENT department, an indirect laryngoscopic examination revealed small swellings at the junction of the anterior one-third and posterior two-thirds of both vocal cords.**

   a. What is the likely diagnosis?

   b. What is the next step in management?

   Answers

   a. Vocal nodules.

   b. Treatment consists mainly of voice therapy where the patient is taught the proper use of the voice without causing additional strain. Other factors that might irritate the vocal cords like allergies, infections, and reflux should be simultaneously treated. If voice therapy fails and the patient is symptomatic, MLS can performed.

2. **A 3-year-old girl was brought to the emergency room (ER) with breathing difficulty and hoarse voice. An urgent ENT examination with a flexible laryngoscope revealed almost complete obstruction of the supraglottis airway by a warty lesion.**

   a. What is the diagnosis?

   b. How will you secure the airway?

   c. What is the treatment required?

   Answers

   a. JORRP.

   b. Tracheostomy may be required as the airway is compromised by the growth.

   c. Relieving the airway obstruction by MLS, using a microdebrider to shave off the tumor with minimal injury to the mucosa, followed by intralesional injection of cidofovir may slow down the rate of recurrence.

Frequently Asked Questions

1. On examination, what are the differences between a vocal cord nodule and a vocal cord polyp?

2. What are the conditions that will produce a white patch on the vocal cord?

3. What are the differences between JORRP and AORRP?

4. What are the advantages of suspension microlaryngoscopic examination?

5. What is the etiology of a laryngocele and which type presents as a neck swelling?

Endnote

Presbylaryngis is a condition in which the voice is altered due to aging. It is similar to presbyopia where age-related changes occur in the eye. The changes in the vocal cord include atrophy of the muscles of the vocal cord, bowing, ossification of the laryngeal skeleton, and arthritis of the cricoarytenoid joint. These changes result in the voice becoming high pitched and breathy. Presbylaryngis makes it difficult for singers to reach the correct pitch as they get older.

55 Malignant Tumors of the Larynx

Arun Alexander and Soorya Pradeep

The competency covered in this chapter is as follows:

EN4.46 Describe the clinical features, investigations, and principles of management of malignancy of the larynx.

Malignancy of Larynx

The larynx is the most common site of head and neck malignancy worldwide. It is most commonly seen in males in the age group of 40 to 70 years. It is 10 times more common in males than in females, although its incidence in women has increased in western countries due to increased smoking in women.

Etiology

Smoking is the most important etiological factor for laryngeal malignancy, but alcohol intake has also been implicated in its pathogenesis. In patients who both smoke and drink, the risk increases 15-fold. Occupational asbestos exposure, polycyclic aromatic hydrocarbons, wood dust, coal dust, and cement dust contribute to laryngeal cancer risk. It is seen more commonly in patients from lower socioeconomic backgrounds, although genetic conditions such as Fanconi anemia and congenital dyskeratosis have also been associated with carcinoma of the larynx.

Anatomical Subsites of the Larynx

The anatomical subsites of the larynx are described in **Table 55.1** and **Fig. 55.1**.

TNM Classification of Carcinoma of the Larynx

The TNM classification of carcinoma of the larynx is described in **Table 55.2**.

■ AJCC Prognostic Stage Groups

The AJCC prognostic stage groups are presented in **Table 55.3**.

Histopathology

Squamous cell carcinoma is the most common type of laryngeal cancer, accounting for 90 to 95%, while

Table 55.1 Larynx: Anatomical subsites

	Supraglottis	Glottis	Subglottis
Extent	From the tip of the epiglottis to a horizontal line passing through the apex of the ventricle	From the ventricle to ~0.5–1 cm below the free margin of the true vocal cord	Extends ~1 cm below the level of the true cords to the inferior rim of the cricoid cartilage
Subsites	Suprahyoid epiglottis (including lingual and laryngeal surfaces)	Vocal cords	
	Aryepiglottic folds (laryngeal aspect)	Anterior commissure	
	Arytenoids	Posterior commissure	
	Infrahyoid epiglottis		
	Ventricular bands (false cords)		

Table 55.2 TNM classification

T staging	Supraglottis	Glottis	Subglottis
Tx	Primary tumor cannot be assessed		
Tis	Carcinoma in situ		
T1	Limited to 1 subsite of the supraglottis, with normal vocal cord mobility T1a: limited to one vocal cord T1b: limited to both vocal cords	Limited to the vocal cord(s) (may involve the anterior or posterior commissure with normal mobility	Limited to the subglottis
T2	Invades • Mucosa of >1 adjacent subsite of the supraglottis or glottis • Region outside the supraglottis (e.g., mucosa of the base of the tongue, vallecula, medial wall of the pyriform sinus) • Without fixation of the larynx	Extends to the supraglottis and/or the subglottis and/or with impaired vocal cord mobility	Extends to the vocal cord(s) with normal or impaired mobility
T3	Limited to the larynx, with vocal cord fixation and/or invades: • Postcricoid area • Preepiglottic space • Paraglottic space • The inner cortex of thyroid cartilage	Limited to the larynx with vocal cord fixation and/or invasion of the paraglottic space and/or the inner cortex of thyroid cartilage	
T4a	Moderately advanced local disease Invades through the outer cortex of thyroid cartilage and/or: • Tissues beyond the larynx • Trachea • Soft tissues of the neck, including the deep extrinsic muscles of the tongue • Strap muscles • Thyroid • Esophagus		
T4b	Very advanced local disease Invades • Prevertebral space • Encases carotid artery • Mediastinal structures		

N staging		Criteria
Nx		Regional lymph nodes cannot be assessed
N0		No regional lymph node metastasis
N1		Single ipsilateral lymph node ≤3 cm and ENE –
N2a		Single ipsilateral lymph node >3 cm but ≤6 cm and ENE –
N2b		Multiple ipsilateral nodes none >6 cm and ENE –
N2c		Bilateral or contralateral lymph nodes none >6 cm and ENE –
N3a		Lymph nodes >6 cm and ENE –
N3b		Any node(s) and clinically overt ENE +

M		Criteria
M0		No distant metastasis
M1		Distant metastasis

Abbreviation: ENE, extranodal extension.

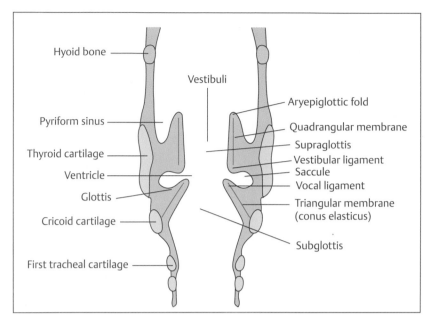

Fig. 55.1 Anatomical subsites of the larynx showing supraglottis, glottis, and subglottis

Table 55.3 Prognostic stage groups established by the American Joint Committee on Cancer (AJCC)

T	N	M	Staging
Tis	N0	M0	0
T1	N0	M0	I
T2	N0	M0	II
T3	N0	M0	III
T1, T2, T3	N1	M0	III
T1, T2, T3, T4a	N2	M0	IVa
Any T	N3	M0	IVb
T4b	Any N	M0	IVb
Any T	Any N	M1	IVc

adenocarcinoma, malignant salivary gland tumors, verrucous carcinoma, spindle cell carcinoma, and sarcomas comprise the remaining 10 to 15%.

Pathways of Spread of Laryngeal Cancer

- Direct spread: There may be direct spread by contiguity along the soft-tissue planes and muscles. Cartilage acts as an effective barrier to spread, but the cribriform (infrahyoid) epiglottis and the anterior commissure where the perichondrium is deficient allow the spread of malignant cells to the preepiglottic and paraglottic spaces. The conus elasticus, the quadrangular membrane, and ligaments such as the hyoepiglottic and glossoepiglottic ligaments act as fibrous barriers to the spread of malignancy (**Fig. 55.2**).

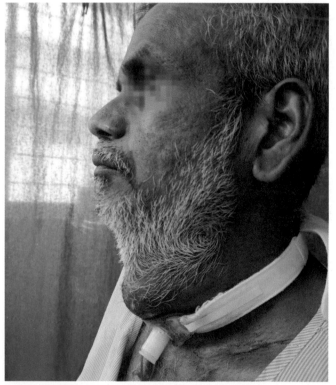

Fig. 55.2 Picture showing tumor coming out of the larynx into the neck (extralaryngeal direct spread).

- Lymphatic spread: The supraglottis is a midline structure derived from the buccopharyngeal primordium and has bilateral lymphatics. Hence, supraglottic tumors tend to be associated with an increased risk of nodal metastasis (60%) with a propensity for bilateral metastasis. In glottic tumors, the lymphatic spread is rare due to the absence of lymphatics. Subglottic tumors may be associated with microscopic nodal metastasis.

Diagnosis

■ Symptomatology

Glottic cancers present early since even carcinoma in situ causes changes in the mucosal wave pattern of the cords and result in hoarseness (**Table 55.4**). In fact, any patient presenting with persistent or progressive voice change for more than 3 weeks needs to undergo a flexible or rigid laryngoscopic examination to rule out laryngeal malignancy.

Subglottic tumors spread caudally and circumferentially; hence, these remain silent until these are advanced enough to encroach on the airway and are often detected only when the patient presents with stridor.

■ Clinical Examination

- Indirect laryngoscopy:
  - Appearance: Lesions may be exophytic, ulcerative, nodular, or may even present as a submucosal bulge.
  - Extent: Extension of the lesion to more than one subsite of the larynx or the involvement of the base of the tongue, the vallecula, or the pyriform fossae upstages the disease and needs to be noted. The adequacy of the laryngeal airway should be documented. Any signs of aspiration should also be noted.
  - Vocal cord mobility: Impairment of vocal cord mobility implies infiltration into the thyroarytenoid muscle, while fixation of the cord indicates involvement of the cricoarytenoid joint, the paraglottic space, or invasion of the recurrent laryngeal nerve and upstages the disease. The bulk of the tumor may also impair mobility.
- Flexible or rigid endoscopic examination: It is done as an office procedure for detailed examination and documentation of the lesion (**Figs. 55.3** and **55.4**).
- Examination of the neck:
  - Laryngeal crepitus: Loss of laryngeal crepitus indicates involvement of the postcricoid space or the prevertebral space.
  - Splaying of the thyroid cartilage: This is indicative of the extralaryngeal spread of disease.
  - Neck swelling: This may represent direct invasion through the thyrohyoid or cricothyroid membrane or may represent metastatic neck nodes. In the case of neck nodes, their number, size, mobility, location, and laterality should be noted.

■ Radiological Investigations

- Neck computed tomography (CT): Contrast-enhanced CT of the neck is the investigation of choice to determine the extent of the lesion, involvement of preepiglottic, paraglottic spaces, cartilage erosion, and to look for nodal metastases.
- Neck magnetic resonance imaging (MRI): MRI of the neck is more sensitive than CT to determine soft-tissue involvement but is more expensive and time-consuming. Hence, it is often used in suspected cases of recurrence.

Table 55.4 Symptoms of the supraglottic, glottis, and subglottic cancers

Supraglottic	Glottic	Subglottic
Globus/foreign body sensation in the throat	Hoarseness	Dyspnoea
Hot potato voice	Progressive dyspnoea	Stridor
Dysphagia/odynophagia	Stridor	
Referred otalgia	Aspiration	
Neck swelling		

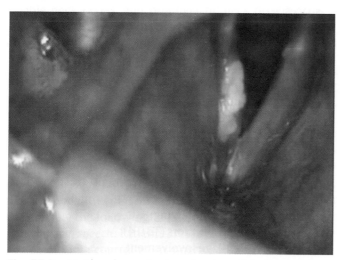

Fig. 55.3 Rigid endoscopic view showing white lesions along the right vocal cord.

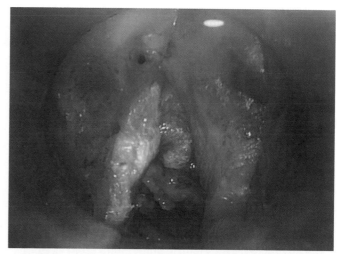

Fig. 55.4 View of transglottic malignancy with growth involving the supraglottis, glottis, and subglottis.

Case-Based Question

1. **A 60-year-old man, a smoker for the past 20 years, presented with a 3-month history of gradual-onset hoarseness of voice. On clinical examination, there is a proliferative lesion along the anterior one-third of the right vocal cord, but bilateral cords are mobile. No neck nodes were palpable.**

   a. What is the probable diagnosis?

   b. What investigations need to be done to confirm the diagnosis?

   c. What are the possible treatment modalities available for this patient?

Answers

a. Malignancy glottis T1N0M0 (stage I).

b. Direct laryngoscopic examination or microlaryngeal surgery and biopsy for histopathology, and contrast-enhanced CT of the neck to determine the extent of the disease and the presence of occult nodes.

c. Transoral laser microsurgery or radiation therapy.

Frequently Asked Questions

1. List the subsites of the larynx.

2. Why are glottic tumors generally associated with favorable prognosis?

3. Enumerate the treatment modalities available for advanced laryngeal cancer.

4. What are the indications for total laryngectomy?

5. What are the options available to rehabilitate a patient post total laryngectomy?

6. What are the risk factors for developing laryngeal malignancy?

Endnote

The first laryngectomy in the world was performed by Theodor Billroth in 1873. The surgery was difficult because of significant bleeding and poor anesthesia, but the patient survived and even received an artificial larynx. The patient lived for 7 months. Billroth was an Austrian surgeon and he was also the first person to do a gastrectomy.

56 Stridor and Congenital Lesions of the Larynx

Deepak K. Mehta and Jonathan Chiao

The competencies covered in this chapter are as follows:

EN4.47 Describe the clinical features, investigations, and principles of management of stridor.

PE28.7 Discuss the etiology, clinical features, and management of stridor in children.

PE28.9 Elicit, document, and present age-appropriate history of a child with upper respiratory problem including stridor.

Introduction

Stridor is described as a harsh, musical sound produced by a turbulent airflow through a partially obstructed upper airway. Pathology of the larynx may disrupt the normal laminar airflow of the upper airway, and the resultant turbulent airflow produces stridor. Stridor is therefore a symptom rather than a diagnosis.

Stridor can be inspiratory, expiratory, or biphasic:

- Inspiratory stridor suggests supraglottic or glottic obstruction.
- Expiratory stridor is typically related to tracheal or bronchial obstruction.
- Biphasic stridor is usually associated with a glottic or subglottic narrowing.

Loudness should not be misconstrued as disease severity, as loudness will change with variables such as respiratory effort and adequate compensation. In fact, soft stridor in a pediatric patient with weak respiratory effort may indicate an impending respiratory collapse.

Management of the stridulous child can range from reassurance to immediate surgical intervention. The goal of this chapter is to understand the physiology, presentation, and assessment of childhood stridor. In addition, one should be able to describe the underlying pathology and principles of disease-specific management.

Airway Physiology

Ventilation and airway dynamics are dependent on the two main principles of airflow resistance and transluminal pressure.

Poiseuille's law describes the relationship between flow of fluid or air through a tube and the cross-sectional radius of the tube:

$$Q = \Delta P \pi r^4 / 8 \mu L.$$

Thus, resistance to airflow is inversely proportional to the radius of the airway. A stenotic segment of the airway thus increases resistance and decreases airflow across the segment by a factor determined by the radius to the fourth power. A small narrowing in the airway diameter of an infant can therefore have a significant effect on the airflow and ventilation.

The Bernoulli principle describes that the reduction in cross-sectional area of an airway causes an increase in velocity of airway flow which decreases the intraluminal pressure along the walls. A higher velocity of airflow exacerbates luminal collapse and worsens underlying laryngo-, tracheo-, and/or bronchomalacia. This collapse also creates turbulent airflow that can be heard as stridor. Depending on the location of collapse, stridor can be inspiratory, expiratory, or biphasic.

Anatomic Locations of Stridor

■ Supraglottis

- The supraglottis is the space between the lingual surface of the epiglottis and the superior margin of the true vocal folds.
- It functions to coordinate safe swallowing and help protect the lower airway.
- Supraglottic collapse may create inspiratory stridor.
- In the newborn, laryngomalacia is the most common cause of stridor. Anatomically, laryngomalacia is

characterized by curling and tethering of the epiglottis secondary to short aryepiglottic folds. This causes the epiglottis and sometimes redundant supra-arytenoid tissue to prolapse into the glottis during inspiration resulting in turbulent airflow.

- Later in childhood, inspiratory stridor is often associated with infections such as epiglottitis that cause enlargement of supraglottic structures leading to increased turbulence.

■ Glottis

- Obstruction at the level of the glottis may present as inspiratory or biphasic stridor.
- Whereas laryngomalacia is a dynamic collapse, glottic obstructions tend to be fixed.
- In the stable child, loudness of stridor with a glottic obstruction can be correlated to the degree of obstruction.
- A small vocal fold cyst or granuloma may have very faint stridor or none at all; a unilateral vocal fold paralysis may have soft stridor at rest; and bilateral vocal fold paralysis may have significant stridor at rest with corresponding cyanosis.
- Clinical symptoms, etiology, and patient stability will guide the aggressiveness and course of management.

■ Subglottis

- Subglottic causes of stridor include pathologies such as subglottic stenosis, subglottic cysts, and airway hemangiomas. These are fixed obstructions that often present as biphasic stridor.
- The pediatric larynx is funnel shaped with the narrowest portion being the cricoid cartilage in the subglottis, which is the *only complete ring of cartilage* within the airway.
- Given its rigid structure, it is susceptible to iatrogenic injury (i.e., intubation) and infection (i.e., croup) that may lead to overlying fibrosis and stenosis.
- An infant's subglottis is normally between 4 and 7 mm. Less than 4 mm in a newborn or less than 3.5 mm in a premature infant is diagnostic of subglottic stenosis.
- The subglottis may be surgically evaluated for fixed obstruction via flexible nasopharyngoscopy, direct laryngoscopy with rigid bronchoscopy (DLB). This allows visualization of the area as well as the ability to measure the diameter of the subglottic airway using known sizes of uncuffed endotracheal tubes.
- The Cotton–Myer grading scale is the most widely used classification of subglottic stenosis severity (**Fig. 56.1**):
  - Grade I is less than 50% obstruction.
  - Grade II is between 51 and 70% obstruction.
  - Grade III is 71 to 99% obstruction.
  - Grade IV is no detectable lumen.

■ Trachea

Tracheal obstruction may present as expiratory or rarely biphasic stridor, and may be subdivided by its extrathoracic or intrathoracic location.

- Extrathoracic tracheal collapse necessitates increased inspiratory effort such as with congenital absence of tracheal rings or external compression from a thyroid goiter, cysts, or tumors.
- Intrathoracic collapse typically leads to increased expiratory effort to overcome the collapsed segment. This is seen in dynamic collapse processes of the trachea or bronchi, for example, tracheobronchomalacia, and is often associated with a chronic cough. As the child inhales, the negative intrathoracic pressure assists in tracheal expansion, but upon expiration the positive intrathoracic pressure collapse leads to collapse of the intrathoracic malacic segment.
- Fixed extrinsic compression of the intrathoracic trachea, such as a vascular ring or innominate compression, must also be considered when evaluating a stridulous child with corresponding cough. Fixed lesions such as tracheal tumors or complete tracheal rings will produce biphasic stridor and one would expect blunted expiratory and inspiratory curves on flow-volume loop.

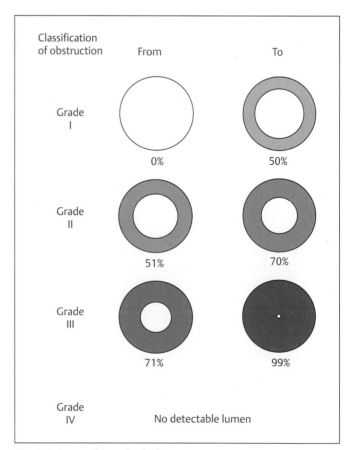

Fig. 56.1 Grading of subglottic stenosis.

Clinical Features and Evaluation of Stridor

■ History

- Children with noisy breathing may present in differing levels of respiratory distress. This may range from an otherwise asymptomatic and intermittent noise to acute respiratory distress necessitating securement of the airway.
- Depending on the presentation, securing a tenuous airway may supersede and postpone taking a complete history.
- For those patients who are clinically stable, one should first begin with a thorough history to determine character, severity, progression, exacerbating factors, and timing of the stridor. One should describe the onset and evolution as well as other associated signs and symptoms such as drooling, fever, cough, weight loss, and cyanosis.
- History of recent infections, feeding difficulty, coughing, or choking with objects such as food or toys in the mouth should be elicited.
- Previous airway interventions the child has needed, such as intubation, should also be explored.
- A thorough birth history including need for supplemental oxygen, noninvasive positive pressure ventilation, and intensive care unit management should be sought. Moreover, recurrence or similar episodes of the current complaint are important diagnostic clues that may change the management.
- Additionally, a past medical history complete with genetic syndromes (**Box 56.1**), neurological deficits, prenatal exposures, cardiac and pulmonary conditions, failure to thrive, and reflux should all be considered when evaluating a child with stridor.

Box 56.1 Syndromes associated with airway obstruction

- Down's syndrome
- Pierre Robin's sequence.
- Chiari malformation.
- DiGeorge's syndrome.
- CHARGE association.
- Goldenhar's syndrome.
- Cerebral palsy.
- Crouzon's syndrome.
- Treacher collins syndrome.
- Opitz's syndrome.
- Pallister–Hall syndrome.
- Beckwith–Wiedemann syndrome.
- Cornelia de Lange syndrome.
- Klippel–Feil syndrome.
- Mucopolysaccharidoses.

- In older children, a preexisting asthma diagnosis unresponsive to bronchodilator therapy may be suggestive of stridor and upper airway disease.
- Past surgical histories may indicate missed intubation history or cardiac procedures that may have injured the recurrent laryngeal nerves.

■ Physical Examination

The physician's initial impression and simple observation of a child can reveal a substantial amount of information. Increased work of breathing at rest, the color of the lips, tracheal tugging, and the use of accessory muscles can quickly aid in the assessment of airway severity. Complete assessment of vital signs and assessment of weight (position on growth curve, maintenance of curve, and trends) should be collected and evaluated.

The remainder of the physical examination should attempt to *localize* the airway obstruction.

- *Positional changes* may reduce the respiratory effort in patients with micrognathia and glossoptosis or laryngomalacia, but would have no effect in fixed lesion such as subglottic stenosis.
- A stridulous child with *cutaneous lesions*, especially large hemangiomas in a beard distribution, should raise the suspicion of an airway hemangioma.
- *Cervical masses* such as lymphadenopathy, goiter, or tracheal deviation may lead you to suspect extratracheal compression.

Awake *nasopharyngoscopy* should be performed by a trained otolaryngologist to examine the upper airway of the stridulous child. This technique can evaluate the anatomy and dynamic function of the airway extending from the nasal cavities into the subglottis in an awake patient at the clinic or bedside setting. An appropriate size endoscope is selected and placed into the nasal vestibule of an awake patient. Infants are often able to be swaddled and occupied with a sugar-coated pacifier to improve tolerance.

The endoscope is passed distally to evaluate the remainder of the nasal cavity, the nasopharynx, the function of the soft palate, the adenoid bed, the tonsils, the base of the tongue, the vallecula, the pharyngeal walls, the epiglottis, the arytenoid complexes, the vestibular folds, the pyriform sinuses, and the true vocal folds. A limited view of the subglottis may also be achieved. Examination should be performed during quiet respiration after the patient calms from insertion, and while crying and swallowing. These findings can aid in providing both the physician and family an immediate diagnosis and outline management strategy.

■ Radiography

The subglottis may be difficult to examine in some children during awake nasopharyngoscopy. Some patients may not tolerate the procedure, or a limited view may not reveal any pathologic abnormalities. In these children, a *lateral neck plain film* can identify epiglottitis, subglottic narrowing, asymmetrical lung patterns, and radio-opaque foreign bodies. While not commonly used as an initial evaluation method, a *dynamic airway computed tomography (CT) of the chest* can assess intrathoracic lesions such as a vascular ring, innominate compression, pulmonary agenesis, tracheal rings, pulmonary sling, and tracheobronchomalacia.

Congenital Lesions of the Larynx

The conditions covered under congenital lesions of the larynx include the following:
- Laryngomalacia.
- Vocal cord paralysis.
- Subglottic stenosis.
- Subglottic hemangioma.
- Tracheomalacia.
- Complete tracheal rings.

■ Laryngomalacia

Laryngomalacia is the most common congenital laryngeal anomaly, and is the underlying etiology in up to 74% of newborns with stridor. There is flaccidity of the supraglottic structures, which may be due to cartilage or neural immaturity, which improves with age.
- Patients with laryngomalacia have intermittent inspiratory stridor that is exacerbated with agitation, crying, supine positioning, and/or feeding. Stridor will begin

and progressively worsen in the first few weeks of life, peak around 6 months, and mild cases will resolve by 24 months of age. The stridor may reduce in the prone position.
- In the cases where laryngomalacia is more severe, coughing and choking are often witnessed after feeding secondary to airway obstruction.
- The resultant increased work of breathing and decreased caloric intake may cause these infants to descend from their projected growth curves leading to loss of weight.
- Awake nasopharyngoscopy in a child with laryngomalacia will often identify curling of the epiglottis (Ω epiglottis), short aryepiglottic (AE) folds, redundant supra-arytenoid tissue, and prolapsing supraglottic tissue with inspiration (**Fig. 56.2a, b**). Types of laryngomalacia are illustrated in **Fig. 56.3**.
- In case there is severe stridor, other coexisting causes should also be sought for by imaging and endoscopy.

While laryngomalacia in most infants will be mild, it is estimated that 20% will need surgical intervention.

Treatment

- Supraglottoplasty is often performed by dividing the AE folds and reducing the amount of supraglottic tissue (redundant tissue over arytenoids) to release the prolapsing supraglottic tissue from being pulled over the glottis on inspiration.
- It is important to note that laryngomalacia is associated with gastroesophageal reflux in up to 70% of cases, and this should be managed with antireflux medications, especially if supraglottoplasty is to be performed.

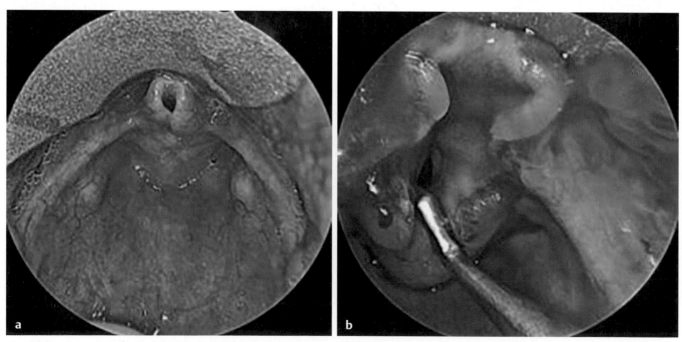

Fig. 56.2 Laryngomalacia. **(a)** Omega epiglottis with short aryepiglottic folds. **(b)** After supraglottoplasty.

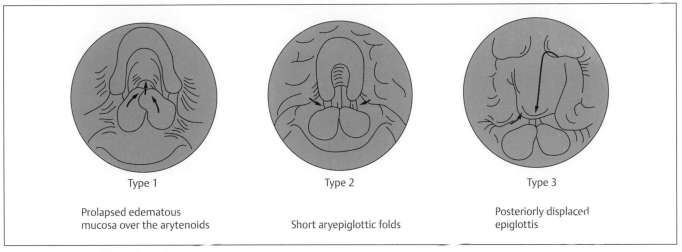

Type 1

Prolapsed edematous mucosa over the arytenoids

Type 2

Short aryepiglottic folds

Type 3

Posteriorly displaced epiglottis

Fig. 56.3 Types of laryngomalacia.

Pearls

- Laryngomalacia is the commonest congenital anomaly of the larynx that can cause stridor.
- Symptoms improve with age.
- Surgical intervention is required only in severe cases.
- Gastroesophageal reflux disease (GERD) should be treated simultaneously.

■ Vocal Fold Immobility or Paralysis

Vocal fold immobility or paralysis is the second most common cause of stridor in infants. These patients, especially with bilateral involvement, may require tracheostomy for airway stabilization.

Etiology

- The recurrent laryngeal nerve is responsible for vocal fold movement and is susceptible to trauma through cardiac surgery, thyroid surgery, or birth trauma.
- Causative neurologic factors should be investigated including the Arnold–Chiari malformation, hydrocephalus, and cerebral hemorrhage.
- Non-neurological causes should also be explored, especially in infants with history of intubation. Traumatic or prolonged intubation may lead to posterior glottic stenosis or cricoarytenoid subluxation/fixation.

Clinical Features

- A weak cry and dysphagia are common symptoms in unilateral vocal fold paralysis (**Fig. 56.4a**).
- Infants with bilateral vocal fold paralysis will have significant stridor, retractions, and cyanotic episodes due to a fixed glottic obstruction (**Fig. 56.4b**).

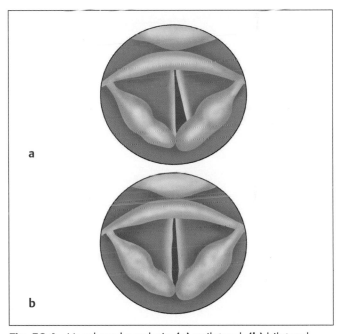

a

b

Fig. 56.4 Vocal cord paralysis. **(a)** unilateral. **(b)** bilateral.

Investigations

- In children, this may be diagnosed with laryngeal ultrasound or flexible laryngoscopy.
- Imaging by CT scan or magnetic resonance imaging (MRI) should be performed to evaluate the course of the vagus nerve from the skull base through the chest to identify lesions or masses. MRI is required to rule out Arnold–Chiari malformation/hydrocephalus.
- Laryngeal electromyogram (EMG) may be employed to further investigate the nerve's integrity and endplate muscle function. It may help differentiate palsy from fixity.

- Careful endoscopic palpation may be used to assess for cricoarytenoid fixation and posterior glottic stenosis.

Treatment

- Tracheostomy is the current gold standard management for symptomatic pediatric bilateral vocal fold paralysis.
- In bilateral vocal cord palsy, procedures either to avoid tracheostomy or to help decannulate a child include vocal fold lateralization and endoscopic arytenoidectomy.
- In cases of recurrent laryngeal nerve damage, such as from iatrogenic cardiac or thyroid surgery, there is reported success in improving bulk and tone via laryngeal reinnervation of bilateral posterior cricoarytenoid muscles with the use of the phrenic nerve.
- Correction of neurological problems by placement of shunt or posterior fossa decompression will help in improving the cord mobility.

Pearls

- Idiopathic and neurological causes of vocal cord palsy can present as unilateral or bilateral palsy. After trauma, it is usually unilateral.
- MRI of the brain is done to rule out Arnold–Chiari malformation in bilateral vocal fold palsy.
- Airway management is required for bilateral cord palsy, as the patient presents with stridor.

■ Subglottic Stenosis

Subglottic stenosis can be acquired, inflammatory, or congenital.

Acquired

- Intubation-related subglottic injury is the most common cause of subglottic stenosis (**Fig. 56.5**).
- Symptoms can develop a few days to a few weeks after intubation and range from dysphonia, stridor, and oxygen desaturations to use of accessory respiratory muscles.
- Treatment with steroids and inhaled racemic epinephrine will often stabilize and improve symptoms temporarily; however, the patient should be monitored for rebound edema and declining status even after treatment.
- Although flexible laryngoscopy can diagnose vocal fold granulomas to explain postextubation dysphonia, a formal operative airway endoscopy is recommended for diagnosis of subglottic stenosis. This allows both a diagnostic and therapeutic intervention via dilation techniques in the operating room.
- Endoscopic balloon dilation of a membranous subglottic stenosis has a very favorable response rate. Refractory cases may benefit from lysis of the membranous band and steroid injection at the time of dilation.
- Patients with grade III and IV subglottic stenoses are less likely to respond to endoscopic balloon dilation and will typically require an open airway procedure.

Inflammatory

The inflammatory conditions producing stridor, that is croup, are discussed in Chapter 52 "Acute and Chronic Inflammation of the Larynx."

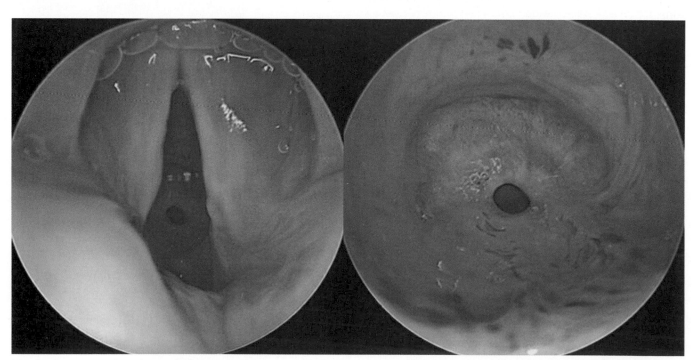

Fig. 56.5 Acquired grade III subglottic stenosis.

Congenital

- Congenital subglottic stenosis often presents with progressive symptoms in an infant who has no history of intubation, trauma, or any other causative insult (**Fig. 56.6**). The cricoid ring is small or elliptical, and may be due to an entrapped first tracheal ring.
- Stridor, poor feeding coordination, and aspiration soon develop as the stenosis matures and the child tries to adapt to an insufficient airway. As caloric expenditure increases to overcome increased airway resistance, children will start to descend on the growth curve and lose weight. Decreased caloric intake secondary to the feeding incoordination puts the child at risk of stunted growth.
- Thickening of the feeds will allow improved timing of the suck–swallow reflex, but a gastric tube may be indicated for those patients who have severe dysphagia and/or aspiration until operative correction can be safely performed.

Treatment

- Early stages, which are an incidental finding or with mild symptoms, can be kept on observation.
- Membranous stenosis can be treated by balloon dilatation.
- Tracheostomy may be required when there is stridor.
- Evaluation using endoscopy should be done in the controlled setting of the operating room where there is provision for airway intervention including tracheostomy.
- Surgical options to improve the subglottic airway are the following:
  - Anterior and/or posterior cricoid split with cartilage (costal, thyroid) grafting.
  - Cricotracheal resection and end-to-end anastomosis.

> ### Pearl
>
> The subglottic region is the only part of the airway that has cartilage all around (cricoid) and stenosis is more commonly acquired due to prolonged intubation.
>
> Lumen <4 mm in neonates and <3 mm in premature is considered as stenosis; grade 1: 0–50%; grade 2: 51–70%; grade 3: 71–99%; and grade 4: complete.

■ Subglottic Hemangioma

- Subglottic hemangioma is rare, yet it represents the most common neoplasm of the infant airway (**Fig. 56.7**).
- Subglottic hemangiomas typically present as biphasic stridor that worsens with agitation or viral upper respiratory infection and/or recurrent "croup" prior to 6 months of age.
- Concurrent cutaneous hemangiomas may be present in up to 50% of children with subglottic lesions. Hemangiomas in a "beard distribution" have been associated with airway hemangiomas in up to 62% of the cases.
- Subglottic hemangiomas may be seen with awake nasopharyngoscopy and appear as a smooth red mass in the posterolateral aspect of the subglottis, but formal operative endoscopic evaluation may be required to identify and characterize lesions.
- Propranolol has become the mainstay of treatment for infantile hemangiomas to disrupt the proliferative phase and promote stabilization of the lesion. Typical dosing starts at 0.6 mg/kg/d, increasing up to 3 mg/kg/d for 6 months for treating infantile hemangiomas.
- In infants who are not responsive to propranolol consider biopsy of the lesion looking for GLUT-1 receptor. In these conditions, open excision of lesion can be considered.

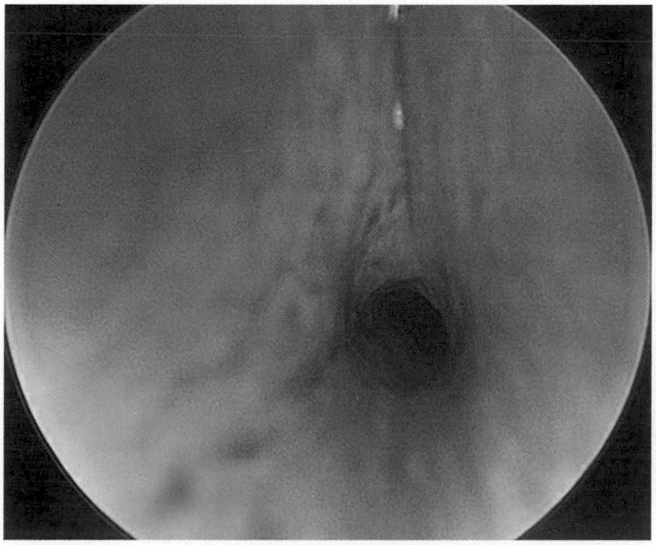

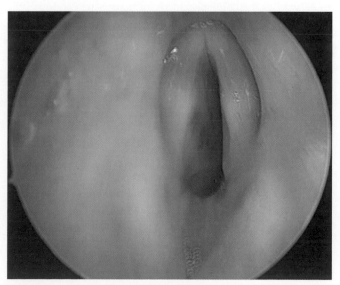

Fig. 56.6 Congenital grade III subglottic stenosis.

Fig. 56.7 Subglottic hemangioma.

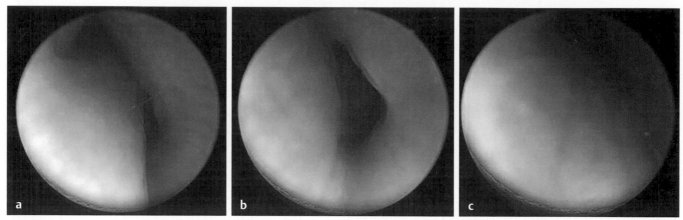

Fig. 56.8 Tracheobronchomalacia. **(a)** At the carina. **(b)** Right main stem bronchus. **(c)** Left main stem bronchus.

■ Tracheomalacia

- Cartilage typically accounts for up to three quarters of the tracheal circumference and is separated posteriorly by the trachealis muscle (**Fig. 56.8**).
- Excessive dynamic collapse of the trachea can arise from extrinsic or intrinsic forces:
  - Tracheomalacia due to extrinsic forces typically arise from masses, vascular compression, or lack of normal tracheal cartilage.
  - Intrinsic tracheomalacia is more common. The collapse occurs with expiration.
- Tracheomalacia will present differently depending on the location:
  - Intrathoracic compression presents with a barking or crouplike cough.
  - Extrathoracic compression will typically present with an inspiratory stridor.
  - Recurrent bronchitis, prolonged recovery, or escalation of care should raise the concern for tracheomalacia.
- Airway endoscopy under spontaneous respiration will identify dynamic airway collapse, location, and severity.
- Tracheomalacia can also be identified on dynamic airway CT scan.

Management

- *Treatment* of tracheomalacia is dependent on the severity.
  - Reassurance is often all that is needed for mild malacia.
  - Tracheostomy may be required for prolonged positive pressure ventilation or to traverse and maintain patency of the malacic segment.
  - There have been a variety of surgical approaches to address severe tracheomalacia, including posterior tracheopexy, tracheobronchoplasty, tracheobronchial stenting, endoluminal stents, extraluminal stents, and aortopexy.

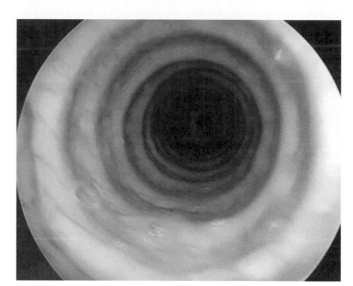

Fig. 56.9 Complete tracheal rings.

■ Complete Tracheal Rings

- When the trachealis muscle fails to develop, a complete tracheal ring is formed (**Fig. 56.9**).
- Varying length and degree of tracheal narrowing result in a fixed obstruction. This may lead to increased work of breathing with retractions and varying distal airway sounds.
- Depending on the location and length of tracheal involvement, stridor may be inspiratory, expiratory, or biphasic. Stridor, a "barking" or brassy cough, and "washing machine"–like breathing sounds may all be present.
- Cyanotic spells and apparent life-threatening events trigger urgent action.
- Bronchoscopy remains the gold standard of diagnosis, either rigid or flexible, to accurately describe the location, severity, and length of the affected segment.
- MRI, CT, and echocardiogram can add additional information about concurrent vascular anomalies, for example, pulmonary sling.

- Approximately 80% of patients with complete tracheal rings will require surgical intervention. Slide tracheoplasty has become the standard procedure.

Points to Ponder

- Stridor is a nonspecific term describing a symptom of underlying turbulent airflow in the upper airway.
- Stridor can be inspiratory, expiratory, or biphasic.
- Stridor can vary in onset, phase, character, and duration, which depend on the etiology.
- A secure and patent airway is of paramount importance.

- Take a thorough history and careful evaluation of the patient to discern the underlying pathology.
- Understanding of the anatomy of the upper and lower airways as well as clinical judgment to assess severity helps determine the appropriate management.
- Laryngomalacia is the most common congenital anomaly of the larynx producing stridor.
- Vocal cord paralysis is the second most common cause of stridor in infants.
- The most common cause of acquired subglottic stenosis is intubation injury.

Case-Based Questions

1. **A 5-month-old infant was referred to the otolaryngology department with history of noisy breathing. There were intercostal and suprasternal retractions. The infant had feeding difficulties. There was inspiratory stridor. The symptoms reduced in the prone position but increased while crying.**

   a. What is the most likely diagnosis?

   b. How would you confirm the diagnosis?

   c. What is the treatment?

   Answers

   a. Laryngomalacia is the most likely diagnosis.

   b. A flexible nasolaryngoscopy with or without bronchoscopy should be done in the operating room to confirm the diagnosis and rule out other causes.

   c. Once diagnosis of laryngomalacia is confirmed, a supraglottoplasty should be done and treatment for GERD should also be initiated.

2. **A 2-month-old infant was brought with a history of noisy breathing of 1-week duration. There was history of intubation at birth. There was a recent failed attempt at intubation following which the stridor increased.**

   a. What is the possible diagnosis?

   b. What is the management?

   Answers

   a. Acquired subglottic stenosis is the most likely diagnosis.

   b. In view of increase in stridor, the airway should be secured by tracheostomy. If the stridor was mild, an endoscopic assessment of the airway could have been done. Balloon dilation can be done for the stenosis. For grade III and IV stenosis, which is thick, an open procedure is required to increase the subglottic airway.

Frequently Asked Questions

1. What is stridor and how will you classify it?

2. What are the symptoms associated with laryngomalacia?

3. What is the surgical management of laryngomalacia?

4. How will you medically manage a patient with subglottic hemangioma?

5. What investigation can be performed in the outpatient clinic to confirm laryngomalacia?

6. What is the Cotton–Myer classification for subglottic stenosis?

Endnote

The sound produced by an obstructed airway in the larynx or trachea is called "stridor." It is high pitched and has a musical quality, whereas obstruction to the airway in the nasopharynx or oropharynx is low pitched and rough, and has a snoring quality to it. This is called "stertor." Obstruction to the bronchial airway in the thorax, seen in asthma, is called wheezing.

57 Tracheostomy and Airway Emergencies

Deepak K. Mehta and Chantal Barbot

The competencies covered in this chapter are as follows:

EN4.48 Elicit, document, and present a correct history; demonstrate and describe the clinical features; choose the correct investigations; and describe the principles of management of airway emergencies.

EN4.50 Observe and describe the indications for and steps involved in tracheostomy.

EN4.51 Observe and describe the care of the patient with a tracheostomy.

EN2.13 Identify, resuscitate, and manage ENT emergencies in a simulated environment including tracheostomy.

EN3.6 Observe and describe the indications for and steps involved in the skills of emergency procedures in the ear, nose, and throat.

Introduction

Tracheostomy is a surgical procedure where an opening is made into the trachea. It allows access to the airway and the lower tracheobronchial tree. It also permits ventilation to occur in conditions where there is an upper airway obstruction.

Definition

Tracheotomy is the operation of "opening the trachea," referring to the surgical procedure itself and carries no implication that it is a permanent procedure. Tracheostomy has an ending derived from the word *stoma* and, strictly speaking, implies an opening in the neck created by suturing skin flaps onto the tracheal walls.

Anatomy and Physiology

The trachea begins at the subglottic larynx extending from the lower border of the cricoid, at the level of the C6, and terminates at the carina and main stem bronchi, corresponding to the sternal angle and the T5 vertebra. The trachea is a set of 18 to 22 incomplete cartilaginous rings (*C*-shaped). In the average adult, the distance from the cricoid to the carina is approximately 11 cm in length, with a range of 10 to 13 cm. The posterior wall of the trachea lies anterior to the esophagus. The trachea lies deep to the sternohyoid and sternothyroid muscles, also called the strap muscles. The thyroid isthmus is adherent to the anterior trachea from the second to the fourth tracheal cartilages. Lateral structures include the recurrent laryngeal nerves, common carotid arteries, inferior thyroid arteries, and lobes of the thyroid gland.

Indications

The indications for tracheostomy are broadly classified into obstructive and nonobstructive conditions (**Boxes 57.1 and 57.2**).

The aim is to bypass the upper airway obstruction. The obstruction can be intraluminal or extraluminal, by occlusion, compression, or infiltration.

The advantages of doing a tracheostomy in nonobstructive indications include the following:

- Prevention of laryngotracheal stenosis due to prolonged intubation.
- Retained secretions can be removed (bronchial toilet).
- The dead space is reduced by 50%.
- There is increase in alveolar ventilation due to reduction in airway resistance.

Box 57.1 Obstructive indications for tracheostomy

- *Congenital*
  - Subglottic stenosis
  - Bilateral abductor palsy
- *Inflammatory/infections*
  - Acute infections: Epiglottitis, laryngeal diphtheria, and Ludwig's angina
- *Trauma*
  - Neck/laryngeal trauma
  - Facial fractures
- *Malignancy*: Larynx, oropharynx, hypopharynx, and thyroid
- *Obstructive sleep apnea*
- *Neurological*: Bilateral abductor palsy following thyroidectomy and cerebrovascular accident
- *Laryngotracheal stenosis*
  - Prolonged intubation
  - Laryngotracheal trauma
  - Corrosive poisoning
  - Granulomatosis with polyangiitis
  - Rhinoscleroma (subglottic involvement)
- *Impacted foreign body in larynx*
- *Angioneurotic edema*
- *Prophylactic* prior to certain head and neck procedures (mainly those involving the base of the tongue and the larynx)

Box 57.2 Nonobstructive Indications for tracheostomy

- *Prolonged mechanical ventilation*
  - Respiratory disease
  - Neuromuscular disease
- *Pulmonary toilet*
  - Inadequate cough
  - Inability to handle secretions
  - Aspiration

- The cuff, when inflated, may protect the lower airway from aspiration.
- The cuff also helps in facilitating intermittent positive pressure ventilation.

Tracheostomy can be broadly divided into two categories:
- Emergent or emergency tracheostomy.
- Elective tracheostomy.

Whenever possible, patients needing tracheostomy should be managed by intubation using an endotracheal tube (ETT). The advantages of endotracheal intubation include the following:
- It is a relatively easier procedure than a tracheostomy.
- It can secure the airway faster when compared to a tracheostomy.

- It is well tolerated by the patient for short periods of 1 to 2 weeks.

However, there are some notable emergency exceptions of acute upper airway obstruction where the patient cannot be intubated. Some examples of this can include foreign body, angioedema, infection, or anaphylaxis. Tracheostomy is the preferred airway for unstable patients with anterior laryngeal trauma, especially for those with obvious laryngeal fracture, stridor, and increased work of breathing.

Emergent tracheostomy may also be necessary in severe facial fractures including comminuted mandibular fractures, midfacial fractures at the Le Fort III level, and panfacial fractures. Urgent tracheostomy may be indicated for head and neck neoplasms, in which oral, oropharyngeal, and laryngeal tumors have enlarged to the point of obstruction of the upper airway. Also, if an emergent cricothyrotomy is performed for any reason, it should be converted into a tracheostomy in the operating room once an airway has been secured.

The most common indication for tracheostomy is acute respiratory failure and the need to provide access for prolonged mechanical ventilation. Other indications for elective tracheostomy include pulmonary toilet, which can be secondary to inadequate cough or aspiration and the inability to handle secretions. It is important to note that tracheostomy *does not completely prevent aspiration* (especially liquids), but it provides an ability to suction the secretions from the airway. In cases of severe obstructive sleep apnea not amenable to continuous positive airway pressure (CPAP) devices, or other less invasive surgery, tracheostomy offers a solution that bypasses the upper airway all together. Elective tracheostomy can also be considered as a prophylactic measure in preparation for extensive head and neck cancer treatment and the base of the tongue procedures.

Timing of Tracheostomy

Although the indications for tracheostomy are well established, the timing of elective tracheostomy for the patient requiring prolonged ventilation is a widely debated subject without a clear consensus. The conventional thinking is that tracheostomy facilitates weaning from mechanical ventilation by reducing dead space and decreasing airway resistance, improving secretion clearance, reducing the need for sedation, and by decreasing the risk of aspiration. It is also noted that the duration of mechanical ventilation increases the risk of ventilator-associated pneumonia, which has a significant morbidity and mortality. Local complications such as subglottic stenosis are more likely if tracheal intubation is continued for more than 2 weeks. *Early tracheostomy*, in critically ill medical patients who undergo more than 14 days of ventilation, may have reduction in the following:

- Mortality rate.
- Frequency of pneumonia.
- Duration of mechanical ventilation.
- Length of time in intensive care.

Contraindications

Although there are no absolute contraindications to tracheostomy, active cellulitis of the anterior neck skin and bleeding disorders can be considered as relative contraindications. Before taking up for tracheostomy, it is important to discuss end-of-life issues when appropriate and the need for continued care. This often requires a multidisciplinary approach.

Tracheostomy Technique

■ Open Tracheostomy

- The head and neck should be extended to bring the trachea as anteriorly as possible. This is accomplished by placing a shoulder roll. Patients with cervical mobility issues as well as Down syndrome patients with atlantooccipital instability can cause additional difficulty in

the procedure due to an inability to fully extend the neck.

- The thyroid notch, cricoid cartilage, and sternal notch are the anatomic landmarks that need to be identified by palpation and are marked on the skin. This can be made difficult in a morbidly obese patient. Palpation at the sternal notch should be performed to evaluate for possible high-riding innominate artery (**Fig. 57.1**).
- A horizontal skin incision is marked in the midline of the neck anteriorly, approximately 1 to 2 cm below the inferior border of the cricoid cartilage, or between the cricoid cartilage and sternal notch. Alternatively, approximately two fingerbreadths above the sternal notch is the site for the incision (**Fig. 57.2**). Occasionally for an emergency tracheostomy, a vertical incision from the cricoid to the suprasternal notch may be used.
- The incision is extended through subcutaneous tissue and then subplatysmally to expose the strap muscles, the sternohyoid, and the sternothyroid. The median raphe is then identified and transected vertically and the strap muscles are retracted laterally to expose the thyroid gland (**Fig. 57.3**).

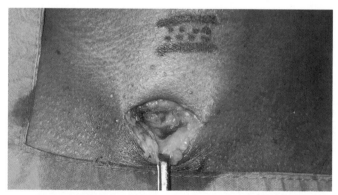

Fig. 57.2 Horizontal incision.

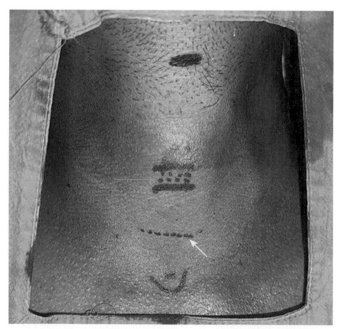

Fig. 57.1 The neck showing the site of cricoid (*blue arrow*), line of incision (*yellow arrow*), and suprasternal notch (*green arrow*).

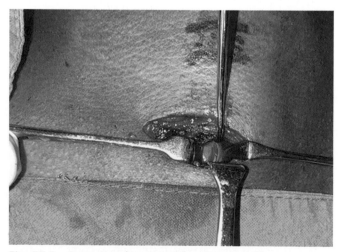

Fig. 57.3 Strap muscles exposed and separated.

- The isthmus generally needs to be ligated to fully expose the second and third tracheal rings. Alternatively, the isthmus can be retracted with a blunt hook.
- The trachea is opened between the second and third rings, and the tracheostomy tube is inserted. There are various modifications to placing an incision in the trachea including removing a window of cartilage, use of a vertical incision (in pediatric tracheostomy), or the creation of a Bjork flap (inferiorly based cartilage flap secured to the subcutaneous tissues). The first tracheal ring is avoided to reduce the risk of subsequent subglottic stenosis (**Fig. 57.4**).
- The tracheostomy tube can then be inserted and the patient can immediately be ventilated through the tube (**Figs. 57.5, 57.6,** and **57.7**). Care is taken for the first 3 to 5 days to avoid accidental decannulation as the tract is not fully mature, creating a potential emergency situation of inability to successfully re-cannulate the patient.

■ Percutaneous Tracheostomy

A percutaneous tracheostomy technique initially described by Ciaglia (1985) utilizes bronchoscopy for visualization

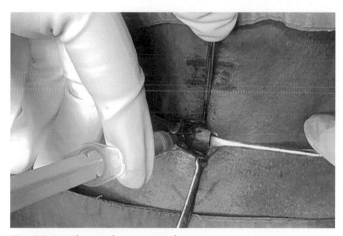

Fig. 57.4 The trachea exposed.

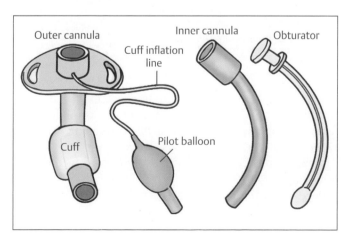

Fig. 57.5 Parts of a tracheostomy tube.

of the puncture followed by a dilatational process (modified Seldinger technique) for tube insertion. Various types of percutaneous techniques are available. All these techniques require puncture of the trachea and insertion of a guidewire into the trachea (**Fig. 57.8**).

■ Surgical Tracheostomy (Open Type) versus Percutaneous Tracheostomy

The percutaneous technique is stated to be more amenable to being performed at the bedside and avoids the transporting of potentially critically ill patients to the operating room. Open tracheostomy can also be easily performed at the bedside overcoming the transport concern although some of the cost-savings of performing the surgery in the intensive care unit (ICU) are lost by using the operating room personnel and equipment in the ICU.

The advantage of the percutaneous technique over the open technique is that there is less blood loss and lower infection rates. The percutaneous technique, however, has been reported to have catastrophic complications like tracheal laceration, injury to the aorta, and esophageal perforation, which are uncommon in the open procedure.

■ Contraindications for Percutaneous Tracheostomy

Contraindications for percutaneous tracheostomy are the following:
- In emergency tracheostomy tube placement.
- A neck in which the anatomical landmarks are difficult to palpate, especially in morbidly obese patients.
- Tracheal deviation.
- Requirement for tracheostomy tubes not designed for percutaneous tracheostomy may make the procedure problematic.

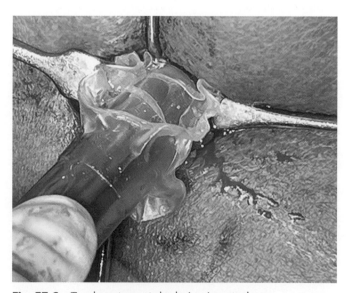

Fig. 57.6 Tracheostomy tube being inserted.

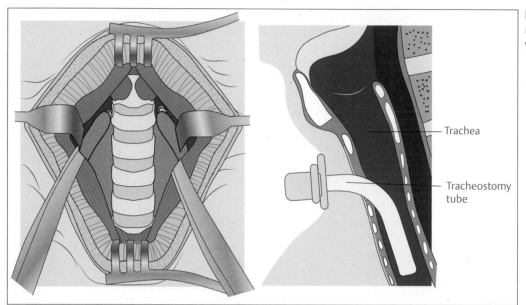

Trachea

Tracheostomy tube

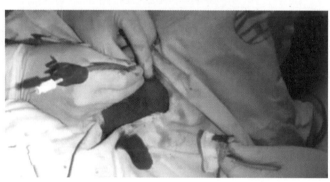

Fig. 57.8 Percutaneous tracheostomy being performed.

- Enlarged thyroid.
- Malignancy at the site of tracheostomy.
- Inability to extend the neck because of lack of cervical spine mobility.
- Previous tracheostomy.

Complications of Tracheostomy

Complications of tracheostomy are listed in **Box 57.3**.

Pearl

When tracheostomy is done for airway obstruction with severe stridor, the carbon dioxide buildup stimulates the respiratory center. Once the trachea is opened, there is a carbon dioxide washout leading to sudden withdrawal of the stimulus, which can lead to respiratory arrest. During tracheostomy, sedation should be avoided as this would affect the respiratory center leading to deterioration of the patient. Desaturation with bradycardia is an ominous sign.

Box 57.3	**Different types of complications of tracheostomy**

- Immediate
  - Hemorrhage
  - Subcutaneous emphysema
  - Apnea
  - Pneumothorax
  - Pneumomediastinum
  - Tracheoesophageal fistula
  - Recurrent laryngeal nerve injury
  - Tube in false tract

- Early
  - Acute obstruction of tube (blood and mucous)
  - Stomal infection
  - Accidental decannulation (false tract)
  - Hemorrhage

- Late
  - Granulation tissue (stomal/trachea)
  - Tracheal stenosis/suprastomal stenosis
  - Tracheomalacia
  - Late tracheoesophageal fistula
  - Tracheocutaneous fistula
  - Tracheoinnominate fistula
  - Difficult decannulation

A good stepwise technique of tracheostomy and careful postoperative care avoids most of the complications. Infections of the stoma can usually be treated with local wound care.

Routine postoperative tracheostomy care include the following:
- Regular suctioning through the tube.
- Use of humidification.
- The inner cannula is cleaned and replaced frequently to reduce the risk of obstruction of the tube. If for some

reason the obstructed tube cannot be cleared, it should be removed and replaced immediately. This is one of the reasons an extra tracheostomy tube should always be readily available at bedside.

Tube Dislodgement and Accidental Decannulation

This can be very problematic and potentially fatal in the immediate postoperative period before a tract has matured around the tracheostomy tube. Displacement into a false passage should be kept in mind if there is sudden respiratory distress in the early postoperative period, especially if a patient who is on the ventilator is suddenly able to phonate.

Because of the potential difficulty in replacing a fresh tracheostomy tube, intraoperative techniques are used to facilitate replacement. This can include placing of stay sutures in the lateral part of the trachea (more common in pediatric tracheostomy) and securing the tracheostomy tube to the adjacent skin with stay sutures (more common in adults), allowing the fistula time to mature. Sometimes reintubation is required when there is difficulty in reinserting a dislodged tracheostomy tube in the immediate postoperative period. There should not be an upper airway obstruction for intubation.

Stenosis of Trachea

One of the reasons a tracheostomy is performed is to avoid prolonged ETT intubation, which can predispose to tracheal and subglottic stenosis. However, tracheal stenosis and tracheomalacia can also be late complications of tracheostomy tube placement. Ischemic necrosis of the tracheal wall can occur due to a high pressure in the cuff of the tracheostomy tube. This can lead to healing by scar formation followed by stenosis. This complication can be avoided by the use of a tracheostomy tube with low-pressure cuff.

The incidence of stenosis can also be decreased by the following:
- Proper placement of the tracheostomy tube intraoperatively between the second and third tracheal rings.
- Use of smaller sized tubes for tracheostomy.
- Minimizing cuff inflation pressures and cuff inflation times.

If mechanical ventilation is no longer required, the cuff on the tracheostomy tube should be deflated, and the tracheostomy tube changed to a cuffless tube. Late tracheoesophageal fistula is rare, but when present it may also be the result of an overinflated or improperly fitted cuff.

Granulation Tissue

Granulation tissue can be problematic and is one of the most common late complications of tracheostomy.

Granulation tissue can bleed, complicate tracheostomy tube changes, and also obstruct the airway. Local care with steroid creams and silver nitrate can be helpful, but granulation tissue sometimes requires surgical excision. Granulation tissue is more commonly seen in children or when a fenestrated tracheostomy tube is used. Regular tracheostomy tube changes can reduce this complication, but not eliminate it.

Tracheocutaneous Fistula

Tracheocutaneous fistula is a persistent opening between the trachea and skin following decannulation, which has been found to be much more common with a long period of tracheostomy, prior to decannulation. When the tracheostomy tube is removed, the stoma is covered by an occlusive dressing. The stoma will usually close within 24 to 48 hours without any additional intervention. A fistula can persist if there is:
- Inward growth of skin to meet the trachea.
- Granulation tissue present preventing closure.
- The fistula remains to compensate for upper airway compromise. Due to this last concern, an endoscopic examination (transnasal flexible laryngoscopy and retrograde endoscopy through the stoma) should be undertaken before any repair of a tracheocutaneous fistula is attempted.

Tracheoinnominate Fistula

Tracheoinnominate fistula (TIF) is rare, but when it does occur, it is catastrophic, with mortality reported as high as 80%. Some patients will present with a small amount of bleeding 24 to 48 hours before the occurrence, which generally stops spontaneously. This bleeding should elicit concern because the bleed can be a harbinger of massive hemorrhage and is called the sentinel bleed and can occur in up to 30% of patients with TIF.

Tracheostomy in Children

With only rare exceptions, tracheostomy in children should be performed in the controlled setting of the operating room under general anesthesia. A notable difference in the operative procedure, is the use of a vertical incision in the trachea in infants and small children. This has been suggested to reduce the instance of suprastomal collapse and tracheal stenosis. With a vertical incision, retention sutures placed in a paramedian position on either side of the incision prior to making the incision helps retract the opening in the trachea intraoperatively. Also, these sutures can facilitate replacement of the tube in case of accidental decannulation in the early postoperative period.

Post Tracheostomy Care

- A chest X-ray is taken to note the position of the tube and to look for pneumothorax and emphysema.
- Tracheostomy tubes are available as a single or a double cannula. The double-cannula tubes require the inner cannula when connected to a ventilator. Dual cannula tubes are more commonly seen in adult tracheostomy tubes and single cannula tubes are more commonly seen in pediatric tracheostomy tubes due to the already smaller diameter of the airway. The presence of the inner cannula allows for retention of the outer tube, and quicker and easier cleaning, which is done once or twice a day. This prevents obstruction of the inner tube by the secretions.
- Cuffed tubes are for short-term use, until a patient is weaned from a ventilator and can manage their own secretions. However, a cuffed tube may be required long term in patients with chronic conditions. Importantly, the cuff pressure on a cuffed tracheostomy tube requires regular checks to ensure it is at an appropriate pressure of between 20 and 30 cm of H_2O. The cuff should be deflated hourly for 5 minutes.
- Normal humidification and filtration of inhaled air is affected. Without this humidification, the epithelium of the trachea and bronchi will become dry and tracheal secretions thicken with crusting, increasing the potential for tube blockage. Tracheal humidification can be provided by a humidifier or heat and moisture exchanger (HME).
- Suctioning of the tracheostomy tube is necessary to remove mucus, maintain a patent airway, and avoid tracheostomy tube blockages. The frequency of suctioning varies and is based on individual patient assessment. Tracheal damage may be caused by suctioning past the length of the tracheostomy tube. Suctioning should be done after deflation of the cuff. Some tubes have a suction cannula, which can remove secretions above the cuff.
- The stoma should be inspected and cleaned daily to ensure the skin is clean and dry to maintain skin integrity and avoid breakdown. A dressing should be placed daily at the stomal site. Tracheostomy ties should also be replaced on a regular basis.
- Tracheostomy tubes should be changed approximately 30 days after placement. It is best that two people who are competent in tracheostomy care are present for tracheostomy tube changes.

Decannulation

Decannulation refers to the removal of the tracheostomy tube and subsequent closure of the tracheal stoma. This can be done by assessing the airway via transoral or transnasal endoscopy and a retrograde endoscopy through the tracheal stoma. X-ray of the neck (anteroposterior [AP] and lateral views) may be helpful. The inner cannula of the tracheostomy tube should be a fenestrated one. The outer tube is blocked for 24 to 48 hours to assess the patency of the upper airway. Once the patient is able to tolerate the "corking," the tube is removed and the stoma is covered by an outer dressing or a formal two-layer closure is done with sutures. Alternatively, the tube can be serially downsized till closure.

Airway Emergencies

Airway emergencies are rare. They include sudden, life-threatening events, which cause disruption in the patency of the natural or artificial airway. Airway emergencies include those conditions in which the airway is blocked, traumatized or failed, or a combination of any of these. Many of these described situations are indications for urgent tracheostomy.

The common cause for an airway emergency is an obstructed airway. The level of obstruction will help in forming a differential diagnosis for upper airway obstruction. The classic sounds and signs of obstruction at the various sites vary and include stertor at a nasal or nasopharyngeal level, possible gurgling at an oropharyngeal level, inspiratory stridor at a supraglottic level, inspiratory or biphasic stridor at a glottic or subglottic level, and expiratory stridor or wheeze at tracheobronchial level.

Airway, breathing, and circulation (ABC) is the initial step in management. Oxygen saturation should be monitored, and oxygen should be delivered via a face mask. At this time, depending on how stable the patient is, imaging studies may be done, and antibiotics may be administered along with obtaining a history. In the unconscious patient, the advanced cardiac life support (ACLS) protocol should be activated.

■ Foreign Body Aspiration

Foreign body aspiration "choking" is an emergency that is more common in children than in adults. When choking is suspected, the Heimlich maneuver (abdominal thrust maneuver) should be performed. This skill is taught in basic life support (BLS) and ACLS classes. It is performed by standing behind the person who is choking and wrapping his or her arms around the upper abdominal region, approximately 2 inches above the umbilicus. The fist made by one hand is grasped by the other hand tightly, and five sharp midline thrusts inward and upward are delivered (**Fig. 57.9**). For an infant, backslaps with the heel of one hand between the shoulder blades are given with the baby prone. If the object does not come out after five backslaps,

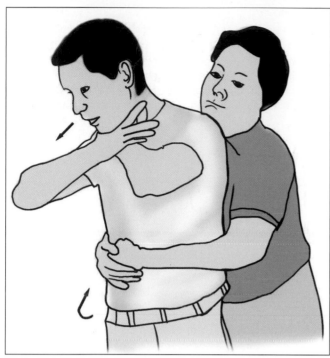

Fig. 57.9 Heimlich's maneuver.

turn the infant over onto his or her back and give five chest thrusts using two fingers. Repeat, giving five backslaps and chest thrusts until the infant can breathe, cough, or cry, or until he or she stops responding, in which case initiate BLS.

■ Fiberoptic Guided Intubation

This is usually done transnasally when orotracheal intubation is not feasible or difficult, for example, in conditions causing trismus (maxillofacial fractures and Ludwig's angina). The flexible endoscope is passed through the ETT. The endoscope is then passed through the nose up to the laryngeal inlet. The glottis is anesthetized with lidocaine, the endoscope passed into the upper trachea, and the ETT guided over the endoscope through the vocal cords and then general anesthesia is induced.

■ Cricothyroidotomy

This is a procedure that can be rapidly done in adults in an emergency situation when other more routine methods, including laryngeal masked airway and endotracheal intubation, are not effective or contraindicated. The technique is often described in three steps:

- The first step is skin incision. The cricothyroid membrane is identified using the nondominant hand, and the index finger stabilizes the larynx. Using the dominant hand, a vertical incision of approximately 4-cm incision is made over the skin overlying the cricothyroid membrane.
- The next step is to make a 5-mm horizontal incision through the cricothyroid membrane. A bougie is placed into the defect and advanced until resistance is felt.
- The last step is to then place an uncuffed ETT over the elastic bougie. A cricothyroidotomy should be converted into a tracheostomy within 24 hours.

Rigid bronchoscopy may help secure the airway in some cases. Maneuvering the rigid scope through the larynx into the trachea is relatively easier than trying to manipulate an ETT.

Points to Ponder

- Tracheostomy is a procedure by which an opening is made into the trachea for the purpose of ventilation.
- Tracheostomy can be of two types: Emergency tracheostomy and elective tracheostomy.
- The indications for tracheostomy is broadly classified into obstructive and nonobstructive conditions.
- A vertical incision is made for an emergency tracheostomy.
- The complications for tracheostomy can be immediate, early, or late complications.
- When making an incision on the trachea, avoid the cricoid cartilage and the first tracheal ring.
- Cricothyroidotomy is a surgical procedure that allows the surgeon to secure the airway faster than in a tracheostomy.

Case-Based Questions

1. **A 67-year-old man was brought to the hospital because of breathing difficulty. A quick examination revealed he had stridor, and a malignant mass was noted in the oropharynx obstructing the airway. After taking due consent for an emergency tracheostomy, the patient was immediately shifted to the operation theater.**

   a. What incision would help reach the trachea faster during tracheostomy?

   b. Where is the cut placed on the trachea?

   c. What are the immediate complications that can be encountered?

   Answers

   a. A vertical incision in the midline can be used for emergency tracheostomy as there is likely to be less bleeding.

   b. A horizontal incision is placed between the second and third rings on the trachea. The first ring is avoided.

c. The immediate complications include hemorrhage, subcutaneous emphysema, injury to the recurrently laryngeal nerve, apnea, and tracheoesophageal fistula.

2. **You are in a restaurant, and you see a customer choking on his food at a nearby table.**

   a. What step would you take to secure his airway?

   b. How would you perform a cricothyroidotomy in an emergency?

Answers

a. Heimlich's maneuver so that the foreign food particle can be expelled out.

b. A transverse incision is made just above the cricoid cartilage in the midline with a knife. Then the knife handle is rotated by 90 degrees so that there is enough airspace around the knife blade for the person to breathe.

Frequently Asked Questions

1. What are the obstructive indications for tracheostomy?

2. Enumerate the nonobstructive indications for tracheostomy.

3. Mention the late complications of tracheostomy.

4. What is cricothyroidotomy?

5. What type of tracheostomy tube is used immediately after the procedure?

6. How would you perform a Heimlich maneuver?

Endnote

Documentation of tracheostomy dates back to 3600 BC with Egyptian artifacts depicting the surgery, making it one of the oldest documented surgical procedures. However, from the 15th to the 19th century, tracheostomy was generally regarded by surgeons as dangerous.

Surgical tracheostomy along with indications, techniques, and aftercare of the tracheostomy patient was presented by Jackson in 1909. These techniques remained essentially the same for over 100 years. Tracheostomy gained even more utility during the poliomyelitis epidemic and was used in conjunction with the iron lung. Percutaneous dilatational tracheostomy was invented by Ciaglia in 1985 and now has become a common place in the ICU.

58 Foreign Bodies in the Air Passage

K.S. Gangadhara Somayaji and A. Rajeshwary

The competencies covered in this chapter are as follows:

EN2.13 Identify, resuscitate, and manage ENT emergencies in a simulated environment. (Removal of foreign bodies from the upper respiratory tract.)

EN4.49 Elicit, document, and present a correct history, demonstrate and describe the clinical features, choose the correct investigations, and describe the principles of management of foreign bodies in the air and food passages.

PE28.8 Discuss the types, clinical presentation, and management of foreign body aspiration in infants and children.

Introduction

Entry of foreign objects into the airway is a life-threatening emergency in clinical practice. It is one of the leading causes of death in the pediatric age group. The details about the foreign bodies in the nose, which is technically the beginning of the air passage, are described in another chapter (Chapter 32). This chapter deals with foreign bodies in the larynx and tracheobronchial tree. Depending on the size, the objects may get lodged at the level of the glottis or descend down into the trachea or the bronchi.

Etiology

In children, most often, the foreign object gets entry into the airway while playing or while talking or laughing with food in the mouth. In addition, lack of molar teeth, poor mastication, immature reflexes of larynx, tendency to put things in the mouth, and lack of parental supervision are contributory factors. More than half of the patients are under the age of 4 years and 70% are under the age of 8 years.

In adults, foreign body aspiration is less frequent. It is commonly seen after the sixth decade. It is often associated with:

- Alcohol ingestion.
- Traumatic intubation.
- Seizures.
- Parkinson's disease.
- Dental procedures.

It can also be due to lack of coordination between swallowing and breathing as seen in unconscious patients, hurried swallowing, paralysis of vagus and glossopharyngeal nerves, or due to a sudden tap on the back while having food.

Classification

- Nonhygroscopic foreign bodies like pins, metallic objects, glass, plastic toys (e.g., whistle), and other such materials which do not cause any local reaction.
- Hygroscopic foreign bodies like seeds of tamarind, pumpkin, watermelon, peanuts, areca nuts, and other such materials which can cause local inflammation.

Clinical Features

Children may not always give a history of keeping a foreign object in the mouth. A history of sudden onset of severe cough with choking spells and occasional gagging is typical of foreign body inhalation, until proven otherwise.

If this episode goes unnoticed, there may be a brief asymptomatic phase depending on the nature of the foreign body. Hygroscopic foreign bodies tend to be more symptomatic than nonhygroscopic objects because of local inflammation.

The symptoms and signs caused by the foreign body depend upon the nature, size, location, and time since lodgement of the foreign body in the tracheobronchial tree. A large foreign body blocking the upper airway may cause sudden death whereas a small foreign body lodged in the distal bronchial tree may cause less severe symptoms.

Laryngeal Foreign Body

A large object completely blocking the glottic chink (space between the two vocal cords) can lead to asphyxia and death before medical intervention is sought. A relatively small object remaining in the larynx can cause hoarseness of voice, croupy cough, irritation in the throat, inspiratory stridor, and blood-stained sputum.

Tracheal Foreign Body

Sharp inorganic objects can cause hemoptysis, throat pain, cough, and expiratory stridor. A hygroscopic object can typically cause "tracheal thud" or "audible slap" due to the movement of the foreign object within the lumen of the trachea in addition to the other symptoms.

Bronchial Foreign Body

The angle made by the main bronchus with the trachea is similar on the right side and left side, until the age of 15 years, resulting in equal incidence of foreign body in either bronchus. However, after the age of 15 years, most of the foreign bodies tend to enter the right bronchus which becomes wider and more in line with the trachea. The presentation can be in any of the ways as shown in **Fig. 58.1**.

Check-Valve Obstruction

Partial obstruction to the bronchus produces check valve type of obstruction allowing only entry of air leading to features of obstructive emphysema. The trachea and cardiac shadow get shifted to the opposite side and the dome of the diaphragm will be depressed.

Stop-Valve Obstruction

Total obstruction to the air entry and exit will cause atelectasis or collapse of that lobe of the lung. This stop-valve effect may occur when a large foreign body causes total occlusion from the time of inhalation, or it may progress from a check-valve type of obstruction after the foreign body swells up. The clinical picture is of collapse and consolidation of the affected bronchopulmonary segment.

Ball-Valve Obstruction

This is associated with organic foreign bodies such as peas and beans, or rounded, smooth, metallic bodies such as pellets. The foreign body is dislodged by the passage of air during expiration but re-impacts during inspiration. This type of obstruction causes an early atelectasis. X-ray picture will be similar to the one seen with stop-valve obstruction

wherein the mediastinal shift will be toward the affected side and the dome of the diaphragm gets elevated.

By-Pass Valve Obstruction

This is associated with partial obstruction of the lumen in both phases of respiration leading to reduced distal ventilation. X-ray shows diminished aeration on the involved side without any marked mediastinal shift.

Small foreign bodies can occasionally move from one segment to another segment of the bronchus or to the trachea, if not swollen by the inflammatory reaction, causing frequent changes in symptoms and signs.

Infections caused by the local inflammatory reaction can lead to features of laryngitis, tracheobronchitis, pneumonitis, bronchiectasis, or abscess. Rupture of an emphysematous bullae can result in spontaneous pneumothorax.

Pearls

- Foreign bodies impact at the level of the vocal cords or subglottis produces a biphasic stridor, where the sound is heard during both inspiration and expiration, when the airway is blocked.
- Inspiratory stridor suggests obstruction above the vocal cords and expiratory stridor indicates obstruction in the lower trachea.

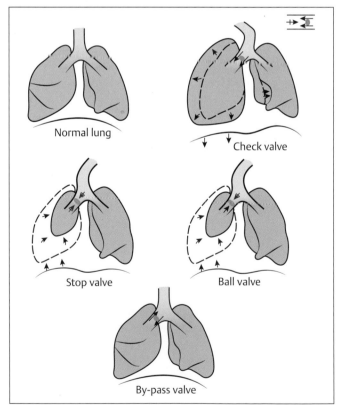

Fig. 58.1 Lung manifestation of bronchial foreign bodies.

Diagnosis

A detailed history and physical examination of the chest are very important.

Sudden cough with choking, wheezing, and reduced air entry into the lung on auscultation should raise the suspicion of a foreign body inhalation. Patients with features of recurrent chest infection not responding to antibiotics also need to be investigated. Radiological investigations are key for diagnosis as they may help in localizing the foreign body and in assessment of any secondary changes:

- X-ray of neck in posteroanterior (PA) and lateral views in the extended position will pick up radio-opaque foreign bodies in the larynx and trachea. Soft tissue views can sometimes help to detect radiolucent objects as well.
- Plain X-ray chest in PA and lateral views will show the radio-opaque foreign body, lobar or segmental atelectasis, or hyperinflation of a lobe, segment, or entire lung. Mediastinal or tracheal shift to opposite side or same side may be seen in hyperinflation (**Figs. 58.2, 58.3, and 58.4**).
- Videofluoroscopy or X-rays taken during inspiration and expiration are helpful in getting a clearer picture. Fluoroscopy is performed to study moving structures of the body. In the case of foreign bodies, lung movements can be studied to see the effect of impact of the foreign body.

- Occasionally, X-rays can be normal if it is taken very early in case of radiolucent object inhalation. High-resolution computed tomography (HRCT) of the chest may be helpful in such cases for the diagnosis.
- Magnetic resonance imaging with T1-weighted images may be useful for the definitive diagnosis and location of peanut fragments in the lower airway, as it appears as a high-intensity signal surrounded by low-intensity lung tissue.
- Flexible laryngoscopy and bronchoscopy can be used for both diagnostic and therapeutic purposes.

Treatment

Removal of the foreign body at the earliest is the treatment of choice. A common cause of death after foreign body inhalation is hypoxia. Hence, adequate pre-oxygenation, quick and smooth induction of anesthesia, laryngoscopy/bronchoscopy, and foreign body removal will save the life of the patient. Instruments appropriate for the age group should be kept ready.

■ Laryngeal Foreign Bodies

A large foreign body above the level of vocal cords may completely occlude the airway, asphyxiating the patient. Establishing breathing becomes the top priority in such cases.

Heimlich's Maneuver

Standing behind the patient, arms of the doctor should be placed around the upper abdomen and five abdominal thrusts are to be given with a fist thrust upwards and backwards below the xiphisternum, in the epigastrium area. The residual air in the lungs is compressed and expels the dislodged foreign body thereby opening up the airway.

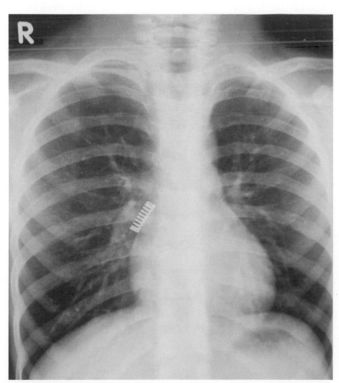

Fig. 58.2 Chest X-ray in posteroanterior (PA) view showing a spring in the right bronchus.

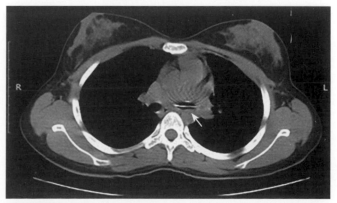

Fig. 58.3 Computed tomography (CT) scan of the chest with foreign body in the left bronchus.

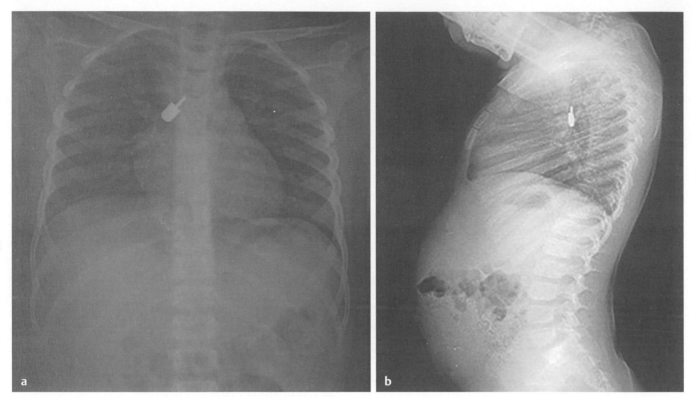

Fig. 58.4 **(a)** Chest X-ray in posteroanterior (PA) view showing a radio-opaque foreign body lying obliquely. **(b)** X-ray in lateral view confirms the location in the airway.

One should be careful while doing this maneuver in partial obstruction of the airway as it may turn into a complete obstruction (**Fig. 58.5**).

Cricothyrotomy or emergency tracheostomy may be needed if Heimlich's maneuver fails (**Fig. 58.6**).

Once the airway is established, the foreign body can be removed by direct laryngoscopy. Impacted foreign bodies may need an open approach through laryngofissure during which the thyroid cartilage is split in the midline to reach the inner larynx.

■ Tracheal and Bronchial Foreign Bodies

Rigid bronchoscopy under general anesthesia is the standard procedure for foreign body removal.

Bronchoscopy might have to be performed as an emergency procedure when there is an airway obstruction or if the object is an organic foreign body. Conventionally, rigid bronchoscopy is performed with a Hopkins telescope (using optical forceps under good illumination and a camera with monitor) for retrieval of the foreign body (**Fig. 58.7**). Some cases may need C-arm fluoroscopy, snares, and basket or a Fogarty's balloon catheter. Retrograde bronchoscopy through the tracheostomy may be done for some tracheal foreign bodies. Thoracotomy and bronchotomy

may be needed for foreign bodies reaching the periphery. Lobectomy or pneumonectomy may be needed in cases of old foreign bodies. For more details on bronchoscopy, see Chapter 62.

Flexible bronchoscopes are now being used with very good results and this has been found to be more useful in removing the peripheral or distal foreign bodies especially if aided by cinefluoroscopy. Fiberoptic bronchoscopy may be easier and safer in adults. Video imaging can provide a clear and magnified view and reduces the risk of residual foreign bodies, and the need for repeat bronchoscopy.

Complications

Anesthesia-related complications are common as both the surgeon and the anesthetist have to work on the airway. However, recent ventilating bronchoscopes and advances in anesthesia techniques allow both the ventilation and the procedure to be carried out simultaneously.

Laryngeal edema, pneumothorax, and cardiac arrests can occur following the procedure. Sharp objects can cause local injury and bleeding. Long-standing foreign bodies cause local granuloma, postoperative pneumonitis, bronchiectasis, and abscess requiring long-term chest care.

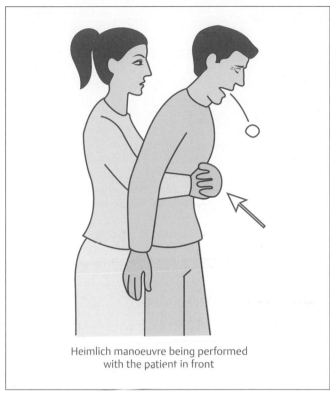

Heimlich manoeuvre being performed
with the patient in front

Fig. 58.5 Position for Heimlich's maneuver.

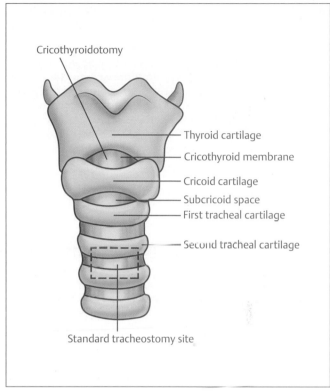

Cricothyroidotomy

Thyroid cartilage
Cricothyroid membrane
Cricoid cartilage
Subcricoid space
First tracheal cartilage
Second tracheal cartilage

Standard tracheostomy site

Fig. 58.6 Comparison of sites for cricothyrotomy and tracheostomy.

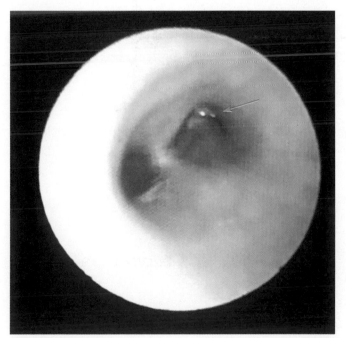

Fig. 58.7 Foreign body with secretions in the right main bronchus.

Points to Ponder

- Foreign bodies in the airway must be ruled out in a child with recurrent respiratory infections not responding to medical treatment.
- History of sudden cough and choking while playing or having food should raise the suspicion of foreign body aspiration.
- Foreign body can enter into any bronchus in children. However, entry into right bronchus is more common in older age groups.
- Heimlich's maneuver should not be attempted in partially obstructed airway.
- Diagnostic bronchoscopy is mandatory on the slightest suspicion of foreign body in the airway.
- Earliest removal of the foreign body with rigid bronchoscope and appropriate instruments is the treatment of choice.

Case-Based Questions

1. **A 5-year-old boy was brought to the emergency department at 10 pm following a choking episode that lasted a few minutes. It was unwitnessed but was heard by his mother who was in the next room. Clinically, the child was looking healthy without any distress but the mother is giving a history that the child makes a whistling sound when he breathes in deeply. Oxygen saturations are 99% on room air and he is speaking normally.**

   a. What could be the diagnosis?

   b. What is the immediate investigation required?

   c. What is the treatment?

   Answers

   a. The child could have a foreign body in the trachea or the bronchus.

   b. X-ray of neck with chest in posteroanterior (PA) and lateral views need to be taken immediately.

   c. (i) If X-ray of chest appears normal, it still doesn't rule out a foreign body. The child needs to be admitted and examined carefully for any chest signs. If everything is normal, the child needs to be observed and started on medical treatment including antibiotics if there is evidence of lung infection. Further treatment is based on the clinical progress.

   (ii) If X-ray shows a foreign body, urgent removal under general anesthesia using rigid bronchoscope is the treatment of choice.

2. **A 35-year-old man was shifted to the operation theater struggling to breathe due to a large bolus of meat impacted in the larynx. There was inspiratory stridor. Laryngeal mask was ineffective, and intubation was ruled out. What is the quickest way to secure the airway?**

   Answer

   The fastest way to secure the airway is to perform a cricothyrotomy or cricothyroidotomy. In this procedure, a quick stab incision is made vertically in the midline over the cricothyroid membrane after palpating and confirming the position of the cricoid cartilage below and the thyroid cartilage above. There are no major blood vessels or nerves in the midline. In children below 12 years, a needle cricothyrotomy is carried out because their cricothyroid membrane is smaller and funnel shaped.

Frequently Asked Questions

1. Which is the commonest site for lodgement of foreign bodies in the lower respiratory tract?

2. What is the nature of the stridor when the glottic chink is obstructed by a foreign body?

3. What is the commonest mode of presentation of a foreign body aspiration in children?

4. How do you perform a Heimlich's maneuver?

5. How do you perform a cricothyrotomy?

Endnote | *Gustav Killian was the first person to remove a foreign body from the lower airways. He removed an aspirated pork bone from the bronchus of a farmer aged 63 years, under local anesthesia (cocaine), using an esophagoscope in 1897.*

59 Direct Laryngoscopy

Krishna Koirala

The competency covered in this chapter is as follows:

EN3.3 Observe and describe the indications for and steps involved in the performance of rigid/flexible laryngoscopy.

Introduction

Direct laryngoscopy is a procedure carried out to visualize the larynx. It can be carried out under general or local anesthesia, but commonly it is done under general anesthesia. Depending on the type of procedure being done, there are various types of rigid laryngoscopes available. Indications for laryngoscopy are listed in **Table 59.1**.

Types of Direct Laryngoscopes

- The Macintosh laryngoscope is mainly used for intubation. It can also be used for introduction of a rigid bronchoscope.
- The Jackson direct laryngoscope (**Fig. 59.1**) is useful for visualizing the laryngeal inlet, supraglottis and glottis, as well as the hypopharynx.
- The anterior commissure laryngoscope is useful in examining the ventricles, anterior commissure, and subglottic region.
- The Kleinsasser laryngoscope is commonly used in microlaryngeal procedures.
- The distending laryngoscope is useful for procedures of the base of the tongue and supraglottis such as biopsies and resection of lesions and tumors.

Position

The patient is positioned supine with flexion of the neck on the chest and extension of the head. This position is referred to as the Boyce position or sniffing position or "barking dog" position (**Fig. 59.2**). In this position, the neck is flexed onto the neck and the head is extended. To obtain this position, the patient is placed supine on the table with a pillow under the head. The head has to be raised by around 7 cm.

Contraindications

- Advanced supraglottic and glottic lesions with respiratory obstruction (tracheostomy is required first to provide airway).
- Blunt trauma to larynx (laryngeal fracture or disruption of the laryngotracheal junction).
- Grade II or III trismus leading to inadequate mouth opening.
- Severe edema and swelling of the larynx (infections/burns/anaphylaxis).
- Diseases or injuries of cervical spine (leading to limited neck extension).

Difficult laryngoscopy is found in the following conditions:
- Micrognathia.

Table 59.1 Indications for direct laryngoscopy

Diagnostic	Therapeutic
Biopsy of lesions including suspected malignancy in the larynx and pyriform fossa	Foreign body removal from the larynx and pyriform fossa
Examination of hidden areas: anterior commissure, laryngeal ventricle, subglottis, infrahyoid epiglottis, and pyriform fossa apex	Excision biopsy of benign or localized malignant laryngeal lesions
Unsuccessful indirect laryngoscopy	Dilatation of laryngeal strictures
Evaluation of hoarseness and dysphagia	

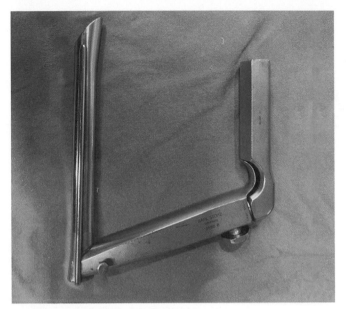

Fig. 59.1 Direct laryngoscope.

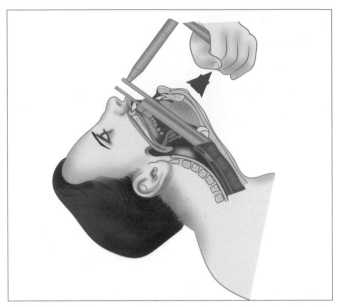

Fig. 59.2 The Boyce position helps allow for clear visualization of the larynx.

- Macroglossia.
- Short, fat neck.
- Higher Mallampati grades.

Pearl

There are some predictors for airway obstruction during the time of intubation for anesthesia. One such airway assessment is known as the Mallampati classification, which assesses the oropharyngeal airway in relation to the tongue.

The patient is seated with the head straight, mouth open, and tongue sticking out.

- Class 1: Soft palate, anterior pillars, and uvula are seen through the oral cavity.
- Class 2: Soft palate and part of the uvula are visible.
- Class 3: Soft palate and only the base of the uvula are visible.
- Class 4: Only the hard palate is visible, not the soft palate.

Anesthesia

General anesthesia with endotracheal intubation is commonly used. Occasionally, general anesthesia is given through a tracheostomy tube in a prior tracheostomized patient. The procedure can be performed under intravenous anesthesia (propofol), if a short-term diagnostic procedure is planned. Direct laryngoscopy can also be done under local anesthesia by laryngeal nerve blocks.

Steps of the Procedure

- Protection of the upper dentition is done by placing a gauze piece or tooth guard over them.
- Lubrication of the laryngoscope with lignocaine jelly is done.
- The laryngoscope is held in the left hand. The right hand is used to stabilize the laryngoscope, retract the lips, guide the laryngoscope, and handle suction and instruments.
- The laryngoscope is then inserted through the right side of the mouth and then guided to the center. The soft palate and uvula are visualized, and the scope is lifted anteriorly toward the base of the tongue.
- The scope is then guided between the epiglottis and the endotracheal tube, lifting the epiglottis anteriorly, to see the interior of the larynx.
- After withdrawing the scope to the level of the aryepiglottic fold, it is guided into the ipsilateral pyriform fossa. From here, it is guided to the postcricoid region and then the other pyriform fossa.
- The following structures are examined in this order:
  - Posterior third of the tongue (tongue base).
  - Vallecula.
  - Epiglottis (tip, lingual, and laryngeal surfaces).
  - Aryepiglottic folds.
  - Arytenoids.
  - False cords.
  - Anterior commissure and posterior commissure.
  - Ventricles.
  - Right and left vocal cords and subglottis.
  - Postcriciod region and pyriform sinuses.

Vocal cord mobility is best visualized during flexible laryngoscopy, but during direct laryngoscopy, it can be observed during extubation.

A microscope with lens of 40-cm (400f) focal length along with Kleinsasser's suspension laryngoscope unit can be used for microlaryngoscopy for better precision, which is dealt with in Chapter 61.

Complications

- *Traumatic*:
  - Injury to the lips, tongue, teeth, pharynx, and larynx.
  - Laryngeal edema and injury to the vocal cords.
  - Dislocation of the cricoarytenoid joint.
  - Sore throat (temporary and usually resolves by 48 hours).
- *Nontraumatic*:
  - Aspiration of blood, bronchospasm, laryngospasm, arrhythmias, and myocardial ischemia or infarction.

The most common complication of this procedure is a sore throat after intubation for anesthesia and it occurs roughly in one-third of patients. This is mild and usually subsides within 48 hours.

Points to Ponder

- Direct laryngoscopy allows visualization of the larynx.
- It is performed during intubation in general anesthesia, for surgical procedures in the larynx and hypopharynx and for resuscitation.
- The Boyce position involves flexion of the neck at the chest and extension of the head.
- Direct laryngoscopy can be performed for diagnostic as well as therapeutic indications.

Case-Based Question

1. **A 65-year-old male patient was seen in the casualty with history of foreign body ingestion. He was found to be an obese, diabetic patient with a short neck. A plain x-ray of the neck revealed a radio-opaque foreign body lodged at the C4 vertebral level, just behind the arytenoids. Further enquiry into the history revealed a possible chicken bone ingestion.**

   a. What is the next step in the management of this patient?

   b. What are the difficulties you will encounter?

   c. What complications can occur?

   Answers

   a. From the history and the x-ray, it is evident that the patient has a chicken bone lodged in the hypopharynx.

   After relevant investigations to see his fitness for the procedure, he will have to undergo direct laryngoscopy to have the foreign body removed under general anesthesia.

   b. It is mentioned that he is an obese patient with a short neck. This has to be taken into account during intubation of the patient for anesthesia as well as for direct laryngoscopy. The short, fat neck will make visualization of the larynx difficult. The Boyce position will help. The patient is kept supine. There should be no sandbag under the shoulder. The head should be elevated with a pillow by 7 cm so that the position is one of extension flexion.

   c. Complications that can occur during the procedure include injury to the tongue, teeth, and lips, and bleeding due to mucosal injury. If the blood sugar is uncontrolled, infections like retropharyngeal abscess can develop.

Frequently Asked Questions

1. What are the indications for direct laryngoscopy?
2. What are the instruments used and how would you perform this procedure?
3. What are the differences between direct and indirect laryngoscopy?
4. What are the complications of this procedure?
5. Describe the Boyce position.

Endnote

Historians generally give credit to Manuel Garcia for having developed the technique to see the vocal cords for the first time in 1854. He is credited with having invented the first laryngoscope. But the first device invented to look into the interior of the human body was by Philipp Bozzini of Germany in 1806. He called his device a "light conductor." It was a tube with angled mirrors that could be inserted into the human body and the source of light was a candle. It was initially used for examining the larynx, but later had applications in gynecology and urology.

60 Hypopharyngoscopy

Inku Shrestha Basnet

The competencies covered in this chapter are as follows:

EN2.10 Identify and describe the use of common instruments used in ear, nose, and throat (ENT) surgery.

EN3.4 Observe and describe the indications for and steps involved in the removal of foreign bodies in ENT.

EN3.6 Observe and describe the indications for and steps involved in the skills of emergency procedures in ENT.

Introduction

The hypopharynx is the gateway into the esophagus. Disorders of the hypopharynx, otherwise known as laryngopharynx, can present as a clinical challenge due to their location. It is the lower portion of the pharynx, a continuation of the oropharynx with the larynx adjacent to it, and merges with the esophagus inferiorly. It forms a part of the upper aerodigestive tract.

The three clinical subdivisions of hypopharynx (**Fig. 60.1**) are the following:
- Pyriform sinus (synonym: Smuggler's fossa).
- Postcricoid region.
- Posterior pharyngeal wall.

A hypopharyngoscope or an esophageal speculum is used to inspect these regions or subsites individually in a more meticulous manner. These scopes are of various lengths and come in different models depending on the manufacturer (**Figs. 60.2** and **60.3**).

Indications

■ Diagnostic

- Examination of the subsites of the hypopharynx in the following situations:
  - Symptoms of persistent feeling of stickiness in throat and pricking sensation on swallowing.

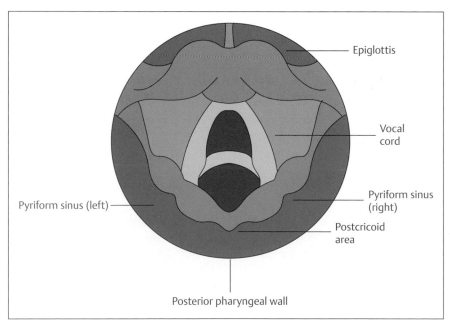

Fig. 60.1 Diagram showing the three subdivisions of the hypopharynx.

Epiglottis

Vocal cord

Pyriform sinus (right)

Postcricoid area

Pyriform sinus (left)

Posterior pharyngeal wall

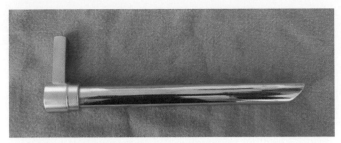

Fig. 60.2 Short rigid hypopharyngoscope.

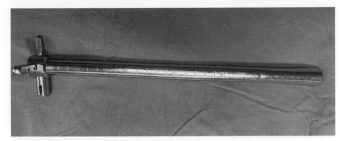

Fig. 60.3 Long rigid hypopharyngoscope with external markings.

- Referred pain to the ear (in view of suspected malignancy).
- Pain on swallowing (odynophagia) and difficulty in swallowing (dysphagia).
- Pooling of saliva in the pyriform sinus on indirect laryngoscopy.
- For biopsy of lesions: benign (e.g., papilloma, hemangioma, adenoma, lipoma, fibroma, and leiomyoma) and malignant.
- For accurate assessment of the extent of growth.
- As a part of panendoscopy (triple endoscopy) to find out the primary site in cervical carcinoma with unknown primary (metastasis with unknown origin).
- To find out any synchronous primary (malignancy) at other sites.
- To find the third or fourth branchial cleft sinus internal opening.
- To detect the diverticula: An upper endoscopy can detect it if the opening is big enough; however, endoscopy in such patients can be risky.
- Check endoscopy for patients with Plummer–Vinson syndrome (to rule out postcricoid malignancy) and post-treatment of hypopharyngeal malignancy (to assess for residual/recurrent disease).

■ Therapeutic

- Removal of ingested foreign bodies.
- Excision biopsy of benign tumors or localized malignant lesions.
- Excision of cystic lesions like ductal cysts.
- Cricopharyngeal myotomy for cricopharyngeal spasm and for diverticulum.
- Cauterization of the fistulous tract.

Contraindications

- Injuries or diseases of the cervical spine.
- Grade 2 or 3 trismus.
- Receding mandible.
- Aneurysm of the aorta.
- Heart, liver, or kidney diseases.

- Hemodynamic instability.
- Coagulopathy.
- Unable to give consent.

Preoperative Management

- A detailed history, including past and current comorbidities, procedures, and medication history.
- Examination with emphasis on the oral cavity, pharynx, and neck. The status of the dentition should be documented. Dentures and glasses should be removed prior to the procedure.
- The patient should be nil per os (NPO) for 6 hours prior to the procedure.
- Prior radiological assessment: Barium swallow, contrast-enhanced computed tomography (CT) scan, magnetic resonance imaging (MRI), etc.

Types of Hypopharyngoscope

■ Rigid Hypopharyngoscope

Hypopharyngoscopy is done preferably under general anesthesia with an endotracheal tube, and with muscle relaxation (**Figs. 60.2** and **60.3**). Under general anesthesia, negotiating the rigid scope is easier and visualization is better with better comfort to the patient. The Weerda's distending laryngoscope can be used for removal of lesions or tumors as it allows for better visualization and more space for instrumentation including lasers.

Advantages

- It allows better visualization of the hypopharynx.
- It is easier access to foreign bodies compared to the flexible endoscope.
- It also allows use of laser for surgery in the subsites.

Disadvantages

- A rigid hypopharyngoscopy is more traumatic.
- General anesthesia is often required.

Position and Anesthesia

The patient is positioned supine on the operation table with the pillow under the head. The surgeon sits on the head end of the table. The head is raised 10 to 15 cm with the pillow under the occiput or by raising the head flap of the operating table with flexion of the neck on the chest and extension of the head at the atlantooccipital joint (posterior sword swallowing position or barking dog position). The upper teeth and lips are protected with a tooth or gum guard and by lubricating the tube, respectively.

Instruments Required

- A rigid hypopharyngoscope (length varies from 22 to 24 cm).
- Suction cannulas of different sizes and adequate length with the suction device.
- Light cable attached to the light source (**Fig. 60.4**).
- Biopsy forceps.
- Grasping forceps.
- Other instruments like laser depend on the procedure being done.

Procedure

The surgeon holds the rigid hypopharyngoscope with the right hand. The forefinger of the left hand is placed on the palate and palatal surface of the incisor tooth, whereas the lower lip is retracted using the third finger. The left hand stabilizes the mandible of the patient and protects the lips and teeth. The hypopharyngoscope is inserted to visualize the soft palate and the uvula. It is then lowered so that it rests on the thumb of the left hand, thus protecting the upper dentition. This thumb is used to advance the scope anteriorly to the base of the tongue and is also used as the fulcrum. The scope is now placed on the left side of the oropharynx. The surgeon can visualize the uvula and then the epiglottis, which is pushed with the beak of the scope. The aim of the observation via the lumen is to maintain the center of the lumen though which it is intended to visualize or pass the scope further. The scope is advanced into the hypopharynx, where it is possible to visualize the right aryepiglottic fold and then the right pyriform sinus. The scope is advanced further to visualize the walls of the right pyriform sinus and the apex of the sinus. Then it is swept into the midline to visualize the posterior pharyngeal wall and the left pyriform sinus with its apex.

The scope is again brought to midline and slightly advanced, so it comes to lie behind the posterior lamina of the cricoid. The surgeon then starts to visualize the posterior pharyngeal wall, the pyriform fossae (right side and left side, in turn), apex of the pyriform fossae, and the postcricoid region. Care should be taken to assess not only the mucosal integrity of the lumen and subsites of the hypopharynx but also for any indenting mass lesion. Examination should be continued during the removal of the endoscope. Particular attention should be given at the apex of the pyriform sinus, the postcricoid region, and the cricopharyngeal inlet, which is the lowermost point of visualization (**Fig. 60.5**).

If suspicion arises, esophagoscopy, laryngoscopy, and bronchoscopy should also be combined with this procedure.

■ Flexible Fiberoptic Hypopharyngoscope

It can be done under local or topical anesthesia using throat spray, with or without sedation. It can also be done by general anesthesia.

Advantages

- It is an outpatient procedure. General anesthesia is usually not required.
- There is less morbidity, and it is safer and less traumatic.
- It can be done in cases of trismus or cervical spine disorders.

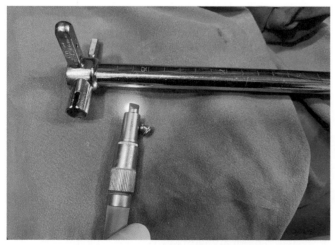

Fig. 60.4   Rigid hypopharyngoscope with light source.

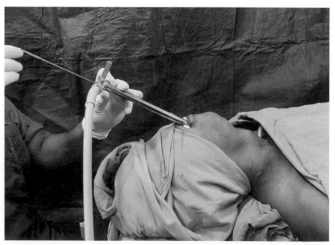

Fig. 60.5   Hypopharyngoscopy in progress.

- It has good illumination and magnification.
- It provides accurate diagnosis of mucosal diseases.

Disadvantages

- It has a narrow channel, which limits the size of instruments and removal of certain foreign bodies.
- Removal of foreign bodies is difficult.
- A detailed examination is difficult, especially of the postcricoid region.

Position: The left lateral decubitus position or supine with neck extension.

Oxygen saturation, pulse, and blood pressure should be monitored throughout the procedure.

The most common position for the examination is the left lateral decubitus position, with the neck flexed. Under general anesthesia, the patient can be supine and intubation aided by the anesthetist providing a chin lift. A dental guard is used to protect the endoscope, which is passed under direct vision over the tongue to the back of the oropharynx where the epiglottis and larynx are visualized. Slight neck flexion and an instruction to swallow, while maintaining the endoscope in the midline, will allow the endoscope to visualize the pyriform fossa, posterior pharyngeal wall, and the postcricoid region. The cricopharyngeal sphincter and upper cervical esophagus can also be visualized, if needed. Gentle pressure should be used and particular care taken in elderly patients with anterior cervical osteophytes or symptoms suspicious of a pharyngeal pouch. The endoscope is advanced under direct vision with gentle air insufflations to provide an optimal view.

The following structures are examined in order:

- The soft palate and the uvula.
- The base of the tongue.
- The epiglottis (tip and lingual surface).
- The right pyriform fossa (with its boundaries and apex).
- The posterior pharyngeal wall.
- The left pyriform fossa (with its boundaries and apex).
- The postcricoid region.
- The cricopharyngeal sphincter.

Complications of Rigid Hypopharyngoscopy

- *Traumatic*:
  - Injury to the lips, teeth, gums, uvula, soft palate, and arytenoids.
  - Mucosal tear with bleeding.
  - Hypopharyngeal perforation.
  - Surgical emphysema.
- *Nontraumatic*:
  - Aspiration.
  - Airway obstruction.
  - Hypoventilation.
  - Infection and retropharyngeal abscess.
  - Cardiopulmonary complications.
  - Adverse reactions to medications.

Points to Ponder

- Hypopharyngoscopy helps in visualizing the various subsites of the hypopharynx for diagnostic and therapeutic purposes.
- The rigid endoscope is better for visualizing the postcricoid region.
- Hypopharyngeal cancers tend to present late and thus have a less favorable prognosis than laryngeal cancers.
- Panendoscopy, a combination of direct laryngoscopy, hypopharyngoscopy, esophagoscopy, and bronchoscopy, along with nasal endoscopy, is performed in cases of metastasis of unknown origin (MUO). It can also be done to rule out a synchronous malignancy.

Case-Based Questions

1. **A 3-year-old boy presented with a 2-day history of inability to take food orally. There was drooling of saliva. The child was afebrile. There was no history of a witnessed foreign body. There was no history of breathing difficulty.**

   a. What investigation would be required if a foreign body in the upper digestive tract is suspected?

   b. What is the method of removing a foreign body in the postcricoid region or cervical esophagus?

   c. Which foreign bodies would require urgent removal?

   Answers

   a. AP and lateral neck X-ray to localize the foreign body, that is, the level, and also the site, that is, the airway or digestive tract. In children, X-rays of the neck, chest, and abdomen are taken to localize the foreign body, to look for multiple foreign bodies, and to see if the foreign body has gone down the digestive tract.

   b. Hypopharyngoscopy and foreign body removal with forceps. Check scopy should be done following removal to assess for a remnant or second foreign body and to look for any mucosal injuries caused by the foreign body or the procedure.

   c. Button batteries can cause a severe local reaction with mucosal loss and can lead to mortality. Sharp foreign bodies can penetrate the mucosa and cause a perforation and migrate extraluminally.

2. **A 57-year-old man, a chronic smoker, presented with a 5-month history of dysphagia, which had progressed**

to absolute dysphagia since the past 1 week. Indirect laryngoscopy showed an ulceroproliferative growth involving the lateral wall of the right pyriform fossa.

a. What is the urgent blood investigation that needs to be done?
b. What radiological investigations can be done?
c. How would you confirm the diagnosis?

Answers

a. Serum electrolytes as there may be an electrolyte imbalance, which will require correction with intravenous fluids.
b. Since the patient cannot swallow, the patient may aspirate if a barium swallow is attempted. A contrast-enhanced CT scan or MRI of the neck is done to assess the primary site.
c. Hypopharyngoscopy and biopsy for histopathological examination will help confirm the diagnosis.

Frequently Asked Questions

1. What are the indications for hypopharyngoscopy?
2. What are the different areas visualized during hypopharyngoscopy?
3. What are the instruments used?
4. What is the position of the patient during the procedure?
5. What are the complications of the procedure?
6. What are the contraindications?

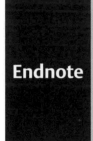

Endnote

The word "endoscopy" comes from the Greek words "endo," meaning "within," and "skopein," meaning "to view." Historically, the first attempts to view the body orifices were made by the Egyptians and Romans when metallic tubes were devised for viewing the vagina and the anus. However, due to poor lighting, they fell into disrepute. During the 1800s, several attempts were made to overcome the illumination inside the tubes, including the use of burning magnesium and platinum wires. This produces good light but also resulted in heat and smoke. It was left to Chevalier Jackson to finally solve the problem with the use of a rigid esophagoscope with a light bulb at the end of the scope in 1890. The power for the bulb came through leads from a battery box. He then went on to devise laryngoscopes and bronchoscopes in spite of struggling with tuberculosis. He is considered the father of scopies.

61 Microlaryngoscopy

Krishna Koirala

> **The competencies covered in this chapter are as follows:**
>
> EN3.5 Observe and describe the indications for and steps involved in the surgical procedures in ear, nose, and throat.
>
> EN4.42 Elicit document and present a correct history; demonstrate and describe the clinical features; choose the correct investigations; and describe the principles of management of hoarseness of voice.

Introduction

The development of new laryngoscopes and application of video endoscopes have provided ear, nose, and throat (ENT) surgeons with a magnified view of the larynx during surgery while minimizing the difficulties caused by conventional techniques. Microlaryngeal surgery (MLS) deals with minimum excision of pathological tissue with maximum conservation of normal tissue, in particular the epithelium of the vocal folds and the lamina propria.

Indications

- Precise staging and anatomic localization of laryngeal malignancy.
- Endoscopic resection of localized laryngeal malignancy.
- Excision of vocal nodules, polyps, cysts, Reinke's edema, and granulomas of the larynx.
- To evaluate dysphonia of unclear etiology.
- For precise resection of recurrent respiratory papillomatosis.
- Management of web and stenosis of the glottic and subglottic region.
- Biopsy from laryngeal lesions.

Contraindications

- Unstable cervical spine.
- Coagulopathy may lead to hemorrhage (stop all antiplatelet and anticoagulation therapies 5–7 days before surgery).
- Conditions leading to difficulty in visualizing the larynx include short fat neck, micrognathia, macroglossia, trismus, and an anteriorly placed larynx.

> **Pearl**
>
> Microlaryngoscopy gives a magnified view of the larynx in comparison to direct laryngoscopy. The illumination is better, and since the scope is suspended, both hands are free. These features make the procedure more precise.

Preoperative Preparation

- Flexible nasopharyngoscopic evaluation of the larynx.
- Consent for surgery.

Instrumentation and Equipment

- Direct laryngoscope with chest piece.
- Operating microscope plus camera unit.

Preparation during Surgery

Position the patient in the reverse Trendelenburg position.

The head of the patient is placed at the end of the bed with head extension and the neck is slightly flexed ("sniffing" position). In some cases, a sandbag is placed below the shoulder blades for extension.

Types of Laryngoscopes

- The Jackson laryngoscope is commonly used in the past.
- The Hollinger anterior commissure laryngoscope is useful when exposure is impossible with other laryngoscopes.

- The Dedo laryngoscope.
- The Lindholm and Weerda laryngoscope is good for supraglottic surgery (expands both proximally and distally to provide excellent exposure of the supraglottic larynx).

The Dedo laryngoscope is the workhorse during MLS and provides adequate exposure of the glottis in most patients.

Anesthesia Considerations

- General anesthesia with endotracheal intubation with a small endotracheal tube (microlaryngeal tube).
- Glycopyrrolate: The drying effect improves exposure (avoided in patients with xerostomia, cardiac disease, glaucoma, or prostatic hyperplasia).

Steps

- The introduction of the scope into the larynx is the same as for direct laryngoscopy.
- The laryngoscope is suspended. This allows both hands to be free for the procedure (**Fig. 61.1**).

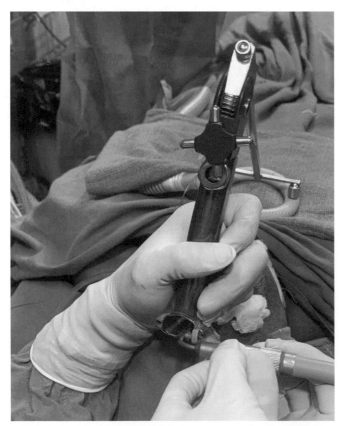

Fig. 61.1 Laryngoscope with light source and a chest piece in place. Sometimes rods are used to suspend the laryngoscope without compression of the chest.

- The operating microscope (400-mm focal length lens) is used to focus on the lesion in the larynx (**Fig. 61.2a, b**).
- Once the lesion is visualized (**Fig. 61.3**), instruments are introduced under direct vision for excision of the lesion (**Fig. 61.4**).

Postoperative Care

- Humidification (bedside humidifier).
- Adequate hydration (drink noncaffeinated fluids).
- Voice rest:
  - Absolute voice rest for 48 hours.
  - Arm's length rule (do not speak to anyone farther away than an arm's length).
  - Ensure voice conservation for 2 weeks postoperatively (a voice professional may require a longer period of voice rest).
- Follow-up:
  - Reevaluate 2 weeks postoperatively.
  - Video endoscopy with speech pathology assessment at 6 weeks postoperatively.

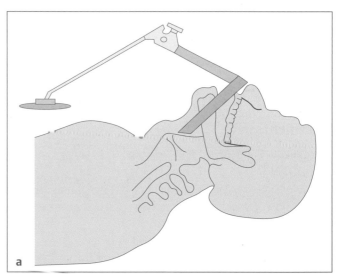

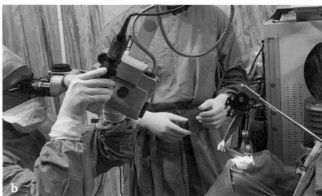

Fig. 61.2 (a) Diagram showing position of laryngoscope with chest piece. (b) Patient positioned with a laryngoscope and a microscope in place for the procedure.

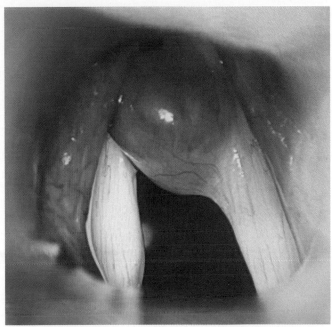

Fig. 61.3 A vocal cord lesion magnified through the microscope.

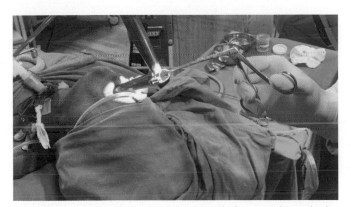

Fig. 61.4 A procedure in progress with forceps through the laryngoscope.

Complications

MLS is a relatively safe procedure. But as with all surgical procedures there are complications that have to be explained to the patient before the procedure. These include the following:

- Injury to the tongue, lips, or teeth due to the laryngoscope.
- Bleeding from the larynx during and after the procedure.
- Hypoglossal nerve injury due to pressure from the laryngoscope.
- Breathing difficulty and possibly stridor postoperatively due to trauma and edema.
- Synechia formation between the vocal cords or glottic web.

Differences between Microlaryngoscopy and Direct Laryngoscopy

The differences between microlaryngoscopy and direct laryngoscopy are presented in **Table 61.1**.

> **Points to Ponder**
>
> - MLS is the procedure whereby the larynx is visualized and magnified with a microscope.
> - Since the laryngoscope is fixed onto the chest of the patient or suspended over the chest, both hands are free for surgical manipulation.
> - It allows for binocular vision.
> - Lasers can be used for surgical resection.
> - Recording is possible for documentation

Table 61.1 Differences between microlaryngoscopy and direct laryngoscopy

Microlaryngoscopy	Direct laryngoscopy
Binocular vision	Monocular vision
Better illumination	Less illumination
Magnification	No magnification
Better precision	Less precision
Both hands are free	One hand holds the scope
Video attachment possible	Video attachment not possible
Can be combined with laser	Cannot be combined

Case-Based Question

1. **A 65-year-old man presented with a 3-month history of voice change. Rigid telescopy of the larynx in the outpatient clinic showed a suspicious irregular mass over the right vocal cord.**

   a. What investigation would you like to proceed with?

   b. What complications can arise from the procedure?

Answers

a. When there is a lesion on the vocal cord, the ideal procedure is MLS. This would allow the extent of the lesion to be assessed and a biopsy to be taken.

b. MLS is an extremely safe surgery. But complications can occur like injury to the lips, teeth, or tongue due to the laryngoscope; bleeding during the biopsy; and voice change due to damage to the vocal cords postoperatively.

Frequently Asked Questions

1. What is suspension MLS?

2. What are the advantages of suspension MLS?

3. Enumerate the indications for MLS.

4. How does it differ from direct laryngoscopy?

Endnote

Victor von Bruns (1812–1883) was a German professor of surgery at the University of Tubingen. He was the first person to perform endolaryngeal surgery in 1861. He did pioneering work in laryngology including removal of vocal cord polyps and tumors. His work was carried on by Gustav Killian who invented the suspension laryngoscopy in 1912 so that both hands of the surgeon are free. The modern-day technique of suspension microlaryngoscopy was popularized by Kleinsasser in 1974 when the microscope was introduced, including the use of fine instruments for surgical precision.

62 Bronchoscopy

Krishna Koirala

The competencies covered in this chapter are as follows:

EN2.10 Identify and describe the use of common instruments used in ear, nose, and throat (ENT) surgery.

EN3.4 Observe and describe the indications for and steps involved in the removal of foreign bodies in the ear, nose, and throat.

Introduction

The tracheobronchial tree comprising the trachea, bronchi, bronchioles, and respiratory bronchioles helps transmit air toward the lung parenchyma. Diseases involving the tracheobronchial tree are varied, including congenital, inflammatory, traumatic, foreign bodies, and neoplastic. Their management, in addition to radiological and laboratory investigations, often requires a flexible or rigid endoscopy. Advances in the instrumentation, endoscopes, and anesthesia have expanded the indications and made the procedure relatively safer. Bronchoscopic evaluation can be done up to the segmental bronchi. Bronchoalveolar lavage, brushings, and transbronchial biopsies taken can be sent for histopathological and microbiological studies.

Endoscopic Anatomy

The trachea extends from the lower border of the cricoid cartilage to the level of the bifurcation at the carina (**Fig. 62.1**). The number of tracheal rings varies from 16 to 22. The trachea is cartilaginous anteriorly and membranous posteriorly (*D*-shaped). The lumen is more circular in a newborn and tends to change toward adolescence.

The length of the trachea is 10 to 13 cm and the diameter is 1.5 to 2 cm in adults; it is slightly shorter and narrower in adult females.

It is 6 cm in children and 4 cm in infants. In infants and younger children, it tends to angulate posteriorly in the mediastinum (creating an angle between the cervical and mediastinal trachea), which relatively straightens with age.

The bronchi start from the T5 vertebral level where it divides into the right and left main bronchi at the carina. The right main bronchus is shorter (2.5 cm), wider, and more vertical when compared to the left main bronchus (5 cm in length). The bronchi divide into secondary or lobar bronchi and then into tertiary or segmental bronchi.

A *bronchopulmonary segment* comprises a part of the lung supplied by a segmental bronchus with adjacent blood vessels (artery, vein, and lymphatics). Most of the bronchi and bronchioles conduct air but do not take part directly in gas exchange and therefore add to the dead space. The respiratory bronchioles have alveoli and branch into alveolar ducts that form the functional respiratory unit.

Types of Bronchoscopes

■ Flexible Bronchoscope

The diameter of the scope can range from 2.2 to 6.4 mm. With the flexible bronchoscopy (**Fig. 62.2**), one has the advantage of visualizing the subsegmental bronchi and at angles like the upper lobe bronchi. It can be used in patients with abnormalities of the jaw and neck and can be done bedside. However, due to problems of ventilation in a relatively smaller airway, it has limited use in children.

It is introduced through the nasal cavity directed to the nasopharynx and then guided inferiorly to the oropharynx. At the laryngeal inlet, topical anesthesia can be used following which it is passed through the larynx and trachea. At the carina, it is guided to either bronchus. During the passage of the flexible laryngoscope, various structures from the nasopharynx to the bronchus can be evaluated and also during the withdrawal of the scope.

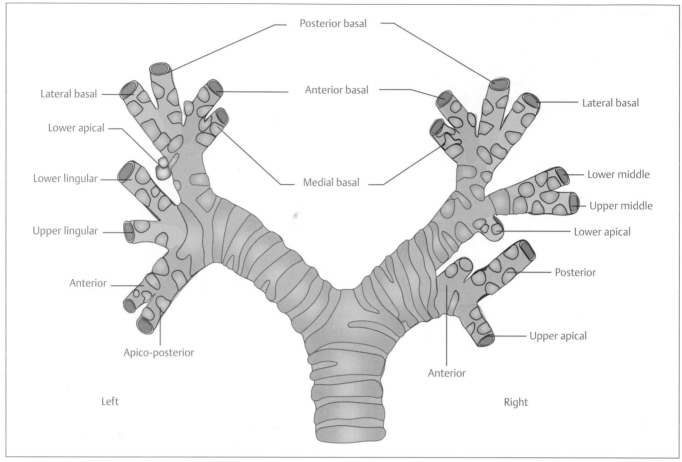

Fig. 62.1 Bronchopulmonary segments as seen during bronchoscopy.

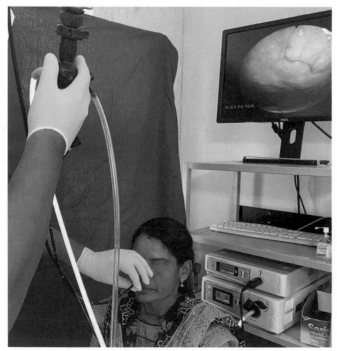

Fig. 62.2 Flexible bronchoscopy.

■ Rigid Bronchoscope

There are various sizes based on age (**Fig. 62.3**). Due to its hollow structure, a variety of instrumentation is possible.

■ Bronchial Telescopes

These are rigid endoscopes that may be angled. Instruments can be used along with them for biopsy and foreign body removal. These can also be passed through the rigid bronchoscope for better visualization, especially at angles and for documentation (camera with monitor; **Fig. 62.4**).

■ Differences between Flexible and Rigid Bronchoscopy

The differences between flexible and rigid bronchoscopy are presented in **Table 62.1**.

■ Size of Rigid Bronchoscope Based on Age

- Premature: 3 mm.
- Age 0 to 6 months: 3.5 mm.
- Age 6 to 18 months: 4 mm.

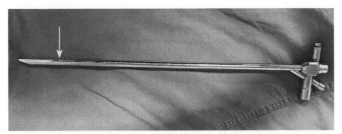

Fig. 62.3 Rigid bronchoscope with vents (*yellow arrow*) for ventilation of the opposite bronchi.

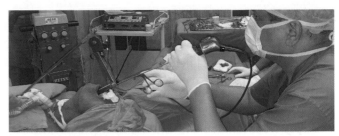

Fig. 62.4 Rigid telescopy with forceps being passed through a microlaryngoscope.

Table 62.1 Contrast between flexible and rigid bronchoscopy

Characteristics	Flexible bronchoscope	Rigid bronchoscope
Constituent	Multiple optical fibers	Hollow tube
Distal/subsegmental bronchi	Can be visualized	Cannot be visualized
Apical bronchi	Visualized	Requires angled bronchial telescope
Site of procedure	Bedside, operating room	Operating room
Position	Upright or supine	Supine; "sniffing" position
Anesthesia	Topical/sedation; rarely, general	General; rarely under sedation
Introduction site	Through the nose; can be transoral	Transoral
Instrumentation	Fine	Based on size, instruments can be larger or more rigid
Foreign body (FB) removal	Small FB can be removed; may have to be broken down	Large FB can be removed
Other equipment: Laser, cryosurgery	Difficult but possible	Easily used, including microdebrider
Transbronchial biopsy	Feasible	Not feasible
Airway	Compromises airway	Maintains airway
Ventilation	Difficult	Possible
Abnormalities in the neck, jaw, and oral cavity	Can be used	Cannot be used
Pediatric use	Difficult due to small airway	Possible
Camera for monitoring/recording	Possible	Needs a bronchial telescope
Hemorrhage	Difficult to control	Easier to control; preferred

- Age 18 months to 3 years: 4.5 mm.
- Age 3 to 6 years: 5 mm.
- Age 6 to 9 years: 5.5 mm.
- Age 9 to 12 years: 6 mm.
- Age 12 to 14 years: 7 mm.
- Adults: 7 to 9 mm.

Indications

■ Diagnostic

- Pulmonary infiltrates with diagnostic dilemma.
- Radiological changes like lung lesions, mass, atelectasis (segment or lobe), and obstructive emphysema.
- Hemoptysis and unexplained cough/wheeze.

- Obtain bronchial secretions for culture and sensitivity, fungal stains, and cytology (malignancy).
- Endobronchial lesions and mediastinal lymphadenopathy.
- Biopsy from or through the bronchus (transbronchial).
- Part of panendoscopy in the head and neck cancer to look for a second primary tumor.
- Evaluation of laryngotracheal or bronchial stenosis, tracheomalacia, and trachea-esophageal fistula.
- Strong suspicion of pulmonary tuberculosis when sputum smears and culture are negative—bronchial aspirate is taken.

For diagnostic purpose, the following can be done:

- *Bronchoalveolar lavage*: Saline is injected into the airway and using suction it is removed and secured in a

■ Complications

- Desaturation.
- Bradycardia and cardiac arrhythmias.
- Trauma to the larynx or vocal cords.
- Hemorrhage from tumors, and tracheal or bronchial wall.
- Bronchial and tracheal tears.
- Pneumothorax.
- Injury to structures during introduction, for example, the lips, teeth, tongue, and soft palate.
- Laryngeal edema.
- Laryngospasm, which can be avoided by spraying the vocal cords with 4% lignocaine.

Points to Ponder

- Bronchoscopy can be performed by both rigid and flexible techniques.
- Rigid bronchoscopy is the gold standard for removal of foreign bodies.
- Flexible bronchoscopy can be used for most of the diagnostic procedures in pulmonary disorders.
- Complications are common in rigid bronchoscopy.

Case-Based Question

1. **A 3-year-old child was brought to the emergency department with history of choking spells following a suspected inhalation of a foreign body 5 hours prior to the visit to the hospital. On examination, the child was not in respiratory distress and his oxygen saturation was being maintained. There was no stridor.**
What is the next step in the management?

Answer

Any suspicion of a foreign body inhalation in a child must be investigated immediately. Since there is no acute emergency,

a computed tomography (CT) scan of the neck and thorax can be taken to confirm the presence of a foreign body and also to detect any lung lesion like lung collapse due to bronchial obstruction.

Once the foreign body is confirmed on CT scan, it must be removed under general anesthesia. A rigid bronchoscope with a telescope can be used for visualizing the foreign body and removal is with the help of optical forceps.

Frequently Asked Questions

1. What are the indications for rigid bronchoscopy?

2. What are the contraindications for rigid bronchoscopy?

3. What is the position for rigid bronchoscopy?

4. What are the differences between flexible and rigid bronchoscopy?

5. Describe the parts of a rigid bronchoscope.

6. Enumerate the complications associated with bronchoscopy.

Endnote

Rigid bronchoscopy has been performed for more than 100 years. It was in 1897 that Gustav Killian performed the first bronchoscopy to successfully remove a foreign body from the airway. He removed a pork bone that was lodged in the right main bronchus of a 63-year-old farmer. This was a major milestone because aspiration of foreign bodies till that time was associated with 50% mortality. Killian prepared for this procedure by practicing on his servant at home. He experimented with cocaine as local anesthesia or ether as general anesthesia.

63 Anatomy and Physiology of the Esophagus

Sajilal M.

Anatomy of the Esophagus

■ Introduction

The esophagus is a fibromuscular tube that connects the pharynx to the stomach. It extends from the lower border of the cricoid cartilage at the C6 vertebral level to the cardia of the stomach at the T11 vertebral level.

■ Dimensions and Course

The length of the esophagus, from the cricopharynx to the level of the diaphragm, is approximately 22.5 to 25 cm (**Fig. 63.1**).

It can be divided into three parts: cervical, thoracic, and abdominal. The cervical esophagus is 5 cm long and the abdominal part is 2.5 cm long. The distance from the upper incisor of the oral cavity to the upper esophageal sphincter of the cricopharynx is 15 cm.

In a newborn, the esophagus extends from C4 or C5 till the T9 vertebral level. At birth, the length of the esophagus is approximately 8 to 10 cm.

> **Pearl**
>
> The recurrent laryngeal nerves are branches from the vagus. The nerve winds around the right subclavian artery on the right side and the aortic arch on the left side to travel up into the neck along the *tracheoesophageal groove*. This nerve supplies the muscles of the larynx. Unless this nerve is identified and protected, it can frequently be injured, especially during thyroidectomy.

■ Curvatures and Constrictions

- One anteroposterior curvature (corresponding to the curvature of the cervical and thoracic vertebrae; **Fig. 63.2**).
- Two lateral curvatures:
  - First: Just below the commencement of the esophagus, to the left and returns to the midline at T5.
  - Second: Below T5, it again courses to the left through the posterior mediastinum before piercing the diaphragm.
- Three constrictions (**Fig. 63.3**):
  - First: At 15 cm from the upper incisor teeth, where the esophagus commences at the cricopharyngeal sphincter (pharyngoesophageal junction).
  - Second: At 23 cm from the upper incisor teeth, where it is crossed by the aortic arch and the left main bronchus (**Fig. 63.4**).
  - Third: At 40 cm from the upper incisor, where it pierces the diaphragm (T10 vertebral level), that is, lower "physiological" esophageal sphincter (**Fig. 63.4**).

Foreign bodies entering the esophagus can be held up at these constrictions.

■ Relations of the Esophagus

The esophagus, though fibromuscular, is a flattened tube due to its anterior and posterior relations.

The *cervical esophagus* has the trachea in front and the vertebra behind with the recurrent laryngeal nerve adjacent to the tracheoesophageal groove. The thyroid is related anterolaterally and the common carotid artery is lateral.

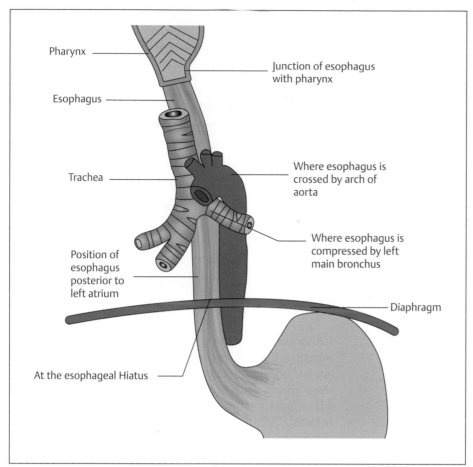

Fig. 63.1 Relations of the esophagus.

Pharynx

Junction of esophagus with pharynx

Esophagus

Where esophagus is crossed by arch of aorta

Trachea

Where esophagus is compressed by left main bronchus

Position of esophagus posterior to left atrium

Diaphragm

At the esophageal Hiatus

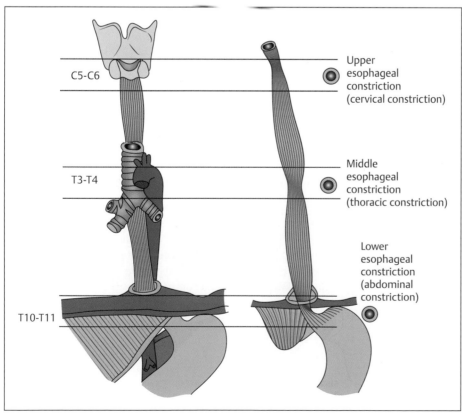

Fig. 63.2 Constrictions of the esophagus.

C5-C6

Upper esophageal constriction (cervical constriction)

T3-T4

Middle esophageal constriction (thoracic constriction)

Lower esophageal constriction (abdominal constriction)

T10-T11

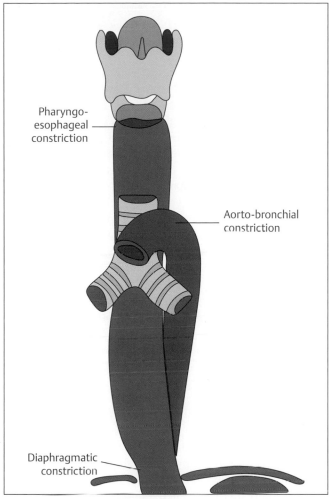

Fig. 63.3 Constrictions of the esophagus at 15, 23, and 40 cm.

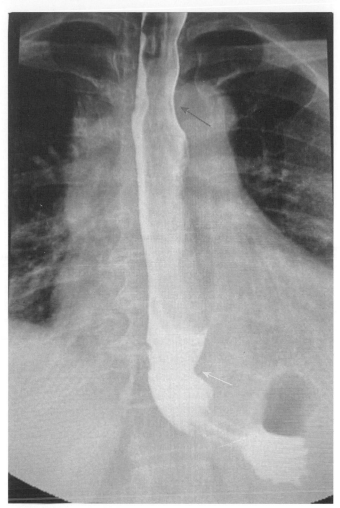

Fig. 63.4 Barium swallow showing constrictions at the aortic arch (*blue arrow*) and at the diaphragm (*yellow arrow*).

In the *superior mediastinum*, the trachea is in front and the vertebra is behind. The aortic arch forms an impression on the left. It courses behind the left main bronchus. The thoracic duct is toward the left.

In the *posterior mediastinum*, it is posterior to the left atrium. It is related to the lung and mediastinal pleura.

■ Layers of the Esophageal Wall

- The mucous membrane is lined by nonkeratinizing stratified squamous epithelium, fibrous connective tissue (lamina propria), and muscularis mucosae.
- The submucosa comprises loose connective tissue that contains large blood vessels, small esophageal glands, and *Meissner's nerve plexus* of the postganglionic parasympathetic fibers. Meissner's plexus controls glandular secretions and local blood flow, and alters electrolyte and water transport.
- The muscular layer is composed of the inner circular and outer longitudinal layers of muscles. The muscle fibers

in the upper one-third are striated muscle fibers (voluntary), the middle one-third are striated and smooth (voluntary), and the lower one-third are smooth. The *myenteric/Auerbach plexus* is located between the longitudinal and circular muscles of the esophagus. This plexus controls esophageal motility.

- The outer fibrous layer is a loose covering of the esophagus made of irregular, dense connective tissue (mainly elastin fibers).

Pearl

The longitudinal muscle fibers of the esophagus diverge at the upper end to attach at the cricoid arch, posteriorly. At this point, only the circular fibers are present in the midline, posteriorly below the cricopharyngeus muscle. This area is called the Laimer–Hackermann area. The importance of Laimer's dehiscence is that it is a site for perforation during esophagoscopy.

Blood Supply

- The cervical esophagus is supplied by the inferior thyroid artery.
- The thoracic part is supplied by the bronchial and intercostal arteries and the thoracic aorta.
- The abdominal part is supplied by the left gastric and left phrenic artery.

Nerve Supply

The nerve supply is through the parasympathetic fibers from the vagus (10th cranial nerve) and sympathetic fibers from the sympathetic trunk.

Lymphatic Drainage

The cervical part drains to the lower deep cervical, thoracic part to the posterior mediastinal and the abdominal part to the celiac group of preaortic lymph nodes.

Physiology of the Esophagus

Physiology of Swallowing (Deglutition)

Swallowing is a complex coordination of voluntary and involuntary movements that results in the transfer of food bolus from the oral cavity to the stomach.

There are three phases of deglutition: oral, pharyngeal, and esophageal. An *anticipatory phase*, which involves the visual and olfactory senses along with prior experience of the food, that is, appearance, consistency, taste, and bolus size, is also considered the initial part of deglutition.

- *Oral preparatory phase* (voluntary phase): It is a voluntary phase of deglutition that starts after the food is placed in the mouth. The lips close by the action of the orbicularis oris. Movement of the mandible is responsible for crushing of solid food (the masseter, medial pterygoid, and temporalis elevate, and the lateral pterygoid depresses the mandible) and shearing of food (rotatory movement due to the masseter and medial pterygoid).

  Food is guided between the teeth by the tongue (intrinsic and extrinsic muscles of the tongue). Mastication and salivation are important for the formation of a food bolus. Sensation (lingual nerve), taste (chorda tympani), and dentition are also important in this phase. The soft palate is pulled downward and forward (palatoglossus) to seal the oral cavity from the nasopharynx. The airway is open during this phase; therefore, any incoordination or loss of control over the bolus can lead to aspiration. In the *oral transfer phase*, food is directed to the posterior part of the oral cavity.

- *Pharyngeal phase* (involuntary phase): This phase lasts for less than 1 second. The soft palate moves upward and backward (tensor veli palatini, levator veli palatini, palatoglossus) and, along with contraction of the palatopharyngeus and formation of Passavant's ridge (superior constrictor), seals the oropharynx from the nasopharynx. Failure of closure of the nasopharyngeal isthmus, that is, velopharyngeal insufficiency, leads to nasal regurgitation.

  The bolus is propelled into the oropharynx by the base of the tongue. The larynx moves superiorly and anteriorly (thyrohyoid and suprahyoid muscles). There is approximation of the vocal cords (by the adductors) and the ventricular bands (false cords). The epiglottis directs the bolus toward the sides. This sequence of movements of laryngeal elevation and closure of the laryngeal inlet with direction of the bolus laterally helps prevent aspiration. Cessation of breathing and closure of the airway during swallowing is called *deglutition apnea*. Vagal palsy can lead to aspiration.

  The cricopharynx opens due to relaxation of the sphincter assisted by laryngeal elevation. Food is allowed to enter the upper esophagus. This is assisted by the sequential contraction of the superior constrictor, middle constrictor, and inferior constrictor. Mobility of the muscles when affected due to surgery, gastroesophageal reflux disease (GERD), radiotherapy, or neurological disorders can lead to residual food, which can get aspirated.

Pearl

The cricopharyngeal bar is a posterior narrowing or indentation of the cricopharynx seen on barium swallow, which occurs due to increase in muscle tone or due to fibrosis (**Fig. 63.5**).

- *Esophageal phase* (involuntary phase): The cricopharynx goes to its resting state, that is, closes, which prevents reflux and also prevents air from entering the esophagus. The peristaltic movement of the esophagus aided by the circular and longitudinal muscles propels food downward till the lower esophageal sphincter, which opens to allow food to enter the stomach.

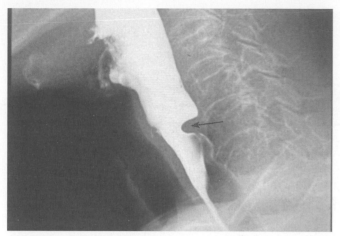

Fig. 63.5 Barium swallow showing the cricopharyngeal bar (*orange arrow*).

Points to Ponder

- The length of the esophagus, on an average, is 25 cm in adults. The distance from the upper incisor of the oral cavity to the upper esophageal sphincter is 15 cm. So to reach the lower end of the esophagus, the distance to be covered during esophagoscopy is 40 cm.
- It is important to remember that the esophagus has three main constrictions: at 15, 23, and 40 cm from the upper incisor. This is taken into consideration during rigid endoscopy.
- There are three phases of deglutition; oral, pharyngeal, and esophageal.
- Elevation of the larynx and closure of the laryngeal inlet prevent aspiration while swallowing.

Case-Based Questions

1. **A 56-year-old man came with a history of swallowing dentures while eating. X-ray showed the dentures impacted in the chest. An urgent esophagoscopy was performed and the denture was found to be impacted at 23 cm from the upper incisor.**

   a. Where is the foreign body impacted?

   b. Why does it get impacted at this site?

   Answers

   a. At 23 cm, the denture is impacted in the thoracic part of the esophagus. The esophagus starts at 15 cm from the incisors, and the upper 5 cm of esophagus is in the neck. So this was impacted in the thoracic part.

   b. There is a constriction at 23 cm where the arch of the aorta and the left main bronchus press on the esophagus.

2. **During the pharyngeal phase of deglutition, the bolus of food is propelled from the oral cavity into the oropharynx. The movement of the soft palate helps prevent nasal regurgitation during this process.**

   a. What are the muscles in the soft plate helping with the pharyngeal phase of swallowing?

   b. What is the nerve supply of the soft palate?

   Answers

   a. There are four main muscles in the soft plate helping with deglutition:
   - Tensor veli palatini.
   - Levator veli palatini.
   - Palatoglossus.
   - Palatopharyngeus.

   b. Nerve supply to these muscles is from the pharyngeal plexus, except for the tensor veli palatini, which is supplied by the medial pterygoid nerve, which is a branch of the mandibular division of the trigeminal nerve.

   The pharyngeal plexus consists of the following:
   - Pharyngeal branches of the glossopharyngeal nerve: sensory.
   - Pharyngeal branches of the vagus: motor.

Frequently Asked Questions

1. What is the length of the esophagus?
2. What are the common sites of constriction?
3. What is the commonest site of perforation during esophagoscopy?
4. Describe the phases of deglutition.
5. How is the airway protected during swallowing?

Endnote

The word "esophagus" comes from the Greek word oisophagos, which means "gullet." It was Galen, a Greek physician, who first described the esophagus as an organ for transporting food from the oral cavity, where it is chewed and broken down, to the stomach, where it was digested. The first esophagectomy, in which the esophagus was removed, was performed by Theodor Billroth in 1872.

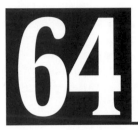

Diseases of the Esophagus

Kailesh Pujary

The competencies covered in this chapter are as follows:

EN4.52 Describe the clinical features, investigations, and principles of management of diseases of the esophagus.

PE14.2 Discuss the risk factors, clinical features, diagnosis, and management of kerosene ingestion.

Introduction

The esophagus, being part of the food passage, can be affected by many conditions as a result of inflammation, trauma, or neoplasm. The symptoms of esophageal disease are often seen initially by the ear, nose, and throat (ENT) surgeon, so it would be useful for the medical students as well as practitioners to be aware of the conditions that can affect the esophagus.

The common presenting symptoms include dysphagia, retrosternal pain, and discomfort. The dysphagia can be due to mechanical obstruction or due to neuromuscular disease. The initial symptoms may be subtle, which may delay diagnosis. Imaging and endoscopy are required for a definitive diagnosis. The relations of the esophagus in the neck and thorax, including its relations with the major blood vessels, can sometimes pose a challenge in the treatment.

Classification of Esophageal Diseases

- Congenital:
  - Esophageal atresia with or without tracheoesophageal fistula.
  - Stricture.
- Esophagitis:
  - Gastroesophageal reflux disease.
  - Caustic injury: Acid and alkali; medications like nonsteroidal anti-inflammatory drugs (NSAIDs) and doxycycline.
  - Infection: Candidiasis and tuberculosis.
  - Radiotherapy.
  - Eosinophilic esophagitis.
- Traumatic:
  - External trauma.

- Iatrogenic trauma (endoscopy, tracheostomy, nasogastric tube insertion, and open neck procedures like thyroidectomy), leading to stricture or perforation.
  - Foreign body.
- Vascular impression:
  - Intrinsic (varices): Portal hypertension and superior vena cava obstruction.
  - Extrinsic (*dysphagia lusoria*): Aberrant right subclavian artery, right aortic arch, double aortic arch, and aberrant left pulmonary artery.
- Esophageal tear (Mallory–Weiss syndrome, Boerhaave's syndrome) and perforation.
- Esophageal web (Plummer–Vinson syndrome), ring (Schatzki's ring), and stricture.
- Esophageal diverticula: Pulsion diverticula and traction diverticula.
- Motility disorders:
  - Incomplete relaxation of the lower esophageal sphincter: Achalasia cardia.
  - Major motility disorder: Absent contractility and diffuse spasm.
  - Minor motility disorder: Ineffective motility and fragmented peristalsis.
- Neoplasms:
  - Benign: Leiomyoma.
  - Malignant: Squamous cell carcinoma and adenocarcinoma.

Esophageal Atresia (with Tracheoesophageal Fistula)

■ Introduction

Esophageal atresia is due to incomplete development of the esophagus and is often associated with an abnormal communication with the trachea as a fistula.

■ Embryology

During development, the esophagus is separated from the trachea by the tracheoesophageal septum, which develops from cranial to caudal. Canalization of the esophagus occurs during the latter part of development. The atresia may occur due to failure to recanalize; due to increased pressure on the thoracic part of esophagus, which disrupts its growth; or due to the differential growth of the trachea and the esophagus. Genetics may play a role. Approximately 50% will have other major abnormalities. The VACTERL syndrome, with three or more defects, that is, vertebral defects, anorectal atresia, cardiac defects, tracheoesophageal fistula, esophageal atresia, renal anomalies, and/or limb defects, is seen in 25% of cases.

■ Types (Fig. 64.1)

- Type I: Pure atresia.
- Type II: Atresia with proximal tracheoesophageal fistula.
- Type III: Atresia with distal fistula.
- Type IV: Atresia with double fistula.
- Type V: H-type fistula with no true atresia.

■ Diagnosis

The condition may be suspected during antenatal ultrasound screening, which will reveal a small stomach of the fetus and polyhydramnios. Fetal magnetic resonance imaging (MRI) may show the lesion. Chest X-ray and a water-soluble contrast esophagogram can be done.

■ Treatment

Treatment includes the following: gastrostomy (for feeding) along with division of the fistula, division of the fistula along with end-to-end anastomosis, and continuous suctioning from the proximal pouch and total parenteral nutrition till the repair heals.

Plummer–Vinson Syndrome

■ Synonym

Synonyms of the Plummer–Vinson Syndrome are Paterson–Brown–Kelly syndrome and sideropenic dysphagia.

■ Introduction

The syndrome consists of a triad of dysphagia, iron deficiency anemia, and esophageal web. It is usually seen in females in the 40- to 60-year age group. It is a premalignant condition.

■ Etiopathogenesis

The exact etiology is not known. It may occur due to iron and nutritional deficiency, autoimmunity, or a genetic predisposition. There may be an increased risk following gastrectomy. There is depletion of iron-dependent oxidative enzymes, which affects the muscles in the pharynx and esophagus. The subepithelial inflammation leads to subepithelial fibrosis and atrophy of the overlying mucosa, and over time the web develops. Squamous cell carcinoma can develop in the postcricoid region or cervical esophagus in these patients.

■ Clinical Features

The patient will have painless, progressive dysphagia. There will be symptoms and signs of anemia. There may be koilonychia, glossitis, and angular cheilitis.

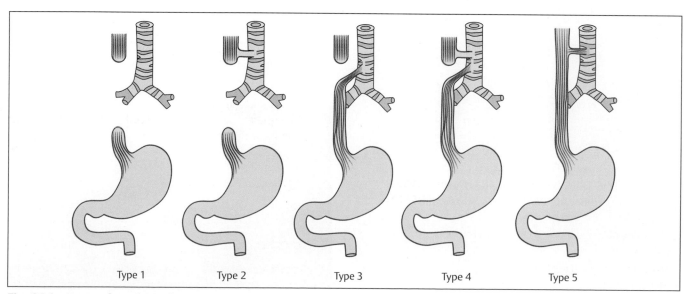

Fig. 64.1 Types of esophageal atresia.

■ Investigations

Blood investigations required are a complete blood count including hemoglobin, peripheral smear and serum iron, ferritin, and iron-binding capacity. Other causes for anemia should be ruled out including gastrointestinal malignancies. Barium swallow will show a smooth shelflike projection into the lumen in the anterior wall of the esophagus usually at the C6 level, which corresponds to the cricopharynx (**Figs. 64.2** and **64.3**). If there is irregularity, it may signify malignant transformation, in which case a biopsy is warranted.

■ Treatment

- Correction of the anemia by iron and vitamin supplements.
- Blood transfusion in case of severe anemia.
- For persistent dysphagia, endoscopy and dilatation of the web with balloon or bougie is done.
- Regular follow-up to assess for malignant transformation in the postcricoid region and cervical esophagus.

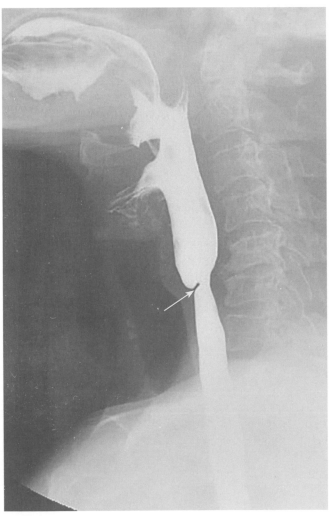

Fig. 64.2 *Yellow arrow* outlining the esophageal web.

Gastroesophageal Reflux Disease

■ Introduction

Gastroesophageal reflux disease (GERD) occurs due to the retrograde flow of gastric contents (gastric acid, pepsin, bile, and trypsin) into the esophagus. When the effect is on the larynx and pharynx, it is referred to as laryngopharyngeal reflux (LPR). Reflux to some degree is considered normal and is seen in many infants up to the age of 4 months.

■ Etiopathogenesis

Esophageal manifestations are related to relaxation of the lower esophageal sphincter for a prolonged time, in the absence of swallowing. An abnormal motility secondary to esophagitis and delayed gastric emptying may contribute.

In infants, the obtuse angle of the esophagus to the stomach, shorter intra-abdominal esophagus, and immature lower esophageal sphincter contribute to this condition.

In conditions like sliding hiatus hernia and laryngomalacia, there is an increased risk of GERD. Risk factors include obesity, alcohol intake, smoking, spicy or oily food, and heavy meals or shorter intervals between meals, especially before lying down. Long-term reflux can change the epithelial lining of the lower esophagus from stratified squamous to columnar epithelium. This is referred to as *Barrett's esophagus* and is a premalignant condition because it can predispose to adenocarcinoma.

LPR disease is due to dysfunction (increased relaxation) of the upper esophageal sphincter.

■ Clinical Features

Symptoms

In GERD, usually there will be an epigastric or retrosternal pain or a burning sensation, especially when lying down.

LPR can occur in the upright position. The presentation may be accompanied with frequent clearing of the throat, chronic cough, globus sensation, sore throat, and change in voice.

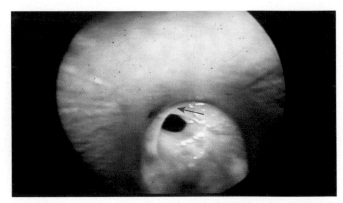

Fig. 64.3 Endoscopic view of the esophageal web.

Signs

GERD can aggravate asthma and asthma can worsen acid reflux. LPR is also associated with subglottic stenosis and vocal cord contact granuloma. It has been considered an etiological factor for chronic rhinosinusitis, otitis media with effusion, and apnea in infants.

Examination findings in the larynx on rigid telescopy include the following:

- Pachyderma laryngis (thickening of the mucosa in the posterior commissure).
- Supraglottic or glottis erythema and edema.
- Pseudosulcus vocalis (due to subglottic edema, there appears a sulcus at the medial margin of the vocal cord).
- Obliteration of the ventricle.
- Signs in the trachea include cobblestone appearance, erythema, and increased secretions.

Pearl

Eosinophilic esophagitis is an idiopathic inflammatory disease of the esophagus that may mimic GERD. It does not respond to treatment with proton pump inhibitors and is diagnosed by biopsy (>15 eosinophils in one high-power field).

■ Investigations

Transnasal, flexible, fiberoptic endoscopy should be done to assess the upper airway and pharynx. Upper gastrointestinal endoscopy must be done to assess the changes in the esophageal mucosa and in long-term cases to rule out Barret's esophagus by biopsy.

Barium swallow with fluoroscopy is useful in detecting structural changes in the esophagus like mucosal thickening, strictures, ulcers, and hiatus hernia; it also helps rule out conditions that may mimic GERD-like achalasia and diffuse esophageal spasm.

Twenty-four-hour ambulatory pH probe testing is done to monitor the pH at the upper and lower esophageal sphincters. Impedance monitoring is done along with pH testing. Esophageal manometry can assess peristalsis and for motility disorders. Reflux symptom index helps assess the quality of life in patients with LPR.

Pearl

A reflux event can be demonstrated by multichannel, intraluminal, impedance pH monitoring. Sensors are kept at the upper and lower esophageal sphincters. An LPR event occurs when the pH at the upper esophageal sphincter goes below 4 and the total acid exposure time is more than 1%. This is the percentage of time in 24 hours when the sensors detected pH less than 4.

■ Treatment

Lifestyle modifications: Stop smoking and use of alcohol, stay in upright position after meals for at least 2 to 3 hours, lose weight (in obesity), elevate the head end of the bed, avoid spicy food, avoid caffeine/aerated drinks/peppermint, and avoid tight clothing and medications like anticholinergics, sedatives, tricyclic antidepressants, and NSAIDs.

Pharmacotherapy

- Drugs to reduce the stomach acid: Proton pump inhibitors (PPIs) and H2 blockers. The commonly used PPIs include omeprazole and pantoprazole.
- Sucralfate.
- Prokinetic agents.
- Baclofen reduces the number of lower esophageal sphincter relaxation.

Surgery

- Nissen's fundoplication, either laparoscopic or open approach.
- Treatment of a hiatus hernia.

Pearl

GERD has to be under control prior to undertaking any surgery for airway disorders like resection of laryngeal lesions, contact granuloma, laryngotracheal reconstruction, and in lung transplant.

Corrosive Burns

■ Introduction

Caustic agents have the ability to cause mucosal burns in the upper aerodigestive tract. In children, it is usually accidental. In teenagers and adults with psychiatric illness and in alcoholics, it is likely to be an attempted suicide. Most of the effects are seen locally on the tissues they come into contact with. The systemic effects are negligible.

Chemicals with extremes of pH can cause the damage. The injury to the tissues will depend on the following:

- Concentration of the chemical.
- Duration of contact of the chemical with the tissues.
- The amount ingested.
- The pH of the chemical.

Solid materials will cause more damage in the mouth and pharynx, whereas liquids pass through the upper aerodigestive pathway and cause more damage to the esophagus and stomach

■ Causative Agents and Their Mode of Action

- Alkalis: Lyes (sodium and potassium hydroxide found in household and farm cleaning products), bleaches, household detergents, ammonia, and disk batteries are the common chemicals in this category. Alkalis cause *liquefaction necrosis*. Their action ends when diluted or neutralized by the tissues.
- Acids: These include toilet and swimming pool cleaners, and rust removers. Acids cause *coagulation necrosis*. Large quantities are required to cause damage to the esophagus.

Strictures occur when there is a circumferential injury (**Figs. 64.4** and **64.5**). The usual sites of injury are the areas of normal constrictions and areas of pooling of saliva.

■ Clinical Features

There will be drooling of saliva, odynophagia, and vomiting. Respiratory tract involvement presents with hoarseness and wheezing with or without stridor. There may be associated burns in the hands and face. Chest pain, abdominal pain, or interscapular pain may signify esophageal perforation with or without mediastinitis. The amount and type of caustic agent with concentration should be noted.

Pearl

Oral medications like NSAIDs, steroids, doxycycline, and oral contraceptives can cause tissue damage due to their acidic properties especially when there is prolonged contact with the esophageal mucosa.

■ Management

Investigations

- Complete blood count, serum electrolytes, and arterial blood gas.

- Chest X-ray (for pulmonary edema/infiltrates, free peritoneal air, and disk battery).
- Transnasal flexible endoscopy to assess the pharynx and the laryngeal airway. Esophagoscopy is done within 12 to 48 hours of injury.
- Barium swallow is done after 3 weeks. It will show the site and extent of stricture. There may be multiple strictures.

Endoscopic Grading of Corrosive Injury

- I: Edema and erythema (superficial first-degree injury).
- IIa: Hemorrhage, erosion, and ulcers (second-degree injury—submucosa).
- IIb: Circumferential ulceration (second-degree injury—submucosa and muscularis).
- III: Multiple deep ulcers with discoloration (third-degree injury—near full thickness).
- IV: Perforation.

Treatment

- Drink milk or water to dilute the agent; irrigate sites of contact and examine oral cavity.
- Secure airway/treat laryngeal edema.
- Intravenous antibiotics and proton pump inhibitors.
- Insert a nasogastric tube or an esophageal stent in circumferential injury.
- Serial dilatations may be necessary after 4 weeks depending on the stricture.

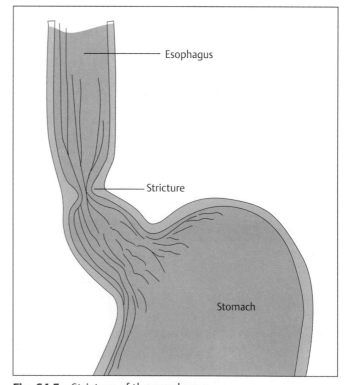

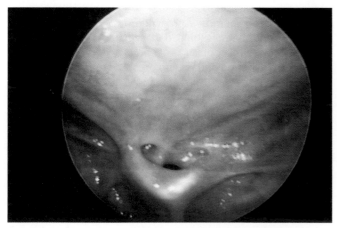

Fig. 64.4 Postcorrosive stricture of the laryngopharynx.

Fig. 64.5 Stricture of the esophagus.

- Large segment or multiple strictures may require resection and reconstruction by jejunal-free graft, gastric transposition, or colonic interposition.
- Psychiatry consultation for the patient. In children, counseling of the parents is also required. and in children and counselling of parents is required.

Kerosene Poisoning

■ Introduction

Accidental ingestion of kerosene is seen in children, usually below 5 years of age, especially in developing countries. The most common age group is from 1 to 3 years.

■ Pathogenesis

Kerosene is a distillate of petroleum consisting of paraffin and naphthenes. It is a form of hydrocarbon used in lamps and for heating, especially in the lower socioeconomic status. It is a chemical substance that is highly volatile and of low viscosity and low surface tension. The low viscosity promotes aspiration. Due to the high-volatility property, oxygen is displaced leading to transient hypoxia. These properties enable the substance to not only cause aspiration but also penetrate the distal airway and involve a large area of lung parenchyma. The decrease in surfactant production will cause alveolar collapse and reduced perfusion. This results in bronchial necrosis, interstitial inflammation, vascular necrosis, and intra-alveolar hemorrhage and edema. The central nervous system symptoms are usually secondary to the hypoxia and acidosis and sometimes directly by crossing the blood–brain barrier.

■ Clinical Features

Symptoms

The child will be found smelling of kerosene with the offending agent nearby. There will be cough and nausea followed by fever with grunting and restlessness. Due to aspiration, the patient may develop chemical pneumonitis, and rarely, pneumatocele, bronchopleural fistula, subcutaneous emphysema, pneumomediastinum, pneumothorax, and pleural effusion. The aspiration may be directly into the lungs or due to vomiting.

In the gastrointestinal tract, it can cause abdominal discomfort, pain, and vomiting.

Signs

The patient will have tachypnea and hypoxia. The child may develop drowsiness and convulsions. It can also, rarely, affect the kidneys and myocardium leading to cardiac dysrhythmias.

■ Investigations

- A complete blood count may show leukocytosis.
- Blood gas analysis is done especially in hypoxic patients.
- Chest X-ray or computed tomography (CT) thorax may show lung field infiltrates, lower lobe consolidation, and/or other pulmonary complications.

■ Treatment

- Prevention is by education regarding the labeling of bottles with their composition and keeping poisonous substances and medications away from the reach of children.
- Remove the clothes and wash the body with soap and water to decontaminate skin and air.
- Supportive management with oxygen through face mask, hydration through intravenous fluids, antipyretics, antiemetics, and intravenous antibiotics.
- Counseling of the parents: in cases of intentional poisoning, the individual will require psychiatry evaluation.

Benign Strictures of Esophagus

■ Introduction

An esophageal stricture is a condition wherein there is narrowing of the lumen of the esophagus (the normal diameter is ~20 mm).

■ Etiology

Narrowing of the esophageal lumen can occur from within due to GERD, caustic ingestion, esophagitis, postradiotherapy, postsurgery, iatrogenic causes, and systemic inflammatory disease. Rarely, it may be congenital. Extraluminal causes for esophageal narrowing are tuberculosis, mediastinal tumors, and vascular conditions like aneurysm and anomalous vessels.

■ Clinical Features

The patient will present with dysphagia. If the stricture is small, there will be dysphagia only to solids. Indirect laryngoscopy or rigid telescopy may show pooling of saliva in the pyriform fossa if the obstruction is in the cervical esophagus. This is also known as Chevalier Jackson's sign.

■ Investigations

Barium swallow is done to assess the site, extent, and number of strictures. Contrast-enhanced CT scan or MRI is done for mediastinal tumors. CT or MR angiography is used for vascular lesions. Flexible or rigid esophagoscopy is used to assess the lesion and take a biopsy if required.

■ Treatment

Initial management is to treat the cause. For persistent intraluminal strictures, serial dilatations are done using rubber bougies or balloon dilators. The main complications of dilatation are bleeding and perforation, especially when the mucosa is vulnerable as in caustic ingestion or when forceful dilatation is done. An ideal lumen should be more than 15 mm in diameter. The patient should avoid NSAIDs. Treatment to prevent reflux with proton pump inhibitors should be started.

Globus Pharyngeus

■ Introduction

Globus pharyngeus refers to a sensation of lump in the throat. Most often, it is a diagnosis of exclusion. This condition is difficult to treat, and although there may be initial improvement, it tends to recur.

■ Etiology

The exact etiology is not known. It has been attributed to gastroesophageal reflux and abnormal upper esophageal sphincter. Other inciting factors are stress and psychiatric disorders. The sensation can also be caused by a retroverted epiglottis, hypertrophied tongue base, pharyngeal inflammation, upper esophageal malignancy, anterior cervical osteophytes, and thyroid lesions.

■ Clinical Features

The typical history is that of a lump or foreign body sensation in the throat or that of something stuck in the throat. There is no true dysphagia because the patient can swallow liquids and solids without discomfort. The symptom can be intermittent or persistent.

■ Investigations

After a detailed history and examination of the throat, a flexible nasolaryngoscopy is done. Endoscopy not only is a diagnostic tool but also can help reassure the patient. Barium swallow and flexible esophagoscopy are done when a lesion is suspected, especially when there is dysphagia, odynophagia, change in voice, or weight loss.

■ Treatment

- Reassure the patient of the benign nature, after evaluation.
- Antireflux treatment, including proton pump inhibitors, is the first line of treatment.
- With reduction of symptoms, further investigations may not be required.

- Exercises for speech and swallowing may help reduce the pharyngolaryngeal tension.
- Some patients, especially those with psychiatric disorders, may benefit from antidepressants.
- Cognitive behavioral therapy (CBT) may be helpful when the symptoms are persistent.

Achalasia Cardia

■ Introduction

The esophagus in achalasia cardia is dilated as the lower esophageal sphincter does not open and food does not pass into the stomach.

■ Etiopathogenesis

The cause for the primary condition is unknown, but it is said to be due to the degeneration of the inhibitory ganglion in the myenteric plexus in the esophagus with resultant unopposed action of the excitatory neurotransmitters. There is poor lower esophageal sphincter relaxation and absent peristalsis in the esophagus. It may be mediated by an autoimmune response or a viral infection.

Secondary causes are Chagas' disease and postfundoplication, which is done for gastroesophageal reflux disease.

■ Clinical Features

This is usually seen in the 30- to 60-year age group. Initially, the patient will have dysphagia. There will be regurgitation of the accumulated food, which when recurrent can lead to aspiration pneumonia. There may be retrosternal discomfort and weight loss in long-standing cases.

■ Investigations

- Flexible endoscopy can be carried out. It will show retained food in a dilated, tortuous lumen. An underlying malignancy of the lower third of the esophagus should be ruled out.
- Barium swallow will show a dilated lower two-thirds of esophagus with abrupt narrowing at the gastroesophageal junction. In early cases, there may be a "bird beak" appearance at the lower end (**Fig. 64.6**).
- Esophageal manometry is the gold standard for diagnosis. It shows incomplete relaxation of the lower esophageal sphincter and poor peristalsis.

Treatment

- Pharmacotherapy with calcium channel blockers and long-acting nitrates, which reduce the lower esophageal sphincter pressure, will give temporary relief.

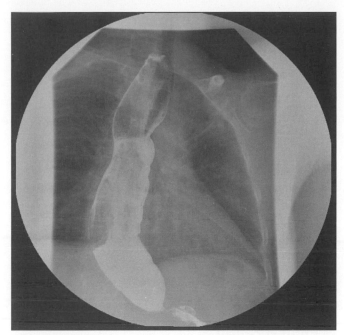

Fig. 64.6 Barium swallow of achalasia cardia showing dilatation of the lower two-thirds.

- Botulinum toxin injection into the lower esophageal sphincter can be used in patients not fit for surgery.
- Endoscopic balloon dilatation will also give relief and will have to be repeated.
- The surgical treatment of choice is cardiomyotomy done by the open (Heller's) or laparoscopic approach. This procedure may be done along with partial fundoplication. Transoral endoscopic myotomy has also been tried with varied results.

Regular follow-up is mandatory to assess malignancy, which may develop at a later stage.

> **Pearl**
>
> *Pseudoachalasia* refers to dilatation of the lower esophagus due to a cause other than primary neuronal denervation. A common cause for this condition is malignancy.

Cricopharyngeal Achalasia

Synonyms of cricopharyngeal achalasia are cricopharyngeal dysfunction/cricopharyngeal spasm. This refers to the inadequate relaxation or opening of the upper esophageal sphincter, which is denoted by a smooth posterior impression at the C6 level on barium swallow. It may be congenital, primary, or secondary (neurological conditions). It is a rare cause for dysphagia.

Botulinum toxin when injected at the site, guided by ultrasound, is both diagnostic and therapeutic. The treatment of choice is an open or endoscopic cricopharyngeal myotomy (**Fig. 64.7**).

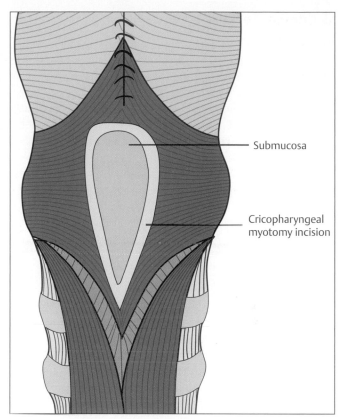

Submucosa

Cricopharyngeal myotomy incision

Fig. 64.7 Open cricopharyngeal myotomy.

Perforation of Esophagus

■ Introduction

Esophageal perforation is not common but has a high mortality if undetected due to the resultant mediastinitis.

■ Etiology

- It can occur, although not common, spontaneously (Boerhaave's syndrome) following a bout of forceful vomiting or due to increased intrathoracic pressure.
- Iatrogenic perforation can occur during endoscopy, especially when there are sites of weakness due to caustic ingestion and malignancy, and during use of force at sites of narrowing.
- Other surgeries like cricopharyngeal myotomy, cervical spine, and thyroidectomy can result in opening of the esophagus.
- Foreign bodies that are large, sharp, or long standing can result in a perforation.
- Button batteries due to their composition can erode the esophageal mucosa with rapid necrosis of tissue.
- External trauma like penetrating injury of the neck can sometimes lead to a perforation.
- During tracheostomy, injury to the posterior wall of the trachea can lead to a tracheoesophageal fistula.

■ Clinical Features

The diagnosis is based on a high degree of suspicion. When the cervical esophagus is involved, there can be crepitus over the neck on palpation. The patient may complain of retrosternal pain, which may radiate to the neck or interscapular pain, which raises the suspicion of mediastinitis. Other symptoms of mediastinitis are fever and chills, cough, and breathing difficulty. There may be a crackling sound on auscultation of the chest (Hamman's sign) when there is mediastinal emphysema. When diagnosis is delayed, there may be signs of sepsis.

■ Management

Early intervention will avoid the high morbidity and high mortality associated with esophageal perforation.

■ Investigations

- A contrast X-ray of the esophagus using a water-soluble medium is used to detect the site of leak.
- A complete blood count will show leukocytosis and thrombocytopenia in mediastinitis and C-reactive protein may be raised. Contrast-enhanced CT scan or MRI of the neck and thorax is taken to assess the extent of mediastinal involvement.

■ Treatment

The patient is not allowed to take anything orally. Immediate treatment is to start on intravenous fluids, antibiotics, and proton pump inhibitors. A nasogastric tube is placed or a temporary feeding jejunostomy is done. A flexible endoscopy may be done to place a temporary stent at the site of leak or to put fibrin glue in case of a small perforation. If conservative measures fail, the patient is deteriorating, or the defect is large, then a surgical intervention is required. Closure of the defect with intervening muscle flap is done.

Leiomyoma

This is a benign tumor arising from the smooth muscles of the esophagus and accounting for less than 1% of esophageal neoplasms. This is the commonest benign tumor to affect the esophagus. It occurs more commonly in the lower one-third of the esophagus. It may be an incidental finding on endoscopy or the patient may have dysphagia, retrosternal discomfort, or regurgitation. Esophagoscopy and biopsy are done to confirm the diagnosis. A CT scan or MRI is useful to assess the lesion. Treatment is by excision or enucleation. The approach is based on the site. A minimally invasive approach or a video-assisted thoracoscopic resection is preferred.

Malignancy of Esophagus

■ Introduction

It is the eighth most common malignancy. It affects the older age group and is more common in males.

■ Etiopathology

Squamous cell carcinoma is the commonest malignancy involving the upper one-third and middle one-third of the esophagus. The risk factors are low socioeconomic group, smoking, alcohol consumption, caustic ingestion, and tylosis. In females, the upper one-third is common and there may be a history of Plummer–Vinson syndrome. Adenocarcinoma affects the lower end of the esophagus. The risk factors are Barrett's esophagus, smoking, and alcohol consumption. There may be a family history of gastrointestinal cancer.

■ Clinical Features

The early symptoms are nonspecific and therefore the presentation is late. The patient presents with progressive dysphagia. There may be a prior history of reflux. In later stages, there will be loss of appetite and weight. Change in voice may occur due to reflux or due to recurrent laryngeal nerve involvement. Cough may be due to regurgitation of food or aspiration or a malignant tracheoesophageal fistula.

■ Investigations

- Barium swallow will show the site and extent of the lesion (**Fig. 64.8**).
- A flexible or rigid esophagoscopy with biopsy will help confirm the diagnosis.

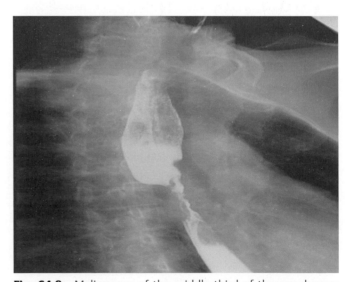

Fig. 64.8 Malignancy of the middle third of the esophagus: Barium swallow.

- Contrast-enhanced CT scan of the thorax, abdomen, and neck or pelvis, depending on the site of the lesion, will help assess the primary tumor especially in relation to the adjacent structures.
- A positron emission tomography (PET) scan will help assess for distant metastasis, especially in advanced lesions.
- Additionally, a bronchoscopy needs to be done.
- In case of an inconclusive histology, an endoscopic mucosal resection can be done for a more representative sample.

■ Treatment

- It depends on various factors like the stage of disease, histology, fitness of the patient, and the choice of the patient after counseling regarding the disease and treatment options.
- For early-stage disease (T1/T2), surgery is the choice of treatment.
- For intermediate stages (T3 or N1 disease), a preoperative chemotherapy with or without radiotherapy followed by surgery and adjunct chemotherapy is an appropriate management approach.

Surgery involves an esophagectomy and lymphadenectomy. The defect is replaced by a conduit either with the stomach (called gastric transposition) or jejunal free grafts depending on the size and site of the defect.

In late stages (grossly advanced local disease and/or distant metastasis), the treatment is mainly palliative. Palliative treatment includes chemotherapy with or without radiotherapy, pain management, and management of dysphagia by placing a stent at the site of the lesion or creating an alternate route for feeding like a gastrostomy or a feeding jejunostomy.

Points to Ponder

- The esophagus is a muscular tube, 25-cm long, connecting the pharynx to the stomach.
- Among the esophageal diseases, GERD is the commonest condition and results in reflux of acid from the stomach into the esophagus. At least 50% of all adults will experience this at some point in their lives.
- Plummer–Vinson syndrome is a premalignant condition consisting of a triad of dysphagia, iron-deficiency anemia, and esophageal web.
- Globus pharyngeus is a functional esophageal disorder where the patient complains of a lump in the throat.
- Corrosive burns are caused by caustic agents. Solid chemicals produce burns in the mouth and pharynx. Liquids produce burns in the esophagus and stomach.
- The commonest malignancy affecting the esophagus is squamous cell carcinoma, and it usually affects the upper two-third. Adenocarcinoma is mainly seen in the lower one-third of the esophagus.
- The commonest benign tumor to affect the esophagus is leiomyoma.

Case-Based Questions

1. **A 42-year-old female patient presented with a 2-year history of dysphagia to solids. There was a recent increase in severity of the symptom leading to absolute dysphagia and mild stridor. She had pallor and glossitis.**

   a. What is the possible diagnosis?

   b. How would you evaluate?

   Answers

   a. The patient probably had Plummer–Vinson syndrome, which has progressed to a postcricoid or cervical esophagus malignancy.

   b. A complete blood count would show anemia. Barium swallow will show the site of obstruction. A contrast-enhanced CT scan will show the site, extent of disease in relation to the surrounding structures, airway involvement, and metastatic lymph nodes (paratracheal). An endoscopy and biopsy are required to confirm the diagnosis.

   If only a web is noted on endoscopy, it can be dilated and iron supplementation should be started.

2. **A 36-year-old obese male presented with a history of cough and change in voice. There was a history of retrosternal burning sensation. Flexible nasopharyngoscopy showed thickening in the region of the posterior commissure of the larynx and pseudosulcus vocalis.**

   a. What is the diagnosis?

   b. What is the treatment?

   Answers

   a. Gastroesophageal reflux disease (GERD).

   b. Lifestyle modifications including weight loss and anti-reflux measures. The patient should sleep with the head end elevated. Proton pump inhibitors, like omeprazole and pantoprazole, are given to reduce the stomach acid. In severe cases, not improving with conservative measures, Nissen's fundoplication can be done.

3. **A 33-year-old man presented with a history of retrosternal discomfort and dysphagia. There was a**

history of regurgitation of food. The barium swallow test showed dilatation of the lower two-thirds of the esophagus with abrupt narrowing.

a. What is the diagnosis?

b. What is the management?

Answers

a. Achalasia cardia.

b. Flexible esophagoscopy should be done to confirm diagnosis and rule out an underlying malignancy. The procedure of choice is an open or laparoscopic cardiomyotomy.

Frequently Asked Questions

1. What is Plummer–Vinson syndrome and what is its importance?

2. What is globus pharyngeus?

3. Discuss the management of corrosive poisoning.

4. Enumerate the causes of esophageal strictures.

5. Enumerate the causes of esophageal perforation.

6. What are the radiological features of achalasia cardia and carcinoma of the middle third of the esophagus?

7. What is the etiology for esophageal malignancy?

Endnote

Chevalier Jackson developed the first illuminated esophagoscope and treated many children with strictures due to lye ingestion. His persistent lobby led to the Federal Caustic Act (United States), 1927. His interest in esophagoscopy began in England and, upon return to the United States, he removed a coin from a child in 1890. Once this was published, inexperienced endoscopists practiced this art, leading to complications and deaths, so he stopped the manufacture of esophagoscope until training was imparted.

Kailesh Pujary

Introduction

Swallowing propels food from the mouth to the stomach. Dysphagia (difficulty in swallowing) is a symptom in which there is an inability to take orally or an impairment of transport of solids or liquids from the oral cavity to the stomach, which is necessary for sustenance of life. The term absolute dysphagia is used when both solids and liquids cannot be swallowed.

Dysphagia can lead to malnutrition, dehydration, aspiration, and weight loss.

Etiology

The different stages of deglutition can be affected separately or in combination based on the etiology (**Fig. 65.1** and **Table 65.1**).

The etiology of dysphagia may also be classified as the following:

- *Congenital*: Choanal atresia, esophageal atresia, laryngeal cleft, vascular rings, vallecular cyst, and cleft palate.
- *Traumatic*: Foreign body, caustic injury, postendoscopy, external trauma, and surgical trauma.
- *Infection*: Deep neck space abscesses, tonsillitis, and epiglottitis.
- *Inflammatory*: Eosinophilic esophagitis, GERD, Plummer–Vinson syndrome.
- *Neurological*: Cerebral palsy, cerebrovascular accident, encephalopathy's, infections, motor neuron disease, Alzheimer's disease, myasthenia gravis, and botulism.
- *Neoplastic*: Benign and malignant tumors of the oral cavity, oropharynx, hypopharynx, and esophagus.
- *Drugs*: Affecting the mucosa (antibiotics and anticancer drugs), striated muscle (sedatives), sphincters (tricyclic antidepressants), and propulsion (calcium channel blockers), and causing xerostomia (antihistamines, diuretics).

- *Psychological*: Globus.
- *Connective tissue/autoimmune*: Systemic lupus erythematosus, scleroderma, dermatomyositis, Sjogren's syndrome, rheumatoid arthritis, and secondary autoimmune disease (Steven–Johnson syndrome).
- *Systemic illnesses* like hepatic failure, renal failure, hyperthyroidism, and diabetic neuropathy.

In the geriatric population, age-related changes in the digestive tract, medications, oral hygiene, nutritional deficiencies, and psychosocial problems can contribute to dysphagia.

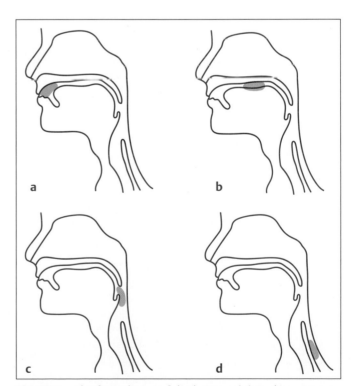

Fig. 65.1 The four phases of deglutition. **(a)** Oral preparatory phase. **(b)** Oral phase. **(c)** Pharyngeal phase. **(d)** Esophageal phase.

Evaluation

History taking is vital to get a clue toward diagnosis.

- If it is acute, the onset of the dysphagia could be an infection or neurological.
- If it is gradual, it could be a tumor.
- Progressive difficulty in swallowing solids and then semisolids and liquids points toward a tumor.
- When it is associated with pain, an infection or advanced malignancy should be suspected.
- Cough on swallowing (Ono's sign) may signify aspiration seen in advanced malignancy and neurological problems as well as in tracheoesophageal fistula.
- History of weight loss, prior head and neck surgery, systemic diseases, sleep apnea, trauma, or caustic ingestion should be elicited.

Table 65.1 Etiology of dysphagia based on deglutition phase

The phase of deglutition affected	Etiology
Oral preparatory phase	• Dental: Age related, trauma, and posttumor resection • Reduced salivation: Age related, postradiation, and Sjogren's syndrome
Oral phase	• Anatomical changes: Oral and oropharyngeal tumors, posttumor resection, and enlarged tonsils • Oropharyngeal incoordination: Neurological conditions like cerebral palsy • Velopharyngeal insufficiency
Pharyngeal phase	• Neurological causes • Anatomical changes: Infections, tumors, posttumor resection, reflux disease, and diverticulum, • Cricopharyngeal dysfunction
Esophageal phase	• Strictures: Benign/malignant • Motility disorders • Inflammation • Plummer–Vinson syndrome

- In children, there may be a failure to thrive.

Clinical assessment for signs of dehydration and the body mass index should be documented. The examination should include the following:

- Nose (nasal mass and choanal atresia in children).
- Oral cavity and oropharynx (tongue, palate, tonsil, and base of the tongue).
- Hypopharynx (tumors and pooling of saliva).
- Larynx (tumors and vocal cord mobility).
- Neck (swelling including thyroid and neck nodes).
- A neurological examination must be performed, including evaluation of the gait, posture, presence of tremors, power of limbs, and cranial nerves.

Bedside evaluation of swallowing includes assessing the posture, positioning, motivation, oral cavity deformities, types of difficulties during oral intake, and cough during swallowing.

Investigations

- Blood investigations include a complete blood count to assess the hemoglobin level (nutritional deficiencies), total count and neutrophil count (infection), serum electrolytes (electrolyte imbalance), renal function tests, and liver function tests.
- A barium swallow demonstrates the site and extent of luminal (**Fig. 65.2**) or extraluminal (**Fig. 65.3**) obstruction. Barium sulfate can be given at various consistencies

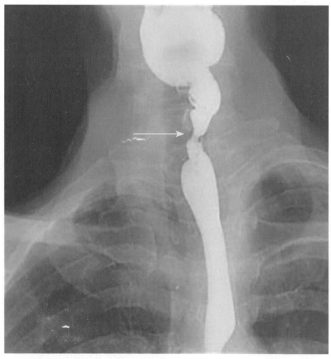

Fig. 65.2 Barium swallow showing narrowing with mucosal irregularity in cervical esophagus suggestive of malignancy.

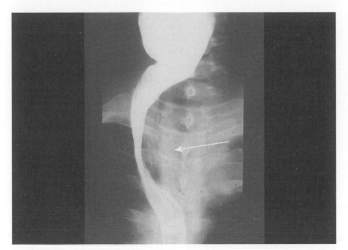

Fig. 65.3 Barium swallow showing extrinsic compression.

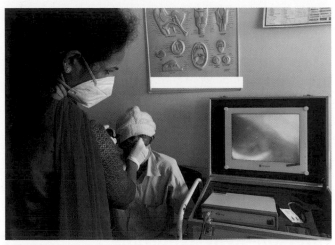

Fig. 65.4 Fiberoptic endoscopic evaluation of swallowing (FEES).

during evaluation. A videofluoroscopy done during the study would be a dynamic evaluation process from the oral cavity to the stomach. It helps in identifying inco-ordination, regurgitation, aspiration, and obstruction. When there is a history of aspiration, there is a risk of aspiration of the contrast material, and gastrografin should be used as it is less toxic to the lung when compared to barium sulfate.

- Flexible nasopharyngolaryngoscopy and bronchoscopy are used to assess structural anomalies in the nose, nasopharynx, oropharynx, laryngopharynx, and tracheobronchial lumen.
- Fiberoptic endoscopic evaluation of swallowing (FEES) is done using liquid or food bolus with a dye for better visibility. This test involves using a flexible scope passed through the nose, and the patient is asked to swallow. With the flexible endoscope tip in the nasopharynx, velopharyngeal insufficiency can be assessed. The endoscope at the nasopharyngeal isthmus does not interfere with swallowing and can study laryngopharyngeal coordination, residual particles in vallecula or hypopharynx, penetration or aspiration through laryngeal inlet, and regurgitation (**Fig. 65.4**).
- Esophageal manometry (motility studies) with or without pH monitoring is used to assess the upper and lower esophageal sphincter function and the movement of the esophageal wall during swallowing. It is helpful in cricopharyngeal dysfunction, achalasia cardia, scleroderma, and gastroesophageal reflux disease (GERD).
- Esophagoscopy (flexible or rigid) is used to assess abnormalities within the lumen and to take biopsy when needed (see Chapter 67).
- Contrast-enhanced CT scan or magnetic resonance imaging (MRI) is useful in assessing whether the lesion is luminal or extraluminal, its extent and spread, and for vascular anomalies compressing the esophagus.

- Angiography is done when there is a vascular anomaly like a vascular ring or an aberrant right subclavian artery.

Treatment

Genetic counselling is essential in syndromic children.
Swallowing therapy encompasses a wide variety of techniques used to initiate and facilitate swallowing, some of which are the following:

- In infants, oral motor stimulation, adjusting the feeding schedule, and pacing the feeds.
- Alterations in the bolus consistency, volume, temperature, and taste.
- Positive reinforcement.
- Postural changes like chin tuck and head rotation.
- Oropharyngeal muscle-strengthening exercises.
- Swallowing manoeuvers like multiple swallows, supraglottic or super supraglottic swallow.
- Manoeuvers to improve elevation of the larynx, reduce aspiration, and open the cricopharynx.

Alternate feeding is done when there is absolute dysphagia and severe aspiration. Alternate feeding methods are through a nasogastric tube, feeding gastrostomy, or feeding jejunostomy. Sometimes, total parenteral nutrition may be required.

Treatment of the lesion often relieves the symptom. This includes dilatation of the web or stricture, cricopharyngeal myotomy, excision of a diverticulum, removal of a tumor, or foreign body removal.

Treatment of neurological conditions often improves swallowing when done along with swallowing therapy. However, treatment of neurological conditions may not be possible in progressive disorders.

Lower airway protection is required in severe aspiration. This includes measures that prevent food from entering the airway while swallowing. This can be achieved by using a cuffed tube after tracheostomy. The cuff, when inflated, will prevent the food from entering the lungs.

Medialization thyroplasty with cricopharyngeal myotomy is done for combined laryngeal nerve palsy. Thyroplasty will prevent the entry of food into the larynx and cricopharyngeal myotomy will relax the upper esophageal sphincter and allow the food into the esophagus.

Plummer–Vinson Syndrome or Paterson–Kelly Syndrome

In Plummer–Vinson syndrome, the patient presents with a classical triad of symptoms that include the following:
- Dysphagia.

- Iron deficiency anemia.
- Postcricoid web.

This syndrome is common in women in countries like India due to widespread nutritional deficiencies. For clinical features and management of this condition, see Chapter 64.

Points to Ponder

- Dysphagia can affect all three phases of swallowing: oral, pharyngeal, and esophageal phases.
- There are a number of causes for dysphagia ranging from congenital lesions to infections and neurological conditions.
- Investigations should include FEES where a bolus of food is given and a flexible endoscope is used to evaluate swallowing in real time.
- Swallowing therapy is carried out by a trained therapist from the speech, language, and swallowing therapy department. It requires multiples sittings.

Case-Based Question

1. **A 45-year-old woman with a tracheostomy tube in situ is seen in the ear, nose, and throat (ENT) clinic with complaints of difficulty in swallowing. How does a tracheostomy tube add to dysphagia?**

   Answer

   The normal upward movement of the larynx, during deglutition, helps in swallowing and prevents aspiration.

The epiglottis covers the laryngeal inlet during swallowing and the esophageal sphincter opens up. A tracheostomy tube fixes the larynx in the neck preventing upward movement of the larynx.

The swallowing process can be aided by downsizing the tracheostomy tube (using a smaller tracheostomy tube) or by using a fenestrated tube to allow airflow through the larynx.

Frequently Asked Questions

1. What are some of the esophageal causes of dysphagia?
2. What is dysphagia lusoria?
3. What are the methods to prevent aspiration in a patient with dysphagia?
4. What is the triad of symptoms in Plummer–Vinson syndrome?
5. How will a cricopharyngeal myotomy help in dysphagia?

Endnote

The term "presbyesophagus" was coined more than 35 years ago to describe the "aging esophagus." Just like the other organs of the human body, the esophagus is subjected to age-related changes, but they are not as drastic as was made out to be initially. Symptoms of dysphagia occur after the age of 80 years. Esophageal peristalsis is reduced in the elderly along with changes in the upper esophageal sphincter.

66 Foreign Bodies in Esophagus

Ashok S. Naik

The competency covered in this chapter is as follows:

EN4.49 Elicit, document, and present a correct history; demonstrate and describe the clinical features; choose the correct investigations; and describe the principles of management of foreign bodies in the air and food passages.

Introduction

Foreign body ingestion is a common condition, especially among children, mentally challenged individuals, and psychiatric patients. Roughly 80% of patients visiting an emergency department for an esophageal foreign body are children. The type of foreign body ingested varies depending on the age group. Foreign bodies impacted in the esophagus need endoscopic removal with either a rigid esophagoscope or a flexible fiberoptic endoscope.

Etiology

Most foreign bodies are swallowed accidentally. Sometimes, it may be due to intentional ingestion, either for suicidal or homicidal purpose.

- The commonest foreign body seen in children are coins. Buttons, toy parts, marbles, safety pins, disk batteries, and magnets are also reported.
- But in adults, it is usually due to food getting impacted, especially a bolus of meat. Loose-fitting dentures and narrowing of the esophagus due to strictures or growth, (benign or malignant) are additional risk factors. Adults in an inebriated state may swallow large boluses of food, sometimes with attached bone, which may get impacted in the esophagus. Other common foreign bodies in adults include dentures and metallic wires.
- Blunt and smooth foreign bodies that have passed beyond the esophagus usually pass uneventfully through the intestinal tract. The foreign bodies tend to get impacted at sites of normal constrictions of the esophagus like the cricopharynx, arch of aorta, left main bronchus, and lower esophageal sphincter. Children and mentally challenged individuals may swallow multiple foreign bodies.

Presentation

- The patient usually presents with a history of foreign body ingestion, following which they have difficulty in swallowing and or pain during swallowing, especially in cases of sharp foreign bodies.
- Sensation of choking, drooling of saliva, and respiratory distress are other symptoms.
- In children, sudden onset of dysphagia without any fever should be evaluated for foreign body unless proven otherwise.
- Chest pain may signify a perforation.
- There may be a history of recurrent impaction of food due to a prior lesion like a stricture.
- On indirect laryngoscopy, pooling of saliva in the pyriform fossa is seen.

Management

■ Investigations

Plain X-Ray: Neck

Anteroposterior and lateral views and chest X-ray posteroanterior and lateral views are taken to localize the site of foreign body impaction (**Figs. 66.1** and **66.2**). It may also show associated changes like abscess formation and surgical emphysema.

Plain X-Ray: Abdomen

The radiograph is also taken to locate a foreign body (especially smooth and blunt) that may have gone down (**Fig. 66.3**). When the radiograph is taken along with neck and chest, it may show multiple foreign bodies.

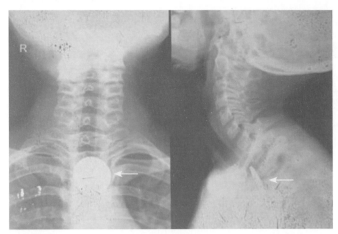

Fig. 66.1 Posteroanterior (PA) and lateral views of the neck showing the radio-opaque foreign body (coin).

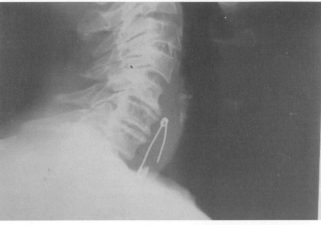

Fig. 66.2 Lateral view of the neck showing a radio-opaque sharp foreign body (safety pin) at the cricopharynx.

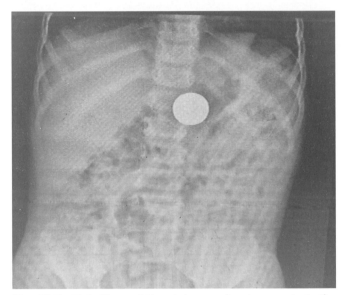

Fig. 66.3 Plain X-ray of the abdomen showing a coin in the stomach.

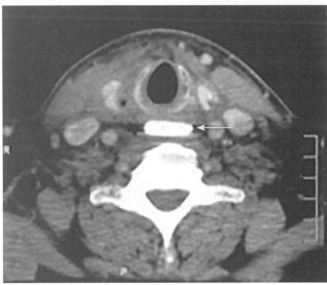

Fig. 66.4 Computed tomography (CT) scan of the neck showing radio-opaque foreign body (*yellow arrow*).

Barium Swallow

It may be helpful in non-radio-opaque foreign bodies. It shows a filling defect. Gastrografin is used (instead of barium) when a perforation is suspected.

> **Pearl**
>
> Gastrografin (sodium amidotrizoate) is a contrast medium that is swallowed by the patient after which an X-ray is taken to delineate the borders of the esophagus and stomach. A barium swallow is not used when a perforation is suspected because it is an irritant. Gastrografin contrast material is less irritating to the surrounding tissues and airway if it leaks out through a perforation.

CT Scan of Neck and Chest

Computed tomography (CT) scan may be needed to locate the foreign body (**Fig. 66.4**). It is the imaging of choice for nonopaque foreign bodies and when a perforation, extraluminal migration, proximal to a major vessel or abscess is suspected.

■ Treatment

Foreign bodies can be removed by using rigid or flexible fiberoptic endoscope. Rigid esophagoscopy is preferably done under general anesthesia, especially in children, as the endotracheal tube protects the airway. After removal of any foreign body, it is good to reexamine the esophagus (check scopy) to find (1) any mucosal erosions/trauma/perforation, (2) the cause for impaction of foreign body–like stricture, and (3) the second foreign body. Impacted dentures with metal wires and safety pins should be removed carefully after disimpacting any sharp parts that have pierced the mucosa, and removed along with the scope. For impacted sharp foreign bodies in the cervical esophagus or extraluminal migration, an open approach (cervical esophagostomy) and removal may be required. For impacted sharp foreign bodies in the thoracic esophagus, a thoracotomy may be needed. Occasionally, use of fluoroscopy (C-arm) may be required to find the exact location of the foreign body and its subsequent removal. The C-arm is a mobile X-ray machine used for taking intraoperative x-rays in the operation theater.

Pearl

Early intervention is required when there is absolute dysphagia, impending airway compromise, sharp foreign bodies, button batteries, magnets, long foreign bodies, and prolonged impaction.

Complications

- Perforation of the esophagus with surgical emphysema (**Figs. 66.5** and **66.6**). This can be caused by sharp foreign bodies, button batteries, and long-standing foreign bodies due to pressure necrosis.
- Periesophageal cellulitis or abscess seen with long-standing, impacted sharp foreign bodies (**Figs. 66.7** and **66.8**).
- Ulceration leading to stricture.
- Respiratory obstruction can occur if there is tracheal obstruction anteriorly or laryngeal edema due to infection.
- Bleeding will occur if the sharp foreign body pierces through the esophageal wall or becomes extraluminal and injure a major vessel. Button batteries can erode through the esophageal wall to involve a major vessel and lead to torrential bleeding and death.

Pearl

Button batteries have a heavy metal cover and contains sodium or potassium hydroxide. The action on the tissues is rapid leading to perforation and mediastinitis, sometimes involving the major blood vessels leading to death (even after removal). Early removal and observation for a few days is mandatory.

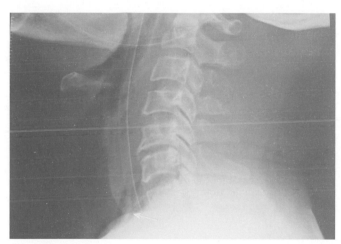

Fig. 66.5 Lateral view of the neck showing surgical emphysema.

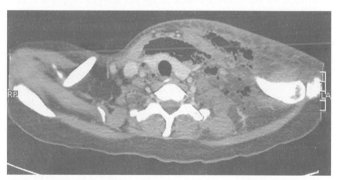

Fig. 66.6 Axial computed tomography (CT) scan showing surgical emphysema (*dark space*) in the neck due to a sharp foreign body of the esophagus perforating the wall.

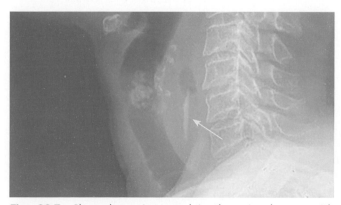

Fig. 66.7 Sharp bone impacted in the cricopharynx with abscess.

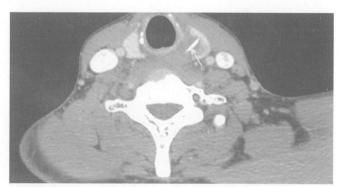

Fig. 66.8 Axial computed tomography (CT) scan with contrast showing extraluminal migration of a sharp foreign body out of the esophagus and into the neck.

Points to Ponder

- Foreign bodies in the esophagus are common and are usually accidental.
- The commonest foreign bodies in children are coins and in adults, bolus of meat or bones, and dentures.
- Dysphagia and odynophagia are two common symptoms.
- Plain X-ray of the neck, chest, and abdomen may have to be taken in order to localize the foreign body as well as to rule out multiple foreign bodies.
- Treatment involves removal as early as possible by either flexible or rigid esophagoscopy (see Chapter 67).
- Complications include perforation, abscess formation, ulceration, and bleeding.

Case-Based Questions

1. A 5-year-old child was brought to the emergency room with a 4-hour history of difficulty in swallowing. The mother observed the child putting something in his mouth followed by a choking sensation and drooling of saliva from the mouth. What is the next step in the management of this child?

Answer

Children are attracted by shiny, bright objects like coins. To rule out a foreign body in the food passage, x-rays of the neck are taken first since the commonest site for impaction is in the region of the cricopharyngeal sphincter, opposite to the C6 vertebra. X-rays may have to be taken of the thorax and abdomen, if the foreign body is not localized in the neck X-ray. Then under general anesthesia, a rigid esophagoscopy is performed to take out the foreign body.

2. A 6-year-old girl was brought to the hospital with a 4-hour history of fever, severe vomiting, and neck and epigastric pain. History revealed an accidental ingestion of a button or disk battery. What is the management of this patient?

Answer

Button batteries contain sodium hydroxide or potassium hydroxide and can lead to necrosis of the walls of the esophagus and subsequent peroration. Therefore, an attempt is made to retrieve the battery as early as possible, ideally within 2 hours of ingestion to avoid esophageal burns. The patient is kept fasting and a flexible esophagoscopy is performed to remove the battery after localizing it by taking an X-ray. If the battery size is greater than 15 mm in diameter, a rigid esophagoscopy may be required rather than a flexible one.

3. A 62-year-old man presented with acute-onset dysphagia with lower neck pain. There was a history of the patient using dentures with wires, which could not be traced. What is the management?

Answer

Dentures with metal wires tend to get impacted. If the wire goes through the mucosa, it can be in close proximity to the major vessels. A CT scan should be done to note the site and the relation to any vessel. Esophagoscopy has to be done under general anesthesia for the removal after disimpaction from the mucosa. Rarely, an external approach may be required.

Frequently Asked Questions

1. What is the commonest foreign body encountered in children?
2. Where is the first site of impaction of a foreign body in the esophagus and why?
3. What are the problems associated with a sharp foreign body?
4. What investigation would you prefer when there is a radio-opaque foreign body lodged at the C6 vertebral level?
5. What is the management of a smooth foreign body that has passed into the stomach?

Endnote

The first person to describe the symptoms of rupture of the esophagus was Herman Boerhaave, a Dutch physician, in 1724. The rupture he described was due to increased esophageal pressure after forceful vomiting. It can also occur during delivery or lifting heavy weights. This type of spontaneous rupture is also known as Boerhaave's syndrome, whereas a tear of the mucosa of the esophagus with subsequent bleeding, but not rupture, is known as Mallory–Weiss syndrome.

67 Esophagoscopy

Ashok S. Naik

The competencies covered in this chapter are as follows:

EN2.13 Identify, resuscitate, and manage ear, nose, and throat (ENT) emergencies in a simulated environment (including tracheostomy, anterior nasal packing, and removal of foreign bodies in the ear, nose, throat, and upper respiratory tract).

EN3.4 Observe and describe the indications for and steps involved in the removal of foreign bodies from the ear, nose, and throat.

Introduction

Esophagoscopy is a procedure to visualize the lumen and mucosal lining of the esophagus for diagnostic and therapeutic purposes. The esophagus starts at the cricopharynx, which corresponds to the lower border of the cricoid cartilage. The cervical esophagus curves to the left. It is again in the midline at T5, turns to left at T7, and follows the anteroposterior curve of the thoracic vertebra. These curvatures along with the normal constrictions, that is, the cricopharynx, the arch of the aorta, the left main bronchus, and at the level of the diaphragm (which are 15, 25, 27, and 40 cm, respectively, from the upper incisors) are important to know and keep in mind while negotiating the esophagoscope.

Types of Esophagoscopy

- Rigid (**Fig. 67.1**).
- Flexible fiberoptic (**Fig. 67.2**).

Indications for Esophagoscopy

■ Diagnostic

- It is done to evaluate the causes of dysphagia and hematemesis. This procedure allows you to evaluate the esophagus to rule out growths, ulcer strictures, or any other mass that may lead to dysphagia or hematemesis.
- Biopsy is taken from a suspicious area to confirm the diagnosis.
- In gastroesophageal reflux disease (GERD), esophagoscopy helps assess the mucosal changes, especially at the lower end of the esophagus. Changes in the mucosa results in a condition called Barrett's esophagus.
- It is done as a part of the panendoscopy procedure in head and neck cancers, especially in cervical metastatic lymph node carcinoma with an unknown primary. This will allow a primary in the esophagus to be ruled out.
- It is done following caustic ingestion and for assessment of esophageal trauma.
- Placement of capsules that monitor pH is done via esophagoscopy.

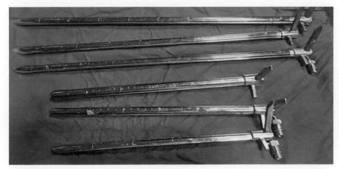

Fig. 67.1 Rigid esophagoscopy set.

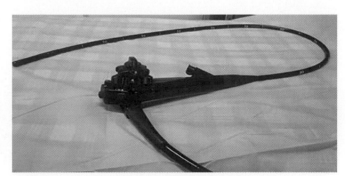

Fig. 67.2 Flexible fiberoptic esophagoscope.

- Following treatment, like radiotherapy for esophageal malignancy, esophagoscopy is done for assessment of the primary site to note the response to treatment.

Pearl

Panendoscopy (peroral) refers to a triple endoscopy performed to make a detailed search of the aerodigestive tract to look for an unknown primary. It includes direct laryngoscopy, esophagoscopy, and bronchoscopy.

■ Therapeutic

- It is commonly done to remove a foreign body. For large foreign bodies, a rigid endoscope is required.
- Dilatation of the esophageal web or stricture (with or without stenting), and in achalasia cardia.
- Removal of benign neoplasms like papilloma and fibroma.
- Resection of a malignant mass leading to obstruction and dysphagia. Palliative resection can be done using laser. Stents are often placed after resection in malignancies to keep the lumen patent.
- During tracheoesophageal puncture (TEP), after total laryngectomy, to visualize the lumen for the site of puncture. TEP is a procedure performed after laryngectomy in order to make a fistula between the posterior wall of trachea and the pharynx behind to allow air to flow up the pharynx and allow vibration and sound production.
- In the treatment of pharyngeal diverticulum and cricopharyngeal myotomy, the endoscopic-guided procedure can be done.
- Treatment of esophageal varices.
- Injection of botulinum toxin.

Contraindications for Esophagoscopy

- Bleeding disorders and aneurysm of the aorta are the main contraindications.
- In severe trauma to the cervical spine, and in lesions like Pott's spine and cervical spondylosis, rigid endoscope cannot be used.
- Rigid endoscope is difficult when the neck movements and mouth opening are restricted. A flexible endoscope is used in these conditions.

Rigid Esophagoscopy

This procedure is performed preferably under general anesthesia along with medications to reduce oropharyngeal secretions. It is useful for the evaluation of the esophageal lumen and mucosal lining, especially the proximal part.

For the postcricoid region and cervical esophagus, a hypopharyngoscope or esophageal speculum is preferred. With the use of the rigid endoscope, larger instruments and suction can be used. Removal of foreign bodies, especially if it is large, is easier with a rigid endoscope. Radiography of the neck and chest should be done prior to a rigid esophagoscopy, particularly for conditions like ingestion of sharp foreign bodies and for tumors. A contrast esophagogram, prior to surgery, will help delineate a lesion if present.

There are two basic types of rigid esophagoscopes based on their site of illumination: the Jackson esophagoscope has distal illumination and therefore less brightness at the site of visualization and the Negus esophagoscope has proximal illumination and although it has good illumination, it gets soiled by secretions easily.

■ Procedure

The patient is placed in the supine position with a pillow placed under the shoulder and neck extended. (The Boyce position or the sword swallowing position can be used.) After placing a head drape, examine the teeth and lips. Teeth guard or wet gauze is inserted to protect the upper teeth. The lubricated esophagoscope of appropriate size is held in the right hand, introduced through the right side of the mouth, and advanced toward midline (**Fig. 67.3**).

The epiglottis, endotracheal tube, and arytenoids are identified. Keeping the tip of the scope in the midline behind the larynx, the hypopharynx is opened up with a slow and gentle movement and the scope is pushed further distally till it reaches the cricopharyngeal sphincter. This may require gentle pressure or deflation of the endotracheal tube cuff or the use of muscle relaxant by the anesthetist in order to relax the cricopharyngeal sphincter, which is normally closed. The tip of the esophagoscope is guided into the upper part of the esophagus, after bypassing the sphincter (**Fig. 67.4**). It is important to always keep the lumen of the esophagus under vision when advancing the scope to prevent perforation of the esophagus.

While advancing through the thoracic esophagus, the shoulders and chest may have to be repositioned to align the scope with the lumen. At the cardiac end of the esophagus (lower end), the mucosa is usually red and velvety (**Fig. 67.5**). During withdrawal of the scope, inspect the esophagus again. Biopsy, if required, is done toward the end to avoid blood from obscuring the view during assessment.

Complications

- Trauma to the lips, teeth, tongue, and palate can occur during introduction of the scope. In the pharynx, there can be injury to the posterior pharyngeal wall and dislocation of the arytenoid.

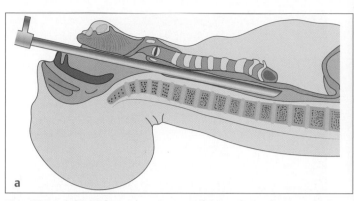
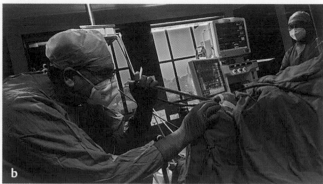

Fig. 67.3 **(a)** Rigid esophagoscopy. **(b)** Rigid esophagoscopy being carried out.

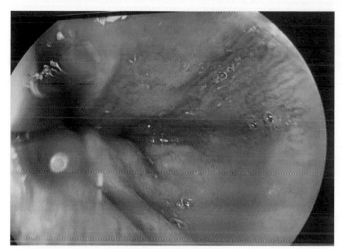

Fig. 67.4 Upper end of the esophagus.

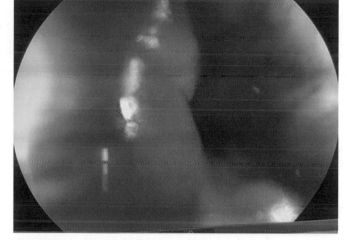

Fig. 67.5 Lower end of the esophagus.

- Within the lumen, esophageal mucosa can be traumatized leading to bleeding or perforation of the esophagus can occur.
- Cardiac stress during the procedure can lead to arrhythmias, ectopia, and bradycardia.

Pearl

Perforation of the esophagus is a dangerous complication with a high mortality if not detected and treated early. The patient will develop vomiting, chest pain or interscapular pain, and subcutaneous emphysema, also known as *Mackler's triad*. Perforation is more common when there is mucosal inflammation (after acid or alkali ingestion), after radiotherapy, poor technique by an inexperienced surgeon, or while trying to maneuver around tumors.

Prevention: Careful, gentle handling of the scope, and advancing only when the lumen is visualized. Catheters are used as guides when the lumen is not visualized.

Flexible Esophagoscopy

It can be done under sedation using topical anesthesia with relatively less morbidity. The diameter of the scope is 10 to 12 mm. There is good magnification and it allows for diagnosis of mucosal diseases including that of the stomach and duodenum. It can be done in patients with spinal abnormalities.

Flexible endoscopy is indicated for the following:
- Assessing esophageal lesions and taking a biopsy.
- Removal of small foreign bodies.
- Dilatation of webs and strictures.
- Injection of a sclerosing agent.

■ Procedure

The patient is placed in the left lateral position (**Fig. 67.6**). The lubricated scope is inserted into the mouth through a plastic mouth gag. The scope is advanced to visualize the epiglottis, pharynx, and postcricoid region. The patient is

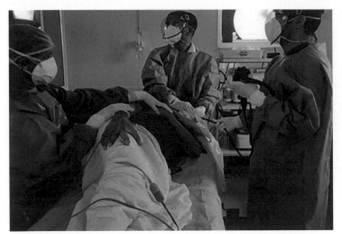

Fig. 67.6 Flexible esophagoscopy being carried out.

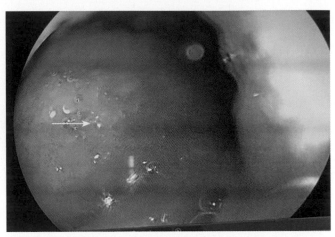

Fig. 67.7 Pseudocyst of the esophagus.

asked to swallow and as the cricopharynx opens, the scope is advanced into the esophagus. Air or water insufflation opens the lumen of the esophagus and the esophagoscope is guided into the lower end. It allows a clear, magnified view of the various lesions (**Fig. 67.7**).

Transnasal Esophagoscopy

It is performed under topical anesthesia of the nose and oropharynx, without sedation and hence is more comfortable for the patient with minimal risk. The diameter of the scope is 4.5 to 5.1 mm. It has channels for insufflation, suction, and instrumentation, including laser.

The patient is in the sitting or 45-degree reclining position. The scope is held using the standard vertical or the fishing pole technique. It can be used even in patients with trismus and restricted neck movements. It can be advanced to visualize the stomach also. Prior to withdrawing the scope from the stomach, excess air should be removed by suction.

Points to Ponder

- Rigid esophagoscopy and flexible esophagoscopy are valuable procedures for evaluation and treatment of esophageal disease.
- The cricopharyngeal sphincter is normally closed, so care must be taken when negotiating this region to avoid perforations.
- Rigid scopies, when being performed, must take into account the four sites of narrowing in the esophagus as well as the curvatures.
- Flexible esophagoscopy is an outpatient procedure, whereas rigid ones are ideally done in a controlled setting such as the operation theater.
- Always assess the limitation of neck movements or any cervical spine abnormalities before positioning for a rigid esophagoscopy.
- The commonest complication of a rigid scopy is perforation.

Case-Based Question

1. **A 45-year-old man reported to the emergency room with a 1-day history of ingestion of a chicken bone. X-ray revealed the bone and a scopy was performed for removal. Postoperatively, he developed neck pain, vomiting, and interscapular pain.**

   a. What is the commonest site for impaction of the bone?

   b. What complication was observed postoperatively?

   c. How will you manage this acute condition that he has now developed?

Answers

1a. The commonest site is at the first constriction of the esophagus, that is, the cricopharyngeal sphincter.

1b. Postoperatively, the patient developed symptoms related to a perforation of the cervical esophagus.

1c. A plain x-ray of the neck and chest will show free air. Antibiotics should be started to control the infection due to the flow of fluid from the esophagus into the tissues of the neck. If possible, a nasogastric tube is to be inserted for feeding. If perforation is confirmed, and it is large, the patient will have to be taken up for repair of the tear. If it is a small perforation, it may be treated conservatively.

Frequently Asked Questions

1. What are the common instruments used for esophagoscopy?

2. What are the indications for rigid esophagoscopy?

3. What are the complications associated with esophagoscopy?

4. Where are the normal sites of constrictions in the esophagus?

5. What are the symptoms of an esophageal perforation?

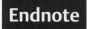

Adolph Kussmaul used a urethroscope for esophagoscopy in 1868. He learned how to position the head for directing the scope after observing a sword swallower. Chevalier Jackson (1908) pioneered the distally illuminated rigid esophagoscope and standardized the technique.

68 Anatomy of the Neck

Amit Kumar Sharma

The competencies covered in this chapter are as follows:

EN1.1 Describe the anatomy and physiology of head and neck.

AN39.2 Explain the anatomical basis of hypoglossal nerve palsy.

Introduction

The neck contains many important structures related to the upper aerodigestive tract and nerves and vessels which if compromised can lead to morbidity and mortality. The upper limit of neck is formed anteriorly by floor of mouth; posteriorly it is formed by the base of skull. The first rib and first thoracic vertebra form the lower limits of the neck.

Triangles of Neck

The sternocleidomastoid muscle divides the neck into anterior and posterior triangles. These are further subdivided by the digastric and omohyoid muscles.

■ Anterior Triangle

It is bounded by:
- The midline of the neck anteriorly.
- The anterior margin of sternocleidomastoid posteriorly.
- The lower border of body of mandible superiorly as the base.

Anterior triangle is further divided into four triangles by the anterior belly and posterior belly of the digastric, and the superior belly of the omohyoid (**Fig. 68.1**).

- *Submental triangle* is bound by anterior belly of digastric on both sides, with the hyoid bone as its base. It contains submental lymph nodes; the tip of tongue drains here (**Fig. 68.2**).
- *Submandibular triangle* is bounded by the anterior and posterior bellies of the digastric muscle along with the lower border of the mandible as its base. Its contents are submandibular salivary gland, submandibular lymph nodes, facial vessels, and marginal mandibular and cervical branches of facial nerve and hypoglossal nerve (**Fig. 68.3**).
- *Carotid triangle* boundaries are formed by the posterior belly of digastric, the superior belly of omohyoid, and the sternocleidomastoid muscle. Its contents are lymph nodes, carotid sheath, and the common carotid artery and its bifurcation into the external carotid artery (ECA) and internal carotid artery (ICA). The bifurcation is the site of carotid body tumor (**Fig. 68.4**).

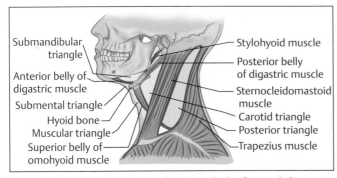

Fig. 68.1 Anterior triangle of neck with the four subdivisions.

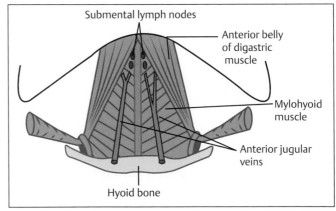

Fig. 68.2 Boundaries and contents of the submental triangle.

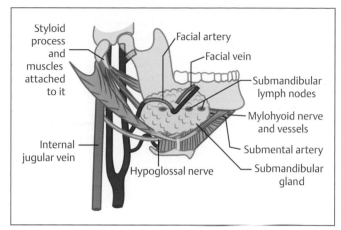

Fig. 68.3 Boundaries and contents of the submandibular triangle.

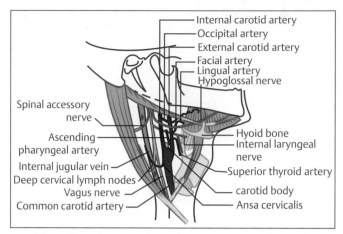

Fig. 68.4 Boundaries and contents of the carotid triangle.

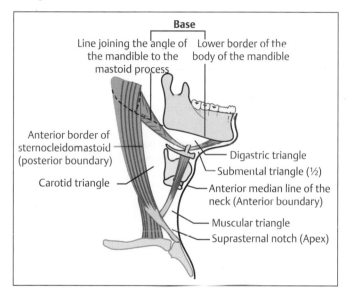

Fig. 68.5 Boundaries and contents of the muscular triangle.

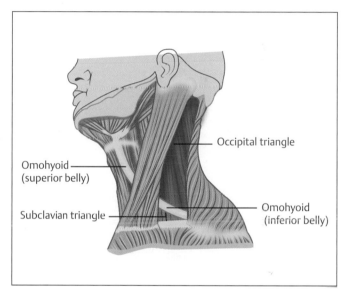

Fig. 68.6 Posterior triangle of neck with the two subdivisions.

- *Muscular triangle* is bounded by the median line of the neck, the anterior margin of the sternocleidomastoid, and the superior belly of the omohyoid. Its contents are infrahyoid muscles (thyrohyoid, sternothyroid, sternohyoid), vessels (superior and inferior thyroid arteries, and anterior jugular veins), and the deeper structures like thyroid and parathyroid glands, larynx, trachea, and esophagus (**Fig. 68.5**).

■ Posterior Triangle

The boundaries of the posterior triangle are formed by:
- Anterior border of trapezius.
- Clavicle inferiorly.
- Posterior border of sternocleidomastoid anteriorly.

The inferior belly of omohyoid divides posterior triangle into two parts—occipital triangle and subclavian triangle (**Fig. 68.6**).

The roof of the posterior triangle is formed by the investing layer of the deep cervical fascia stretching from the trapezius to the sternocleidomastoid muscle anteriorly. The structures piercing the roof include four cutaneous branches of the cervical plexus and the external jugular vein. This is depicted in **Fig. 68.7.**

The floor of the posterior triangle is formed by four muscles (**Fig. 68.8**):
- Semispinalis capitis.
- Splenius capitis.
- Levator scapulae.
- Scalenus medius.

There is a layer of deep cervical fascia which covers the muscular floor of the posterior triangle and forms a sheath around the subclavian artery and the brachial plexus.

The contents of the posterior triangle are shown in **Fig. 68.9.**

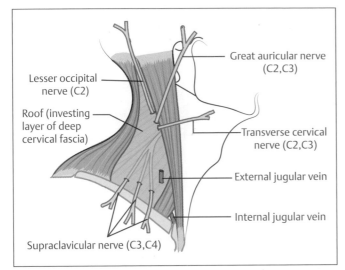

Fig. 68.7 Structures piercing the roof of the posterior triangle.

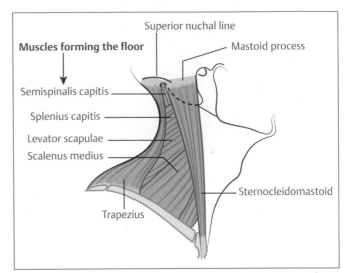

Fig. 68.8 Floor of the posterior triangle formed by four muscles.

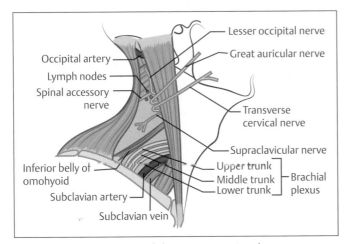

Fig. 68.9 The contents of the posterior triangle.

The two subdivisions of the posterior triangle are:
- *Occipital triangle*: It is bound by the posterior border of sternocleidomastoid, the anterior border of trapezius, and the inferior belly of omohyoid. Its contents are spinal accessory nerve, external jugular vein, subclavian artery, lymph nodes, nerves of cervical plexus, and brachial plexus trunks.
- *Subclavian triangle*: It is bound by the posterior border of sternocleidomastoid, the inferior border of omohyoid, and the clavicle. Its contents are the third part of the subclavian artery, the brachial plexus trunks, the nerve to subclavius, and the lymph nodes.

Erb's Point

The midpoint of the posterior border of the sternocleidomastoid muscle is known as Erb's point. From this point, five nerves emerge from behind the muscle:
- Lesser occipital nerve.

- Great auricular nerve.
- Transverse cervical nerve.
- Spinal accessory nerve.
- Supraclavicular nerve.

Surgical implication: Erb's point is made use of to identify the spinal accessory nerve during neck dissection.

Cervical Fascia

■ Superficial Fascia

It is the subcutaneous layer of connective tissue present just beneath the skin. It contains the platysma, cutaneous nerves, blood, and lymphatic vessels. There is varying amount of adipose tissue within it. There is space present between the superficial fascia and investing layer of deep cervical fascia, which has the following structures present within:
- Adipose tissue.
- Sensory nerves.
- Vessels: External and anterior jugular veins.
- Superficial lymphatics.

■ Deep Cervical Fascia

It has three layers (**Fig. 68.10**):
- *Superficial investing layer* which encapsulates the parotid gland and submandibular gland. It also encloses two spaces: The supraclavicular space and suprasternal space of Burns.

  It has following attachments:
  – External occipital protuberance and superior nuchal line superiorly.

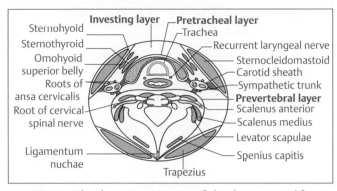

Fig. 68.10 The three components of the deep cervical fascia.

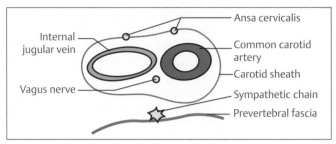

Fig. 68.11 Carotid sheath and its contents.

- Mastoid process and zygomatic arch laterally.
- Spine of scapula, acromion, clavicle, and manubrium of sternum inferiorly.
- Middle visceral (*pretracheal*) layer begins superiorly at the hyoid bone and end inferiorly in the upper thoracic cavity.
  - Anteriorly, it crosses the neck just posterior to the infrahyoid muscles and covers the trachea and thyroid.
  - Laterally, it covers the thyroid gland and esophagus.
  - Posteriorly, it is referred to as the buccopharyngeal fascia which separates the pharynx and esophagus from the prevertebral layers.
- Deep *prevertebral layer* is attached posteriorly to the ligamentum nuchae and cervical spine. It divides into two divisions at the transverse processes of cervical vertebra:
  - Prevertebral division: It extends from the skull base up to the coccyx, extending laterally as the axillary sheath. It helps in gliding movement of pharynx during the swallowing. It splits and encloses various structures like muscles (vertebral, deep posterior triangle, and scalene), vessels (vertebral and subclavian), and nerves (phrenic and brachial plexus).
  - Alar division: It lies between the visceral layer of middle layer and prevertebral division of deep layer of deep cervical fascia. Visceral layer of middle layer fuses posteriorly with the alar division of prevertebral fascia at T2 level, forming the anterior wall of retropharyngeal space.

Carotid sheath is a column of fascia receiving contribution from the investing fascia, pretracheal fascia, and prevertebral fascia. It encloses the common carotid artery, the ICA, the internal jugular vein, and the vagus nerve (**Fig. 68.11**).

Lymph Nodes of the Neck

The lymph glands of the neck consist of:
- Horizontal chain.
- Vertical chain.

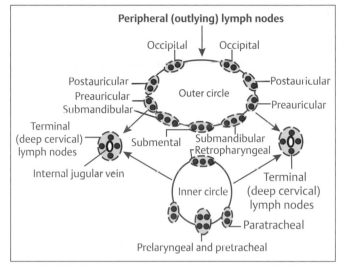

Fig. 68.12 Horizontal group of lymph nodes divided into an outer and inner ring.

■ Horizontal Chain

It is divided into outer and inner circles and includes the following (**Fig. 68.12**):
- Occipital lymph node situated midway between the mastoid process and the external occipital protuberance.
  - Drains the back of the scalp.
- Posterior auricular group situated on the mastoid process behind the pinna.
  - Drains temporal region of the scalp, back of the pinna, and external auditory meatus.
- Preauricular node situated immediately in front of the tragus.
  - Drains outer surface of the pinna and side of the scalp.
- Parotid group situated both in the substance of the parotid gland and deep to it.
  - Drains eyelids, front of the scalp, external auditory meatus, tympanic cavity, and nasopharynx.
- Facial group has three nodes:
  - Infraorbital situated below the orbit; drains the conjunctiva and eyelids.
  - Buccinator situated near the angle of mouth; drains the nose.
  - Supramandibular situated in front of Masseter; drains the cheek.

- Submandibular or submaxillary situated in close contact with the submandibular gland.
  - Drains side of nose, inner angle of eye, cheek, whole of upper lip, outer part of lower lip, the gums, and side of tongue.
- Submental situated in the submental triangle.
  - Drains central part of lower lip, floor of the mouth, and tip of tongue.
- Superficial cervical situated on the outer surface of the sternomastoid around the external jugular vein.
  - Drains parotid region and part of the pinna.
- Anterior cervical consists of:
  - Infrahyoid situated near the midline of neck—drains larynx.
  - Prelaryngeal situated in front of larynx—drains thyroid.
  - Pretracheal situated in front of trachea—drains trachea.

All the lymph from the glands enumerated above drain to the deep cervical chain.

■ Vertical or Deep Chain of Lymph Nodes

The deep chain is classified into:
- Anterior—related to the anterior border of the sternomastoid.
- Posterior—related to the posterior border of the sternomastoid.

Each is further subdivided into upper and lower depending upon the relationship to the point of bifurcation of the common carotid artery (hyoid bone) and to the inferior belly of the omohyoid muscle.

The cervical lymph node levels are discussed in Chapter 73 "Cervical Lymphatic System and Neck Dissection."

Points to Ponder

- The neck can be divided into anterior and posterior triangles.
- The anterior triangle is further subdivided into submental, submandibular, carotid, and muscular triangles.
- The posterior triangle is further divided into occipital and subclavian triangles.
- The deep cervical fascia has three layers: the investing layer, pretracheal, and prevertebral layers.
- Cervical neck nodes are arranged into circular and vertical chains.

Case-Based Question

1. **A 59-year-old man was admitted with complaints of painful swallowing and loss of weight with a mass over the right side of neck. Investigations revealed a pyriform malignancy of the right side with lymph node metastasis in the upper part of the right neck.**

   a. If the lymph node metastasis is in the anterior triangle, which subdivision is commonly affected?

   b. What are the boundaries of this triangle?

   c. If the lymph node metastasis is found in the posterior triangle, which subdivision is commonly affected?

   d. What are the contents of the occipital triangle?

Answers

a. Carotid triangle. This is where the Level II lymph nodes are situated, and they are commonly affected by pyriform malignancy.

b. Submandibular triangle is bound by the anterior and posterior bellies of the digastric muscle along with the lower border of the mandible as its base.

c. Occipital triangle.

d. The contents of the occipital triangle are spinal accessory nerve, external jugular vein, subclavian artery, lymph nodes, nerves of cervical plexus, and brachial plexus trunks.

Frequently Asked Questions

1. What are the components of the carotid triangle?
2. Name the structures within the carotid sheath.
3. What are the contents of the submandibular triangle?
4. Name the parts of the deep cervical fascia.
5. Which muscles form the floor of the posterior triangle?

Endnote

The importance of spread of malignancy to the cervical lymph nodes has been known for over 100 years. In the 19th century, metastatic nodes were generally considered as a sign of incurability. But in 1846, John Collins Warren proved that theory wrong. Till that time the general belief was that neck dissection was impossible. He demonstrated a neck mass excision at Massachusetts General Hospital under anesthesia using ether. The wide publicity surrounding this landmark event gave birth to modern general anesthesia, longer operating time, and better vascular control.

Examination of the Neck

Amit Kumar Sharma

The competency covered in this chapter is as follows:

EN2.7 Demonstrate the correct technique of examination of the neck including elicitation of the laryngeal crepitus.

History

A detailed history is necessary to evaluate various swellings and lesions involving the neck.

- *Age*: Some swellings are age specific, for example, a sternomastoid tumor is congenital, cystic hygroma is seen in infants, and malignant swellings are common in the older age group.
- *Swelling*: Onset and duration of swelling should be sought. A swelling with a long history is more likely to be benign. Rapidly growing swellings are usually malignant. Swellings due to acute inflammation also have a short duration.
- *Pain*: Inflammatory swellings are painful and malignant swellings are painless unless there is nerve involvement, seen in advanced stages. A swelling in the submandibular region seen, during meals with pain, can be suggestive of calculi within the submandibular gland duct.
- Related history like throat pain, dysphagia, odynophagia, breathing difficulty, change in voice, and cough should be sought.
- History of trauma and prior surgery should be taken.
- Family history of thyroid swellings including medullary carcinoma should be noted.

Local Examination (Video 69.1)

■ Inspection

There should be proper exposure of neck during examination, that is, till the level of nipples.

- *Attitude of the neck*: The neck in the neutral position has lordosis (mild anterior curve). Straightening can occur in retropharyngeal abscess and malignancy with prevertebral involvement.
- *Laryngeal framework* is normal. Look for splaying of the thyroid cartilage and fullness of the thyrohyoid membrane.

- It should be observed whether the trachea is central or deviated.
- It should be observed whether dilated veins are present.
- Presence of scars from a previous surgery or trauma should be noted.
- *Swelling*: Note the number, size, shape, location, and surface of the swelling. Based on site, one can get a differential diagnosis, for example, a branchial cyst swelling is in relation to the anterior border of the upper part of the sternomastoid muscle, submandibular gland tumors and plunging ranula are found in the submandibular triangle, the dermoid is always found in the midline of the neck, cystic hygroma is found in the lower part of the posterior triangle, and carotid body tumor is found at the level of the upper border of the thyroid cartilage. A swelling that moves with deglutition is attached to the larynx and trachea, for example, thyroid swelling, thyroglossal cyst, and subhyoid bursa. Multiple swellings are usually suggestive of lymph nodes.
- *Skin*: Look for a sinus, fistula, scar, or ulcer. In tuberculous lymphadenitis, a lymph node may burst to form a discharging sinus; it has undermined edges. On healing, it forms a puckered scar. Look for redness and edema, which indicate acute inflammation. Skin can be adhered to the underlying swelling indicating malignancy.

■ Palpation

This is done to confirm the inspection findings:

- *Swelling*: A neck swelling should be palpated from behind the patient. The head should be flexed toward the side of swelling to be palpated (**Fig. 69.1**).
  - Note the size, shape, surface, margin, and consistency.
  - The reducibility and change with cough impulse should be noted.
  - Mobility should be checked in the horizontal and vertical axes. A carotid body tumor can be moved in the horizontal axis but not along the length of the carotid artery.

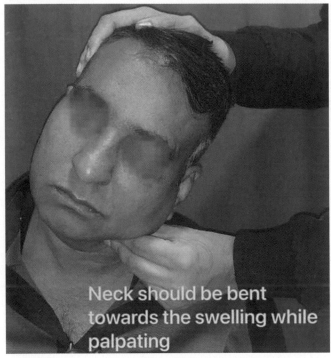

Fig. 69.1 Palpation of neck swellings with the head flexed.

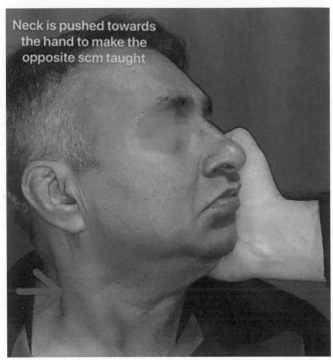

Fig. 69.2 Contracting the sternocleidomastoid muscles to find its relation to a neck swelling.

- Relation of the swelling with the sternocleidomastoid can be determined by contracting the muscle. If the swelling lies beneath the muscle, the swelling decreases in size and its mobility is reduced, whereas if the swelling lies above the muscle, it becomes more prominent and is mobile (**Fig. 69.2**).
- Try to pinch the skin above the swelling. In a malignant swelling adherent to the skin, the skin is not pinchable and cannot be glided over the swelling. Nonmalignant swellings with similar findings are sebaceous cysts, acute lymphadenitis, or cold abscesses.
- *Pulsatile or not*: If it is pulsatile, it should be checked whether it is transmitted or expansile. A swelling like an aneurysm that arises from an artery is expansile, whereas a swelling that lies above an artery gives transmitted pulsations.
- Cystic hygroma is brilliantly transilluminant. All cystic swellings including abscesses are fluctuant.
- *Lymph nodes*: A sequence should be followed in palpation. It should start from the supraclavicular group, followed by palpating the nodes of the posterior triangle, jugulo-omohyoid, jugulodigastric, submandibular, submental, preauricular, and the occipital groups. Examine the drainage area in case of enlarged nodes for inflammatory or neoplastic lesions. In case of multiple enlarged lymph nodes, examine the lymph nodes of the other parts like axillary and inguinal lymph nodes to rule out lymphoma.
- *Laryngeal crepitus*: For laryngeal crepitus, the thyroid cartilage is held and moved from one side to another

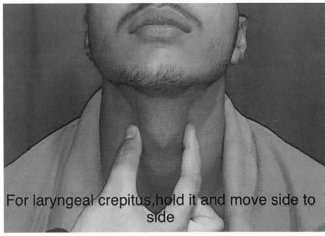

Fig. 69.3 Laryngeal crepitus being elicited during palpation.

horizontally (thyrovertebral) to feel the crepitus. It is absent in case of laryngeal/hypopharyngeal malignancies, trauma, and postradiation cases. The cricoid cartilage can also be moved horizontally against the vertebra (cricovertebral) to assess for crepitus (**Fig. 69.3**). Absence of laryngeal crepitus is called *Bocca's sign*.

■ Percussion

Although it is not very important in neck examination, it can be used in laryngocele where percussion gives a tympanic note. Percussion can also be carried out over the sternum to see if there is any retrosternal extension of a thyroid.

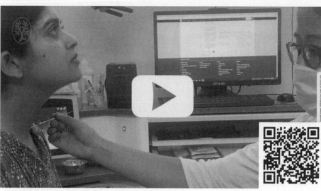

Video 69.1 Examination of neck.

■ Auscultation

A bruit may be heard on auscultation over a carotid body tumor.

Case-Based Question

1. **A 55-year-old man presented with 5-month history of difficulty in swallowing. It was gradual in onset and mainly toward solid food. He also complained of weight loss with a neck swelling developing in the upper part of the left side of the neck of 1-month duration.**

   a. What are the important clinical details to be elicited when examining the neck swelling?

   b. How will you elicit the laryngeal crepitus? What is its significance?

   Answers

   a. When a neck swelling is being examined, go through the standard process of inspection and palpation. Look at the site, size, shape, and surface of the swelling. Note the skin over the swelling. On palpation, see if there is any local rise in temperature, which can denote inflammation. Confirm your inspection findings. Look for consistency and mobility and determine the plane of the swelling. Hard swellings are a sign of metastatic disease in the lymph nodes.

   b. Move the larynx, with slight pressure posteriorly, from side to side. Feeling of a grating sensation is considered normal. If it is absent, it is a sign of soft tissue intervening between the laryngeal cartilage and the cervical vertebra behind.

Frequently Asked Questions

1. How will you determine the plane of a swelling in relation to the sternocleidomastoid muscle?

2. How will you elicit the laryngeal crepitus?

3. In which condition will you auscultate the neck?

4. What is the role of percussion of the neck?

5. Where does the examiner stand when palpating a neck swelling?

Endnote *A scabbard trachea is a tracheal deformity where the lateral walls are flattened and opposed to each other, resulting in tracheal compression. This can result in tracheal stenosis. It is called scabbard because, radiologically, the trachea looks like the sheath of a sword. Kocher's test is performed during thyroid examination to rule out scabbard trachea, which can be caused by tracheomalacia. The test is carried out by compressing the lateral lobes of the thyroid with the fingers. Kocher's test is positive if there is stridor. This is seen in multinodular goiter or malignancy of the thyroid.*

70 Diseases of the Salivary Glands

Bini Faizal

The competency covered in this chapter is as follows:

EN4.36 Describe the clinical features, investigations, and principles of management of diseases of the salivary glands.

Introduction

The parotid, submandibular, and sublingual glands are the three major pairs of salivary glands in the human body. In addition to this, numerous minor salivary glands are present in the mucosa of the oral cavity and pharynx. Over a 24-hour period, 1 to 1.5 L of saliva are secreted. The saliva is essential for taste, swallowing, speech, and maintenance of oral immunity through lysozymes and immunoglobulins. Saliva is 99% water and contains electrolytes, urea, lipids, amino acids, and proteins, including digestive and other enzymes and immunoglobulins. Saliva draining into the oral cavity is isotonic.

Stenson's duct (parotid duct) drains into the oral cavity adjacent to the upper second molar tooth. The submandibular duct (Wharton's duct) opens in the floor of the mouth at the sublingual papilla. Multiple sublingual ducts open into the submandibular duct. The sublingual glands secrete mucous saliva, the parotid glands secrete serous saliva, and the submandibular glands secrete both mucous and serous saliva (**Fig. 70.1**).

The neural control of salivation is a complex interaction of the sympathetic and parasympathetic nervous systems. Histologically, the salivary glands are composed of acinar cells (80%) and ductal cells (15%), along with nerves, connective tissues, and blood vessels. The inflammatory conditions of the salivary glands could be due to infective or inflammatory causes. The most common infective conditions are acute and chronic sialadenitis. These occur due to obstruction or other granulomatous conditions.

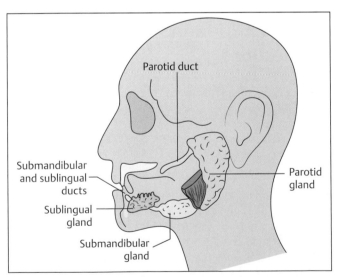

Fig. 70.1 Diagrammatic representation of the three major salivary glands.

Inflammatory Conditions of the Salivary Glands

■ Acute Viral Parotitis (Mumps)

Viral parotitis or mumps is an acute, self-limiting viral infection of the salivary glands, most commonly of the parotid. It is the commonest cause of salivary gland infection in children and is usually caused by paramyxovirus. The incidence has reduced with the universal measles, mumps, and rubella (MMR) vaccination. There is an incubation period of 2 to 3 weeks followed by a period of viremia when it localizes in the parotid gland, germinal tissues, and central nervous system. It spreads by droplet infection.

Clinical Features

The child will have fever, malaise, headache, trismus, and dysphagia. It may start from a single parotid gland and later may involve the other major salivary glands (**Fig. 70.2**).

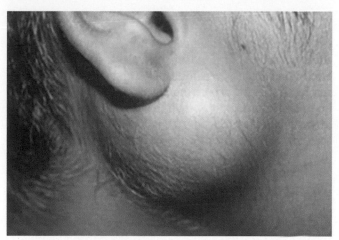

Fig. 70.2 Mumps affecting the right parotid gland.

The patient is infective 3 days before and 4 days after the onset of parotitis. After the prodromal period, one or both parotid glands will enlarge. In 80% of children, there is bilateral parotid swelling. It resolves spontaneously in about a week.

The swelling is associated with pain over the parotid due to stretching of the parotid fascia. There may be referred pain to the ear. The opening of the duct is inflamed, but there will be no pus emanating from it.

The blood picture may show leukocytopenia and the serum amylase may be raised.

Complications

- Orchitis can develop in 20 to 30% of males with mumps. This is the most common complication in adult males. Usually it appears during the first week of parotitis.
- Oophoritis can occur in 5% of females.
- It can cause sterility.
- Aseptic meningitis or meningoencephalitis may occur in 10% of cases. Indications of the central nervous system (CNS) involvement include headache, fever, nausea, and vomiting.
- Pancreatitis can occur in 5% of cases.
- Sensorineural hearing loss has been reported in 0.5 to 4% of cases. The sensorineural hearing loss is of rapid onset, unilateral, profound, and usually permanent. Tinnitus, ataxia, and vomiting precede hearing loss.

Treatment

- Supportive with analgesics like acetaminophen or ibuprofen.
- Adequate oral hydration and sialogogues are prescribed. Sialogogues promote secretion of saliva.
- Antibiotics are usually not required since this is a viral infection. Antivirals are not required as this is a self-limiting condition.
- Oral hygiene should be maintained.

Prevention

Routine administration of MMR vaccine is advisable. This is ideally given after the first year. It is advisable not to administer before that because of the presence of maternal antibodies, which can interfere with the seroconversion. A second dose should be given at age 4 to 6 years.

> **Pearl**
>
> Other viruses like influenza, parainfluenza, coxsackie, and echovirus can cause sialadenitis mimicking mumps. Cytomegalovirus and adenovirus can affect the salivary glands in human immunodeficiency virus (HIV) patients.

■ Acute Bacterial Sialadenitis

Acute bacterial infections have a similar clinical presentation to viral sialadenitis. The parotid gland is commonly involved. Multiple glands are rarely involved. *Staphylococcus aureus* is the most common organism. The other organisms involved are β-haemolytic streptococcus, *Haemophilus influenzae*, *Pneumococcus*, and gram-negative organisms.

Infection may reach the gland due to retrograde transmission of disease from oral cavity or due to stasis of salivary flow due to obstruction. Elderly patients on medications like diuretics, antidepressants, beta-blockers, anticholinergics, and antihistamines, which reduce the salivary flow, are also at high risk.

Clinical Features

The clinical presentation is with pain and swelling of the gland. Chewing becomes painful. On gentle pressure over the gland, pus may be seen extruding from the duct opening, which is usually inflamed. In parotitis, pus may be seen in the ipsilateral external auditory canal due to the communication via the fissures of Santorini.

Treatment

Antibiotics are started by the intravenous or oral route, depending on the severity. Depending on the virulence of the organism and the immune status of the patient, the sialadenitis may progress to abscess formation. This may lead to sepsis and multi-organ dysfunction in debilitated patients.

■ Chronic Sialadenitis

Chronic inflammation of the salivary glands is known as chronic sialadenitis. It presents as recurrent episodes of pain and swelling of the salivary glands, usually at mealtime.

It is more common in the parotid gland.

Etiology

- It is thought to be due to repeated attacks of acute sialadenitis, which leads to destruction of the acinar cells and lymphocytic infiltration, or due to obstruction of the duct by calculi or strictures.

Streptococcus viridans are the usual offending organisms. The causes for obstruction or inflammation have to be ruled out by investigations.

Inflammatory sialadenitis is due to immune-mediated disorders like Sjogren's syndrome, Wegener's granulomatosis (also known as granulomatosis with polyangitis or GPA), cat-scratch disease, sarcoidosis, tuberculosis, actinomycosis, toxoplasmosis, HIV, and lymphoma (**Fig. 70.3**).

■ Obstructive Sialadenitis

Sialolithiasis is the presence of stones or calculi within the salivary glands or ducts. These account for 50% of the causes for obstructive sialadenitis. It is seen in 1.2% of general population. Calculi are mostly seen in the submandibular gland (80%) followed by the parotid glands, and very rarely in the sublingual glands.

Reasons for increased frequency of stones in the submandibular gland are the following:
- Antigravity drainage of the submandibular gland.
- High mucin content of saliva.

- Greater concentration of calcium and phosphate in the saliva.
- High alkalinity.
- Superior, longer course of the submandibular duct.
- Kinking of the course of the submandibular duct as it hooks over the mylohyoid muscle.

Clinical Features

The patient presents with a *mealtime syndrome* characterized by pain and swelling of the salivary gland while having food. Later, the gland can get infected and abscess may develop. On examination, the gland is swollen and tender. The calculus may be palpable near the orifice of the salivary ducts. Pus is extruded on massaging the salivary gland.

Investigations

X-rays can detect submandibular stones in 80 to 95% of cases and parotid stones in 70% of cases (**Fig. 70.4**). The X-rays commonly taken are the submandibular occlusal view, a lateral oblique view of the mandible, and an orthopantomogram.

Ultrasound of the neck is useful in detecting a calculus if it is more than 2 mm.

A *computed tomography (CT) scan* can detect a calculus. It is useful in multiple calculi and when the calculi are in the deep part of the gland (**Fig. 70.5**).

Sialography, the conventional technique to define the ductal system by injecting dye into the ducts, is outdated.

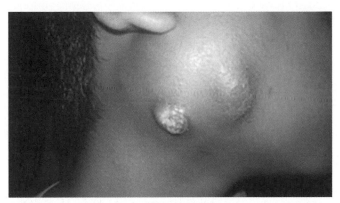

Fig. 70.3 A case of recurrent parotitis that on evaluation turned out to be Sjogren's syndrome.

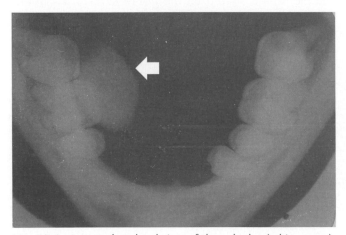

Fig. 70.4 Intraoral occlusal view of the calculus (*white arrow*).

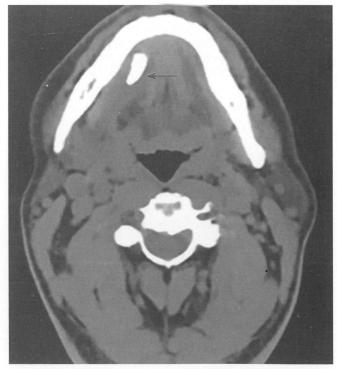

Fig. 70.5 Computed tomography (CT) scan showing a large calculus in the right submandibular duct.

A *magnetic resonance imaging (MRI) sialography* is preferred. An *MRI scan* is mainly used to evaluate the ductal system, especially strictures (MRI sialography), and to rule out glandular pathology and tumors.

Sialendoscopy is an endoscopic examination performed through the natural ostium of the parotid and submandibular glands to visualize the ductal system (**Fig. 70.6**). The procedure helps diagnose ductal pathology and treat obstructive pathology like calculus and stenosis.

Treatment

Treatment requires removal of the calculi. Some calculi may spontaneously extrude. If the calculus is accessible and palpable, it can be easily removed by slitting the salivary duct open (sialodochotomy) and delivering the calculus (**Fig. 70.7**). If the stone is not accessible, sialendoscopy can be done.

Sialendoscopy is a technique developed to visualize the ductal system through the natural ostium of the salivary gland. The calculi, if visualized, can be removed with the help of a basket or broken down with laser. It will be difficult to remove calculus if it is not visualized with a sialendoscope (**Figs. 70.8** and **70.9**). When the stone is embedded in the parenchyma, excision of the salivary gland is indicated if the patient is symptomatic (**Fig. 70.10**).

■ Sjogren's Syndrome or Sicca Syndrome

This is an autoimmune disorder characterized by recurrent inflammation of the salivary glands. Patients may present with dry mouth, dry eyes, and uveitis. The condition is diagnosed by autoimmune markers like SS-A and SS-B. Salivary tests using protein biomarkers and mRNA biomarkers are also useful in diagnosis. Schirmer's test to detect dryness of eyes and a biopsy of minor salivary gland from the lips (labial biopsy) aid in the diagnosis.

Sjogren's syndrome is classified into primary and secondary syndromes.

In primary Sjogren's syndrome, there is no other underlying rheumatic disease, whereas secondary Sjogren's syndrome is associated with another rheumatic disorder like systemic lupus erythematosus or SLE, rheumatoid arthritis (RA), or scleroderma.

■ Ranula

This is a cystic mass in the floor of the mouth due to obstruction of the minor salivary gland or the sublingual gland. It can also occur in ductal abnormality and following trauma or transposition of the duct. The term was derived from the Latin word *rana*, meaning frog. The sublingual glands secrete continuously unlike the other major salivary glands.

Clinical Features

Obstruction leads to bluish, cystic, translucent swelling in the sublingual space or under the tongue (**Fig. 70.11**). It resembles the belly of a frog. It may grow into the mylohyoid muscle.

A *plunging ranula* results from extravasation of mucus below the mylohyoid, from ectopic tissue or from a duct communicating with the submandibular gland. It may also

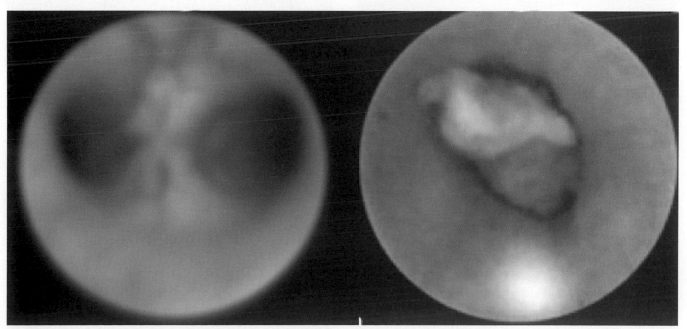

Fig. 70.6 A sialendoscopic image of the hilar area of the salivary gland. The second image shows a calculus obstructing the lumen of the duct.

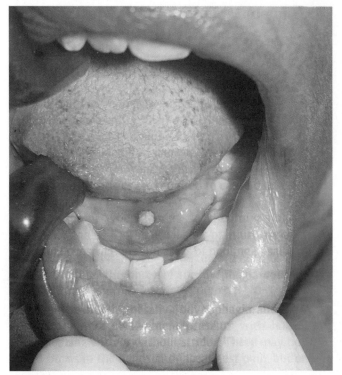

Fig. 70.7 Calculus at the opening of Wharton's duct.

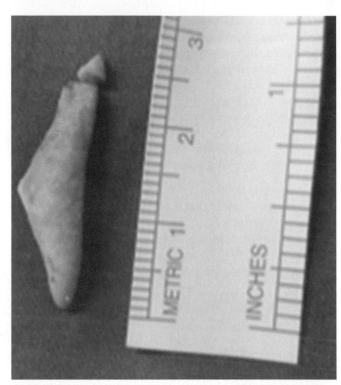

Fig. 70.8 A giant calculus delivered by sialendoscopy.

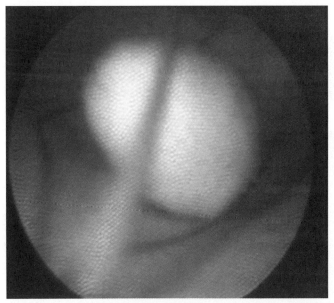

Fig. 70.9 A sialendoscopic image of a calculus being retrieved by a basket.

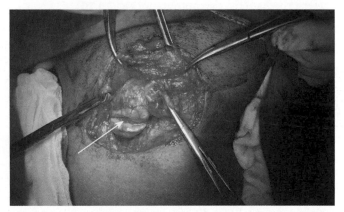

Fig. 70.10 A submandibular sialadenectomy (excision of the gland).

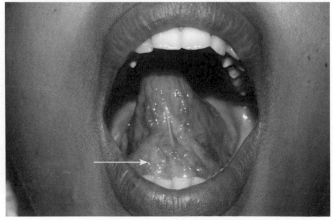

Fig. 70.11 A ranula in the floor of the mouth.

arise from an ectopic sublingual gland tissue. It may present as a painless cystic neck swelling. It usually presents in the second and third decades of life.

Investigations done are an ultrasound, a CT scan with contrast, or an MRI with contrast.

Treatment of a ranula is marsupialization, especially for smaller cysts of ≤1.5 cm. It may recur. Excision along with removal of the sublingual gland can reduce recurrence, especially for a plunging ranula.

Complications of surgery include a high recurrence rate, approximately 50%, if the sublingual gland is not excised, and only 2% if it is removed. Lingual nerve injury can cause paresthesia of the tongue. Wharton's duct injury may cause obstructive submandibular sialadenitis. The marginal mandibular branch of the facial nerve may be injured in the surgery of a plunging ranula.

> **Pearl**
>
> A mucocele can occur due to injury to a minor salivary gland leading to extravasation of mucous, which gets walled off as a pseudocyst.

■ Necrotizing Sialometaplasia

This is a benign, self-limiting, rare inflammatory disease of the minor salivary glands. The exact etiology is not known, but it is thought to be due to ischemia of local blood supply in the salivary gland lobules due to local trauma, ill-fitting dentures, smoking, drinking, allergy, and/or infection. It may be found in any site where there is minor salivary gland tissue, but it is commonly seen in the hard palate. It may present as a nodule or as a painful deep-seated ulcer. The appearance may mimic malignancy. The lesion heals spontaneously by secondary intention within 4 to 10 weeks. A biopsy is indicated if there is suspicion of malignancy. Histopathology shows coagulation necrosis of the glandular acini, inflammatory response, maintenance of the lobular architecture, and pseudoepitheliomatous hyperplasia.

■ Sialadenosis

It is characterized by unilateral or bilateral enlargement of the parotid glands. It is usually seen in metabolic syndromes, nutritional deficiencies, alcoholism, and obesity. It is a noninflammatory, non-neoplastic condition.

■ Differential Diagnosis of Swellings in the Parotid Region

- Neoplasms of the parotid gland.
- Mandibular tumors.
- Enlarged masseter muscle.
- Nonparotid cysts.
- Facial nerve schwannoma.
- Lymph nodes.
- Temporomandibular joint lesions.

Neoplasms of the Salivary Glands

Salivary malignancies make up 5% of all head and neck cancers, and less than 0.5% of all cancers. In adults, the vast majority of salivary gland tumors are benign. Salivary gland tumors are far less common in the pediatric population. Unlike adults, hemangiomas and lymphatic tumors are the most common pediatric salivary gland tumors. In the parotid gland, 80% of the tumors are benign. About 50 to 60% tumors in the submandibular gland and 25% of the tumors in the minor salivary glands are benign.

> **Pearl**
>
> Rule of 80:
> - 80% of all salivary tumors are in the parotid gland.
> - 80% of the parotid tumors are benign.
> - 80% of the benign parotid tumors are pleomorphic adenomas.
> - 80% of the pleomorphic adenomas occur in the superficial lobe of the parotid gland.
> - 80 to 90% of the sublingual swellings are malignant.
>
> The commonest benign tumor in children is hemangioma.
>
> The commonest malignant tumor in adults is mucoepidermoid carcinoma.

■ Etiopathogenesis

- Low-dose radiation exposure has been implicated as an etiological factor for salivary gland neoplasms.
- Other risk factors include occupational silica dust (from blast furnaces and cement, glass, ceramic, and clay industries).
- Nitrosamine (rubber and tire industries).
- Warthin's tumor is associated with smoking.
- Epstein–Barr virus is implicated in bilateral Warthin's tumor.

■ Classification

Tumors may arise from epithelial or mesenchymal tissues. The classification of these tumors is shown in **Table 70.1**.

■ Clinical Evaluation

Typically, patients with parotid neoplasms will present with a painless, unilateral mass in front of the tragus or below the pinna (**Fig. 70.12**). Rapid change in size may be the result of obstruction of Stensen's duct, from cystic degeneration, or a malignant transformation. Onset of facial nerve palsy may be associated with a malignant tumor.

Benign neoplasms of the submandibular gland are generally painless. Malignant submandibular neoplasms may invade the lingual and hypoglossal nerves, mandible, floor of the mouth, and tongue. These are the hallmarks of an advanced disease.

Symptoms arising from neoplasms of the minor salivary glands depend on their location. Intraorally, the first signs may be poorly fitting dentures, loose teeth, and

Table 70.1 Classification of salivary gland tumors

Benign tumors	Malignant tumors
Epithelial	
Pleomorphic adenoma	Mucoepidermoid carcinoma
Warthin's tumor	Adenoid cystic carcinoma
Oncocytoma	Acinic cell carcinoma
Other adenomas	Adenocarcinoma
	Malignant mixed tumor
	Squamous cell carcinoma
	Undifferentiated carcinoma
Mesenchymal	
Hemangioma	Lymphoma
Lymphangioma	Sarcoma
Lipoma	
Neurofibroma/schwannoma	

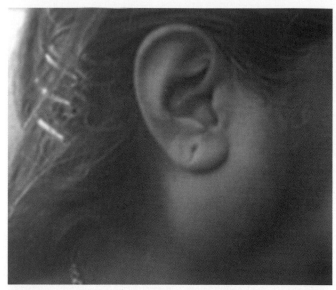

Fig. 70.12 The ear lobe is raised where there is enlargement of the parotid gland.

malocclusion. A comprehensive head and neck examination should be performed to assess the extent of the neoplasm. Intraoral examination may reveal bulging of the pharyngeal wall arising from deep lobe involvement of the parotid gland or from a minor salivary neoplasm in the parapharyngeal space. A submandibular gland neoplasm will be palpable by bidigital palpation. Cranial neuropathies may indicate neural involvement from adenoid cystic carcinoma (ACC). Examination of the neck may reveal cervical lymph node metastasis in malignancy. Other sites of involvement from minor salivary gland neoplasms include the palate, lacrimal gland, sinonasal region, and larynx.

■ Investigations

MRI with contrast is the investigation of choice to differentiate between malignant and benign lesions and to evaluate the extent of disease within the gland and in relation to surrounding structures (**Fig. 70.13**).

Ultrasound may be a preliminary investigation and can be utilized for an ultrasound-guided fine-needle aspiration cytology (FNAC). The accuracy of FNAC is 80 to 90%.

■ Benign Tumors

The tumors discussed here are pleomorphic adenomas and adenolymphomas.

Pleomorphic Adenoma

It is the commonest benign tumor in the salivary glands. In the parotid gland, it usually involves the lower part of the superficial lobe. If it occurs in the deep lobe, it may present as a parapharyngeal tumor (dumbbell tumor passing through the stylomandibular tunnel). This is seen

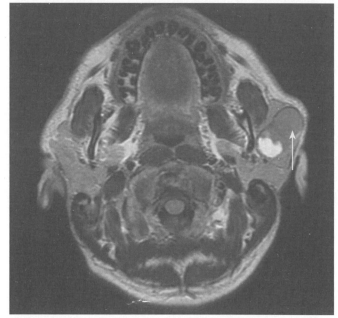

Fig. 70.13 Magnetic resonance imaging (MRI) showing a left parotid tumor (pleomorphic adenoma).

clinically as a medial bulge of the tonsil and lateral wall of the oropharynx.

These are slow-growing tumors occurring in the third or fourth decade of life. The malignant potential is 1 to 5% in 10 years. It can also occur in the oral cavity (**Fig. 70.14**), larynx, pharynx, and nasal cavity.

Histologically, it shows the epithelial elements and nonepithelial elements like chondroid, fibroid, and myxoid elements, and hence is also known as a mixed tumor. The encapsulated tumor may extend to surrounding tissue through pseudopods. Large tumors are bosselated. If a wide

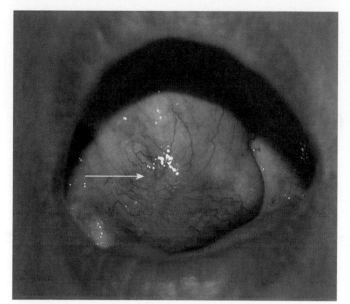

Fig. 70.14 Pleomorphic adenoma of the palate.

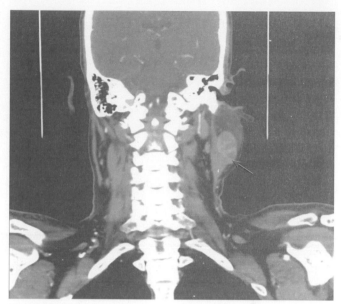

Fig. 70.15 Computed tomography (CT) scan with contrast showing a tumor toward the tail of the left parotid (Warthin's tumor).

resection is not done during surgery, recurrence can occur. Hence, a cuff of tissue is retained around the nodule during surgery. Rupture of the tumor during removal is another cause for recurrence.

Warthin's Tumor (Adenolymphoma, Papillary Cystadenoma Lymphomatosum)

This tumor, seen in smokers, usually occurs in the sixth to seventh decade of life and can be bilateral in 10% of patients. It is seen in the tail of the parotid gland and is a well-rounded, cystic tumor. Histopathology shows epithelial elements, and variable lymphoid tissue with germinal centers.

Contrast-enhanced CT scan will delineate the lesion (**Fig. 70.15**). Since it is a multicentric tumor, imaging by MRI is mandatory. Malignant transformation is rare. It can be treated by a superficial parotidectomy.

■ Malignant Tumors

Mucoepidermoid carcinoma is the commonest malignant tumor. It may be a high-grade or a low-grade tumor. Low-grade tumors are least aggressive and may behave like a benign tumor, but high-grade tumors are very aggressive and behave like ACC. High-grade tumors are treated aggressively with surgical resection of the primary along with neck dissection and postoperative radiotherapy.

ACC infiltrates tissue planes and is notorious for perineural spread and spread through lymphatics. Early involvement of the nerves is a feature of this malignancy.

Carcinoma ex pleomorphic adenoma (malignant mixed tumor) occurs in a preexisting pleomorphic adenoma. Rapid change should arouse suspicion of malignant transformation. It can also occur de novo.

Treatment

Removal of the salivary gland alone is curative for all benign and most malignant salivary gland neoplasms. The surgery may be a superficial parotidectomy or a total parotidectomy, depending on the location and type of neoplasm, with tracing and preservation of the facial nerve when it is not involved (**Fig. 70.16**).

Aggressive tumors may need a radical parotidectomy with sacrifice of the facial nerve. Radiation therapy along with surgery has improved locoregional control and survival in patients with advanced high-grade malignant disease.

Radiotherapy is usually indicated in the following:
- High-risk malignant neoplasms.
- Presence of cervical lymph node metastasis.
- Recurrent disease.
- Primary radiotherapy is indicated as a palliative measure in inoperable disease and in patients who are not fit for surgery.

Prognosis is dependent on tumor grade, stage, and histology of the tumor.

A superficial parotidectomy is the surgical removal of the gland superficial to the facial nerve. Total parotidectomy is the removal of the whole gland (superficial and

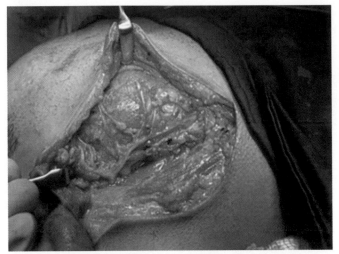

Fig. 70.16 Demonstration of a parotid tumor deep to the branches of the facial nerve.

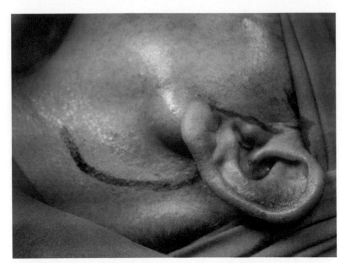

Fig. 70.17 Modified Blair incision or the lazy "S" incision.

deep). Superficial parotidectomy can be partial in relatively small tumors that are removed with a cuff of clinically normal parenchyma without removal of the entire superficial portion of the gland. Special care is taken to preserve the integrity of the facial nerve using anatomical landmarks. The incision used for parotidectomy is the modified Blair (lazy "S") incision (**Fig. 70.17**).

Complications of Parotid Gland Surgery

- Hematoma formation.
- Infection.
- Scar and retromandibular hollowing.
- Temporary or permanent facial nerve weakness.
- Sialocele.
- Permanent numbness of the earlobe associated with great auricular nerve transection.
- Frey's syndrome.

Frey's Syndrome (Gustatory Sweating)

This results from damage to the autonomic innervation of the salivary gland with inappropriate regeneration of the postganglionic parasympathetic nerve fibers of the auriculotemporal nerve that aberrantly stimulate the sweat glands of the overlying skin.

The clinical features include sweating and erythema (flushing) over the region of surgical excision of the parotid gland by the smell or taste of food.

The symptoms are clinically demonstrated by starch iodine test. This involves painting the affected area with

iodine, which is allowed to dry before applying dry starch, which turns blue on exposure to iodine in the presence of sweat.

Frey's syndrome can be treated by antiperspirants, usually containing aluminum chloride, tympanic neurectomy, or by the injection of botulinum toxin into the affected skin.

Complications of Submandibular Gland Surgery

- Marginal mandibular nerve injury.
- Lingual nerve injury.
- Hypoglossal nerve injury.

Points to Ponder

- Mumps is the commonest infection of the salivary glands seen in children.
- The commonest complication due to mumps seen in adult males is orchitis.
- Sialolithiasis is commonly seen in the submandibular glands.
- Sjogren's syndrome can be primary or secondary depending on associated rheumatic disease.
- Plunging ranula appears in the neck due to extension below the mylohyoid muscle.
- Pleomorphic adenoma usually affects the parotid and is the commonest benign tumor. The second most common benign tumor is Warthin's tumor.
- The earlobe is raised in a classical parotid tumor.
- Superficial parotidectomy is removal of the parotid gland above the level of the facial nerve.

Case-Based Questions

1. **A 4-year-old girl presented with a history of right-sided painful facial swelling just in front and below the pinna. There was fever and malaise. The mother noticed that the child did not respond well when called from the right side and needed to be louder. The vaccination schedule was not followed.**

   a. What is the primary illness of the patient?

   b. Why is the child not able to hear well?

   c. What are the complications of this condition?

   d. What is the treatment of the primary condition?

   Answers

   a. Mumps or parotitis.

   b. Right-sided sensorineural hearing loss.

   c. Orchitis, oophoritis, meningoencephalitis, pancreatitis, and sensorineural hearing loss.

   d. Supportive with oral hydration, antipyretic with analgesics, and oral hygiene.

2. **A 28-year-old man presented with a history of swelling and occasional pain in the left submandibular region while taking food. The symptoms have been present for 2 months. A small hard lesion was palpable in the left floor of the mouth. There was minimal pus emanating through the duct opening on applying pressure on the gland in the neck.**

   a. What is the diagnosis?

   b. How would you confirm the diagnosis?

   c. What is the treatment?

   Answers

   a. Left submandibular duct calculus.

   b. An X-ray submandibular occlusal view or ultrasonography.

   c. Sialodochotomy, that is, opening of the duct in the floor of the mouth, removing the calculi and marsupialization of the duct. Alternatively, a sialendoscope can be used for extraction of the calculi.

3. **A 42-year-old woman presented with a right-sided painless swelling in front and below the pinna, which displaced the ear lobule. The swelling has been present for 3 years. The facial nerve function was clinically normal. An FNAC done showed epithelial and nonepithelial elements.**

   a. What is the most likely diagnosis?

   b. What are the investigations required?

   c. What is the treatment?

   Answers

   a. Pleomorphic adenoma.

   b. CT scan or MRI with FNAC.

   c. Superficial parotidectomy.

Frequently Asked Questions

1. What is a plunging ranula?

2. Which gland is usually affected by sialolithiasis? What are the reasons for this?

3. What is the commonest malignancy affecting the salivary glands? What are the treatment options for this tumor?

4. What is Frey's syndrome?

5. Write a short note on pleomorphic adenoma.

6. What are the complications of mumps?

Endnote

Wharton's duct is a thin tube that is 5 cm long and carries saliva from the submandibular gland to the floor of the mouth. It is named after Thomas Wharton (1614–1673), an English anatomist who did extensive studies on the salivary glands. He wrote a book called "Adenographia," which described the glands of the human body. He described the ovaries, the testes and the production of sperms, and the breast and the production of milk. He was responsible for naming the thyroid gland and described "Wharton's jelly" of the umbilical cord.

71 Trauma to the Face and Neck

Thripthi Rai

The competency covered in this chapter is as follows:

EN4.31 Describe the clinical features, investigations, and principles of management of trauma to the face and neck.

Trauma to the Face

Introduction

The face is the front part of the head and extends from the forehead superiorly to the chin inferiorly, and the auricle on either side. It includes the mouth, nose, cheeks, and eyes. It is made up of the facial skeleton, parotid gland, and superficial fascia containing the facial muscles, the vessels, nerves, fat, and skin. The facial skeleton is composed of 14 bones. These are the following:

- **Paired:**
  - The maxilla, zygomatic, nasal, lacrimal, palatine, and inferior nasal concha.
- **Unpaired:**
  - The mandible and vomer.

Any of these structures can be disrupted in a case of trauma to the face. It can cause soft-tissue as well as bony damage. There can be associated damage to the eye, brain, and cervical spine as well as other skull bones like the frontal, ethmoid, sphenoid, and temporal bones.

Etiology

Facial trauma can be caused by a number of events, namely the following:

- Road traffic accidents.
- Assault.
- Sports injuries.
- Falls.
- Explosions.
- Burns.
- Penetrating injuries from gunshot, shrapnel, and glass.

General Management

■ Airway

This is evaluated and secured by endotracheal intubation. A cricothyrotomy or immediate tracheostomy is performed when required. Any fractures compromising airway like mandibular or maxillary fractures are reduced immediately.

■ Breathing

Adequate ventilation is provided.

■ Circulation

Facial hemorrhage can be profuse and needs to be controlled by pressure or ligation. Anterior/posterior nasal packs can stop nasal bleed. Fluid replacement/blood transfusion is given when required.

■ Disability

The level of consciousness and neurological dysfunction is assessed by the Glasgow Coma Scale (GCS). Abdominal, pelvic, orthopaedic, spinal, orbital, dental, or thoracic injuries have to be excluded. Immediate advice/intervention from the concerned department must be sought.

■ Exposure

All other injuries are identified. Cerebrospinal fluid (CSF) rhinorrhea must be identified and prophylactic antibiotic therapy started to prevent meningitis.

■ Tetanus Prophylaxis

It is given in a previously nonimmunized patient.

■ Radiographic Evaluation

All major trauma patients should have chest, cervical spine, and pelvic X-rays as soon as possible. Computed tomography (CT) scan is preferred and is done for a patient with multiple injuries. It is also important as a documentation in medicolegal cases.

Soft-Tissue Injuries

Facial soft-tissue injuries can be classified as open or closed wounds. A closed wound is one where the overlying skin is intact. These can be contusions, hematomas, and crush injuries. Open wounds include abrasions, punctures, lacerations, and avulsions. These can also have retained foreign body.

■ Clinical Features

The presentation may be pain, hemorrhage, edema, visual disturbances, and/or respiratory obstruction. On examination, there may be facial swelling, contusion/hematoma, abrasion, laceration, facial nerve paralysis, and, in the eye, chemosis, hyphema, and/or absent light reflex.

■ Treatment

Facial soft-tissue injuries require careful in-depth evaluation and treatment in order to avoid poor cosmetic outcome and loss of function. In abrasions, burns, and exposed cartilage, the wound is cleaned thoroughly with saline, any foreign body present is removed, and dressing is done with an antibiotic-soaked gauze. Lacerations are ideally closed within the first 8 hours. Wounds are meticulously cleaned of any debris/foreign body and devitalized tissues are debrided. Any underlying bony injury (**Fig. 71.1**) is repaired to enable correct support and soft-tissue draping. Primary closure is done in layers without tension under local anesthesia. Identification and alignment of key landmarks, such as the vermillion border of the lip, eyebrow, and alar margin of the nose, ear, and eyelids, is essential for a good cosmetic result. Larger defects might require flaps or skin grafts. For parotid injuries (**Fig. 71.1**), the wound is explored to identify the damaged parotid duct, which is cannulated intraorally at the level of second maxillary molar. Facial nerve is the easiest to find and repair within the first 48 hours, whereas the peripheral branches can still be stimulated. The cut ends are identified and epineural repair is done. Cable grafting is done in case of nerve loss. Vascular injury (facial or internal maxillary artery) is identified and ligated. For eyelid avulsion, an antibiotic ointment is applied and an occlusive eye shield is placed to prevent exposure keratitis.

Bone Injuries

■ Upper Third Facial Fractures

Frontal sinus fractures involving the frontal sinus can involve the anterior and/or posterior table and the nasofrontal duct and may be treated conservatively if there is no cosmetic deformity. Displaced fractures require reduction and fixation (**Fig. 71.2**). Fractures of the posterior table

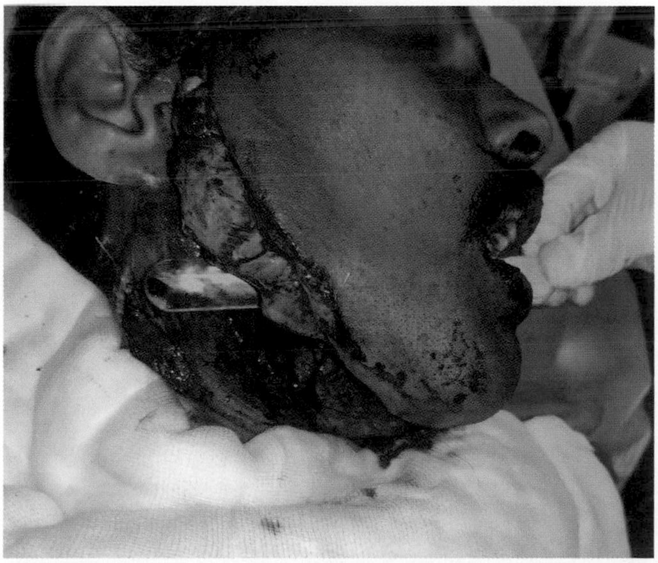

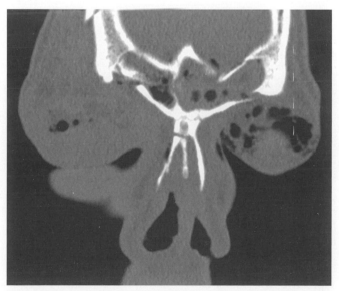

Fig. 71.1 Soft-tissue injury of the face (parotid gland and facial nerve were involved) with underlying mandibular fracture and communication of the wound with the oral cavity (as depicted by the spatula).

Fig. 71.2 Computed tomography (CT) scan, coronal cut, showing fracture involving the frontal bone and the frontal sinus.

require a neurosurgical opinion and may need an obliterative procedure or cranialization of the frontal sinus with obliteration of the frontonasal recess and its lining. It may be associated with brain injury. Fracture repair may be done via a brow or an osteoplastic flap incision.

Middle Third Facial Fractures

Fractures of the midfacial skeleton can be subdivided into central (nasal, naso-orbito-ethmoid, and maxillary) or lateral (zygomatic) fractures.

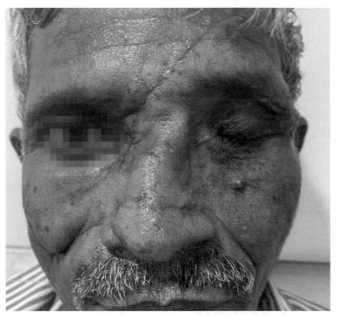

Fig. 71.3 Nasal bone fracture and other associated soft-tissue injuries.

Fracture Nasal Bones

Introduction

The nose is a prominent structure on the face and hence more prone to injuries. Nasal bone fractures commonly occur at the transition zone between the proximal thicker and distal thinner portions. This zone corresponds to the lower third of the nasal bone area (**Fig. 71.3**).

Fractures can be depressed or angulated. Depressed fractures occur in frontal blows and results in an open book fracture. Angulated fractures occur in lateral blow resulting in unilateral or bilateral nasal bone and septum fracture with an external deviation of the nose (**Fig. 71.4**). The septum may be buckled, dislocated, or fractured into several pieces and may be associated with a septal hematoma.

Harrison's Classification

Class 1 (Chevallet) fractures (**Fig. 71.5**) occur when mild to moderate degree of force is used. This can be due to a frontal or frontolateral trauma. It is a vertical fracture. There is minimal deformity. In simple variants, there is a depressed nasal bone, but the nasal septum is not involved. In more severe variants, both nasal bones and septum are fractured.
Class 2 (Jarjavay) fractures (**Fig. 71.6**) require greater force and are due to a lateral trauma. It causes significant cosmetic deformity and involves the nasal bones, septum, and the frontal process of the maxilla. There is a **C**-shaped fracture of septum involving the perpendicular plate of the ethmoid and septal cartilage.
Class 3 fractures are a more severe nasal injury due to high-velocity trauma. It involves a naso-orbito-ethmoid fracture with fracture of the maxilla. A "piglike" appearance

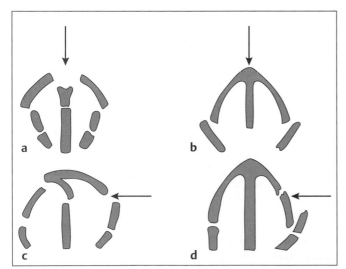

Fig. 71.4 **(a)** Frontal blow resulting in open book fracture. **(b)** Lateral blow resulting in angulated fracture of the bilateral nasal bone and the septum. **(c)** Frontal blow leading to depressed fracture. **(d)** Lateral blow leading to unilateral nasal bone fracture.

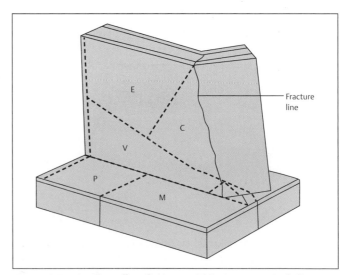

Fig. 71.5 A Chevallet fracture. This is a vertical fracture through the nasal septum. C, cartilage; E, perpendicular plate of the ethmoid; M, palatine process of the maxilla; P, horizontal process of the ethmoid bone; V, vomer.

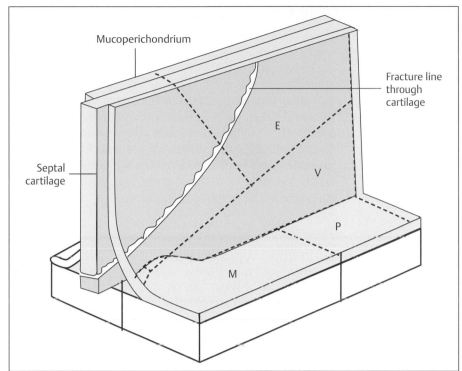

Fig. 71.6 A Jarjavay fracture is a C-shaped fracture of the nasal septum. E, perpendicular plate of the ethmoid; M, palatine process of the maxilla; P, horizontal process of the ethmoid bone; V, vomer.

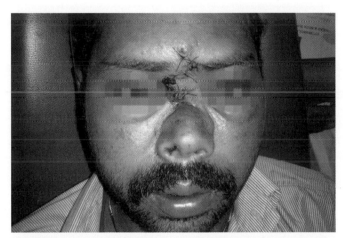

Fig. 71.7 Pig nose deformity. Depression of the upper third nasal bones and anterior projection of the nostrils. Telecanthus is present.

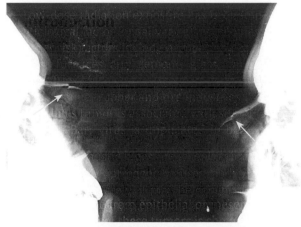

Fig. 71.8 X-ray (lateral view) showing nasal bone fracture.

of the face is noted due to a saddle nose deformity and the nostrils facing more anteriorly. Telecanthus may be present (**Fig. 71.7**).

Clinical Features

The presentation is with symptoms of pain, external deformity, hemorrhage/epistaxis, edema, CSF rhinorrhea, nasal obstruction, anosmia/hyposmia, diplopia, visual disturbances, epiphora, altered bite, loose teeth, and/or trismus.

On examination, there may be ecchymosis, saddle/crooked nose deformity, laceration with exposure of underlying bone/cartilage, tenderness, crepitus, instability, surgical emphysema, septal deviation/perforation, and septal hematoma/abscess.

Investigations

X-ray of the nasal bones (right and left lateral view) and X-ray of the paranasal sinuses (Waters' view) are done for assessment and for documentation of the fractures especially for medicolegal cases (**Fig. 71.8**). CT scan would be a better imaging modality and would be useful to assess for associated intracranial injuries. Nasal discharge, if present, is tested for beta-2 transferrin to rule out CSF rhinorrhea.

Treatment

Reassure the patient. Simple undisplaced fractures do not require any active intervention. Analgesics are given for pain relief.

In case of displaced or compound fractures, either closed or open reduction can be done. This is done before the edema appears or after it subsides, which takes about 4 to 7 days. Fractures heal within 2 to 3 weeks, after which reduction is difficult. Topical vasoconstrictor drops, unless contraindicated, can alleviate congestion and obstructive symptoms.

Septal hematoma is managed by incision and drainage followed by anterior nasal packing.

Delayed management is by closed reduction. Firm digital pressure is used to dis-impact the fragments. Elevators (Freer or Howarth), Walsham forceps (for nasal bones), and Asch forceps (for septum) are used to place the nasal bones and septum in the normal position. Anterior nasal packing and an external nasal splint are used to immobilize the bones so that they heal in the corrected position. Open reduction is done if results are not satisfactory by the above maneuver. For depressed tip or flail lateral fractures that are unstable despite closed reduction techniques, Kirschner's (K) wires can be used.

Septal correction can be done using a Killian or hemitransfixion incision. Elevation of mucosal flaps is done to expose and replace or remove cartilaginous and bony fragments. Quilting sutures and/or anterior nasal packing are done to prevent collection of hematoma in the dead space.

Rhinoplasty or septorhinoplasty is done after 6 months if required for cosmetic and functional correction.

Complications

- External deformity.
- Epistaxis (treated by ligation or prolonged nasal packing).
- Nasal obstruction.
- Septal hematoma.
- Septal abscess.
- Septal perforation.
- Cavernous sinus thrombosis.

Zygomatic Complex Fractures

These form the second most common facial fracture. These are also termed tripod fracture, or more recently quadripod fracture. The following articulations are disrupted:
- Frontozygomatic.
- Infraorbital rim.
- Zygomaticomaxillary buttress.
- Zygomatic arch.
- Zygomaticosphenoid.

Clinical Features

The symptoms include pain, swelling, bruising of the soft tissue, subconjunctival hemorrhage, and diplopia.

On examination, there may be restricted eye movements, reduced zygomatic prominence, step deformity of the infraorbital margin, tenderness at the frontozygomatic suture, depression and restricted mouth opening (arch fractures), and altered cheek sensation (zygomaticotemporal or zygomaticofacial nerves). There will be flattening of the malar prominence and over the zygomatic arch. There may be ecchymosis in the superior buccal sulcus. The lateral palpebral fissure may be displaced.

Investigations

X-rays of the paranasal sinuses (Waters' view), submentovertex (jug-handle) view, and Hirtz view are done. CT scan with or without 3D reconstructed images is preferred specially to assess other associated facial bone and soft-tissue injuries including the orbit. Hess charting is done if diplopia is present. The forced duction test (FDT; as described later) should be done.

Management

Minimally displaced fractures are managed conservatively. The patient is instructed not to blow their nose for a period of 2 to 3 weeks. The patient is reviewed after 10 days once swelling has resolved. Displaced fractures are reduced with or without fixation using the Gillies temporal approach (incision just anterior to the ear down to the superficial temporal fascia), Poswillo hook (applied at the intersection of a line drawn vertically from the lateral orbital margin and a horizontal line drawn from the inferior margin of the nose), or intraoral/Keen approach (mucogingival incision at the molar/premolar region). The zygoma may be plated at the frontozygomatic suture, infraorbital margin, zygomatic buttress, and zygomatic arch.

Blowout Fractures of the Orbit

The term "blowout fracture" was first used by Smith and Regan in 1957, describing the inferior rectus entrapment with decreased ocular motility in the setting of an orbital floor fracture.

Pathophysiology

Blowout fracture occurs when a blunt object greater in diameter than the orbital rim (such as a fist, tennis ball, or cricket ball) strikes the orbital cavity.

The mechanisms proposed for blowout fracture are the following:
- *Direct injury theory*: Sudden compression and backward displacement of the globe raise the intraorbital pressure, leading to fracture of the orbital floor (**Fig. 71.9**).

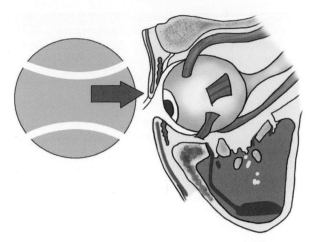

Fig. 71.9 The impact of a direct injury on the eyeball.

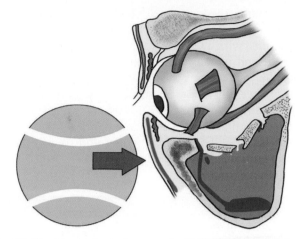

Fig. 71.10 The impact of trauma to the inferior orbital rim.

- *Indirect injury theory*: External force to the inferior orbital rim is transmitted along the orbital walls causing a ripple effect leading to fracture at the weakest point in the posterior medial region of the floor (**Fig. 71.10**).

Types

- *Pure blowout fracture*, which is a fracture of the orbital floor with intact orbital rim.
- *Impure blowout fracture*, which is an associated fracture of the orbital rim.

Clinical Features

The patient presents with epistaxis (due to bleeding into the maxillary sinus) and diplopia.

On examination, there may be periorbital hematoma, emphysema, paresthesia over the ipsilateral lower lid, cheek, and upper lip, enophthalmos, orbital rim deformity and crepitus, and absent pupillary reflex (relative afferent pupillary defect [RAPD] in case of optic nerve injury).

Due to entrapment of orbital contents and inferior rectus muscle, there is motility restriction, especially in upward gaze.

The FDT is a test to differentiate extraocular muscle paralysis from muscle entrapment or fibrosis. Topical anesthesia is instilled on the conjunctiva where the eye is grasped using forceps. The nontest eye is covered. In the test eye, the patient is asked to look in the direction of the muscle that is impaired. The conjunctiva is held with a toothed forceps and attempt is made to move the eye. In blowout fracture with inferior rectus entrapment, the eye will not move freely and FDT is "positive." The eye will move freely during FDT if there is nerve paralysis.

Investigations

- X-ray of the paranasal sinuses (Waters' view) will show a bony discontinuity in the orbital floor with herniation

of soft tissue in the maxillary antrum seen as "hanging drop" or "*teardrop*" sign.
- CT scanning is preferred to outline the fracture and soft-tissue entrapment.
- Magnetic resonance imaging (MRI) can be done.
- Evaluation of the orbit is mandatory.

Treatment

Early intervention is required in case of diplopia associated with a nonresolving oculocardiac reflex (i.e., bradycardia, heart block, nausea, vomiting, or syncope), white-eyed blowout fracture, and early enophthalmos/hypoglobus causing facial asymmetry.

Patients can be managed conservatively (observation) in case of minimal diplopia (not in primary or downgaze), good ocular motility, and no significant enophthalmos or hypoglobus.

Medical Treatment

- Oral steroids are given to reduce edema of soft tissue and extra ocular muscle.
- Oral antibiotics are given on empirical basis.
- The patient is advised not to blow the nose as it can worsen orbital emphysema.
- Nasal decongestants are prescribed, if not contraindicated.

Surgical Technique

The principal approach is to assess the orbital floor, release soft-tissue and muscle entrapment, and strengthen the floor with the use of implants. The various approaches are the following:

- *Subciliary approach*: Incision is made 2 to 3 mm below the lash line.
- *Subtarsal approach*: Incision is below tarsal the plate over the orbital rim giving direct access to the floor.

- *Transconjunctival approach*: Incision is made in the lower fornix 3 mm below the tarsal plate and can be combined with a lateral canthotomy.
- *Transantral approach*: The orbital floor is reached via the maxillary sinus using the Caldwell-Luc incision.
- *Endoscopic approach*: Transmaxillary and transnasal endoscopy gives better visualization of fractures.

The various implant materials used in orbital floor repair are membranous bone, cartilage, titanium mesh, porous polyethylene (Medpore) sheets, silicon sheet, and Silastic sheet (Teflon).

> ### Pearl
> *White-eyed blowout fracture*: In young patients with history of periocular trauma, there is little ecchymosis or edema (white eye) but marked extraocular motility restriction. This occurs as bones are more elastic resulting in anteroposterior buckling with overlapping fracture segments leading to "trapdoor-type" fracture.

Fractures of Maxilla

Le Fort Fractures

Le Fort fractures are complex fractures of the midface due to blunt trauma. They are classified into three groups depending on the direction of the fractures. The fracture lines may be horizontal, pyramidal, or transverse.

Le Fort Classification

Le Fort I (Guerin's fracture): This is a horizontal fracture. The fracture line runs above the floor of the nasal cavity, through the nasal septum, maxillary sinuses, and inferior parts of the medial and lateral pterygoid plates (**Fig. 71.11**). Referred to as the floating palate (**Fig. 71.12**), it occurs due to force of the trauma above the level of the teeth.

Le Fort II (pyramidal fracture): This is a fracture that runs from the floor of the maxillary sinuses superiorly to the infraorbital margin and through the zygomaticomaxillary suture (**Fig. 71.13**). Within the orbit, it passes across the lacrimal bone to the nasion. The infraorbital nerve is often damaged by involvement in this fracture. It occurs due to force of the trauma at the level of the nasal bones.

Le Fort III (craniofacial dysjunction): This transverse fracture traverses the medial wall of the orbit to the superior orbital fissure and exits across the greater wing of the sphenoid and zygomatic bone to the zygomaticofrontal suture (**Fig. 71.14**). Posteriorly, the fracture line runs inferior to the optic foramen, across the lesser wing of the sphenoid to the pterygomaxillary fissure and sphenopalatine foramen. The arch of the zygoma is also broken. It occurs due to force of the trauma at the level of the orbit.

> ### Pearl
> In high-velocity injuries, as in road traffic accidents, there can be multiple Le Fort level fractures together with zygomatic and nasal or naso-ethmoidal fractures.

Clinical Features

In Le Fort I, the patient will have a "floating" maxilla with malocclusion (anterior open bite) and ecchymosis of the upper buccal vestibule and palate. The upper lip will be swollen.

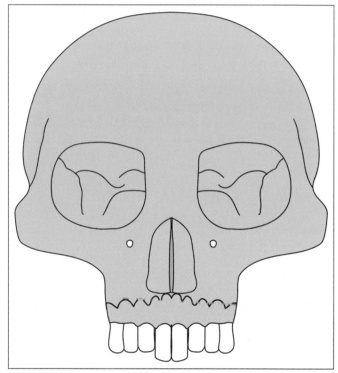

Fig. 71.11 Fracture line in Le Fort I.

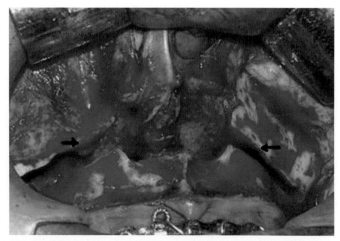

Fig. 71.12 Le Fort I. A horizontal fracture (*black arrows*) seen above the level of the teeth.

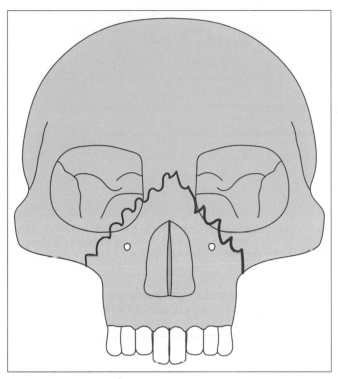

Fig. 71.13 Fracture line in Le Fort II.

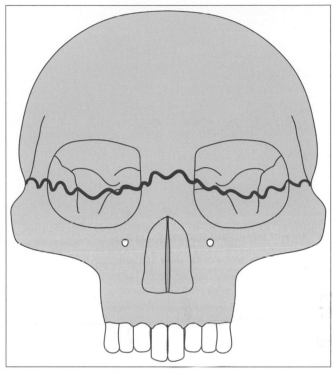

Fig. 71.14 Fracture line in Le Fort III.

In Le Fort II, there will be epistaxis and intercanthal widening. There may be infraorbital anesthesia and CSF rhinorrhea.

In Le Fort III, there will be lengthening of the face with posterior displacement of the maxilla (referred to as dish face deformity; **Fig. 71.15**). There may be enophthalmos, CSF rhinorrhea/otorrhea, hemotympanum, and ecchymosis over the mastoid (Battle's sign).

In Le Fort II and III, there will be bilateral periorbital edema and ecchymosis (referred to as "raccoon eyes" or "panda facies"; **Fig. 71.16**), malocclusion (anterior open bite), and ecchymosis of the upper buccal vestibule and palate.

In addition, the patient may have nasal obstruction, epistaxis, and visual problems.

Investigations

X-rays of the paranasal sinuses (Waters' view) and skull (posteroanterior [PA] and lateral views) may be done. CT scan is the preferred imaging modality to delineate the fractures. In addition, a CT scan or MRI of the brain has to be done to assess an associated intracranial injury. Evaluation of the orbit is mandatory as ocular movements may be affected, and the fracture may involve the optic canal.

Treatment

Epistaxis is arrested by using the anterior and posterior nasal packs.

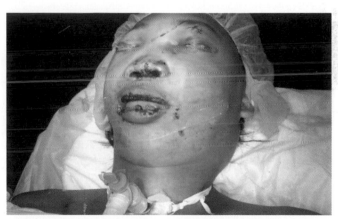

Fig. 71.15 Le Fort III fracture. Clinical appearance.

If a retropositioned maxilla is present, it is pulled forward using the index and middle fingers placed behind the patient's soft palate. Reduction is done by mobilizing the maxilla by a combination of digital pressure and traction on arch bars or interdental wires. Rowe maxillary disimpaction forceps is used, if the maxilla is impacted. Fixation is done via access by a gingivobuccal incision ensuring that there is an adequate cuff of unattached mucosa to isolate the plates from the mouth at closure. Internal fixation is done with 1.3- or 1.5-mm low-profile mini-plates placed along the buttresses for stabilization of the fractured segments.

The infraorbital rim needs to be reduced and fixed in Le Fort II fractures, nasomaxillary fractures, zygomatic injuries, and orbital floor fractures.

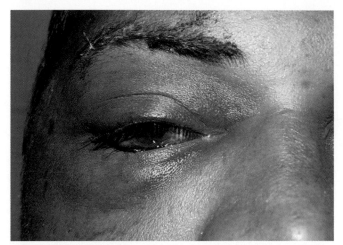

Fig. 71.16 Raccoon eyes, also known as periorbital ecchymosis. A sign of anterior skull base fracture.

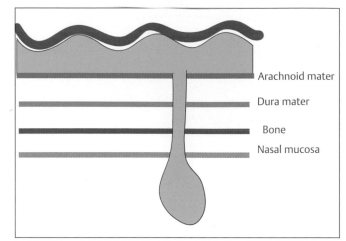

Fig. 71.17 Cerebrospinal fluid (CSF) rhinorrhea due to defect in the arachnoid mater, dura mater, bone, and nasal mucosa.

Pearl

Guerin's sign is bruising and ecchymosis in the palate in the region of the greater palatine vessels.

Note: Dish face deformity is also seen in other conditions where the midface is maldeveloped like in Alport's syndrome and Crouzon's disease. Donkey-face due to lengthening of the face that can occur in Le Fort III fracture.

Cerebrospinal Fluid Rhinorrhea

Introduction

It is defined as the leakage of CSF through the nose. There is disruption of arachnoid mater, dura mater, bone, and nasal mucosa (**Fig. 71.17**). Rhinorrhea itself is a troubling symptom, but more dangerous is the risk of meningitis or other intracranial complications. Endoscopic techniques have demonstrated tremendous benefits in the treatment of CSF leaks.

CSF leaks can be classified as traumatic and nontraumatic leaks. The common causes are outlined in **Table 71.1**.

Etiology

CSF leaks can arise from the anterior, middle, or posterior cranial fossae.

The various sites of CSF leak are outlined in **Table 71.2**.

Clinical Features

The patient presents with watery nasal discharge. There may be headache and/or hyposmia/anosmia.

There may be signs of recent trauma/surgery.

On diagnostic nasal endoscopy, a stream of clear fluid may be seen, which signifies the site of leak. The *reservoir*

Table 71.1 Ommaya's classification system for CSF leak (1964)

Classification of leak	Etiology
Traumatic	Accidental: • Craniomaxillofacial fractures
	Iatrogenic: • Neurosurgical • Endoscopic sinus procedures
Nontraumatic	High-pressure leaks: • Tumors • Hydrocephalus • Benign intracranial hypertension
	Normal pressure leaks: • Congenital anomaly • Focal atrophy • Osteomyelitic erosion

Abbreviation: CSF, cerebrospinal fluid.

sign, that is, sudden gush of clear fluid on bringing the patient to upright from supine position, is positive. The double ring (*halo or target sign*), a clear fluid outer area with central blood stain, is formed when the nasal discharge is allowed to drip on a filter paper, if the CSF is mixed with blood. The Stiff handkerchief test can be done.

Pearl

Tea pot sign: In case of defect in the sphenoid sinus, there will be CSF leak on tilting the head forward.

CSF is a clear watery fluid. Sometimes nasal secretions can mimic CSF. The differences between the two are outlined in **Table 71.3**.

Congenital CSF leaks are uncommon. They are usually seen in association with encephalocele or meningoencephaloceles. MRI helps in the diagnosis.

Table 71.2 Sites of CSF leak

Anterior cranial fossa	Middle cranial fossa	Posterior cranial fossa
• Cribriform plate • Roof of ethmoid air cell • Frontal sinus	• Sphenoid sinus • Temporal bone: CSF otorhinorrhea	• Sphenoid sinus

Abbreviation: CSF, cerebrospinal fluid.

Table 71.3 CSF versus nasal secretion

Features	CSF	Nasal secretion
History	History of trauma, surgery, or intracranial tumor	History of itching, sneezing, and nasal obstruction
Flow	Cannot be sniffed back	Can be sniffed back
Posture	Gushes down on bending forward or straining	No effect
Nature	Watery	Slimy
Handkerchief test	No stiffening	Handkerchief soaked in nasal secretion stiffens on drying due to the presence of mucin
Glucose content	>30 mg/dL	<10 mg/dL
Beta-2 transferrin	Present	Absent

Abbreviation: CSF, cerebrospinal fluid.

CSF leaks associated with tumors are due to substantial erosion of the skull base. Treatment is by surgical management of the tumor.

Spontaneous leaks are seen as a variant of benign intracranial hypertension where the intracranial pressure is elevated due to poor CSF resorption by the arachnoid villi. There occurs thinning of bone and CSF leaks in the weakest areas of the skull base.

CSF leaks following sinus surgery is a serious complication. Small leaks may heal spontaneously, but the patient can develop delayed meningitis. If leak is diagnosed intraoperatively, it should be repaired in the same sitting using local intranasal tissue. The most common site of injury is the lateral lamella of the cribriform plate where it is weakened by entry of the anterior ethmoidal artery.

Investigations

- Glucose oxidase test.
- Nasal discharge chloride estimation: It was higher in CSF than in serum.
- Beta-2 transferrin test: There was excellent sensitivity and specificity for CSF leak.
- High-resolution CT (HRCT) scan of the paranasal sinuses.
- CT cisternography.
- MRI—T2-weighted images.
- *Intrathecal fluorescein study*: Diagnostic nasal endoscopy is done to detect the sites of leakage, which are stained bright-green color under blue filter. The fluorescein dye is injected intrathecally.
- Tests for olfaction—if smell sensation is deranged.

■ Treatment

Conservative treatment is by bed rest and head end elevation. Advice the patient not to blow their nose, and to sneeze with their mouth open. Stool softeners, prophylactic antibiotics, and acetazolamide are given. Insertion of a lumbar drain is done sometimes. Pneumococcal vaccination is done (prophylaxis against pneumococcal meningitis).

Surgical treatment by transnasal endoscopic approach is commonly done. For small defects, free fat grafts are used. For medium-sized defects, bone or cartilage grafts and fascia lata are used with fibrin glue to reinforce the closure. Large defects require vascularized septal or turbinate flaps like the "Hadad–Bassagasteguy" flap (septal mucoperiosteum and mucoperichondrium based on the nasoseptal artery).

An open approach, that is, neurosurgical intracranial, is used in massive head trauma with complex comminuted and displaced fractures of the skull base. An extradural approach like external ethmoidectomy or osteoplastic flap is used for large defects or for defects difficult to access endoscopically.

■ Lower Third Facial Fractures

Mandibular Fractures

The mandible will fracture when subjected to direct and indirect force like trauma to the chin or the opposite side of the body. Fracture of the condyles are the most common followed by the angle, body, and symphysis in decreasing

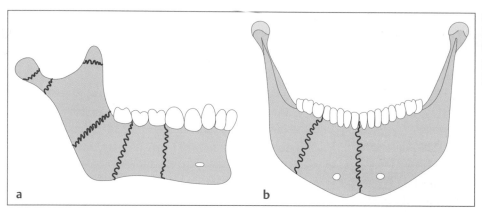

Fig. 71.18 **(a, b)** The Dingman and Natvig classification of mandibular fractures: Symphysis, body, alveolar process, angle, ramus, condylar process, and coronoid process.

order of frequency. The mandible can fracture at more than one site (**Fig. 71.18**).

Clinical Features

The symptoms are pain, blood-stained saliva, anesthesia of the lower lip, trismus, and/or deviation of the jaw.

On examination, a step deformity with crepitus is palpable either externally or intraorally. An asymmetry of the lower dental arch and derangement of the occlusion is present. There may be hematomas in the buccal sulcus or the floor of the mouth. There may be tenderness over the temporomandibular joint. The patient will be unable to move the mandible to the side opposite the fracture. The fracture may be an open fracture with involvement of the parotid and the facial nerve (**Fig. 71.1**).

Compression Test

If doubt exists regarding mandibular fracture, gentle compression of the mandible in two different directions will elicit pain in an undisplaced fracture.

Pearl

Trauma to the mandible can result in fracture of the anterior wall of the external auditory canal. It can be diagnosed by visualizing narrowing of the deep external auditory meatus and movement of the anterior canal wall with opening and closing of the jaw.

Investigations

- X-ray of the skull, PA view (for the condyles).
- Mandible (right and left oblique views) and an orthopantomogram.
- CT scan will help delineate the fractures. The images can be 3D reconstructed (**Fig. 71.19**).

Treatment

Closed reduction techniques include holding the fracture segments in normal occlusion and plating. A simple tie wire placed around the teeth either side of a displaced fracture

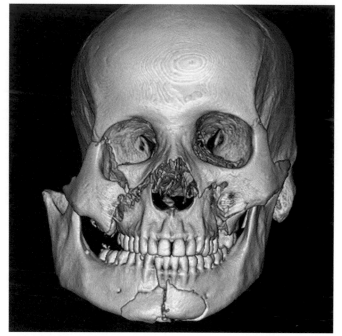

Fig. 71.19 Computed tomography (CT) scan with 3D reconstruction of a mandibular fracture.

reduces pain and bleeding. Intermaxillary fixation is done in undisplaced fractures with no neural deficits and in those with unilateral condylar fractures. Intermaxillary bone pins are placed through the mucosa between the canine and the first premolar on each side and jaw. The screws are then wired together or connected with elastic bands. External fixation is done in gross tissue loss or in pathological fractures. It is achieved by placing cortical screws and then connecting them with an external bar made of acrylic.

In open reduction techniques, the site is exposed and fragments fixed by direct interosseous wiring.

Temporal Bone Fractures

These fractures occur more commonly in males due to a severe blunt head injury. It usually is associated with intracranial, cervical spine, and/or maxillofacial injuries. The most common cause for these fractures is road traffic accidents. Other causes are sports injuries, assaults, and accidental falls. They can occur even with penetrating injuries like gunshot and stab wounds. Important structures like the vestibulocochlear apparatus, facial nerve, internal jugular vein, and internal carotid artery can be involved in the injury.

Classifications

- *Longitudinal and transverse fractures*: Temporal bone fractures were first classified by Ulrich in 1926. These may be oblique or mixed rather than pure longitudinal or transverse. It is a simple classification that is more commonly used.
- *Otic capsule sparing and otic capsule involvement*: Fractures involving the otic capsule can present with severe symptoms and signs.

Clinical Features

Longitudinal

Longitudinal fractures account for 70 to 90% of the fractures. It occurs due to a trauma in the temporoparietal region. These fractures occur parallel to the long axis of the petrous temporal bone.

Bleeding (otorrhagia) can occur due to laceration of skin of the external auditory canal, traumatic perforation of the tympanic membrane, injury to the jugular bulb, or, rarely, due to injury to the internal carotid artery. Hemotympanum (bluish black appearance of the tympanic membrane due to blood in the tympanic cavity) can occur.

Hearing loss may be conductive due to hemotympanum, tympanic membrane perforation, or ossicular chain disruption. Sometimes, a mixed loss can occur when the inner ear is also involved.

Vertigo and tinnitus are not common but can occur due to labyrinthine concussion. These usually subside within a few days.

CSF leak can occur with fracture of the roof of the external auditory canal and tegmen tympani. Meningocele or meningoencephalocele can occur when the gap is significant.

Facial palsy (partial or complete) can occur in 20% of cases.

Transverse

Transverse fractures account for 10 to 30% of the fractures. It occurs due to a trauma in the occipital or frontal region. These fractures run perpendicular to the long axis of the petrous temporal bone.

Hearing loss is usually sensorineural or mixed. Fluctuating hearing loss can occur due to a perilymph fistula.

Vertigo and tinnitus last for a longer duration (weeks to months).

Facial palsy is more common (50% of cases). It can occur due to partial or complete transection of the nerve or due to a bone piece impinging on the nerve. Delayed palsy can occur due to edema of the nerve in an intact facial canal.

Delayed vertigo can occur due to benign paroxysmal positional vertigo or secondary endolymphatic hydrops. The central cause of vertigo may be due to injury in the region of the brainstem.

Management

The trauma may cause multiple injuries. Management of serious injuries like intracranial/spinal injuries, chest injuries, and abdominal injuries may take precedence over temporal bone injuries unless there is profuse bleeding. The initial management of other injuries, including securing the airway and circulation, is done by the emergency department physician/trauma surgeon. Neurosurgical intervention when required should be performed.

Assessment

Cleaning the ear canal (irrigation should not be used especially when a CSF leak is suspected—to avoid meningitis) is done to visualize the canal and the membrane.

An HRCT of the temporal bone (**Fig. 71.20**) is done to assess the site of fracture of the temporal bone, ossicular status, and facial canal. CT of the head and spine is required to assess intracranial and spinal injuries. Angiography is done when a vascular injury is suspected.

Pure tone audiometry is done to assess the hearing. BERA (brainstem evoked response audiometry) may be

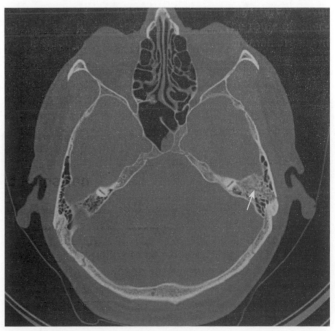

Fig. 71.20 High-resolution computed tomography (HRCT) scan (axial cut) showing longitudinal fracture of the temporal bone on the left side.

required to objectively document the hearing loss, especially in medicolegal cases.

Electrodiagnostic tests (like electromyography) are done when surgical intervention for facial palsy is being contemplated.

Treatment

Bleeding usually stops and rarely requires intervention. Exceptions are when the internal jugular vein or the internal carotid artery is injured. Hemotympanum along with associated conductive hearing loss usually resolves within a few weeks.

Conductive hearing loss due to tympanic membrane perforation resolves when the perforation heals. Ossicular discontinuity requires surgical correction (ossiculoplasty). Sensorineural hearing loss can be managed by a hearing aid or cochlear implant depending on the degree of hearing loss.

Vertigo resolves over few weeks in a longitudinal fracture but may take a few months in a transverse fracture.

Facial palsy can be treated with a tapering dose of steroids, end-to-end anastomosis of the nerve, nerve grafting, or decompression depending on the type of injury.

CSF leak usually resolves with conservative management consisting of bed rest with head end elevation, avoidance of strain, and intermittent lumbar puncture when required. Persistent leaks, especially with herniation of dura, with or without brain matter, require repair as it can lead to recurrent meningitis.

Trauma to the Neck

Etiology

Neck injuries can be due to penetrating (stab and gunshot wound), blast, or blunt trauma (**Fig. 71.21**).

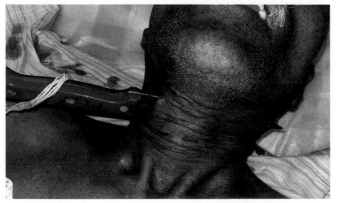

Fig. 71.21 A suicidal stab injury to the neck with a knife.

Zones of the Neck

Roon and Christensen classified the anatomic zones of the neck into the following:
- Zone I: The area between the sternal notch/clavicle and the cricoid cartilage.
- Zone II: The area between the cricoid cartilage and the angle of the mandible.
- Zone III: The area between the angle of the mandible and the base of the skull.

The Trauma Patient: General Principles

■ Primary Survey

The primary survey is an initial assessment of factors that cause early deaths in trauma patients like hypoxia, hypovolemia, tension pneumothorax, and head injury.

Airway and Cervical Spine Protection

The neck should be stabilized with a cervical collar or sandbags. Stridor may be present secondary to hematoma or airway edema. A chin lift and jaw thrust procedure is performed to overcome the obstruction. If the GCS scores are ≤8, endotracheal intubation is done. A cricothyroidotomy/tracheostomy is performed if intubation is not feasible.

Breathing

Chest wall movement and air entry are checked to rule out tension pneumothorax and hemothorax, which have to be managed immediately.

Circulation and Perfusion

If the patient is in shock, crystalloids and/or O negative blood is transfused via two high-flow lines. Active bleeding is controlled by compressive dressing, digital pressure, or ligation. The patient should remain recumbent, or the neck wound must be covered with an occlusive dressing when the patient sits up, to prevent air embolism.

Disability

Assess the GCS, check the pupillary size and light reflex, and assess the power in the limbs.

Exposure

Check for any other associated injuries. The patient is kept warm. An electrocardiogram (ECG), pulse oximetry, and blood pressure monitoring are done.

Investigations

- The complete blood counts (including hemoglobin level), blood glucose, and arterial blood gas analysis are done.
- Cross-sectional CT or MRI with contrast is done to look at the depth of the injury and involvement of the airway, vessels, and other injuries. X-ray of the cervical spine is done to check for spinal column injury and prevertebral air (pharyngeal or esophageal injury). Chest X-ray is done to rule out a hemo- or a pneumothorax, a pneumomediastinum (tracheal or esophageal injury), and a widened mediastinum.
- CT angiography is done in case there is a widened mediastinum to rule out major intrathoracic injury. Pelvic X-ray is done when required.

■ Secondary Survey

Check for the following:
- Large cervical hematoma.
- Subcutaneous emphysema.
- The jugular venous pressure.
- Tenderness over the mandible.
- Peripheral pulses for discrepancy or absence.
- Any neurological deficits.
- Signs of esophageal injury: hemoptysis, hematemesis, dysphagia, and odynophagia.
- Signs of recurrent laryngeal nerve or laryngeal injury: dysphonia, stridor.

All injuries are documented and definitive care is initiated.

Specific Injuries

Pharyngeal injury is seen in zone II penetrating injuries. Dysphagia, odynophagia, voice change, hemoptysis, hematemesis, and surgical emphysema may be present. A flexible nasopharyngoscopy done to visualize edema, blood in the pharynx, or perforation. Upper hypopharyngeal injuries can be managed conservatively. The lower hypopharyngeal injuries should be explored, repaired, and drained like esophageal injuries.

Esophageal injury requires early recognition and treatment.

Vascular injuries are present with deep lacerations. Bleeding from the branches of the external carotid artery can be controlled by embolization or exploration and ligation. The external jugular vein may be ligated if injured. The internal jugular vein may be repaired by lateral venorrhaphy, or ligated. Chylous injury is managed by early ligation via thoracotomy.

Neurological injury like significant brachial plexus nerve injury should be repaired within 24 to 72 hours.

Laryngotracheal Trauma

Laryngotracheal trauma is relatively common. Appropriate early management is required to restore a safe airway and upper aerodigestive tract function for both voice and swallow (**Fig. 71.22**).

Etiology

It is broadly classified into external and internal causes. External injuries can be due to blunt or penetrating trauma, and internal can be due to inhalational or iatrogenic injuries.

Blunt injuries are seen:
- Motor vehicle accidents when a hyperextended neck strikes with objects in front (crush injury).
- Clothesline (high-velocity impact of the larynx with a stationary object).
- Strangulation (hanging or strangulation by a soft object).
- Penetrating injuries are low-velocity gunshot wounds (handguns), high-velocity gunshot wounds (rifles), or stab wounds (knives).

Inhalational injuries are from toxic gases, exposure to fires, or ingestion of toxic substances.

Iatrogenic injuries are due to oro- or nasotracheal intubation, cricothyroidotomy, or during elective operations such as laryngeal surgery, laryngoscopy, or routine tracheostomy.

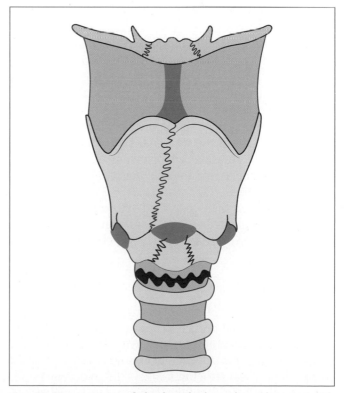

Fig. 71.22 Fracture of the hyoid, thyroid cartilage, cricoid, and laryngotracheal separation.

Pathophysiology

There may be damage to mucosa, nerves (superior and recurrent laryngeal nerves), soft tissue (intrinsic and extrinsic muscles, ligaments), cartilages (arytenoid dislocation and thyroid or cricoid cartilage fracture), and trachea (tracheal rings and trachealis muscle). In an acute injury, the airway can be compromised. Chronic injury like scarring, subluxation, and ankylosis of the arytenoids and cricoarytenoid joints, fibrosis of the laryngeal muscles, anterior and posterior glottic web, and supraglottic and subglottic scarring, muscle palsy with glottic incompetence, dysphonia, aspiration, and dysphagia can occur.

Classification

Fuhrman et al classified the laryngotracheal injuries into the following:
- Group 1: Minor endolaryngeal hematoma without detectable fracture.
- Group 2: Edema, hematoma, minor mucosal disruption without exposed cartilage, and nondisplaced fractures are noted on CT scan.
- Group 3: Massive edema, mucosal tears, exposed cartilage, and cord immobility.
- Group 4: Same as group 3, but with more than two fracture lines or massive trauma to the laryngeal mucosa.
- Group 5: Complete laryngotracheal separation.

Clinical Features

The presentation is with dyspnoea, dysphonia/aphonia, dysphagia, neck pain, hemoptysis, neck wounds, and/or bleeding.

On examination, there may be stridor, tachypnoea, tachycardia, and sweating.

The patient may be in shock. One should look for ecchymosis in the skin of the neck and subcutaneous emphysema and assess abrasions or open wounds.

Check for tenderness, tracheal deviation, cartilaginous, and bony fractures.

On indirect laryngoscopy/rigid telescopy, the following signs may be noted: edema, hematoma, mucosal tears, vocal cord palsy, dislocated cricoarytenoid joint, and exposed cartilage.

Investigations

After establishment of a safe airway, microlaryngoscopy, esophagoscopy, and bronchoscopy are done to assess the extent of injury. A preliminary CT with 3D reconstruction is required for information about injuries to larynx, cervical spine, and vascular structures. MRI is the gold standard for radiological assessment of the larynx and its framework.

Chest X-ray is done to rule out aspiration pneumonia and polytrauma.

Treatment

The management of laryngotracheal injuries may be nonsurgical or surgical depending on the type and extent of injury. It follows a thorough assessment of the patient.

Airway stability is integral to nonoperative management and assumes protection by the patient's own reflexes or by an endotracheal tube as in group 1 and 2 laryngeal traumas. The patient should be admitted to an intensive care unit for airway monitoring for at least 24 hours. The patient is intubated, if required, and nothing is given orally. The head end is elevated. Voice rest is advised. Steroids will help resolve edema and reduce scarring. Antibiotics are given to prevent perichondritis and secondary wound infection. Anti-inflammatory drugs are given for pain. Antireflux medications are given to prevent further irritation of the injured laryngeal mucosa.

Surgical intervention is required in patients in whom nonoperative management options are unsuccessful in improving airway function or in those who continue to deteriorate despite these measures. Intubation may be difficult and may cause disruption of the traumatized laryngotracheal framework. In these cases, tracheostomy is done to secure the airway.

Endoscopic management like aspiration of hematoma, re-approximation of torn margins, placement of stents/keels may be required. Rigid esophagoscopy is done to exclude any injury to the integrity of the esophageal wall.

Open surgical procedures are done in group 5 injuries, namely, emergency tracheostomy, surgical exploration, and immediate repair with nonabsorbable sutures (knots are placed extraluminally). In groups 3 and 4, exploration is done within 24 hours of injury. A laryngofissure (or midline thyrotomy) approach is used. Debridement of devitalized tissues is done, and fractured segments are stabilized with sutures or metal plates. A keel is placed between the cords or a stent in the lumen to prevent adhesions and stenosis. In a grossly injured larynx that is irreparable or incompetent, a laryngectomy can be done.

Complications

The common complications are laryngotracheal stenosis, perichondritis, vocal cord palsy, and granuloma formation.

Pearl

The first successful total laryngeal transplant was performed by Marshall Strome et al in 1998 in a 40-year-old with irreparable traumatic injury to the larynx.

Points to Ponder

- Traumas to the face and neck are on the rise due to increased road traffic accidents.
- Since most of these are medicolegal in nature, careful evaluation and meticulous documentation is of utmost importance.
- The management is according to the Advanced Trauma Life Support (ATLS) guidelines.
- Nasal bones are one of the most common bones to be fractured in the human body.
- Nasal bone fractures are divided into classes I, II, and III.
- Zygoma fractures are also called tripod or quadripod fractures depending on the number of fracture sites.
- Blowout fractures involve the floor of the orbit with a radiological "teardrop sign."
- Le Fort fractures are complex fractures of the midface and classified as Le Fort I, II, and III.
- Target sign is seen on filter paper and is specific for traumatic CSF leak.
- Beta-2 transferrin test is a specific test to identify CSF.

Case-Based Questions

1. **A 35-year-old man was brought into the trauma center with a history of facial trauma after a road traffic accident. He was found to have a clear watery leak from the nose. His airway was patent, blood pressure was stable, and there were no overt signs of internal bleeding. He was conscious and oriented.**

   a. What is the cause of the clear watery fluid from the nose? What other conditions produce this type of discharge from the nose?

   b. What investigations would you like to do to confirm this condition?

   c. What is the treatment?

   Answers

   a. Clear watery fluid from the nose after facial or nasal trauma may be due to CS leak. This type of discharge may also be seen in allergic rhinitis, vasomotor rhinitis, and early stage of viral rhinitis.

   b. Traumatic CSF leak will produce a "halo or target sign" on filter paper. The single best test to identify CSF is to look for beta-2 transferrin protein in the fluid. You need a minimum of 0.5 ml of the fluid and the sensitivity is 92% and specificity is 100%. An HRCT scan is the imaging of choice to detect skull base fractures to determine the location of the leak. CT cisternography will also help in localization through the intrathecal injection of a contrast dye.

   c. A conservative treatment policy has been advocated in cases of CSF leak following trauma. This involves a 7- to 10-day bed rest with the head end elevated 15 to 30 degrees to reduce the CSF pressure. Avoid coughing and sneezing. Prescribe stool softeners to prevent straining. Antibiotics and diuretics are administered. If CSF leak persists, surgery is performed to close the leak. Surgical repair consists of intracranial and transnasal endoscopic approaches and can be done depending on the location and severity of the injury.

2. **A 25-year-old woman was brought into the trauma center after a high-velocity impact injury to the face following a road traffic accident in which there was a two-car collision.**

   On examination, she was drifting in an out of consciousness with profuse bleeding from the nose. She was noted to have bilateral raccoon eyes and dish-shaped deformity of the face.

   a. What does profuse epistaxis and raccoon eyes indicate?

   b. What type of fracture would produce a dish-shaped deformity?

   c. How will you treat this condition?

   Answers

   a. These signs indicate a skull base fracture.

   b. Le Fort III midface fractures. Dish-shaped deformity is due to the posterior displacement of the maxilla. It is also known as craniofacial dysjunction.

   c. Surgery has to be performed after stabilization of her life-threatening condition. Le Fort fractures require fixation with miniplates and screws of the fractured bones to ensure stability.

3. **A 32-year-old male patient was involved in a sports injury with trauma to the nose. On examination, there was gross edema over the nose. What is the management in the following situations?**

   a. Undisplaced fracture of the nasal bones.

   b. Displaced fracture with deformity.

   c. Fracture with deformity presenting after 8 weeks.

   Answers

   a. Conservative treatment with analgesics.

   b. Reduction of the fracture once the edema subsides.

   c. Rhinoplasty for correction of the external deformity.

4. **A 24-year-old man presented with diplopia following an injury from the front, over the right orbit by a cricket ball.**

   a. What is the most likely fracture that has occurred?

   b. What is the typical finding on X-ray?

   c. What is the clinical test done to differentiate it from nerve palsy?

   d. What is the treatment?

   Answers

   a. Blowout fracture.

   b. Teardrop sign.

   c. FDT.

   d. Oral steroids to reduce edema. If the diplopia is persistent or when the FDT is positive, then surgical release of the entrapped muscle with strengthening of the orbital floor with an implant or graft is done.

5. **A 52-year-old man presented to the emergency department following a road traffic accident. The injury was at the level of the teeth. The CT scan done showed the fracture extending along the floor of the nasal cavities and lower part of the maxillary sinuses up to the inferior part of the medial and lateral pterygoid plates.**

   a. What is this type of fracture known as?

   b. What will be the presentation?

   c. What is Guerin's sign?

   Answers

   a. Le Fort I fracture.

   b. Anterior open bite (malocclusion), ecchymosis in the upper gingivobuccal sulcus and palate, and edema of the upper lip.

   c. Ecchymosis of the palate in the region of the greater palatine vessels.

Frequently Asked Questions

1. How do you classify nasal bone fractures?

2. Describe the management of a class I nasal bone fracture.

3. What is a tripod fracture? What are its clinical features?

4. Enumerate the cause of CSF leak.

5. What are the relevant investigations that should be carried out to determine the site of a CSF leak?

6. Describe the various type of Le Fort fractures.

7. What is a blowout fracture?

8. Describe the different types of temporal bone fractures.

9. What are the clinical features of a patient with a transverse fracture of the temporal bone?

10. What is Panda facies?

11. What is forced duction test?

12. What is a teardrop sign?

13. What is a halo sign in CSF rhinorrhea?

Endnote

Rene Le Fort, a French surgeon (1869–1951), was well known for his classification of the fractures of the face. In 1901, he published a paper on his experiments with fractures of the middle one-third of the face. For his experiments, he used cadavers, which were placed on the floor. He would then ascend a ladder and drop stones and other hard objects of different weights from different heights and study the fracture lines that develop on the face. He called these lines the "lines of weakness." From these tests, he concluded that there were three types of fractures: the horizontal (Le Fort I), the pyramidal (Le Fort II), and the transverse (Le Fort III). These were induced by simple blunt trauma. Nowadays, trauma is more complex due to high-velocity impacts from vehicles, but his classification is still widely used in medicine.

L. Sudarshan Reddy

The competencies covered in this chapter are as follows:

EN4.37 Describe the clinical features, investigations, and principles of management of Ludwig's angina.

EN4.41 Describe the clinical features, investigations, and principles of management of acute and chronic abscesses in relation to the pharynx.

AN36.4 Describe the anatomical basis of tonsillitis, tonsillectomy, adenoids, and peritonsillar abscess.

Introduction

Neck space infections are common and potentially life-threatening conditions in both adults and children. The occurrence has been declining since the advent of antibiotic therapy. However, they still do occur and pose a challenging diagnostic and treatment problem. Aggressive monitoring and management of airway is the primary concern followed by appropriate antibiotic therapy and surgical drainage when needed.

Anatomy

The neck is divided into several compartments by the fascia. The fascia is the term used to describe broad sheets of dense connective tissue that separate structures that may run over each other during movement. Understanding these interfascia spaces helps in determining the etiology, pathogenesis, clinical manifestations, and course of spread of infection. Infections that transgress the fascial boundaries and extend along vertically oriented spaces have higher risk of complications.

The cervical fascia is divided into the following:
- Superficial fascia, which is part of the superficial musculoaponeurotic system (SMAS).
- Deep cervical fascia.

The deep cervical fascia is further divided into the following (**Fig. 72.1**):
- The superficial layer (investing layer) envelops the trapezius and sternocleidomastoid muscle along with the parotid and submandibular salivary glands.

- The middle layer is further divided into the following:
  - A muscular layer that envelopes the strap muscles.
  - A visceral layer that surrounds the pharynx, larynx, trachea, esophagus, and thyroid.
- The deep layer includes the alar fascia and the prevertebral fascia.

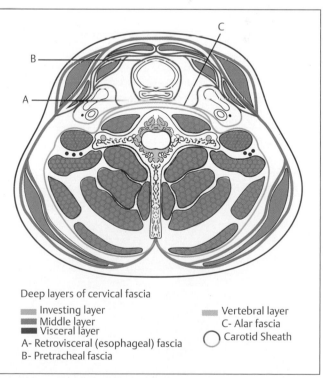

Deep layers of cervical fascia

Investing layer
Middle layer
Visceral layer
A- Retrovisceral (esophageal) fascia
B- Pretracheal fascia

Vertebral layer
C- Alar fascia
Carotid Sheath

Fig. 72.1 Diagrammatic representation of the deep layers of the cervical fascia.

Spaces of Neck

The various spaces of neck are mentioned in **Table 72.1**.

Table 72.1 Various spaces of the neck

Suprahyoid spaces	Infrahyoid spaces	Spaces extending through the entire length of the neck
Mandibular spaces: • Submandibular space • Submental space • Sublingual space	Pretracheal space	Superficial spaces
Masticator space		Deep neck spaces
Lateral pharyngeal space		Retropharyngeal space
Peritonsillar space		
Parotid space		

The neck spaces that traverse the entire length of the neck include the following (**Figs. 72.2, 72.3,** and **72.4**):
- Retropharyngeal space.
- Danger space.
- Prevertebral space.
- Carotid space.

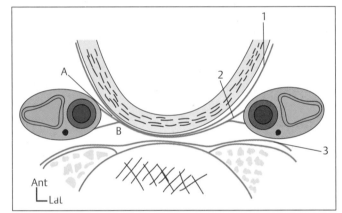

Fig. 72.2 Line diagram showing the retropharyngeal and danger spaces. 1, The visceral fascia; 2, the alar fascia; 3, the prevertebral fascia; A, the retropharyngeal space; B, the danger space.

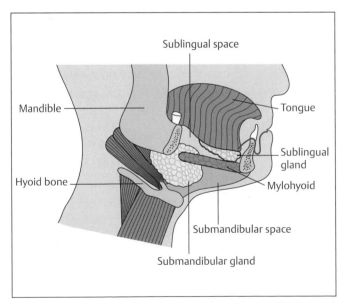

Fig. 72.3 Line diagram depicting the submandibular and sublingual spaces.

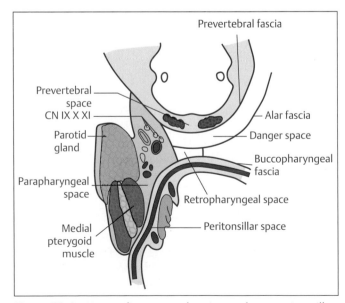

Fig. 72.4 Line diagram showing the peritonsillar, parapharyngeal, and prevertebral spaces.

Deep Spaces of the Neck

The deep spaces are potential spaces in the neck occupied by loose connective tissue between the superficial, middle, and deep layers of the deep fascia.

■ Microbiology

Most neck infections are polymicrobial; only 5% are purely aerobic and 25% are with isolated anaerobes. *Streptococcus viridans*, *Staphylococcus aureus*, and *Klebsiella pneumonia* are the most common aerobic organisms. Bacteroids, *Peptostreptococcus*, *Fusobacterium*, and *Prevotella* are the most prevalent anaerobes. The incidence of methicillin-resistant *S. aureus* is higher in the younger age group. Dental cause for neck infections are usually associated with anaerobes.

Superficial Neck Space Infections

These infections usually present with cellulitis of the skin of the neck. They are divided into the following:
- *Non-necrotizing infections*: impetigo, erysipelas, and nontuberculous cervical fascia lymphadenitis.
- *Necrotizing infections*: *Cervical necrotizing fasciitis* is a rare and rapidly progressive infection with necrosis of subcutaneous tissue. It is seen in the older age group (above 60 years), with diabetes mellitus and in immunocompromised conditions. It can progress to necrotizing mediastinitis, sepsis, and eventually into toxic shock syndrome. It is usually caused by beta-hemolytic streptococci. Treatment includes broad-spectrum intravenous antibiotics, surgical fasciotomy, and early debridement. Hyperbaric oxygen and poly-specific immunoglobulins act as adjuvant therapy.

Deep Neck Infections

■ Introduction

Deep neck infections (DNIs) involve the neck structures surrounded by multiple layers of deep cervical fascia. Clinical features appear due to mass effect of inflamed tissues or abscess cavity on surrounding structures or by direct involvement of structures in the inflammation process. It is more common in patients with poor oral hygiene and with lack of dental care.

Deep neck space infections are serious infections that can rapidly progress to cause airway compromise.

■ Etiology

- Pharyngitis.
- Tonsillitis.
- Odontogenic infection.
- Salivary gland infection.
- Penetrating injury.
- Iatrogenic perforation of the esophagus.
- Fish bone ingestion.
- Suppurative lymph nodes.
- Infected congenital (like branchial cleft cyst) or acquired lesions.
- Intravenous drug abuse.
- Acute mastoiditis.

Peritonsillar Abscess (Quinsy)

The peritonsillar space is bounded medially by the capsule of the palatine tonsil, and laterally by the superior pharyngeal constrictor muscle covered by a layer of the pharyngobasilar fascia. Peritonsillar abscess is the collection of pus between the tonsillar capsule and the surrounding tissues.

Quinsy is usually unilateral; only 3 to 7% of cases are bilateral. It is seen more commonly in young adults. Classically, it is caused by a virulent tonsillar infection that breaks through the tonsillar capsule. This space communicates with the retropharyngeal and parapharyngeal spaces.

■ Etiology

It occurs following recurrent attacks, partially treated or untreated, of suppurative tonsillitis. It can rarely occur without any prior history of tonsillitis. The route of infection is through crypts of the tonsil. The common organism isolated is beta-hemolytic streptococci. Other organisms being *Haemophilus influenzae*, *S. aureus*, and *Neisseria* spp. Anaerobes noted are *fusobacterium*, *Peptostreptococcus*, and *bacteroides*. Bacteriology of acute tonsillitis differs from that of quinsy.

The infection from the crypts can spread through the capsule to the peritonsillar space leading to peritonsillitis. When there is pus formation within this space, it leads to an abscess.

■ Clinical Presentation

Symptoms

The patient presents with the following:
- Fever, chills, and rigors.
- Nonresolving progressive severe throat pain.

- Associated difficulty in opening the mouth or trismus due to spasm of the pterygoid muscles.
- Drooling of saliva and halitosis.
- Ipsilateral referred otalgia.

Signs

On examination, the following may be noted (**Fig. 72.5**):
- Erythema, edema, and bulging of the soft palate with the uvula pushed to the opposite side.
- Anterior, inferior, and medial displacement of the ipsilateral tonsil.
- ipsilateral tender and enlarged jugulodigastric lymph nodes.
- Muffled speech with the classically described "hot potato" voice.

If left untreated, it can lead to a submandibular space abscess, parapharyngeal abscess, laryngeal edema, and/or septicemia.

> **Pearl**
>
> With this presentation, one should rule out peritonsillitis, infectious mononucleosis, neoplasms (including malignancy and salivary gland tumors), impacted foreign body, and aneurysm of the internal carotid artery.

■ Management

Investigations

- The patient requires hospitalization.
- A computed tomography (CT) scan or ultrasound of the neck can confirm the diagnosis.
- A complete blood count will show leukocytosis with neutrophilia.

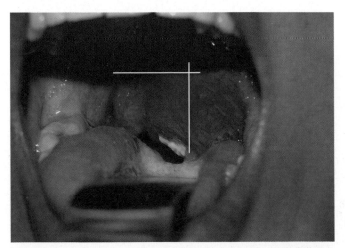

Fig. 72.5 Left peritonsillar abscess (quinsy). There is fullness and inflammation pushing the tonsil medially and the uvula to the opposite side. The intersection of the horizontal line (from base of uvula) and vertical line (along anterior pillar) is the site for incision and drainage.

- Serum electrolytes are done to assess for electrolyte imbalance secondary to inadequate oral intake.
- The monospot test may be done if infectious mononucleosis is suspected.

Treatment

- Systemic, parenteral broad-spectrum antibiotics (covering gram-positive and gram-negative aerobic bacteria, and anaerobic organisms) are started.
- The dehydration is corrected.
- Aspiration can be done with a wide bore needle and syringe.
- Incision and drainage is done (with Quinsy forceps) at the point of intersection of an imaginary horizontal line along the base of the uvula (or the third molar) and a vertical line along the anterior tonsillar pillar. It can also be done at the point of maximum prominence of the abscess. Postdrainage, mouth gargles are used (**Fig. 72.6**).
- Hot (or abscess) tonsillectomy can be done during the acute phase after draining the abscess, but it is usually associated with an increased risk of intraoperative hemorrhage. Interval tonsillectomy is usually done 6 weeks after the initial infection.

Ludwig's Angina

■ Introduction

It is a rapidly progressive, polymicrobial, cellulitis involving bilateral submaxillary, sublingual, and submental spaces. It is a potentially life-threatening infection that can lead to airway compromise.

Before the advent of antibiotics, the mortality from Ludwig's angina was 50%. Currently, it is around 8%.

The primary site of infection in Ludwig's angina is the submandibular space. This space is further divided into the

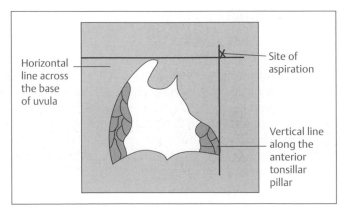

Fig. 72.6 The site of aspiration and the site of incision for drainage of quinsy.

sublingual space above and the submaxillary space below by the mylohyoid muscle. Odontogenic infections are responsible for over 90% of cases and those who are immunocompromised are at risk.

■ Etiology

Although it is a polymicrobial infection, beta-hemolytic streptococci and *staphylococcus* are the common causative organisms. Other organisms are *peptostreptococcus, fusobacterium, bacteroides*, and *actinomyces*. A common source of infection is from a dental root abscess in which there is extension of infection from the root of the mandibular teeth (**Fig. 72.7**).

Depending on the mylohyoid line (i.e., site of the root of teeth above or below the line):

- The submental space is involved from the incisors.
- The sublingual space from the premolars and the first molar.
- The submandibular space from the second and third molars. The second and third molars are the common source (**Fig. 72.8**).

Other causes include the following:

- Floor of the mouth or tongue trauma.
- Following dental extraction.
- Following mandibular fractures or osteomyelitis.
- Salivary gland infection.
- Peritonsillar abscess.
- Oral piercing.
- Infected thyroglossal cyst.

The contributing factors are uncontrolled diabetes, immunocompromised states, poor oral hygiene, and alcoholism.

■ Criteria for Diagnosis

- A rapidly progressive cellulitis, and not abscess, which does not involve the submandibular gland and the lymph nodes.
- It develops along the fascial planes by direct spread and not lymphatic spread.
- It is usually bilateral in presentation.

■ Clinical Presentation

Symptoms

The patient will present with a diffuse neck swelling. They will complain of dysphagia and odynophagia along with fever, malaise, and pain.

Signs

- There will be drooling of saliva, neck rigidity, and trismus.
- In the suprahyoid region, the neck will have a "woody" or brawny induration (**Fig. 72.9**).
- The floor of the mouth is raised due to edema or underlying pus and the tongue is pushed posterosuperiorly, compromising the airway (**Fig. 72.10**).
- Oral hygiene will be poor with associated halitosis.
- There may be tachypnea and dyspnea with impending airway compromise.

> ### Pearl
> If there is crepitus on palpation, it may be a necrotizing fasciitis.

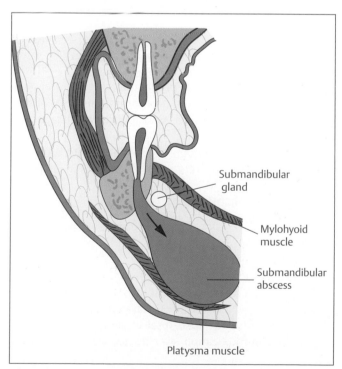

Fig. 72.7 Infection spreading to the submandibular space from the roots of the teeth.

Submandibular gland

Mylohyoid muscle

Submandibular abscess

Platysma muscle

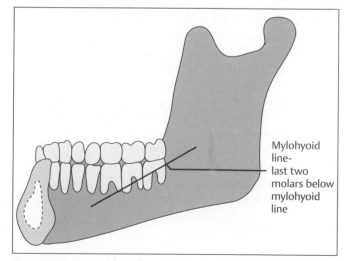

Fig. 72.8 Root of molars below the mylohyoid line helps infection to spread to the floor of the mouth.

Mylohyoid line- last two molars below mylohyoid line

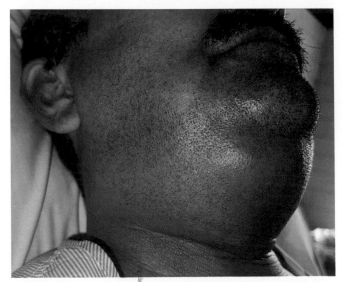

Fig. 72.9 Ludwig's angina showing the typical "bull neck" appearance.

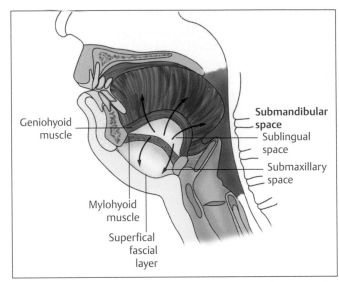

Fig. 72.10 Ludwig's angina showing spread of infection in the sublingual and submaxillary spaces.

■ Investigations

- A complete blood count is done and it will show leukocytosis.
- Dental X ray is done to rule out tooth (apical) infection.
- A CT scan with contrast of the neck is done to assess the extent of spread, especially to the adjacent spaces and laryngeal airway.

■ Treatment

- If the patient has respiratory obstruction due to the infection, the airway must be secured through a tracheostomy.
- *Intravenous antibiotics*: A third-generation cephalosporins or a combination of clindamycin + metronidazole should be started.
- Intravenous fluids are started because the patient will be dehydrated due to odynophagia.
- Surgical decompression is by incision and drainage. Oral endotracheal intubation may be difficult for the anesthetist due to pain, trismus, and edema of the floor of the mouth with upward and posterior displacement of the tongue. There is a possibility of airway compromise during attempts at oral intubation. Therefore, a flexible, fiberoptic endoscopy-guided transnasal intubation is preferred. Tracheostomy is done when the airway is difficult to access.
- Control of diabetes should be done in diabetics.
- Dental extraction is done if a tooth as a source of infection is present.

Parotid Space Infections

The parotid space is a closed space occupied by the parotid gland, facial nerve, external carotid artery, and the posterior facial vein. Its walls are formed by a split in the superficial layer of the deep cervical fascia, which completely encloses the space except for a frequent medial dehiscence adjacent to the pharyngomaxillary space. The fascia is reinforced inferiorly manifesting as a strong band that separates the parotid gland from the submaxillary space.

■ Etiology

It is seen in the older age group, especially with poor oral hygiene, decreased saliva production, recent oral surgery, dehydration, or immunocompromised states. There may be a preceding parotitis or suppurative intraparotid lymphadenitis.

The most common organism associated with a parotid abscess is *S. aureus* in adults and *Streptococcus* in children.

■ Clinical Presentation

- There is a marked swelling at the angle of the jaw with associated pain.
- The patient may be febrile.
- The skin over the swelling is red.
- On palpation, there will be tenderness and induration over the involved region. Occasionally, there will be discharge from the ipsilateral external auditory canal due to communication via the fissures of Santorini.

On pressure over the swelling, pus may be seen emanating from Stensen's duct opening opposite the upper second molar. Deep lobe abscess presents with dysphagia and odynophagia, and the tonsil is pushed medially.

■ Investigations

A complete blood count and blood sugar levels are done. A contrast-enhanced CT scan or magnetic resonance imaging (MRI) will show the site and extent of the abscess (**Figs. 72.11** and **72.12**).

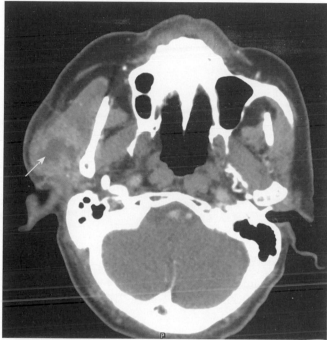

Fig. 72.11 Contrast-enhanced computed tomography (CT) scan axial cut showing the central hypodense area with peripheral enhancement—a right parotid abscess.

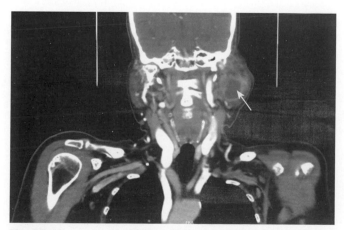

Fig. 72.12 Contrast enhanced CT scan showing a left parotid abscess.

■ Treatment

- Intravenous antibiotics (broad spectrum for aerobic and anaerobic pathogens) are administered.
- Intravenous fluids (for hydration) are given.
- An incision over the prominence of the parotid swelling, parallel to the branches of the facial nerve, is done to drain the abscess. If the swelling is extensive, a modified Blair incision is preferred.
- Oral hygiene is improved with frequent gargles and adequate hydration.

> ### Pearl
> Surgical parotitis is a condition in which there is acute inflammation of the parotid gland after surgery. It is a postoperative complication. It can be unilateral or bilateral. It is seen in patients with dry mouth and decreased salivary production after surgery due to inadequate fluid intake resulting in dehydration. The maximum incidence is seen after abdominal surgery.

Parapharyngeal Abscess

■ Anatomy

The parapharyngeal space is an inverted pyramid–shaped space that extends from the skull base superiorly to the lesser horn of the hyoid inferiorly. It is divided into the prestyloid (muscular) and poststyloid (neurovascular) compartments. It communicates with the retropharyngeal space posteromedially, the submandibular space inferiorly, and the masticator space laterally. It is also related to the carotid space and infection can spread through this space into the mediastinum. This is known as Lincoln's highway. Infection can also spread to the parotid space (**Fig. 72.13**).

■ Etiology

Infection in this space can be due to spread of infection from the surrounding spaces like the peritonsillar, submandibular, parotid, retropharyngeal, or masticator spaces. Spread of infection from the middle ear cleft (acute otitis media) via the mastoid tip (Bezold's abscess) or the peritubal cells can present in this space.

Other sources of infection are from the lower third molar, intravenous drug abuse, and penetrating neck injury.

Uncontrolled diabetes and immunocompromised states are risk factors. It can also be seen in children and adolescents.

■ Clinical Presentation

- There may be associated fever, odynophagia, sore throat, torticollis, signs of toxemia, and stridor.

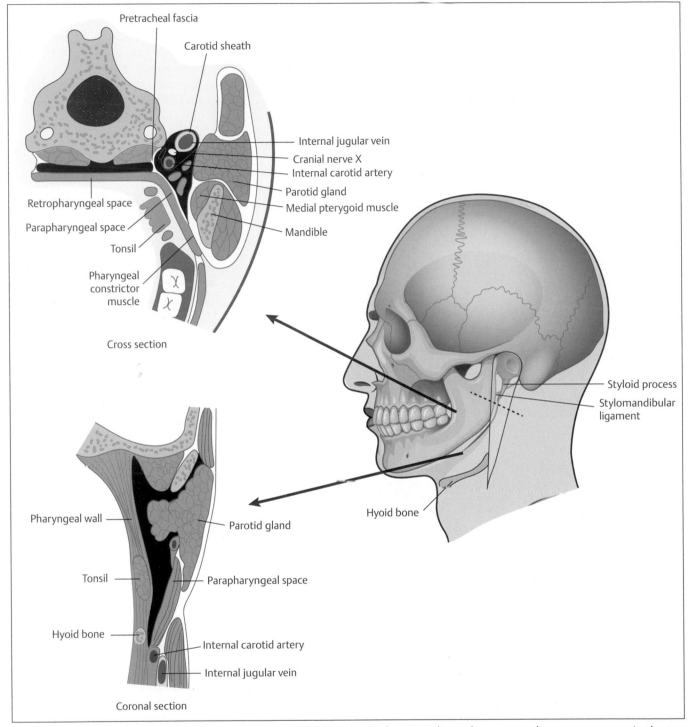

Fig. 72.13 Cross section of the parapharyngeal space dividing it into the muscular and neurovascular compartments in the top diagram and the sagittal section showing the inverted pyramid shape in the lower diagram.

- In prestyloid compartment infection, there is marked trismus and dysphagia. There will be induration at the angle of the mandible and medial displacement of the tonsil. Trismus is due to spasm of the pterygoid muscles. The tonsillar bulge in the oropharynx is more prominent toward the anterior pillar.

- In poststyloid compartment infection, there is medial displacement of the lateral pharyngeal wall behind the posterior tonsillar pillar.
- There may be paralysis of cranial nerves IX–XII.
- Horner's syndrome may be present.

- It can cause internal jugular vein thrombosis with septicemia or a pseudoaneurysm of the internal carotid artery.
- There may be a swelling in the parotid region, or adjacent to the angle of the mandible.

■ Investigations

- A contrast-enhanced CT scan or MRI is done to assess the extent of disease, spread to surrounding spaces, and vascular involvement (**Fig. 72.14**).
- The diabetic status of the patient is monitored.
- A complete blood count and blood culture are also done.
- Chest X-ray or CT scan of the thorax is done to rule out mediastinitis.

■ Treatment

An incision and drainage of the abscess must be carried out. The incision is made at the level of the hyoid bone just below the angle of the mandible. Blunt dissection is used to avoid trauma to the neurovascular structures.

Intravenous (broad-spectrum) antibiotics are administered.

> ### Pearl
>
> Lemierre's syndrome is thrombophlebitis of the internal jugular vein due to infection by anaerobic bacteria like *Fusobacterium necrophorum*. It is secondary to a throat infection. The infection spreads from the throat by retrograde thrombophlebitis of the tonsillar vein to the internal jugular vein. The infection can then spread to distant sites like the lungs, joints, and bone through septic foci.

■ Complications

A parapharyngeal abscess produces morbidity and mortality due to complications.

The following are some of the important complications produced by this condition.
- Airway obstruction due to laryngeal edema.
- Thrombophlebitis of the internal jugular vein (Lemierre's syndrome).
- Spread to the carotid space (Lincoln's highway).
- Mediastinitis.
- Carotid blowout.
- Spread of infection to the retropharyngeal space.

Retropharyngeal Abscess

■ Acute Retropharyngeal Abscess

An acute retropharyngeal abscess is more commonly seen in children younger than 5 years.

Anatomy

Retropharyngeal space lies between the buccopharyngeal fascia anteriorly and the alar fascia posteriorly (**Fig. 72.15**). It extends from the skull base to the level of the tracheal bifurcation. It communicates with the posterior mediastinum inferiorly and the parapharyngeal spaces anterolaterally on both sides. A median raphe divides the space into right and left compartments.

The contents of this space include fat and lymph nodes. The lymph nodes have a medial group (nodes of Krause) and a lateral group (nodes of Rouviere).

Etiology

- In children, suppuration of the lymph nodes in this space can occur following infection in the nose, posterior

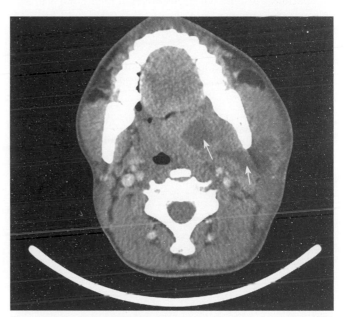

Fig. 72.14 Contrast-enhanced computed tomography (CT) scan showing a left parapharyngeal abscess.

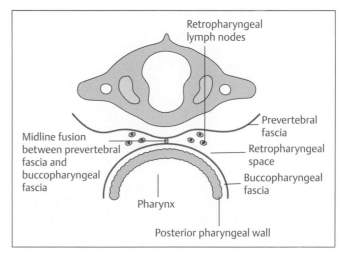

Fig. 72.15 Retropharyngeal space and contents.

paranasal sinuses, and nasopharynx. This may be due to an upper respiratory tract infection with suppurative cervical lymphadenitis.

The retropharyngeal lymph nodes in children generally atrophy by 5 years of age.

In adults, the causes may be due to the following:
- Trauma (including iatrogenic during endoscopy).
- Foreign body in the pharynx.
- Fracture or osteomyelitis of the cervical vertebra.
- Diabetes mellitus and immunocompromised states may be contributing factors in the older age group.

Clinical Presentation

Symptoms

The patient presents with symptoms of fever, malaise, sore throat, odynophagia, and dysphagia. There will be neck stiffness or torticollis. The patient will prefer to keep the neck flexed.

Drooling of saliva and breathing difficulty may be seen.

Chest pain signifies extension to the mediastinum.

Signs

On examination of the oropharynx, bulging of the posterior pharyngeal wall is limited to the right or the left side of the midline due the presence of the midline raphe in the parapharyngeal space.

The voice will be muffled.

Stridor with tachypnea and intercostal retractions may be present.

The overlying pharyngeal mucosa is inflamed.

Investigations

- X-ray of the neck soft tissue, lateral view, with neck extension (taken during inspiration) will show increased prevertebral soft-tissue shadow. This should be > 50% of the width of the corresponding vertebral body, or > 7 mm at C2 level, and > 14 mm in children/> 22 mm in adults at C6 level to be considered as prevertebral widening. Loss of cervical lordosis and presence of air shadow (or air–fluid level) in the prevertebral region is another sign (**Figs. 72.16** and **72.17**).
- The preferred radiological investigation is a contrast-enhanced CT scan or MRI of the neck and thorax. However, if there is an airway compromise, the scan should be done after securing the airway (**Fig. 72.18**).
- A complete blood count will show leukocytosis with neutrophilia. Blood culture may be required.

Treatment

The patient should be hospitalized. The airway must be secured when there is respiratory distress. Broad-spectrum intravenous antibiotics and intravenous fluids should be started. A surgical drainage via a transoral approach should

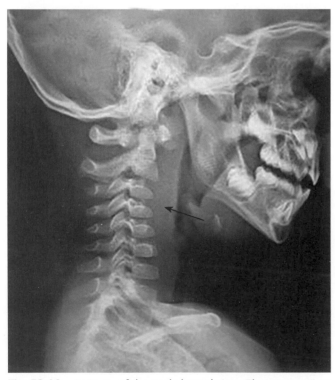

Fig. 72.16 An X-ray of the neck, lateral view. The *arrow* points to the prevertebral widening in a child with retropharyngeal abscess.

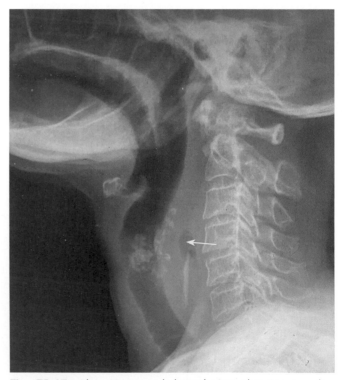

Fig. 72.17 Plain X-ray neck lateral view showing a radio-opaque foreign body with an adjoining small air pocket suggestive of an abscess.

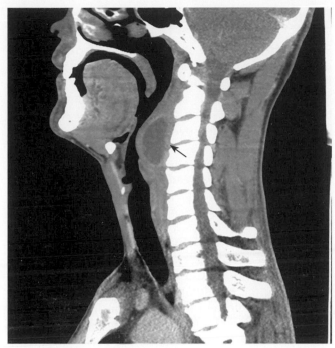

Fig. 72.18 Contrast-enhanced computed tomography (CT) scan (sagittal view) showing a retropharyngeal abscess (straightening of the cervical vertebra can be noted).

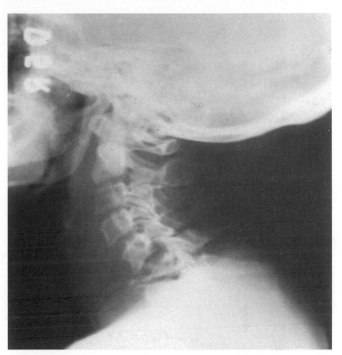

Fig. 72.19 Plain X-ray lateral view of the neck showing prevertebral widening with loss of lordosis and erosion of the lower cervical vertebral bodies with reduced intervertebral disk space suggestive of tuberculosis.

be done with the patient in the Trendelenburg position to avoid aspiration. Suction should be kept ready. The pus should be sent for culture and sensitivity. If intubation is attempted, it should be done by an experienced anesthetist as rupture of the abscess can lead to aspiration pneumonia. An external approach is used if the abscess extends below the level of the hyoid.

Complications

Complications include the following:
- Meningitis.
- Laryngeal spasm.
- Septicemia.
- Rupture with aspiration pneumonia.
- Mediastinitis.
- Esophageal perforation.
- Bronchial erosion.
- Spread to the parapharyngeal space can lead to involvement of the neurovascular bundle there.

The immediate serious complication is an airway compromise.

■ Chronic Retropharyngeal Abscess

Etiology

It is due to spread of infection to this space from tuberculosis of the cervical vertebra (also known as Pott's disease). The spread of tuberculosis to the vertebra is via

a hematogenous route. Occasionally, it can involve the persistent retropharyngeal lymph nodes via a lymphatic spread. HIV infection and immunosuppressant medications can be predisposing factors.

Clinical Presentation

The patient will have dysphagia, odynophagia, and neck pain. There may be a swelling in the neck and neck rigidity. On examination of the throat, there will be a midline swelling in the posterior pharyngeal wall.

An anterior expanding abscess can cause airway compromise, while a posterior expanding abscess can compress the spine leading to neurological deficits.

Investigations

X-ray of the cervical spine (lateral view) will show the following (**Fig. 72.19**):
- Prevertebral widening.
- Straightening of the cervical spine.
- Erosion of the vertebral body anteriorly.
- Reduced/loss of intervertebral disk space.
- In advanced cases, the vertebral collapse with anterior wedging will lead to progressive kyphosis and gibbus deformity.
- Ivory vertebra is noted in later stages due to reactive sclerosis.

A contrast-enhanced CT scan is preferred to an X-ray as it details the abscess and also shows early features like erosion of the endplate. The abscess will show as a central hypodense area with peripheral enhancement.

An MRI can help in early detection of a paraspinal abscess and epidural involvement.

The aspirated pus can be sent for acid-fast bacillus staining and culture. A polymerase chain reaction test can also be done for diagnosis, and to detect drug resistance.

X-ray of the chest (posteroanterior view) is done to rule out pulmonary tuberculosis.

Treatment

- Antitubercular treatment for 9 to 12 months (rifampicin, isoniazid, ethambutol, and pyrazinamide for 2 months, followed by rifampicin and isoniazid for 8–10 months).
- Aspiration of the pus can be done (ultrasound guided).
- If the abscess is large and there are compressive symptoms, drainage using an external incision is done.
- In advanced cases, the spine should be stabilized.

Prevertebral Abscess

■ Anatomy

This space lies immediately anterior to the spinal column bounded anteriorly by the danger space. It extends from the skull base to the coccyx.

■ Etiology

Infection in this space occurs due to direct extension of infection from the vertebrae (osteomyelitis), trauma to the vertebrae, or extension of infection from contiguous deep neck spaces.

Tuberculosis of the spine (Pott's spine) can affect this space. Infections of this space usually does not perforate the prevertebral fascia or extend to the danger space.

■ Clinical Presentation

The patient presents with torticollis and reduced neck movements. It can lead to spinal instability.

■ Investigations

A contrast-enhanced CT scan or MRI is done (**Fig. 72.20**).

■ Treatment

Treatment includes the following:
- Surgical drainage and intravenous antibiotics.
- Antitubercular treatment in case of tuberculosis.
- Postoperatively, the spine should be stabilized especially in Pott's spine.

Danger Space Abscess

It is the infection of the alar space. It is referred to as the danger space as any infection of this space can extend into the thorax, that is, the posterior mediastinum, and affect the major blood vessels and airway causing a potential threat to the patient's life.

It is bound anteriorly by the alar fascia and posteriorly by the prevertebral fascia. It extends from the skull base to the posterior mediastinum up to the T1 level. Infection of this space is due to spread from the retropharyngeal or parapharyngeal space.

Carotid Space Abscess

The carotid space is also called *Lincoln's highway*. It is bounded by the carotid sheath, which is formed by the superficial, middle, and deep layers of the deep cervical fascia. The main constituents of the carotid space include the carotid artery, internal jugular vein, and vagus nerve. Because of the compact nature of this compartment, there is a very little tendency for spread of infection.

■ Clinical Presentation

There will be fever with chills. On palpation, there will be persistent tenderness and induration deep to the sternocleidomastoid. There will be associated torticollis.

■ Treatment

- Drainage of abscess and intravenous antibiotics should be started.
- Anticoagulants should be started.
- The internal jugular vein may need to be ligated.

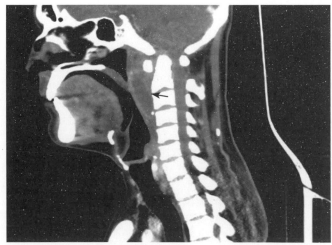

Fig. 72.20 Contrast-enhanced computed tomography (CT) scan showing a prevertebral abscess.

Points to Ponder

- The cervical fascia is divided into the superficial and deep layers. The deep cervical fascia is further divided into an investing layer, middle layer, and a deep layer.
- The fascia encloses potential neck spaces, which are clinically important as they allow for spread of infection into adjacent spaces.
- Quinsy is a collection of pus in the peritonsillar space, which is found between the capsule of the tonsil and the superior constrictor muscle covered by the pharyngobasilar fascia.
- The primary site of infection in Ludwig's angina is the submandibular space and 90% of the cases are due to dental infections, mainly of the lower second or third molar teeth.
- The parapharyngeal abscess can involve the prestyloid or poststyloid compartments. The bulge in the oropharynx is more toward the anterior pillar in the prestyloid abscess and behind the posterior tonsillar pillar in the poststyloid abscess.
- The retropharyngeal space is divided into two compartments by a midline raphe. The contents of the space include fat and lymph nodes.
- Acute retropharyngeal abscess is common in children and is due to suppuration of the lymph nodes in this space due to upper respiratory infections.
- Acute retropharyngeal abscess in adults is mainly due to trauma caused by ingestion of foreign body.
- Chronic retropharyngeal abscess is mainly caused by tuberculosis of the spine.
- The prevertebral space extends down into the coccyx.

Case-Based Questions

1. A 35-year-old man was brought to the ear, nose, and throat (ENT) clinic with complaints of severe pain over the right side of the throat with referred pain to the right ear for the last 3 days. He had fever and difficulty in swallowing, so saliva was drooling from his mouth. Examination of his throat revealed trismus. There was a diffuse bulge over the right side of the soft palate and his right tonsil was pushed medially. The palate was congested. He did not give history of any prior episodes of tonsillitis.

   a. What is the diagnosis?
   b. What is the reason for his trismus?
   c. How will you manage this patient?

   Answers

   a. Right side peritonsillar abscess or quinsy.
   b. Trismus is due to inflammation of the pterygoid muscles.
   c. A contrast-enhanced CT scan can confirm the diagnosis. The patient is hospitalized. Intravenous (IV) fluids are started as these patients will be dehydrated. IV antibiotics are administered, which will cover gram-positive, gram-negative, and anaerobic organisms. Analgesics and antipyretics are given. This will be the requirement for peritonsillar cellulitis. If there is a frank abscess, it should be drained.

2. A 2-year-old boy was referred from pediatrics because of fever and difficulty in swallowing for the last 2 days. The patient was irritable and febrile. On examination, there was a bulge to the right of the midline on the posterior pharyngeal wall. On enquiring about the history, the mother said he suffered from an upper respiratory tract infection 1 week prior to admission.

   a. What is the diagnosis?
   b. What is the reason for this condition in this age group?
   c. How will you treat this condition?

   Answers

   a. Acute retropharyngeal abscess.
   b. There are lymph nodes present in the retropharyngeal space in the pediatric age group. These regress or involute by 5 years of age. An acute infection of the upper respiratory tract will spread to the lymph nodes in children causing suppuration.
   c. Once the abscess is confirmed, either with a neck X-ray or CT scan (ideal), drainage of the pus has to be attempted under general anesthesia through the intraoral route.

Frequently Asked Questions

1. What is the danger space?
2. Enumerate the various spaces of the head and neck.
3. What are the clinical features of quinsy?
4. What is the site of drainage in a peritonsillar abscess?
5. What is Lincoln's highway?
6. Describe the compartments of the parapharyngeal space.
7. What is the prevertebral space? What is the etiology of an abscess in this region?
8. What are the findings on a plain X-ray lateral view in a patient with retropharyngeal abscess?
9. What is the etiology of Ludwig's angina?

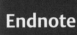

Endnote

*Ludwig's angina was named after the German physician Wilhelm Frederick von Ludwig (1790–1865), who described this condition in 1836. He encountered five patients who had acute swellings in front of the neck between the hyoid and the floor of the mouth. They had minimal inflammation of the throat and did not have lymph node enlargement. The word angina comes from a Latin word meaning strangling or suffocation. At that time, it was described by the 3Fs: it was to be **feared**, it was **fluctuant**, and it was **fatal**. Before the advent of antibiotics, in the early 1900s, the mortality rate was 50% for this condition. Now it is less than 10%.*

In 1929, Mosher called the carotid sheath the Lincoln Highway because the sheath was formed by all three layers of the deep cervical fascia. This was in remembrance of the first transcontinental highway that had been built in the United States, 16 years earlier in 1913.

Cervical Lymphatic System and Neck Dissection

Arun Alexander and Soorya Pradeep

The competencies covered in this chapter are as follows:

EN2.11 Describe and identify by clinical examination malignant and premalignant ear, nose, and throat (ENT) diseases.

SU20.1 Describe the etiopathogenesis of oral cancer, symptoms and signs of pharyngeal cancer. Enumerate the appropriate investigations and discuss the principles of treatment.

Introduction

Cervical lymph nodes comprise 30% of the 800 lymph nodes present in the entire human body, that is, approximately 300 nodes are present in the head and neck region alone. Cervical lymph node enlargement may be reactive in response to local inflammation or infection, or it may be far more ominous and may be the representation of a lymphoma or nodal metastasis from a head and neck carcinoma.

Metastatic lymph nodes may be differentiated from benign nodes clinically as these tend to be hard with irregular margins, are usually nontender, may be fixed to skin or underlying structures, and rapidly increase in size.

Nearly 20% of the head and neck squamous cell carcinomas (HNSCCs) are associated with nodal metastasis. The risk of nodal metastasis is determined by the primary tumor site, size of the primary, degree of differentiation of the tumor, and presence of perineural and perivascular invasion.

The presence of malignant lymph nodes is an important prognostic marker for head and neck cancers. Unilateral metastatic cervical node decreases the 5-year survival rate by 50%, whereas the presence of bilateral nodes reduces it by 75%. The presence of extranodal invasion (skin or soft-tissue involvement and fixity to adjacent structures or neural involvement) also detrimentally affects the prognosis.

Classification of Cervical Lymph Nodes

Anatomically, cervical lymph nodes may be classified as superficial, deep, or visceral (**Fig. 73.1**).

- The superficial group of lymph nodes are present superficial to the investing layer of the cervical fascia and consist of a horizontal and a vertical chain. The horizontal chain consists of the occipital, mastoid, parotid, submandibular, and submental group, and the vertical chain consists of nodes along the external jugular vein.
- The deep group of lymph nodes are more consistent and form a triangular arrangement, bound anteriorly by the nodes along the internal jugular vein (IJV) and posteriorly by the spinal lymph nodes and supraclavicular lymph nodes.

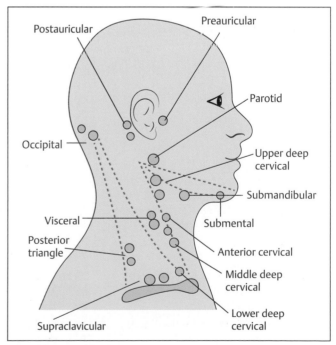

Fig. 73.1 Anatomical classification of the cervical lymph nodes.

- The visceral group comprises nodes surrounding the median visceral structures, namely, the pretracheal, paratracheal, prelaryngeal, and retropharyngeal nodes.

However, this classification was based on the anatomical landmarks encountered during dissection and was inadequate to address lymph node involvement encountered in cases of malignancies. Hence, the Memorial Sloan Kettering Cancer Center proposed a classification system based on the first echelon sites for metastasis from head and neck primary sites, which is now widely accepted (**Fig. 73.2**). Lymph node distribution in the neck are listed in **Table 73.1**.

Level II may be divided into level IIa and IIb by the vertical plane defined by the spinal accessory nerve: anteromedial to the nerve is level IIa and posterolateral to the nerve lies level IIb. Similarly, level V is also divided by the lower border of the cricoid into level Va superiorly and level Vb inferiorly.

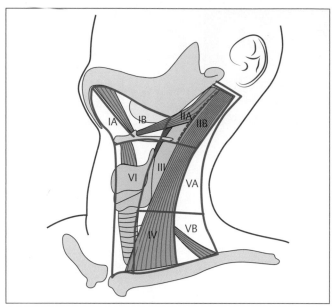

Fig. 73.2 Memorial Sloan Kettering Cancer Center classification of cervical lymph node levels.

Table 73.1 Levels of lymph node distribution in the neck

Levels	Clinical location	Surgical boundaries
Level Ia	Submental triangle	• Symphysis of the mandible • Body of the hyoid • Bilateral anterior belly of the digastric muscle
Level Ib	Submandibular triangle	• Body of the mandible • Anterior belly of the digastric muscle • Posterior belly of the digastric muscle
Level II	Upper jugular	• Level of the lower margin of the jugular fossa • Level of the lower border of the hyoid • Stylohyoid muscle • Posterior border of the sternocleidomastoid muscle
Level III	Mid jugular	• Level of the lower border of the hyoid • Level of the lower border of the cricoid cartilage • Lateral border of the sternohyoid muscle • Posterior border of the sternocleidomastoid muscle
Level IV	Lower jugular	• Level of the lower border of the cricoid cartilage • Clavicle • Lateral border of the sternohyoid muscle • Posterior border of the sternocleidomastoid muscle
Level V	Posterior triangle	• Anterior border of the trapezius • Posterior border of the sternocleidomastoid muscle • Clavicle
Level VI	Anterior compartment	• Hyoid bone • Sternal notch • Bilateral common carotid artery
Level VII	Superior mediastinum	• Sternal notch • Innominate artery • Bilateral common carotid artery

Region-Specific Lymph Node Metastasis

Based on the site of the primary tumor, the pattern of nodal metastasis may be predicted in most cases (**Fig. 73.3** and **Table 73.2**). Certain tumors such as primaries in the tongue exhibit skip metastasis. Midline structures may drain to the contralateral or bilateral neck nodes.

Metastasis of Unknown Origin or Carcinoma of Unknown Primary

It refers to a disease entity characterized by clinical overt metastatic nodal disease without clinical or radiological obvious primary. In other words, metastatic nodal disease without a known primary, after extensive investigation (**Fig. 73.4**).

Metastasis of unknown origin (MUO) is believed to occur due to the presence of a microscopic primary tumor that is too small to be detected by conventional techniques or because the primary tumor was removed by the patient's immunity at an early stage, but not before nodal metastasis had already occurred. With advances in technology, it is now possible to identify the primary in many cases previously categorized as "unknown primary." Hence, the incidence of MUO has been steadily declining and is believed to be around 5% of HNSCCs. Diagnostic workup for MUO is given in **Flowchart 73.1**.

> **Pearl**
>
> If the FNAC is diagnostic of adenocarcinoma, other than from the parotid, then a search should be made for a primary site in the thorax and abdomen.

> **Pearl**
>
> If the FNAC is reported as undifferentiated or poorly differentiated, an immunohistochemistry is required to confirm squamous cell carcinoma or to diagnose other malignancies like lymphoma, melanoma, and sarcoma. P16 positivity points toward an oropharyngeal primary. Detection of Epstein–Barr virus may signify a nasopharyngeal primary.

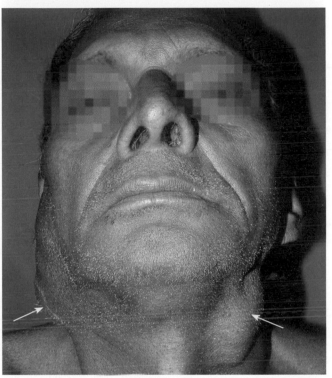

Fig. 73.3 Bilateral metastatic upper deep cervical lymph nodes seen in nasopharyngeal, base of the tongue, supraglottic, and soft palate malignancies.

Table 73.2 Pattern of tumor metastasis to regional lymph nodes

Region	First echelon nodes	Levels
Nasopharynx, nasal cavity, and paranasal sinuses	Retropharyngeal nodes Level Ib	II and III
Oral cavity	Anterior: Ia Posterior: Ib	II–IV II and III Tongue primaries exhibit skip metastasis to level IV
Oropharynx	Retropharyngeal nodes	II–IV
Hypopharynx		Bilateral levels III, IV, VI, and VII
Supraglottis		Bilateral levels II and III
Glottis	Lymphatic spread is rare	
Subglottis	Level VI	III, IV, and VI

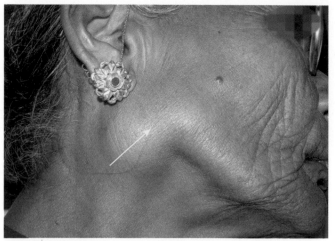

Fig. 73.4 Metastasis of unknown origin (MUO) at the right level II lymph node.

■ Management of MUO

For a single neck node <3 cm with no extracapsular spread, a selective or modified radical neck dissection (MRND) will suffice. There are some who advocate radiotherapy for early cases as it covers the potential primary site. The results are the same with surgery or radiotherapy for early-stage disease. For nodes >3 cm, multiple neck nodes or nodes with extracapsular spread, the neck dissection should be followed by radiotherapy or combined chemoradiotherapy.

Neck Dissection

Radical neck dissection was first described in 1906 by George Washington Crile. *Neck dissection*, also known as *cervical lymphadenectomy*, is the surgical procedure for

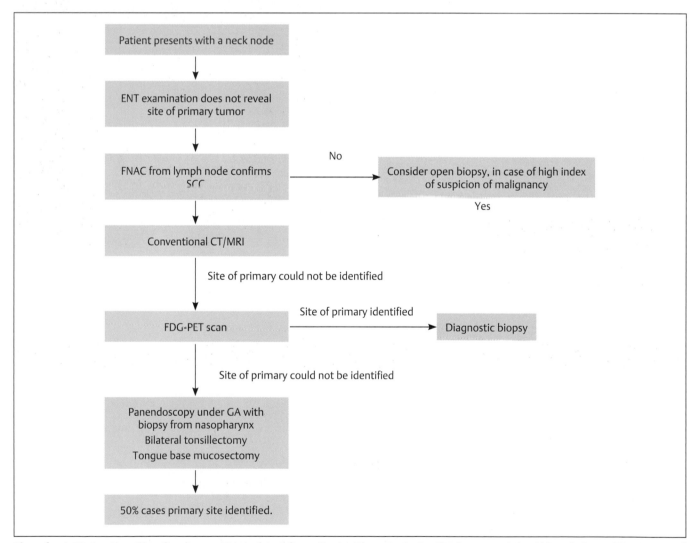

Flowchart 73.1 Algorithm for diagnostic workup of a patient with metastasis of unknown origin. Abbreviations: CT, computed tomography; ENT, ear, nose, and throat; FNAC, fine-needle aspiration cytology; FDG-PET: fluorodeoxyglucose-positron emission tomography; GA, general anesthesia; MRI, magnetic resonance imaging; SCC, squamous cell carcinoma.

treating *metastatic cervical lymphadenopathy*. During neck dissection, extranodal structures like veins, nerves, muscle, and salivary glands may be removed. With new insights into lymphatic drainage patterns and metastasis patterns, surgical management of neck metastasis has shifted from a radical to a functional neck dissection with the removal of only those groups of neck nodes that have the highest likelihood of containing metastatic deposits. This shift in approach is based on the rationale that no head and neck primary metastasizes to all five levels of the neck, and a more conservative approach helps in reducing the morbidity and improves the quality of life after neck dissection. **Table 73.3** enlists the classification of neck dissection techniques.

Pearl

Radical neck dissection has been modified depending on the structures preserved, taking into consideration the IJV, spinal accessory, and the sternocleidomastoid muscle.

Types of MRND:

- Type I: Spinal accessory is preserved. Other two structures are removed.
- Type II: Spinal accessory and IJV are preserved.
- Type III: Spinal accessory, IJV, and sternocleidomastoid are preserved.

■ Complications of Neck Dissection

- Hemorrhage from the IJV, carotid artery, or the other vessels can be avoided by careful dissection. Meticulous hemostasis reduces blood loss.
- Nerve injury and neuroma: Marginal mandibular nerve, hypoglossal nerve, vagus nerve, lingual nerve, and brachial plexus can be injured during neck dissection. Preservation of the spinal accessory nerve should be attempted to avoid morbidity. Neuroma may occur from the stump of a cut nerve.
- A chyle leak can occur during dissection on the left side.

- Wound dehiscence occurs when there is a trifurcate junction of the incision or in postradiotherapy cases.
- Salivary leak/seroma can occur when the tail of the parotid gland (inferior part) is resected.
- Carotid blowout, that is, rupture of the carotid artery can occur in the postoperative period, especially in postradiotherapy cases.
- Pneumothorax can occur when dissecting in the lower part of the neck close to the pleura of the apex of the lung.
- Air embolism can occur when the IJV is opened inadvertently.
- Facial edema can occur due to ligation of the IJV. The intracranial pressure may also increase.

Pearl

The incidence of complications has reduced with fewer radical procedures being performed. Neck dissection is also being done by minimally invasive surgery, through endoscopic and robotic surgery.

Points to Ponder

- The presence of nodal metastasis detrimentally affects the prognosis and is associated with a decrease in survival rates.
- Cervical lymph nodes have been classified into seven levels based on the first echelon sites for metastasis from head and neck primaries.
- Based on the site of the primary tumor, the pattern of nodal metastasis can be predicted. Midline structures tend to involve bilateral neck nodes.
- MUO refers to clinically overt neck metastases in the absence of a clinically or radiologically obvious primary. With advances in technology, the incidence of MUO is decreasing.
- Surgical management of neck nodes has shifted from a radical approach to a selective one where only the involved levels of neck nodes are removed.

Table 73.3 Classification of neck dissection techniques

Types of neck dissection	Structures removed
Radical neck dissection	Removal of levels I–V, spinal accessory nerve, sternocleidomastoid muscle, and internal jugular vein (IJV)
Modified radical neck dissection	Removal of levels I–V with preservation of one or more structures, i.e., the spinal accessory nerve, IJV, or sternocleidomastoid muscle
Selective neck dissection	Removal of one or more levels of lymph nodes, e.g., • Supraomohyoid neck dissection (levels I–III) • Central neck dissection (level VI) • Lateral neck dissection (levels II–IV) • Posterolateral neck dissection (levels II–V)
Extended radical neck dissection	Radical neck dissection + removal of one or more lymphatic/nonlymphatic structures (bone, muscle, nerve, skin, and vessel), e.g., level VII or retropharyngeal nodes, hypoglossal nerve, mandible, and digastric muscle

Case-Based Question

1. **A 56-year-old male patient presents with 2-month history of a right-sided neck swelling. On examination, there is a 3 × 3 cm hard nontender level II node. Ear, nose, and throat (ENT) examination was otherwise unremarkable.**

   a. What is the next step in the management of this patient?

   b. If imaging modalities, including a positron emission tomography (PET) scan, do not reveal the primary tumor site, what are the sites to be biopsied

   c. If the primary site cannot be identified, how will you proceed with the management of this patient?

   Answers

   a. FNAC from the lymph node.

   b. Blind biopsies from the nasopharynx, bilateral tonsillectomy, and the base of the tongue in case the FNAC is reported as squamous cell carcinoma.

   c. MRND with or without radiotherapy depending on the histopathology report.

Frequently Asked Questions

1. Explain the classification of neck nodes in HNSCC.

2. Enumerate the types of neck dissection.

3. What is MUO? How do you work up a patient with suspected MUO?

4. What are the types of MRND?

5. What are the probable sites of biopsy that should be attempted in a patient with MUO?

Endnote

George Washington Crile (1864–1943) was a prominent American surgeon who in the early 1900s performed the first radical neck dissection for laryngeal cancer. Since he performed major head and neck surgeries, his interest shifted to fluid loss and blood pressure fluctuations during surgery. He has many achievements to his credit. He is considered the father of radical neck dissection. He investigated the cause and treatment of shock, performed over 25,000 thyroidectomies, introduced blood pressure monitoring during surgery, was the first to give blood transfusion during surgery, and was the founder of the American College of Surgeons.

Monika Pokharel

The competencies covered in this chapter are as follows:

EN1.2 Describe the pathophysiology of common diseases in the ear, nose, and throat (ENT).

EN2.1 Elicit, document, and present an appropriate history in a patient presenting with an ENT complaint.

EN2.11 Describe and identify by clinical examination malignant and premalignant ENT diseases.

Introduction

Neck swellings are abnormal lumps in the neck. These can occur in any age group and can be situated in the midline or laterally. The classification of neck swellings is given in **Table 74.1**.

Management

- Detailed history of the duration and associated symptoms are elicited. If a metastatic lymph node is suspected, a history of symptoms of the corresponding sites should be elicited.
- Radiology is an important investigation as it gives information of the type (cystic/solid), site, extent, and relation to surrounding structures:
  - Chest X-ray.
  - Barium swallow.
  - Ultrasound.
  - Contrast-enhanced computed tomography (CT) scan or magnetic resonance imaging (MRI).
  - Positron emission tomography.
  - Digital subtraction angiography.
- Fine-needle aspiration cytology (FNAC) gives a possible tissue diagnosis and would help plan further evaluation and treatment.
- Biopsy.
- Panendoscopy.

Treatment is based on the cause.

Midline Neck Swellings

■ Thyroglossal Duct Cyst

A thyroglossal cyst is a common developmental anomaly presenting as a midline neck swelling. The thyroglossal duct is the communication from the foramen cecum to the developing thyroid gland as it descends into the neck. If the duct persists, cystic degeneration can occur, leading to the formation of the thyroglossal cyst. The cyst can present anywhere from the foramen cecum to the mediastinum. The majority present around the level of the hyoid bone. A thyroglossal fistula usually may arise following a spontaneous drainage of an abscess or due to inadequate surgical excision, which may be seen if the body of the hyoid is not resected along with the cyst and the tract.

Clinical Features (Fig. 74.1)

- Midline neck swelling are common in the pediatric population below the age of 5 years, but these can also present in adults.
- It can present as an asymptomatic cystic lump at, above, or below the level of the hyoid bone.
  - Sixty-five percent are at the subhyoid.
  - Twenty percent are at the suprahyoid.
  - Fifteen percent are at the level of the hyoid.
  - Rarely, it can present in the tongue.
- It is smooth, soft, and fluctuant.
- It moves on swallowing and on protrusion of the tongue.
- The cyst can get infected.

Table 74.1 Classification of neck swellings

	Midline	Lateral	Posterior
Congenital	• Thyroglossal cyst • Dermoid • Ectopic thyroid • Bronchogenic cyst	• Branchial cyst	• Lymphangioma
Inflammatory Acute	• Thyroiditis • Abscess • Ludwig's angina	• Lymphadenitis • Bacterial • Viral • Reactive • Abscess: parapharyngeal • Sialadenitis	• Lymphadenitis • Bacterial • Viral
Chronic		• Granulomatous	• Granulomatous (tuberculosis)
Neoplastic			
Benign	• Thyroid adenoma	• Salivary: pleomorphic adenoma, Warthin's tumor • Neurogenic: schwannoma	• Schwannoma
Malignant	• Thyroid malignancies • Local spread from laryngeal or hypopharyngeal malignancy • Metastatic submental lymph node	• Vascular: carotid body tumor • Metastatic lymph node from head and neck • Lymphoma	• Metastatic lymph node from head and neck • Supraclavicular metastatic node due to breast, prostrate, kidney, gastrointestinal tract, or lung malignancy • Lymphoma
Trauma		• Sternomastoid hematoma • Pseudoaneurysm	
Miscellaneous	• Plunging ranula	• Pharyngeal pouch • Laryngocele	

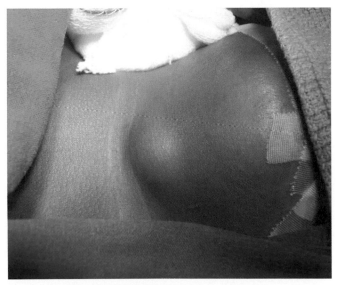

Fig. 74.1 Thyroglossal cyst.

• The thyroglossal fistula presents as a skin fold covering the opening of the fistula, (hood sign), around the region of the hyoid bone.
• Rarely, a thyroglossal duct carcinoma can develop.

Differential diagnosis includes submental lymph node, subhyoid bursa, dermoid cyst, ectopic thyroid, sebaceous cyst, and lipoma.

Diagnosis

• Ultrasound of the neck will delineate the cyst and the normal thyroid gland.
• FNAC, if done, may show colloid.
• Isotope scan with Tc-99m is done if the diagnosis is in doubt in order to exclude an ectopic thyroid.
• A CT scan is useful to delineate the relation of the cyst with the hyoid bone and an MRI is useful when the presentation is within the tongue.

Treatment

The standard treatment is the Sistrunk operation.

Excision of the cyst with the central portion of the hyoid bone along with a core of tissue from the cyst up to the foramen cecum.

■ Ranula

Ranula is a rare mucocele that occur on the floor of the mouth. A plunging ranula occurs due to obstruction of the sublingual gland forming a mucous retention pseudocyst that tracks adjacent to the edge of the mylohyoid or through a dehiscence in the mylohyoid into the submandibular region where it presents as a swelling. These are discussed under diseases of the salivary glands.

■ Submental, Prelaryngeal, and Paratracheal Lymph Nodes

The submental lymph nodes located in the submental triangle drain the chin, the middle part of the lower lip, gingiva, the anterior part of the floor of the mouth, and the tip of the tongue. These can be enlarged by inflammation or malignancy (metastatic lymph nodes). The prelaryngeal and paratracheal nodes lie in front of the larynx and the trachea. These can be involved in malignancy of the thyroid, the subglottis, the postcricoid region, and the upper esophagus.

■ Dermoid Cyst

Types

- Epidermoid.
- True dermoid (congenital or acquired).
- Teratoid cysts.

Epidermoid cysts contain only skin, and no adnexal structures. This is the most commonly encountered type. It contains keratinous material and is lined by the squamous epithelium.

The true dermoid cyst is lined by the squamous epithelium and contains skin along with appendages like hair follicles and sweat and the sebaceous glands. These occur during fetal development due to sequestration of skin at the sites of embryonic closure. These are subcutaneous cysts that usually present at birth.

Teratoid cysts are lined by either the respiratory or the squamous epithelium. These contains ectodermal, mesodermal, and endodermal elements such as the teeth, nails, muscle, cartilage, and glandular tissue. These are a rare occurrence.

Radiological evaluation is by ultrasound, CT scan, or MRI of the neck.

Treatment is by excision biopsy.

■ Thyroid Swelling/Goiter

A goiter may present in the anterior midline of the neck as a swelling that can be diffuse, multinodular, or a solitary nodule (**Figs. 74.2** and **74.3**). It can be euthyroid, hypothyroid, or hyperthyroid.

Goiter can be classified into the following:

- Simple nontoxic goiter: It can be a diffuse hyperplastic (physiological, pubertal, pregnancy) or a multinodular goiter.
- Toxic goiter: It can be diffuse (Graves' disease), multinodular, and toxic adenoma.
- Neoplastic: It can be benign or malignant.
- Inflammatory: It can be autoimmune, granulomatous, infective, fibrosing, and iatrogenic.

A solitary nodule may be a colloid nodule, follicular adenoma, Hürthle cell adenoma, dominant nodule of a

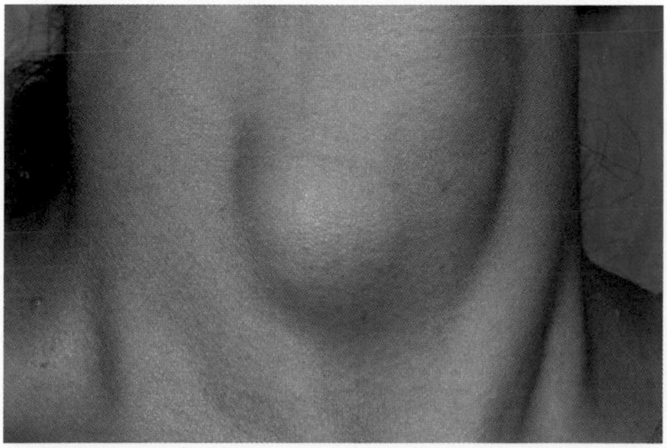

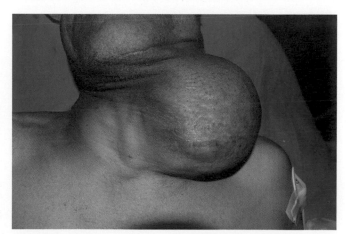

Fig. 74.2 Solitary nodule of thyroid gland involving the right lobe.

Fig. 74.3 Follicular carcinoma of the thyroid gland.

multinodular goiter, autonomous toxic nodule, thyroid cyst, or malignancy. The risk factors for malignancy are listed in **Box 74.1**.

Thyroid malignancy can be classified into the following:
- Follicular cells:
  - Differentiated: Papillary carcinoma, follicular carcinoma, and Hürthle cell carcinoma
  - Undifferentiated: Anaplastic carcinoma (**Fig. 74.4**).
- Parafollicular C cells:
  - Medullary carcinoma.
- Others: Lymphoma and sarcoma.
- Metastatic: From the breast, lung, and kidney.
- Spread from surrounding structures like laryngeal malignancy and esophageal malignancy.

Evaluation of a Thyroid Swelling

- A thyroid profile (serum T3, T4, and thyroid-stimulating hormone [TSH]) is done to check the status of the thyroid, that is, euthyroid, hypothyroid, or hyperthyroid.
- Ultrasound of the neck is done to see the type of swelling, that is, cystic, solid, or mixed, and look for features of malignancy. The TIRADS (thyroid imaging reporting and data systems) has categorized a thyroid swelling into five types based on the risk of a ≥1 cm thyroid nodule being malignant.
- CT scan or MRI is done in case of large goiters, especially with evidence of invasion.
- Thyroid scintigraphy is useful in thyroiditis (Technetium-99m scan) and for follow-up in malignancy after thyroidectomy. Iodine-131 can be used to assess the need for radioiodine ablation.
- FNAC (preferably ultrasound guided) may give a possible tissue diagnosis using the Bethesda classification.

Box 74.1 Solitary nodules with high risk of malignancy

- Age <20 and >45 years.
- Male gender.
- Compressive or invasive features such as change in voice, cough, stridor/dyspnoea, and dysphagia.
- History of prior irradiation to the neck.
- Prior history of Hashimoto's thyroiditis.
- Family history of thyroid cancer.
- Size of nodule >4 cm:
  - Fixed and hard lesion.
  - Rapid growth or recent increase in size.
  - Pain.
- Presence of lymph nodes.
- Nodule in the background of Graves' disease.
- Recurrent or rapidly filling cyst after aspiration.

Pearl

Ultrasound features of thyroid malignancy include the following:
- Solid/mixed lesion with absence of a halo sign.
- Ill-defined margins.
- Irregular shape.
- Hypoechogenic.
- Fine calcifications.
- Invasion of the surrounding structures.
- Presence of lymph nodes.

Pearl

The Bethesda classification in reporting cytology for thyroid is as follows:
- I: Nondiagnostic inadequate.
- II: Benign.
- III: Follicular lesion of undetermined significance/atypia.
- IV: Follicular neoplasm.
- V: Suspicious of malignancy.
- VI: Malignant.

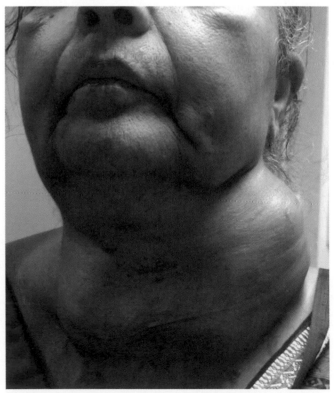

Fig. 74.4 Anaplastic carcinoma of the thyroid.

Treatment (Based on Disease)

- Wait-and-watch policy: Regular follow-up with ultrasound and thyroid profile in benign conditions including small nodules and cysts.
- Antithyroid drugs for hyperthyroidism.
- Thyroid hormone treatment: Supplementation in hypothyroidism, suppression (low dose) for benign goiter, suppression (high dose) for malignancy, that is, post-treatment, and replacement in post total thyroidectomy.
- Thyroidectomy: Hemithyroidectomy may be done for benign lesions (commonly for cosmetic reasons, toxic nodule, or to allay fear of malignancy) and total thyroidectomy is done for large symptomatic goiters and malignancy. In malignancy, the central compartment or modified neck dissection may be required, especially in papillary and medullary carcinomas.
- Radioiodine ablation using I-131 is done for Graves' disease and residual malignancy of differentiated carcinoma of the thyroid.
- Radiotherapy has been used for anaplastic carcinoma and for residual thyroid malignancies not responsive to I-131.

Pearl

When there is a doubt in the FNAC, that is, suspicious, a frozen section can be asked for intraoperatively. If malignant, it can be proceeded with total thyroidectomy ± neck dissection. In the frozen section, it is difficult to distinguish between follicular adenoma and follicular carcinoma in which case the final histopathology should be awaited before considering further treatment.

■ Ectopic Thyroid

Aberrant thyroid tissue may be found at three different sites:
- In relation to the tongue (lingual and sublingual).
- Thyroglossal ectopic thyroid.
- Struma ovarii.

Lingual thyroid is an ectopic thyroid tissue found at the base of the tongue. An ectopic thyroid can also present in the sublingual or anterior midline of the neck at or below the level of the hyoid bone.

Symptoms

Most often these are asymptomatic. There may be muffled voice, hemorrhage, respiratory obstruction, or dysphagia. It may present as an incidental finding during endotracheal intubation.

Signs

It appears as a smooth swelling in the midline of the base of the tongue with prominent vessels on its surface.

Investigations

Evaluation includes an ultrasound to assess for the presence of normal thyroid tissue in the neck, a radionuclide scan (technetium-99m) to confirm the ectopic thyroid and presence or absence of the normal thyroid, and/or an MRI to assess the size, location, and type of mass (cystic or solid). A thyroid profile (serum T3, T4, and TSH) is done. An FNAC may be done to assess for changes including malignant transformation.

Treatment

Treatment is by suppressive dose of thyroxine. If the mass is large and symptomatic, it can be excised by a midline, tongue-splitting approach or an anterior pharyngotomy approach. When the anterior pharyngotomy approach is used, the tissue can be transposed into the lateral part of the neck with its blood supply or transplantation into the rectus abdominis can be done.

Lateral Neck Swellings

■ Branchial Cysts

Branchial cysts appear as a result of developmental failure of the branchial apparatus. These usually occur in young adults with a peak incidence in the third decade of life.

It presents as a smooth, soft, fluctuant swelling usually located in the upper one-third of the lateral part of the neck, at the anterior margin of the sternocleidomastoid muscle. These can occur in any site of the neck including the parotid gland. A branchial cyst can get infected. Increase in size of cysts can cause pressure symptoms, and an obvious cosmetic deformity (**Fig. 74.5**).

An ultrasound-guided FNAC yields acellular fluid with cholesterol crystals. A CT scan or MRI is done for presurgical planning of large cysts.

Treatment is by surgical excision biopsy.

■ Branchial Fistulas and Sinus

Branchial fistulas are congenital defects consisting of a skin-lined tract.
- The *first branchial cleft fistula* is rare and can present from the tragus to the hyoid bone. The upper opening may be in the ear canal, whereas the lower opening can be above or below the angle of the mandible.
- The *second branchial cleft sinus/fistula* is located at the junction of the middle and lower one-third of the anterior border of the sternocleidomastoid muscle. The upper end may open internally as a slit on the anterior aspect of the tonsillar fossa. The tract can also ascend just deep to the deep cervical fascia along the carotid artery. The tract passes deep to the external carotid

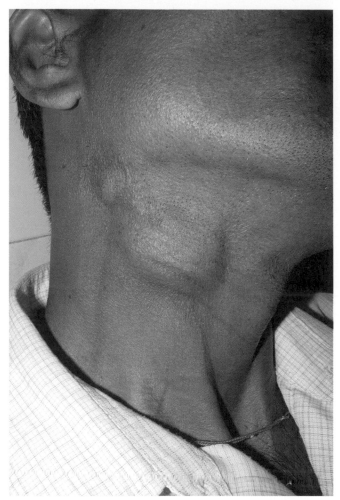

Fig. 74.5 Branchial cyst in the right upper neck.

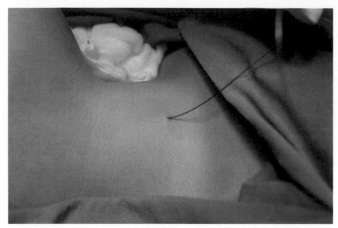

Fig. 74.6 Second branchial arch sinus cannulated and injected with methylene blue to outline the tract.

artery, the posterior belly of the digastric muscle and stylohyoid, superficial to the internal carotid artery and the hypoglossal nerve (between the internal and external carotid arteries; **Fig. 74.6**).

- The *third branchial cleft fistula* has an external orifice at the same site as the second, but the internal opening is located at the pyriform fossa. The tract passes behind both the internal and external carotid arteries, but lies superficial to the vagus and the hypoglossal nerves.
- The *fourth branchial arch sinus/fistula* extends from the apex of the pyriform fossa to the region of the thyroid gland and can present mimicking a recurrent thyroid abscess. The opening of the third and fourth branchial sinuses may be seen on rigid hypopharyngoscopy. A thin barium swallow may help delineate the tract.

Treatment

The treatment is to excise the whole tract to avoid recurrence. The tract that opens onto the skin can be traced by cannulating with a thin catheter or injecting methylene blue. In the second branchial arch fistula, in addition to removal of the tract, an ipsilateral tonsillectomy is done. For a fourth branchial arch sinus, excision of the ipsilateral lobe of the thyroid may be required.

■ Lymphangioma

These are malformations of the lymphatic system which can occur during development and may be due to poor connectivity between the lymphatic channels and the main lymphatic duct. The congenital form usually occurs before 5 years of age. It can also occur due to interruption in drainage of the lymph channels following surgery, trauma, or radiotherapy.

These can be classified based on depth and size into the following:

- Superficial (lymphangioma circumscriptum and acquired lymphangioma).
- Deep based on depth and size.

These can also be classified into congenital and acquired.

Cavernous lymphangioma and cystic hygroma are the congenital, deep forms.

Clinical Features

Lymphangiomas of congenital origin are seen in neonates, infants, or in childhood. These can appear anywhere in the head and neck region. The common sites are the cheek, tongue, and the floor of the mouth in the suprahyoid region and the anterior or posterior triangle in the infrahyoid region. Posterior triangle lesions may be associated with Turner's syndrome or other congenital abnormalities.

On palpation, lymphangiomas are soft and cystic. These are brilliantly transilluminant. These lymphangiomas can involve or remain static, but sometimes increase in size, especially after an infection or hemorrhage, which can lead to life-threatening airway compromise.

Investigation

An MRI will aid in the diagnosis.

Treatment

- Treatment is by repeated aspiration when there is rapid increase in size of the swelling.
- Injection of sclerosants like 3% sodium tetradecyl sulfate or alcohol will help reduce the size. Intralesional injection of Picibanil (OK-432) leads to an inflammatory reaction and thrombosis with subsequent necrosis. Multiple sessions may be required for sclerotherapy to be effective.
- Surgical excision is done for localized lesions in the neck. Debulking/partial glossectomy of oral lesions are done to avoid airway compromise. Use of coblation during the procedure is helpful.

■ Carotid Body Tumors

Synonyms of carotid body tumors are carotid paraganglioma and chemodectoma.

Carotid body tumors are rare neuroendocrine neoplasms arising from the chemoreceptor cells at the carotid bifurcation. These tumors are slow growing and benign. These present as gradually progressive, painless, pulsatile swelling in the lateral neck. There may be pain, dysphagia, and autonomic dysfunction. Large lesions can involve the hypoglossal nerve, glossopharyngeal nerve, vagus nerve, or sympathetic chain.

Diagnosis can be confirmed by a color Doppler, contrast-enhanced CT scan or MRI. A contrast-enhanced CT scan will show an enhancing mass at the carotid bifurcation with splaying of the internal and external carotid arteries (*Lyre's sign*), and also provide information regarding the grade of the tumor, that is, extent of encasement of the carotid artery (**Fig. 74.7**).

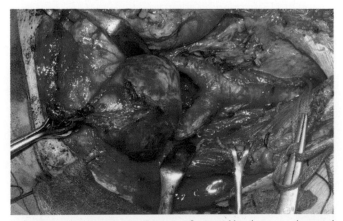

Fig. 74.7 Intraoperative picture of carotid body tumor located at the bifurcation of the carotid arteries.

Treatment

Common treatment is surgical excision. Some small tumors without significant symptoms can be observed for progression, especially in the elderly.

For tumors encasing or infiltrating the carotid, stenting or reconstruction may be required.

■ Pseudotumor of the Sternocleidomastoid

A synonym of pseudotumor of the sternocleidomastoid is fibromatosis colli.

It is a non-neoplastic condition involving the sternocleidomastoid muscle. It is seen in infants usually 2 to 4 weeks after birth. It is associated with diffuse enlargement of the sternocleidomastoid muscle with torticollis probably due to a hematoma following breech, vacuum, or forceps delivery, which can cause necrosis and fibrosis in the muscle. An ultrasound or MRI will show the extent of muscle involvement and the surrounding structures. It can be managed with physiotherapy to prevent the development of fibrosis and shortening of the sternocleidomastoid muscle. If left uncorrected, it may lead to asymmetry of craniofacial growth, compensatory cervical scoliosis, and squint.

■ Benign Cervical Lymphadenopathy

The causes of benign cervical lymphadenopathy are mainly inflammation.

Acute conditions producing lymphadenitis include the following:
- Acute bacterial tonsillitis.
- Reactive nonspecific lymphadenitis.
- Infectious mononucleosis.
- Rosai–Dorfman disease.
- Dental infections.

Chronic diseases like tuberculous lymphadenitis are more common in the posterior triangle, but can affect the lymph nodes in the submandibular, and upper, middle, or lower deep cervical region.

■ Metastatic Lymph Nodes

Cervical lymph nodes may be involved depending upon the primary site of malignancy. The sites and management are discussed in Chapter 73 "Cervical Lymphatic System and Neck Dissection."

■ Parapharyngeal Space Tumors

The parapharyngeal space is divided by the styloid process and its attachments into a prestyloid and a poststyloid compartment.

The poststyloid compartment contains important structures like the internal carotid artery, internal jugular vein, cranial nerves IX–XI, hypoglossal in the lower part, and the sympathetic chain.

The parapharyngeal space can be affected by inflammation (abscess) and tumors.

The tumors of the parapharyngeal space present as a mass in the upper part of the neck just below the angle of the mandible. These may also be seen intraorally displacing the tonsil, soft palate, and the lateral pharyngeal wall medially. The prestyloid compartment lesions are commonly salivary in origin arising from the deep lobe of the parotid. The common poststyloid compartment lesion is a vagal schwannoma. Other tumors like paragangliomas, lymphoma, or metastatic lymph node can also occur.

Investigations include a contrast-enhancing CT scan or MRI, which will help delineate the lesion. It will provide information regarding the type, size, location, (whether prestyloid or poststyloid), and delineate the adjacent structures. For highly enhancing lesions, a digital subtraction angiography should be done. An FNAC may give a possible tissue diagnosis.

Treatment is often surgical excision for benign tumors.

In case of prestyloid tumors, a transcervical–transparotid approach can be used. For poststyloid tumors, a transcervical approach with or without mandibulotomy is used.

◼ Salivary Gland Inflammatory Conditions and Tumors

These present as a neck mass. These are covered under diseases of the salivary glands (**Figs. 74.8** and **74.9**).

◼ Posterior Triangle

Tuberculous Cervical Lymphadenopathy

The synonyms of the tuberculous cervical lymphadenopathy are scrofula and king's evil.

The cervical lymph nodes are a common site for extrapulmonary tuberculosis. It is commonly caused by mycobacterium tuberculosis, although in immunocompromised individuals (like in a human immunodeficiency virus [HIV] positive patient), atypical mycobacteria can be the causative agent. It occurs in children and young adults with a slight female predilection. Most often, there will not be an associated pulmonary tuberculosis. The route of infection that has been proposed is lymphohematogenous or via the adenoid and tonsils.

Tuberculous cervical lymphadenitis can affect any group of lymph nodes but is more common in the posterior triangle followed by the upper deep cervical lymph nodes (**Fig. 74.10**). It usually presents as a painless swelling. Systemic symptoms like evening rise of temperature, night sweats, cough, and lethargy will be absent.

Stages of Tuberculous Cervical Lymphadenitis

The stages of the tuberculous cervical lymphadenitis are the following (**Fig. 74.11**):
- Stage I: Adenitis (firm, mobile, and discrete node).
- Stage II: Periadenitis (matted nodes).
- Stage III: Cold abscess (nodes coalesce with central necrosis).
- Stage IV: Collar stud abscess (abscess tracks through the deep fascia into the subcutaneous tissue).
- Stage V: Discharging sinus (abscess drains out through the skin).

Diagnosis

- Mantoux test or tuberculin skin test (TST): An intradermal injection of tuberculin purified protein derivative (PPD) is given and the size of the induration is measured.
- Chest X-ray to rule out pulmonary tuberculosis.
- Ultrasound of the neck will show matting of the nodes and mild surrounding edema.

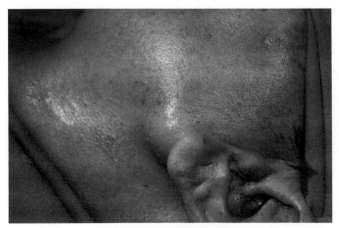

Fig. 74.8 Tumor of the left parotid gland.

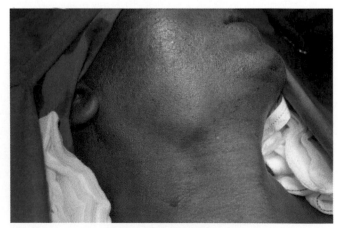

Fig. 74.9 Right submandibular swelling.

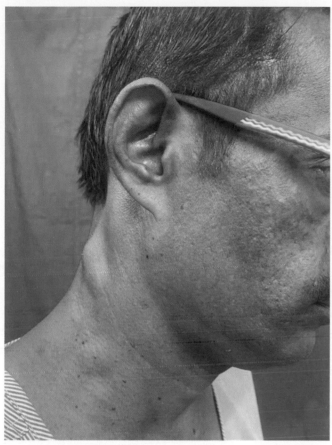

Fig. 74.10 Matted posterior triangle (tuberculous), lymph nodes, right side.

- Doppler may show prominent hilar vascularity (malignant node will show more peripheral and capsular vascularity).
- Contrast-enhanced CT scan may show low attenuation at the center with rim enhancement. There may be calcification within the node.
- FNAC may show epithelioid granuloma and caseation. An acid-fast bacilli staining can be done.
- Biopsy of the node is done when the FNAC is inconclusive. It will show caseation necrosis, multinucleated giant cells (Langerhans giant cells and histiocytes), granuloma, and calcification.
- A cartridge-based nucleic acid amplification test (GeneXpert) is also done on the tissue sample for rapid detection of tuberculosis and for detection of rifampicin resistance.
- Polymerase chain reaction (PCR), a nucleic acid amplification test, is a rapid test that is sensitive and specific for mycobacterium tuberculosis. It can be done from the FNAC aspirate. It is also helpful in detecting rifampicin resistance.

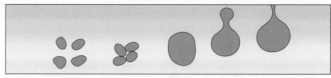

Fig. 74.11 The five stages of tuberculous cervical lymphadenitis are graphically represented.

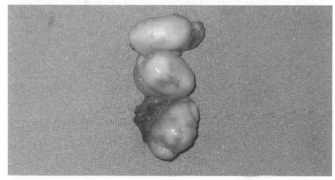

Fig. 74.12 Matted lymph nodes.

Treatment

- Antitubercular treatment (ATT) for a minimum period of 6 months.
- Persistent nodes can be excised (**Fig. 74.12**).
- Incision and drainage should not be done to avoid fistula formation.

Points to Ponder

- A thyroglossal duct cyst is a common cervical midline developmental anomaly. The treatment is by Sistrunk's procedure, to avoid recurrence.
- Th tests commonly done for a solitary nodule of the thyroid are thyroid function tests, ultrasound of the neck, and FNAC.
- A branchial cyst presents along the anterior border of the sternocleidomastoid in the upper neck.
- A second branchial cleft fistula may require an ipsilateral tonsillectomy along with resection of the tract.
- In the parapharyngeal space, the common tumor in the prestyloid compartment is of salivary gland origin, and in the poststyloid compartment, it is a vagal schwannoma.
- Tuberculous cervical lymphadenitis can occur without pulmonary tuberculosis. On palpation, in the initial stages, the nodes are matted.
- In neck swelling, radiology will help assess the size and site of the swelling, and FNAC will help give a tissue diagnosis.

Case-Based Questions

1. **A 6-year-old girl presented with an upper midline painless swelling that was noticed by the mother a few months after birth. On examination, it moved with deglutition and protrusion of the tongue. Ultrasound showed it to be a cystic swelling.**

   a. What is the most likely diagnosis?

   b. Where are the sites of presentation?

   c. What is the hood sign?

   d. What is the treatment?

   Answers

   a. Thyroglossal duct cyst.

   b. At, above, or below the level of the hyoid. Rarely it can occur in the tongue and the suprasternal region or the mediastinum.

   c. When it presents as a thyroglossal fistula, there is a fold of skin in the upper part of the fistula, which is referred to as the hood sign.

   d. The Sistrunk operation.

2. **A 10-month-old male infant was brought to the outpatient department with a swelling in the posterior triangle of the neck. The swelling was soft, cystic, and brilliantly transilluminant. There has been no increase in size.**

   a. What is the most likely diagnosis?

   h What are the investigations required?

   c. What is the treatment?

   Answers

   a. Lymphangioma.

   b. MRI of the neck, and assessment for other congenital anomalies, especially since the lesion is in the posterior triangle.

   c. Wait and watch. If it is increasing in size, plan for surgical resection or injection of sclerosants.

3. **A 42-year-old man presented with multiple posterior triangle neck masses of 5 months' duration. On examination, there were multiple, nontender, matted lymph nodes. There was no history of fever, cough, or hemoptysis.**

   a. What is the possible diagnosis?

   b. How would you confirm the diagnosis?

   c. What are the other investigations required to be done?

   d. What is the treatment?

   Answers

   a. Tuberculous cervical lymphadenitis.

   b. FNAC can give the diagnosis. Biopsy is done if FNAC is inconclusive. A cartridge-based nucleic acid amplification (Gen-Xpert) is done on the specimen for early diagnosis and to check for rifampicin resistance.

   c. X-ray chest (posteroanterior view) and sputum acid-fast bacilli to rule out pulmonary tuberculosis.

   d. ATT for a minimum period of 6 months. The nodes are excised if they persist despite ATT.

Frequently Asked Questions

1. What is the Sistrunk operation?

2. What is the Bethesda classification in thyroid cytology?

3. What are the features of thyroid malignancy on ultrasound?

4. What are the compartments of the parapharyngeal space and the common tumors in each compartment?

5. What are the stages of tuberculous cervical lymphadenitis?

6. How will you manage a patient with lingual thyroid?

7. Enumerate the various midline neck swellings.

Endnote

There are roughly 800 lymph nodes in the human body, out of which 300 are found in the neck. These are organized into seven levels. The Delphian lymph node is one of the lymph nodes in level 6. It is located above the thyroid isthmus, on the cricothyroid membrane. It is called the "Delphian lymph node" because metastasis in this lymph node is a sign or predictor of malignancy of the thyroid. It is named after the Oracle of Delphi, a priestess in Greece, who could make predictions of the future.

75 Viral Infections in the Ear, Nose, and Throat

Chandrakiran C.

Introduction

Infections in the human body can be caused by microorganisms that are either endogenous or exogenous. Those relevant to the ear, nose, and throat (ENT) are most commonly bacterial, viral, or fungal in origin. This chapter helps understand the pathophysiology, clinical manifestations, and management of viral infections in ENT practice. There is also a large amount of clinical research on the ENT manifestations of human immunodeficiency virus (HIV) infection, as many of its presenting symptoms can lead a patient to the ENT clinic.

Viruses Causing ENT Infections

Viruses are the smallest of infective agents visible under the electron microscope. The International Committee on Taxonomy of Viruses classified them according to the molecular composition of the genome: the structure of the virus capsid and whether or not it is enveloped, the gene expression program used to produce virus proteins, host range, pathogenicity, and sequence similarity.

Those that cause ENT-related infections are listed in **Box 75.1**.

Pathophysiology of Viral Infections and Natural History

The pathophysiology of viral infections and natural history are shown in **Fig. 75.1**.

Box 75.1 Viruses with a potential to cause ENT-related infections

- Rhinovirus.
- Adenovirus.
- Coronavirus.
- Influenza A and B viruses.
- Parainfluenza virus.
- HIV.
- Respiratory syncytial virus (RSV).
- Cytomegalovirus (CMV).
- Epstein–Barr virus (EBV).
- Herpes simplex virus (HSV) 1 and 2.
- Coxsackie virus.

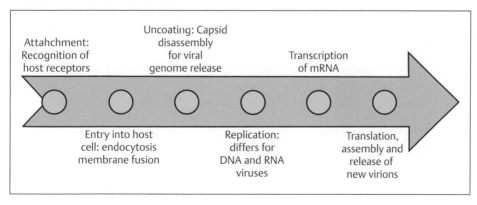

Fig. 75.1 Pathophysiology of viral infections.

Routes of Spread

- Droplets and fomites.
- Airborne transmission.
- Blood and blood products.
- Use of unsterile needles and other sharp objects.
- Unprotected sexual contact.
- Vertical mode of spread from mother to child.

ENT Manifestations of HIV Infection

The ENT surgeon may be the first to identify and assess the initial symptoms of HIV infection (**Table 75.1**). These symptoms could give a clue to disease progression or may suggest the possibility of an underlying immunocompromised state. Hence, it is important to be well versed in its variable presentation. Up to 80% of HIV-infected patients develop ENT manifestations, among which oral diseases are the most common, that is, in around 40 to 50%.

Acute HIV infection can often present persistent generalized lymphadenopathy (especially the posterior group of cervical nodes) and accompanying symptoms of fever, night sweats, weight loss, fatigue, and intractable diarrhea. Certain factors such as a low CD4 count <200/μL, plasma HIV-RNA levels >3,000 copies/mL, xerostomia, poor oral hygiene, and smoking make individuals more susceptible to these manifestations.

Differential Diagnosis of Oral Ulcers

- Aphthous ulcers.
- Syphilis.
- Varicella.
- Herpangina.
- Behçet's disease.
- HIV infection.
- Traumatic ulcers.
- Verrucous carcinoma.
- Inflammatory bowel disease.
- Stevens–Johnson syndrome.

Oral, Oropharyngeal, and Laryngeal Manifestations

■ Candidiasis

It can be found in the oral cavity, oropharynx, larynx, and hypopharynx. It can present in four forms:

- *Pseudomembranous candidiasis* (**Fig. 75.2**): This is the most common type, which presents as curdy-white plaques on the mucosal surfaces that are involved. If peeled away, it leaves red or bleeding surfaces beneath it. *Candida albicans* is the most common causative organism, but other candida species such as *C. glabrata* and *C. dubliniensis* have also been found to have a role.

Table 75.1 Manifestations of HIV that are relevant to ENT practice

Oral and oropharyngeal manifestations	Laryngeal manifestations	Nasal and sinus manifestations	Otologic and audiological manifestations	Head and neck masses
Oral ulceration	Laryngeal candidiasis	Nasopharyngeal lymphoid hypertrophy (early stages)	Otitis Externa and Polyps of the external ear	Lymphadenopathy
Candidiasis	Kaposi's sarcoma of the larynx	Allergic rhinitis (twice as common in HIV infection)	Kaposi's sarcoma of the external ear	Parotid enlargement Malignant lymphoma Kaposi's sarcoma Lymphoepithelial cyst
Oral hairy leukoplakia	Laryngeal tuberculosis	Nasopharyngeal Kaposi's sarcoma	Chronic otitis media with effusion	Lymphomas
Neoplastic growths	Laryngeal histoplasmosis	Non-Hodgkin's lymphomas	Sensorineural hearing loss	Squamous cell carcinomas
Periodontal and gingival disease	Squamous cell carcinoma of the larynx	Extranodal sinus histiocytosis (Rosai–Dorfman disease)	Ramsay Hunt syndrome	
		Sinusitis: recurrent acute and chronic	Isolated facial nerve paralysis	

Abbreviations: ENT, ear, nose, and throat; HIV, human immunodeficiency virus.

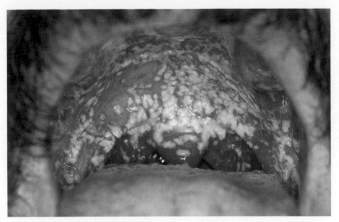

Fig. 75.2 Pseudomembranous candidiasis.

- *Erythematous candidiasis*: This type of candidiasis presents as a red, flat, subtle lesion on the dorsal surface of the tongue, hard or soft palate. It involves two opposing raw surfaces with matching lesions
- *Angular cheilitis*: It appears as red, flaky lesions at the angles of the mouth.
- *Hyperplastic candidiasis*: This is the least common type of candidiasis with HIV infection. It appears as thick, white plaques on the mucosa.

Candidal esophagitis can present with dysphagia and requires esophagoscopy and biopsy in case of failure of medical therapy. Involvement of the pharynx, larynx, or esophagus with candidiasis indicates a late stage of disease, with CD4 counts below 200 cells/mm^3.

Treatment

Depending on the severity of infection, the routes of administration of the antifungal agent can be topical, oral, or intravenous. Topical medications include the following:
- Clotrimazole.
- Miconazole.
- Nystatin.

They are applied like a paint, inside the mouth for 1 to 2 weeks. Clotrimazole lozenges may be used. Fluconazole, oral or intravenous, can be administered in the following:
- Patients who do not respond to topical therapy.
- In recurrent cases.
- Patients with esophageal involvement.

EBV, HSV, human papilloma virus (HPV), and varicella-zoster virus, which are more likely to cause lesions in HIV-infected individuals, are described separately in this chapter.

■ Chronic Hepatitis Infection

It commonly presents with oral pathology in the icteric stage of illness with signs of a yellow-brown hue in the oral mucosa. Lichen planus and lymphocytic sialadenitis can develop due to autoantibody production.

■ Periodontal and Gingival Disease

It is a common oral manifestation of HIV infection. It presents with tender, bleeding, and erythematous gums. It is usually managed with medicated gargles such as chlorhexidine.

■ Kaposi's Sarcoma

It is a common neoplasm that is included in the Centers for Disease Control and Prevention (CDC) classification of acquired immunodeficiency syndrome (AIDS), which usually presents on the skin, hard palate, gingiva, buccal mucosa, dorsum of the tongue, and mucosa of the nose and nasopharynx. Human herpes virus 8 (HHV-8) is found in these lesions. Its characteristic appearance is that of a raised, reddish to purple plaque, which can ulcerate. Mucosal lesions are frequently painful and bleed on touch. The malignant lesions can form in lymph nodes and other organs as well.

Management options include the following:
- Highly active antiretroviral therapy (HAART) along with chemotherapy (intralesional or systemic).
- Immunotherapy.
- Excision/cryotherapy.
- Radiotherapy.

In the pediatric age group, Kaposi's sarcoma tends to be more progressive and disseminated.

Nasal and Paranasal Sinus Manifestations

■ Nasopharyngeal Lymphoid Hypertrophy

It can present with mouth breathing, nasal obstruction, or as serous or acute otitis media. In cases of adenoid hypertrophy in adults, one of the differential diagnoses to be kept in mind is HIV infection.

■ Sinusitis

Infection of the sinuses, acute or chronic, follows a long course in HIV-positive patients, making it more severe and difficult to treat. The symptoms are often nonspecific with a diagnosis being made based on incidental computed tomography (CT) or magnetic resonance imaging (MRI) findings. The prevalence of fungal sinusitis in these cases is also higher than that in immunocompetent persons.

The opportunistic pathogens causing sinus disease are the following:
- CMV.
- Fungi such as *Alternaria*, *Aspergillus*, Cryptococcus, *Candida*, and *Rhizopus*.
- Rarely, bacteria such as *Cutibacterium acnes* and *Pseudomonas aeruginosa* and anaerobic bacteria have been implicated.

Otological manifestations

■ External Ear

in the external ear, it can present as otitis externa, aural polyps, and neoplastic growths such as Kaposi's sarcoma involving the auricle or tympanic membrane.

■ Middle Ear

Serous otitis media leading to a conductive hearing loss could be the mode of presentation of the patient to the ENT clinic. The common organisms responsible are *Streptococcus pneumoniae*, *Haemophilus influenzae*, and *Moraxella catarrhalis*. *Pneumocystis carinii* may also be implicated in otitis media and mastoiditis.

■ Inner Ear

In the inner ear, it can present as sensorineural hearing loss due to opportunistic infections, for example, CMV affecting the inner ear or the cochlear nerve. It could also be due to the use of ototoxic drugs such as azidothymidine, pentamidine, acyclovir, and aminoglycoside antibiotics.

Head and Neck Masses

■ Lymphadenopathy

Persistent generalized lymphadenopathy is commonly seen in the early stages of the disease, which on examination are soft, nontender, and symmetrical in distribution, with posterior cervical nodes being the most common. Although most commonly it is due to a benign reactive process, it could also be indicative of tuberculosis, cryptococcosis, squamous cell carcinoma, or non-Hodgkin's lymphoma.

■ Parotid Enlargement

Presenting unilaterally or bilaterally, it could be an early initial presenting sign of HIV infection. The parotid gland appears bulky, mildly tender on palpation, and fine-needle aspiration cytology, usually reveals a benign lymphoepithelial cyst.

> **Pearl**
>
> *Extranodal sinus histiocytosis (Rosai–Dorfman disease)* is a rare disorder characterized by overproduction of histiocytes in the lymph node, presenting with lymphadenopathy, most commonly cervical. An association with HIV infection has been noted.

Other Viruses Causing Oral Lesions

■ Hairy Leukoplakia

It is caused by EBV (**Fig. 75.3**). It presents as a white lesion at the lateral border of the tongue with an irregular, shaggy surface. It is often asymptomatic and it is seen commonly in immunocompromised patients and its presence indicates a strong possibility of HIV infection. A high viral load, a low CD4 count, and the concomitant presence of oral candidiasis are important risk factors for its development.

Due to its similarity to lesions such as leukoplakia, carcinoma in situ, lichen planus, and hypertrophic candidiasis, a biopsy must be taken to confirm the diagnosis.

Relevant findings on biopsy include hyperkeratosis, acanthosis, and the presence of EBV in the basal epithelial cells.

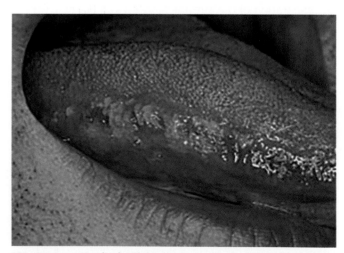

Fig. 75.3 Hairy leukoplakia seen on the lateral border of the tongue.

Management options include topical application of acyclovir with podophyllin cream, or systemic antivirals such as valacyclovir and ganciclovir.

Herpes Simplex Virus

It characteristically presents as small round ulcers without an erythematous halo. These "fever blisters" are seen in the keratinized and attached mucosa of the gums, hard palate, and dorsum of the tongue. It can cause pain and discomfort on chewing and swallowing.

Diagnosis is made based on the characteristic appearance of lesions and by culturing the organism by taking cell scrapings of the base of the ulcer.

The condition is treated with oral famciclovir, valacyclovir, or acyclovir (15 mg per kg five times daily for 7 days). In some cases, depending on the severity of the lesions, intravenous acyclovir may be required. In cases of acyclovir-resistant HSV, the treatment of choice is intravenous foscarnet.

Human Papilloma Virus

It is a double-stranded DNA virus that causes mucosal lesions described as whitish or pink, cauliflower-like growths with a sharp border and irregular surface.

The ace-to-white staining technique used to identify latent genital warts can identify HPV in the uncharacteristic flat lesions in the oral cavity as well (**Box 75.2**).

On light microscopy, koilocytes or balloon cells with hyperchromatic nuclei surrounded by a clear halo is seen.

The morphological lesions induced by HPV in the oral cavity include the following:
• Papillomas of the oral cavity and condyloma acuminata.
• Focal epithelial hyperplasia.
• Oral lichen planus.

Treatment options include surgical excision, chemical ablation, and cryotherapy. However, despite the use of these, recurrence is common.

Varicella-Zoster Virus Infection

This is caused by reactivation of varicella-zoster virus leading to herpes zoster. The virus lays dormant in the dorsal root ganglion alongside the spine, after the initial infection. It presents as unilateral distribution of vesicles on the skin and mucous membrane, localized to a dermatome, that is,

Box 75.2   HPV-induced oral cavity lesions
Squamous papilloma: HPV 6 and HPV 11: Exophytic, cauliflower-like growth
Condyloma acuminata: HPV 2, HPV 6, and HPV 11: Lesions have a wider base and absent hyperkeratosis
Squamous cell carcinoma: HPV 16

the ophthalmic, maxillary, or mandibular divisions of the trigeminal sensory nerve (**Fig. 75.4**). By involving the cranial nerves within their dermatomal distribution, this condition can also present with blindness, hearing loss, vertigo, and facial weakness.

It is treated with acyclovir (200 mg five times a day for 1 or 2 weeks) or valacyclovir (1 g three times daily for 7–10 days). In patients who are immunocompromised, intravenous acyclovir (10 mg/kg every 8 hours for 7 days) is given.

> **Pearl**
>
> HPV is also associated with oropharyngeal carcinoma and laryngeal papillomatosis.

Epstein–Barr Virus

It is a double-stranded DNA virus from the herpes family. It is associated with various diseases in the head and neck region. It spreads through body fluids like saliva, semen, and blood, and can occur by sharing toothbrush and drinking glass; it can be transmitted by organ transplant or blood transfusion as well.

Diseases produced by the EBV include the following:
• Inflammatory: Infectious mononucleosis and chronic fatigue syndrome.
• Autoimmune: Higher risk of developing Sjogren's syndrome and rheumatoid arthritis.
• HIV related: Oral hairy leukoplakia.
• Malignant: Hodgkin's lymphoma, Burkitt's lymphoma, and nasopharyngeal carcinoma.

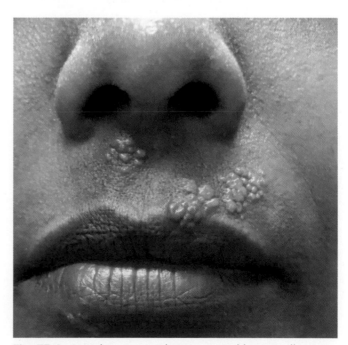

Fig. 75.4 Vesicles seen in clusters caused by varicella-zoster virus.

Treatment of HIV Infection

Classes of drugs used in the treatment of HIV infection are listed in **Box 75.3**.

Box 75.3   Classes of drugs used in HAART regimens

- **Nucleoside/nucleotide reverse transcriptase inhibitors (NRTIs):** Abacavir, didanosine, lamivudine, stavudine, tenofovir, and zidovudine
- **Non-nucleoside reverse transcriptase inhibitors (NNRTIs):** Delavirdine, efavirenz, nevirapine, and rilpivirine
- **Protease inhibitors (PIs):** Atazanavir, darunavir, and indinavir
- **Integrase strand transfer inhibitors (INSTIs):** Dolutegravir, elvitegravir, and raltegravir
- **Fusion inhibitors:** Enfuvirtide
- **Chemokine receptor antagonists (CCR5 antagonists):** Maraviroc

---

Pearl

HAART is a regimen comprising a combination of three or more drugs, aimed at inhibiting viral replication by different mechanisms so that the propagation of the virus with resistance to one agent will be inhibited by the action of the other two agents.

ENT Manifestations of COVID-19 Infection

The novel coronavirus (2019-nCoV), an RNA virus that started in Wuhan, China, was declared as a pandemic on March 11, 2020 by the World Health Organization (WHO). Apart from the lower respiratory tract symptoms, the clinical presentation includes a variety of otolaryngologic manifestations, the most common of which is sore throat.

The other common ENT-related manifestations include a loss of taste and smell, nasal obstruction, nasal discharge, and otological symptoms such as bilateral ear fullness and itching, which were the complaints of a few patients. The sense of smell usually returns within a few weeks but some of these patients develop parosmia later.

In India, there has been a sharp rise in cases of rhino-orbito-cerebral mucormycosis in the COVID-19 era (**Figs. 75.5, 75.6,** and **75.7**). The predisposing factors to developing the invasive fungal infection are uncontrolled diabetes mellitus, transplant recipients, patients undergoing chemotherapy, HIV infection, and other immunocompromised states. It can present as unilateral nasal obstruction, facial pain or fullness, loss of sensations over the face, and swelling around the eyes with blurring of vision.

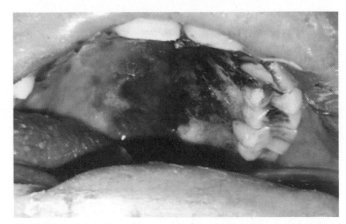

Fig. 75.5   Palatal involvement in mucormycosis.

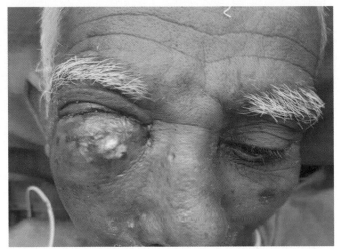

Fig. 75.6   Rhino-orbital mucormycosis with right orbital abscess.

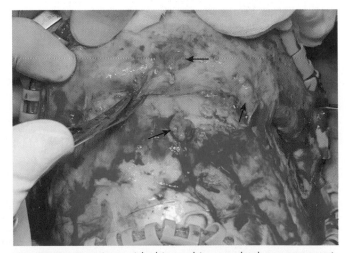

Fig. 75.7   A patient with rhino-orbito-cerebral mucormycosis undergoing debridement of necrotic bony and soft tissue through an osteoplastic flap approach. The *black arrows* point to the necrotic tissue.

On examination, any black, necrotic tissue visualized on anterior rhinoscopy or endoscopy should be sent for microbiological testing to confirm the presence of broad, aseptate hyphae seen in mucormycosis (**Fig. 75.8**). The patient is treated via a combined medical and surgical approach, with regular debridement of necrotic tissue and intravenous liposomal amphotericin B injections.

There are many ongoing studies on the possible long-term side effects that COVID-19 infection could have on ENT. Over the course of the pandemic, various strains of the virus have presented with different virulence and symptomatology. The omicron variant spreads rapidly and has mainly upper respiratory symptoms like nasal discharge and sore throat, along with fever and body ache. There is low morbidity.

Diagnosis of Viral Infections in ENT Practice

Diagnosis of viral infections in ENT practice is presented in **Box 75.4**.

Safety Practices for the ENT Surgeon

- Goggles, N95 masks, and head shields should be used to avoid splashes of blood and fluids during surgeries on HIV-positive persons and limiting exposure to infected aerosols.
- Sharps and waste generated in the outpatient department (OPD) or in the operating room should be carefully disposed.
- Recapping needles should be avoided and the staff should be educated about safe sharp disposal methods.

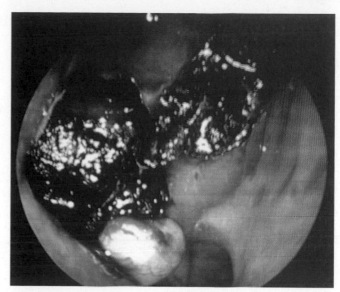

Fig. 75.8 Endoscopic picture of the nasal cavity showing black, necrotic middle turbinate of the lateral wall in a patient with mucormycosis.

- The blood, bone, tissue fragments, and middle ear bone debris/fluid released during drilling in mastoid surgery has also been found to contain HIV virus and hence adequate personal protective equipment must be used by surgeons, assistants, and nurses.
- Wearing gloves during routine examination is a safety measure when the HIV status of the patient is unknown. Double gloving is a reasonable way to provide additional protection.

Box 75.4 Diagnostic techniques for evaluation of viral infections in ENT practice

- HIV:
  - Western blot
  - CD4 counts
  - P24 antigen assays
  - Enzyme-linked immunosorbent assay (ELISA)
- COVID-19:
  - Viral tests: Nucleic acid amplification tests and antigen tests
  - Antibody test/serology test

Points to Ponder

- Viral infections cause a variety of ENT diseases.
- Up to 80% of HIV-infected patients develop ENT-related diseases.
- Oral manifestations of HIV include oral ulcers and candidiasis.
- The most common type of candidiasis is pseudomembranous candidiasis.
- EBV can cause malignancies like Hodgkin's lymphoma, Burkitt's lymphoma, and nasopharyngeal carcinoma.
- Treatment of HIV infection is HAART.
- Covid-19 is an ongoing pandemic with ENT manifestations being common. Black necrotic tissue seen on anterior rhinoscopy over the middle turbinate in a patient, post-Covid, should be sent for microbiological examination to rule out mucormycosis.

Case-Based Questions

1. A 35-year-old man presented to the ENT clinic with a white lesion over the lateral border of the tongue. On examination, there were white, irregular lesions with prominent folds along the lateral border of the tongue. A routine blood workup revealed a low CD4 count.

   a. What is the possible diagnosis?

   b. How will you proceed to investigate this patient?

   c. What is the treatment?

   Answers

   a. Oral hairy leukoplakia (OHL). In most cases, OHL diagnosis is made on clinical grounds.

   b. A biopsy must be done to make a histopathological diagnosis. The EBV can be demonstrated within the epithelial cells of the lesion. A low CD4 is a sign of infection with HIV.

   c. It is a benign lesion with low morbidity. It does not require specific treatment in all cases. There is a tendency for the disease to resolve after some time. Systemic therapy, if required, consists of antiviral agents like acyclovir, 800 mg five times a day. This will lead to resolution of the disease in 1 to 3 weeks. Topical podophyllin resin 25% can also be tried.

2. A 60-year-old man developed right-sided facial pain, nose block of the same side, and periorbital swelling around the right eye. His vision was normal. There was a history of COVID-19 infection 1 month back for which he was hospitalized. He is also a known diabetic. On examination, there was black, necrotic tissue over the middle turbinate.

   a. What is the diagnosis?

   b. How will you arrive at a diagnosis in this patient?

   c. What is the treatment?

   Answers

   a. Mucormycosis of the nose.

   b. Biopsy can be taken to look for the fungus and evidence of tissue and vascular invasion. A KOH (potassium hydroxide) mount is done for fungal staining.

   c. Treatment consists of intravenous antifungal therapy with liposomal amphotericin B and surgical excision. A careful examination of the eye is crucial and active intervention with antifungal must be started as early as possible to save and protect the eye and prevent intracranial involvement.

Frequently Asked Questions

1. Enumerate the oral manifestations of HIV.

2. What are the ENT-related presentations of COVID 19?

3. Enumerate the safety practices required by an ENT surgeon when dealing with a seropositive or COVID patient.

4. What are the malignant lesions associated with the EBV?

5. What are the routes of spread of viral infections in ENT?

6. What is Kaposi's sarcoma? What is its relationship to HIV?

Endnote

HIV was identified in 1983 by Francoise Barre-Sinoussi and Luc Montagnier as the cause of AIDS; it was initially known as lymphadenopathy-associated virus.

Anthony Epstein and Yvonne Barr discovered the EBV, along with Bert Achong.

Burkitt's lymphoma was described by Denis Parsons Burkitt as an endemic pediatric variant of non-Hodgkin's lymphoma in Uganda.

76 Patient Counseling

Kailesh Pujary

The competencies covered in this chapter are as follows:

EN2.12 Counsel and administer informed consent to patients and their families in a simulated environment.
DE4.4 Counsel patients to risks of oral cancer with respect to tobacco, smoking, alcohol, and other causative factors.

Introduction

Hospital visits can be stressful for the patient and their family. When provided in an empathetic setting, counseling helps patients understand and cope with such situations. The role of a health care professional in this setting would be to reduce the patient's fears and improve compliance to treatment for their psychological and physical well-being. Patient counseling requires a health care professional to discuss the disease status, evaluation, treatment process, and outcomes with the patient, preferably using a two-way communication.

The Doctor–Patient Relationship

Mutual trust is an integral part of a relationship between a doctor and a patient. The health care provider should be able to allocate time to interact with the patient without interruptions. An authoritarian attitude would be a one-way communication that denies the patient control over themselves, whereas collaboration encourages a two-way communication.

There are various models of a doctor–patient relationship that have been described:

- *Di Aratteo (1991)*: In an *active-passive* model, the patient does not participate; in the *guidance-cooperation* model, the doctor takes the decisions in management; and in a *mutual participation*, there is a combined decision in all aspects.
- *Emanuel and Emanuel (1992)*: In the *paternalistic* model, the doctor takes decisions and encourages the patient to consent; in the *informative* model, the doctor gives relevant information and the patient decides; in the *interpretive* model, the doctor gives information and counsels

the patient through the process of decision-making; and in the *deliberative* model, the doctor is like a friend and allows the patient to empower themselves to make their own decision.

Barriers to Effective Counseling

The primary *physician factor* that limits effective counseling is poor communication skills. Good communication is quite often learnt over time. Counseling can be time-consuming, and the physician with a busy practice may not have the time or interest. But if not appropriately counseled, the time taken later to counsel again would be more. When a multidisciplinary team is treating the patient, confusion about who does the counseling may arise or can sometimes lead to conflicting remarks that the patient can misinterpret.

Distracted doctoring is when intrinsic or extrinsic factors cause reduced focus on a particular health facility task. Electronic health records can be cumbersome if not used appropriately and may cause less focus while interacting with a patient. Communication between health care providers, especially regarding patient-related matters, should be purposeful to share information to improve care, refocus attention, and collaborate. Nonpurposeful communication can impair performance and contribute to errors. The use of personal electronic devices including mobile phones by the health care provider or others in the vicinity can be distracting while dealing with the patient whether in the outpatient clinic or the operating room.

The central *patient-related factor* is often the distress in dealing with the disease. The inability of the patient to understand the disease, treatment, or outcomes can lead to unrealistic expectations. The cost of treatment can cause undue stress on the family. For the patient, the hospital is an alien environment, which adds to the feeling of insecure and stress. The burden on the caregivers increases with relation to time, money, effort, and sometimes loss of work days. In some places, language can be a limiting factor in effectively communicating with the patient.

The *organizational factors* would be that accreditation agencies' additional paperwork, and documentation can be time-consuming and distracting. Lack of trained personnel to counsel the admission process, financial matters, and hospital facilities can burden the treating physician.

Counseling: Why Should It be Done?

The hospital setting can be a stressful experience for the patient, especially when they are in physical and mental distress regarding the illness. Counseling would also help gather the relevant details from the patient, improve compliance, reduce stress, improve healing, and possibly reduce malpractice suits. Counseling would reduce patient dissatisfaction with the outcome, especially if there were a change in care.

Counseling: When Is It Required?

It is done to explain their disease, the treatment options, and the possible outcomes to the patient. It is also done before doing any procedure in the outpatient department wherein the patient is informed of the reason for the investigations and their necessity.

For a surgical procedure, counseling is done in various stages. *Preadmission counseling* is done to outline the importance of the surgical intervention, the procedure itself, and possible complications. The patient and the caregiver are informed of the hospital facilities and approximate cost by the paramedical or hospital staff. *Presurgical counseling* is done to reduce the patient's fears, and understand the procedure and its complications, and the prognosis of the disease. Counseling is done so that the patient does not have any unrealistic expectations. The role of anesthesia should also be emphasized. *Preoperatively*, if there is a deviation from the plan, unexpected findings, or help from other specialties is sought, this should be informed to the patient's bystander before proceeding and the same should be documented, and the patient should be informed after the surgery. *Postoperative counseling* is done to appraise the patient of the duration of healing, suture removal, wound care, any changes in the outcomes, compliance to medications, possibility of a second surgery, and follow-up. The caregiver should also be involved. *Predischarge counseling* is done to ensure continuity of care and must always include the emergency numbers for contact.

Counseling: Where Should It be Done?

It should be done in a separate room. Counseling in other areas, especially in the presence of others, should be strongly discouraged. The room ideally should have a video-recording facility. For a child, the parent or legal guardian should be present. For a mentally challenged individual or debilitated individual, the caregiver should be present. Ensure the presence of a nurse or female colleague when examining or counseling a female patient. The patient can decide who they would want from the family or a friend during the counseling.

Counseling: Who Should Do It?

The counseling should ideally be done by the treating doctor or a team member managing the patient. Matters like the admission process, cost, and resources of the hospital can be handled by the paramedical staff. Managing the distress of the patient and their family members requires a trained psychologist along with the physician. When a multidisciplinary approach for treatment is required, the lead consultant should gather the necessary data and counsel the patient preferably in the presence of the other team members. However, in some instances, due to the specificity of the treatment, the concerned consultant present can give the necessary information.

Counseling: How Can It be Done?

The art of good counseling starts with showing warmth, courtesy, and empathy. Speaking with a reasonable tone of voice and maintaining eye contact during communication are necessary. Encourage questions, clarify doubts, and summarize the discussion. Allow the patient to take charge of the decision-making process. Do not ridicule the patient's questions including their superstitions.

Consent can be taken in *verbal, written, or videographed form*. The written consent form should have the name of the organization (hospital), treating doctor's name, name of the procedure, complications of the procedure, the signature of the doctor and patient, and the name and signature of a witness. Consent is individualized to the procedure. A separate consent for anesthesia should be taken.

Breaking the Bad News

Certain acute illnesses with poor prognosis and diseases like cancer can be a distressing experience for the patient and their family. The place of counseling should be comfortable with privacy to allow for the patient's emotions. Interruptions should be avoided. The patient can determine who should be there with them. For a child, the parent should be present. The family may request that the patient is not made aware of the illness. The family needs to be explained the benefits of informing the patient and the possible harmful consequences of not telling. Find out what the patient knows and how much they want to know as different patients handle information differently. Share the information regarding the illness and wait for the patient to understand or respond. Be realistic about the severity of the illness to avoid undue expectations. Give the patient and family time to respond and ask if they have any queries. Plan and discuss the next few steps in management in sequence and discuss the support system available. Repeat the salient part of the discussion in subsequent visits.

The initial reaction is usually *denial*, that is, the patient may not accept the illness. They then get *angry* as to why they had to get the illness. The patient *bargains* regarding the possibility of another more favorable diagnosis or outcome. Before coming to terms with the illness and possible outcome, they go into *depression*. *Acceptance* of the illness by most patients is with either hope or reluctance. Being supportive during these stages can be beneficial to the patient and their caregivers.

Informed Consent

Informed consent is a communication process that can lead to a mutual agreement or permission for the care, treatment, or services between the patient and the health care provider.

Two or more persons can consent when they agree upon the same thing in the same sense (Indian Contract Act, Sec. 13). Consent is when permission is given voluntarily without coercion for an investigation or procedure after the details of the purpose, benefit, nature, risks, and alternatives are explained, which gives legitimacy for what is going to be done. The patient can decide to give or withhold consent based on the information provided. Providing information is the legal duty of the doctor, which results in shared decision-making and patient education. Any informed refusal should be documented.

■ Types of Consent

Informed consent requires giving all the information to a competent person for understanding and obtaining a voluntary agreement following a decision-making process.

Implied consent is based on the actions of the patient. In history-taking and clinical examination of the patient in the clinic, a separate written consent is not required as the action of the patient to come to the clinic to seek treatment forms the basis of implied consent.

Expressed consent is in the written or verbal form (both need to be documented). Any consent other than implied consent falls in the category of expressed consent.

Proxy consent is given by the relative or guardian when the patient is not competent to give the consent.

■ Age for Giving Consent

In India, anyone above the age of 18 years is considered a major/adult and when in sound mind can give consent (Indian Penal Code, Sec. 87). A person below the age of 12 years cannot give consent (Indian Penal Code, Sec. 90). A person between 12 and 18 years of age can give consent only for examination, not for procedures (except in case of emergency). Therapeutic privilege (therapeutic exception and therapeutic nondisclosure) is when the physician does not disclose certain health information to the patient as it may cause serious psychological harm or violate the patient's personal, social, or cultural needs.

The consent should encompass diagnosis (including the nature of disease), reason for the procedure (including details of what is going to be done), benefits and complications of the procedure, risk of not undergoing the procedure, and alternate treatment modalities. Any comorbidities (and their medications), allergies, and addictions should be documented. If an opinion has been taken from a colleague, document the same.

■ Exceptions to Informed Consent

In certain situations, informed consent is not necessary. These include the following:
- When a patient is incapacitated and therefore unable to give consent.
- In life-threatening emergencies with very little time to obtain consent.
- When the patient is suffering from a notifiable disease and there is a need to protect the public against the spread of the disease.

Special Situations Requiring Counseling

Disclosing medical errors due to iatrogenic injury or adverse events that can lead to a prolonged stay requires counseling. A medical error is a failure of a planned action to be completed as intended or a wrong plan to achieve an aim. It may be due to investigative procedures, treatment, or equipment failure. Counseling is important to relieve the anxiety of the patient, take early remedial measures, and avoid legal problems. State the problem and the possible corrective measures. Do apologize but do not procrastinate or speculate. Give the initial information and later give the facts after the evaluation.

Blood transfusion requires an informed consent. The responsibility of the doctor is to assess the patient for timely transfusion along with monitoring the progress, volume, and rate of transfusion required.

Implants like a cochlear implant require counseling and consent as a device is placed by surgery into the inner ear. The additional aspects other than the surgery is rehabilitation and cost, which need to be brought to their understanding.

Head and neck cancer and its treatment often affects swallowing, breathing, and speech, and can be disfiguring, which affects the quality of life. The morbidity, additional treatment, posttreatment rehabilitation, and the outcomes should be delicately discussed with the patient and their caregivers.

Orbital exenteration done as a part of paranasal sinus tumor removal or for acute invasive fungal sinusitis requires counseling. This requires two ophthalmologist to concur and document the same after evaluation of the patient.

Laryngeal transplant, although it is not a commonly performed procedure as it is an organ transplant of a nonvital structure, requires counseling as there are ethical issues. It requires vascular anastomosis and reinnervation for the functions of the larynx, that is, respiration, protection of the lower airway, and phonation. There are chances of rejection. Postoperatively, lifelong immunosuppressive medication is required. The ethical issue that needs to be considered is that the immunosuppressive treatment, which is nephrotoxic and hepatotoxic, can also cause a secondary malignancy.

Risk Factors for Oral Cancer and Preventive Counseling

There is a relatively high incidence of oral cancer in the Indian subcontinent. This is mainly due to the addiction to tobacco-related products and alcohol. These addictions are more common in vulnerable individuals. This vulnerability may be genetic or a consequence of a physical or emotional trauma, or a combination of both. Primary prevention, that is, prior to the use of the substance, has a major role especially in the younger age group. This can be done by having sessions for groups in schools and colleges. Secondary prevention, that is, in the early stages of addiction, needs frequent counseling and family support. Tertiary prevention, that is, in addicts, needs a more strategic approach. Further management based on the level of addiction will require gradual reduction of the substance, pharmacotherapy at home, or short hospital stays. Relapses can occur.

Frequent use of tobacco-related products in smoked or smokeless (dry and wet) forms increases the risk of cancer of the oral cavity, oropharynx, larynx, hypopharynx, esophagus, and lungs. In addition, the smoked tobacco can lead to chronic obstructive pulmonary disease and increase the risk of stroke, myocardial infarction, and peripheral vascular disease.

Frequent consumption of large quantities of alcohol, especially when consumed along with the use of tobacco, has also been shown to increase manifold the risk of cancer (oral cavity, oropharynx, hypopharynx, and esophagus). It is also known to increase the risk of cardiac disease (myocardial infarction, cardiomyopathy, and arrhythmias), neurological diseases (memory problems, stroke, Wernicke's encephalopathy, cerebellar degeneration, and peripheral polyneuropathy), liver diseases (portal hypertension and cirrhosis), and pancreatitis.

Other effects of abuse of alcohol and tobacco are social (tends to keep away and be aggressive), psychological (sleep disturbances, anxiety, and memory problems), financial (tends to spend money on the substances and at times selling valuables), family (disturbed family life and may lead to divorce), career (difficulty in concentrating at work, aggressive behavior, and loss of job), and suicidal tendencies.

■ Steps in Counseling

- The patient and the counselor should be seated in a room away from distractions and interruptions. The family members should be counseled separately as frequent interruptions or "blame games" can derail the counseling process.
- The counselor should show interest in the patient and should encourage a two-way conversation, which should be motivational.
- After introductions of the counselor and others in the room, the patient should be asked about the amount of substance consumed and its effects.
- Find out the reasons for the use of substance. Ask whether the substance is used for the taste or effects and whether there are any stressors at home or at work.
- The patient may deny addiction/substance abuse. With empathy, the conversation should be continued with gentle emphasis on the effects of substance abuse.
- Once the initial information has been acquired, the counselor can proceed to inform the patient of the risks of use of substance. The possibility of cancer should be emphasized.
- The other effects on the body/organs should be explained.
- The implications on the family and at workplace should also be emphasized.
- The patient should be encouraged to interrupt if there are any doubts, and also to ask questions.

- At the end of the session, the patient should be asked whether they have understood the risks involved and if any repetition is required.
- The patient should be referred to a psychologist/psychiatrist for further counseling and to discuss the options for de-addiction.
- At the subsequent visit, reinforcement of the points should be done after checking on the changes the patient was able to make.
- Counseling of the family members/caretaker is also vital. Their patience and support, especially during relapses, is imperative in the de-addiction process

Points to Ponder
- Hospital visits can be stressful.
- Understanding of the disease and its course should be conveyed to the patient in an empathetic manner.
- Counseling should be done by a member of the team who has good communication skills.
- Counseling should be personalized to the patient with regard to the disease.
- Reinforcement of what has already been explained is necessary.
- Addictions like alcohol and tobacco use can lead to cancer.
- Early interventions are required to manage addictions.

Case-Based Question

1. **Mr. Kumar is undergoing a tympanoplasty in the right ear. What are the pertinent points he would have to state and sign in the informed written consent form?**

   Answer
   - I hereby give consent to Dr. ... to perform surgery on me.
   - I understand that it will be performed under general anesthesia.
   - The benefits of this procedure have been explained to me.
   - I have been informed of the risks and potential complications of this procedure.
   - I understand that unforeseen conditions may require additional treatment and procedures.
   - I certify that I have read this form and that all the possible risks and complications have been explained to me in the language I understand.

Frequently Asked Questions

1. What is informed consent?
2. What is the minimum age for giving consent?
3. What are the situations where consent is not required?
4. What are the different types of consent?
5. What is the importance of counseling in a hospital setting?
6. What do you understand by the term "Breaking Bad News"?
7. What are the pertinent steps in counseling a patient with tobacco addiction?
8. Counsel a 48-year-old man with early-stage cancer of the oral tongue.

Endnote

The history of counseling can be traced back to ancient times when tribes roamed the earth. They would come together in groups to find solace or comfort in their common problems. Medical counseling and the need to alleviate patient fears developed during the late 1890s under Sigmund Freud. Counseling of patients gathered momentum after the Second World War. In counseling, "empathy" is practiced as a sign of respect and regard the counselor holds for the patient. In that respect, it may be worth quoting Bill Bullard and his views on empathy.

"Opinion is really the lowest form of human knowledge. It requires no accountability, no understanding. The highest form of knowledge is empathy, for it requires us to suspend our egos and live in another's world. It requires profound purpose larger than the self-kind of understanding."

77 Microbiology and Pathology in Ear, Nose, and Throat

Kiran Chawla and Deepak Nayak M.

The competency covered in this chapter is as follows:

EN2.9 Choose correctly and interpret radiological, microbiological, and histological investigations relevant to ENT disorders.

Introduction

Microbiology and pathology form the foundation for investigations which can lead to diagnosis in ear, nose, and throat (ENT)-related diseases. Advances in techniques and use of special tests like immunohistochemistry have helped to increase the accuracy of clinical diagnosis.

Microbiology in ENT

Microbiology in Evaluation of Pharyngeal Pathologies

Sore throat and change in voice can occur due to pharyngitis, tonsillitis, and laryngitis.

■ Common Causative Organisms

Pharyngitis

- Viral causes: Influenza virus (A and B), Epstein Barr virus, herpes simplex viruses, adenoviruses, coronavirus.
- Bacterial causes: *Streptococcus pyogenes* (group A), *Corynebacterium diphtheriae*, *Arcanobacterium hemolyticum*, beta hemolytic streptococci other than group A (group C and group G).

Tonsillitis

- Viral causes: Adenovirus, measles virus, herpes simplex virus, coronavirus, parainfluenza virus.
- Bacterial causes: *S. pyogenes*, *Staphylococcus aureus* (**Fig. 77.1**), *C. diphtheriae* (**Fig. 77.2**).

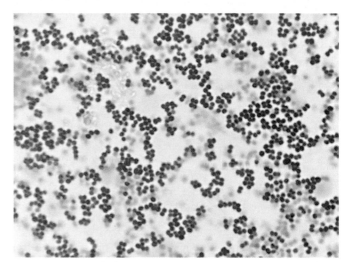

Fig. 77.1 *Staphylococcus aureus*: Gram-positive cocci in clusters.

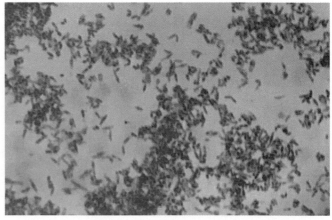

Fig. 77.2 *Corynebacterium diphtheriae*: Gram-positive, club-shaped bacilli with cuneiform arrangement.

Laryngitis

- Acute laryngitis is usually due to viral etiology.
- Epiglottitis is predominantly caused by *Hemophilus influenzae* (**Fig. 77.3**).

Samples Needed

Throat swab from the faucial area and posterior pharyngeal wall. Avoid touching tongue and uvula to prevent gag/cough reflex.

Things to Remember

- Confirmation of viral etiology is not needed in case of sore throat. Throat swabs are sent to lab mainly to confirm or rule out streptococcal sore throat. In the current scenario, though, such swabs are processed to rule out SARS-CoV-2.
- Direct swabbing of inflamed epiglottis is contraindicated because it may lead to laryngospasm and total airway obstruction.
- Use of sterile Dacryon swab is recommended. Cotton swabs are inhibitory for bacterial growth.
- Two swabs should be collected—one for microscopy and the other for culture.
- Collect the sample preferably before antibiotics are prescribed.
- In case of delay in transportation (>2 hours), use Amies' or Stuart's transport media.

Investigations

- Microscopy (Gram staining; Albert staining for *C. diphtheriae*) (**Fig. 77.4**).
- Culture and sensitivity.

Culture Media Used for Bacterial Causes

- Sheep blood agar (for all swabs).
- Crystal violet blood agar (if available).
- Loeffler's serum slope (if *C. diphtheriae* is suspected).
- Blood tellurite agar (if *C. diphtheriae* is suspected).

In case of isolation of *C. diphtheriae*, performance of toxigenicity test is important to label the isolate as pathogenic.

Point of care testing for streptococcal sore throat: Commercial kits (Alere) are available for direct antigen detection of *S. pyogenes* from throat swabs collected.

Microbiology in Evaluation of Ear Pathologies

- Otitis externa.
- Otitis media.

■ Common Causative Organisms

Otitis Externa

- *Pseudomonas aeruginosa* (swimmer's ear, malignant otitis externa).
- Otomycosis.

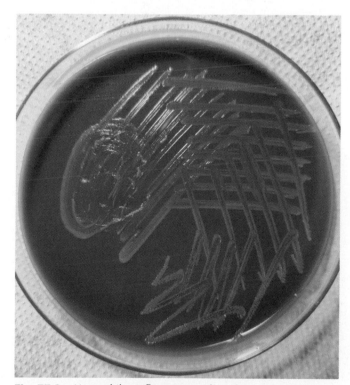

Fig. 77.3 *Hemophilus influenzae* on chocolate agar medium.

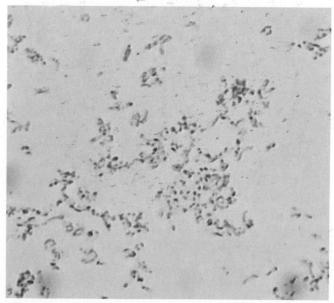

Fig. 77.4 *Corynebacterium diphtheriae*: Albert stain showing faint green bacilli with bluish-black metachromatic granules.

Otitis Media

- *Streptococcus pneumoniae*.
- *S. pyogenes*.
- *H. influenzae*.
- *S. aureus*.
- *Moraxella catarrhalis*.
- Enteric Gram-negative bacilli.
- Anaerobes.
- *Nocardia* spp.
- Fungal cause like *Aspergillus* spp.

Samples Required

- Ear swabs.
- Tympanocentesis (aspirate from middle ear infection).

Investigations Needed

- Microscopy.
- Bacteriological culture.
- Fungal culture.

Transportation

All swabs should reach the lab within 2 hours of collection.

Culture Media

- McConkey agar.
- Sheep blood agar (**Fig. 77.5**).
- Sabouraud's dextrose agar (for fungus).

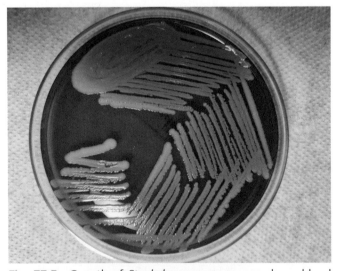

Fig. 77.5 Growth of *Staphylococcus aureus* on sheep blood agar. Golden yellow colonies with beta hemolysis.

Microbiology in Evaluation of Nasal Pathologies

- Sinusitis.
- Nasal carriers of methicillin resistant *Staphylococcus aureus* (MRSA) or *Neisseria meningitidis*.

■ Sinusitis

Sample Collected

Sinus aspirates. Nasal or nasopharyngeal swabs or sinus lavage fluid is *not* recommended.

Common Organisms Associated

- *S. pneumoniae*.
- *H. influenzae* other than group B.
- *M. catarrhalis*.
- *Neisseria* spp.
- Anaerobes.
- Aerobic streptococci.
- Occasionally Gram-negative bacilli or *S. aureus*.
- Fungal causes like Mucorales and *Aspergillus* spp.

Investigations Needed

- Microscopy.
- Aerobic, anaerobic, and fungal culture.

Sample Processing

Gram staining, culture on sheep blood agar, chocolate agar, Sabouraud's dextrose agar (suspected fungus), anaerobic culture.

■ Detection of Nasal MRSA (Methicillin Resistant *S. aureus*) Carriers

Sample Needed

Nasal swabs from vestibule of nose.

Processing of nasal swab: Culture on sheep blood agar or Mannitol salt agar.

■ Detection of Neisseria meningitidis Carriers

Sample collected: Nasopharyngeal swab (better yield) and throat swab.

Culture media required: Sheep blood agar and modified Thayer-Martin medium.

Microbiology in the Evaluation of Oral Cavity Pathologies

- Oral candidiasis.
- Vincent's angina.

■ Oral Candidiasis

- It is usually seen in bottle-fed infants and children, long-term use of steroid inhalers, and in debilitated adults.

Processing of Oral Swabs

- Microscopy.

Microscopy

- Gram staining shows Gram-positive oval budding yeast cells with presence of pseudohyphae or direct potassium hydroxide (KOH)mount can show the yeast cells under microscope.

■ Vincent's Angina

- It is associated with poor oral hygiene and other systemic diseases in adults.

Causative Pathogens

- *Borrelia vincenti* and *Fusobacterium* spp.

Investigation Needed

- Microscopy of oral swabs.
    - Gram staining shows presence of many pus cells with many Gram-negative spirochetes (*B. vincenti*) and fusiform bacilli (*Fusobacterium* spp.).

Pathology in ENT

Fine-Needle Aspiration Cytology

Fine-needle aspiration cytology (FNAC) is a technique whereby cells are obtained from a lesion using a thin bore needle and smears are made for microscopic diagnosis. The technique is based on the premise that the cells are loosely cohesive and can be aspirated easily.

■ Advantages

- Simple and minimally invasive, can be performed in an outpatient setting.
- Economical.
- Multiple sites can be sampled in the same sitting.

- High diagnostic accuracy.
- Allows rapid onsite evaluation (ROSE) of the material for adequacy.
- Ancillary tests such as bacterial culture, cytogenetics, immunophenoptying and polymerase chain reaction (PCR) can be performed using the same source material.

■ Equipments

- A 22- to 23-gauge needle.
- 20-mL syringe.
- Pistol handle.
- Sterile container.
- Glass slides: clean, dry, and free of grease.
- 0.4-mm coverslip for smearing pressure and even spread of the material.
- Fixatives (70–90% ethanol).
- Stains (Toluidine blue for ROSE) and Papanicolaou stain in laboratory.

■ Techniques

The test is performed using a radiologically guided source (for deep-seated and minute lesions) or nonguided method (for superficial and larger, more accessible lesions).

Aspiration Method

It is a popular method where negative pressure is exerted to aspirate material from the tissue of interest. This is used for lymph node and salivary gland lesions.

Nonaspiration Method

The capillary pressure in the needle bore is sufficient to aspirate the cells of interest. It is used in thyroid lesions where hemorrhage can obscure the cellular details (**Fig. 77.6**).
Causes of false-negative aspirate results:
- When the lesion has a cystic or a necrotic core, the needle can miss the solid representative areas and aspirate the nondiagnostic elements.
- Poor operating technique or inexperience.
- When the tissue is fibrotic, the cells may not be aspirated.

■ Stains Used in FNAC

- Papanicolaou stain: Used as a gold standard in most laboratories as it provides excellent nuclear detailing, especially in malignancies (**Fig. 77.7**). In a case of papillary carcinoma of thyroid, the pathognomic nuclear details such as nuclear grooves and pseudoinclusions are appreciated in Papanicolaou-stained smear. In a pleomorphic adenoma of salivary gland, the biphasic nature of the lesion is highlighted by the stain (**Fig. 77.8**).

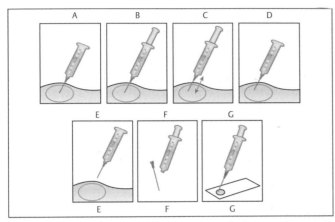

Fig. 77.6 Nonaspirated material is expelled on a glass slide and smears are prepared.

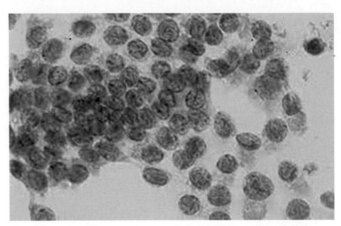

Fig. 77.7 Papillary carcinoma thyroid with nuclear details.

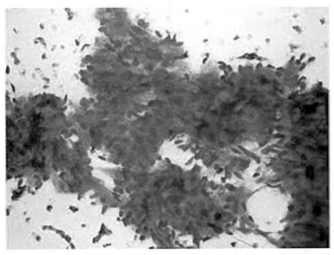

Fig. 77.8 Pleomorphic adenoma with cellular and stromal components.

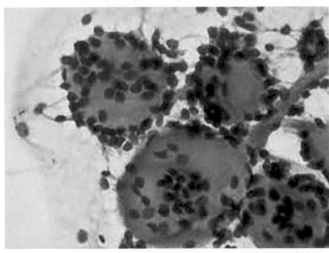

Fig. 77.9 Adenoid cystic carcinoma with pink matrix production.

The disadvantage is that Papanicolaou stain is expensive and many laboratories resort to cheaper stains.

- May-Grunwald Giemsa (MGG): It is used in case of an air-dried smears and is also inexpensive. Especially in matrix producing tumors, the material is highlighted by this stain. In adenoid cystic carcinoma of the salivary gland, the pink basement membrane-like is highlighted by MGG stain (**Fig. 77.9**).
- In nodal nonneoplastic lesions such as in tuberculosis, the granulomas which are noted on a Papanicolaou-stained smear can be confirmed using a Ziehl-Neelsen stain (**Fig. 77.10**).

Pearl

In case of mixed lesions (with solid and cystic areas), an ultrasound-guided FNAC can be done more specifically from the solid area which will improve the accuracy.

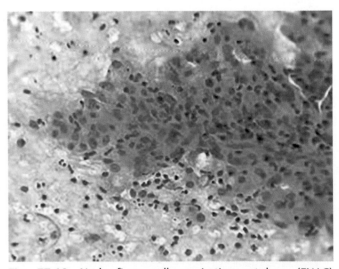

Fig. 77.10 Node fine-needle aspiration cytology (FNAC) showing a granulomatous lesion.

Stains Used in Head and Neck Lesions (Specimens) Analysis

◼ Hematoxylin and Eosin (H&E)

This is a near-universal stain used in tissue analysis. As its name suggests, H&E stain makes use of a combination of two dyes, namely, hematoxylin and eosin. This combination deferentially stains various tissue elements and make them easy for observation.

It is the primary diagnostic stain used in histopathology including application in the fine-needle aspiration biopsies and paraffin fixed embedded tissue.

Principle

The principle behind H&E stain is the chemical attraction between tissue and dye. Hematoxylin, a basic dye, imparts blue-purple contrast on basophilic structures, primarily those containing nucleic acid moieties such as chromatin, ribosomes, and cytoplasmic regions rich in RNA. An acidic eosin counter stains the basic elements such as RBCs, cytoplasm, muscle, and collagen in varying intensities of pink, orange, and red (**Fig. 77.11**).

◼ Special Stains Used in Histopathology

Periodic Acid Schiff

The Periodic Acid-Schiff (PAS) stain is a widely used technique in histopathology for the demonstration of carbohydrates and carbohydrate-rich compounds in tissues. PAS stain demonstrates polysaccharides, mucin, glycogen, certain glycoproteins and glycolipids, basement membrane, and certain fungus in tissues.

Principle

Glycol group of carbohydrates are oxidized by periodic acid to release dialdehydes. These dialdehydes on subsequent combination with Schiff's reagent results in the formation of magenta-colored complex, localized at the site of aldehyde formation.

Applications

- The hyphae and morphology of fungal elements such as in aspergillosis and mucormycosis are highlighted by PAS-positive reaction (**Figs. 77.12** and **77.13**).
- Cytoplasmic PAS-positive material in Ewing sarcoma and PAS-positive cells in acinic cell carcinoma of salivary gland.

Mucicarmine Stain

This stain is intended for staining mucin. Mucin is produced by a variety of epithelial cells and connective tissue cells.

Principle

- The principle of mucicarmine staining is based on the presence of aluminum that forms a chelating complex with carmine. This changes the charge of the carmine molecule to a positive charge, which allows it to bind to low-density acidic substrates such as mucins.

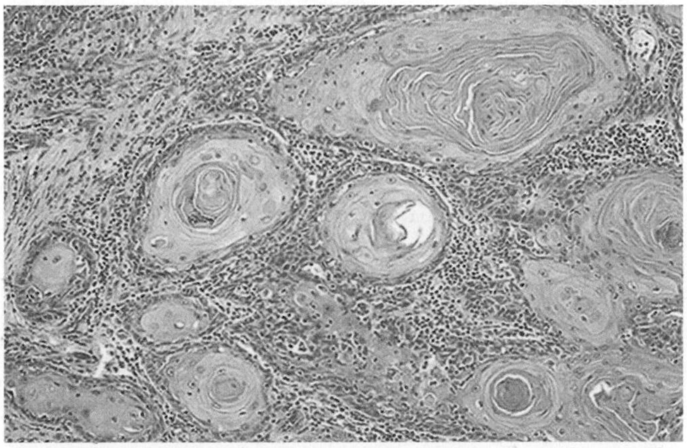

Fig. 77.11 Hematoxylin and eosin (H&E) stain demonstrates a differential staining of cellular components in a squamous cell carcinoma.

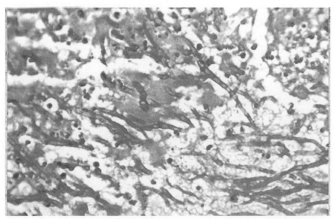

Fig. 77.12 Periodic Acid-Schiff (PAS) stain demonstrates acute angled septate branching in aspergillosis.

Applications

- Demonstration of mucin in mucous retention cyst and mucoepidermoid carcinoma (MEC) (**Fig. 77.14**).
- Demonstration of capsule in cryptococcosis (**Fig. 77.15**).

Grocott Methenamine Silver (GMS)

This is commonly used for the identification of fungi on cytosmears and tissue sections. It imparts a black color to the fungal profiles and a pale green color to the background. It stains all pathogenic and nonpathogenic fungi (**Fig. 77.16**).

Congo Red

The staining principle is based on the formation of hydrogen bridge bonds with the carbohydrate component of the substrate. Congo red is an anionic dye and is capable of depositing itself in amyloid fibrils, which then exhibit a conspicuous dichroism under polarized light. The tissue stained with Congo red appears orange-red under the transmitted-light microscope; under polarized light, however, the amyloid deposits show up as brilliant green, double-refraction images against a dark background. However, other structures also stained by Congo red, for example, collagen, are not visualized under polarized light (**Fig. 77.17**).

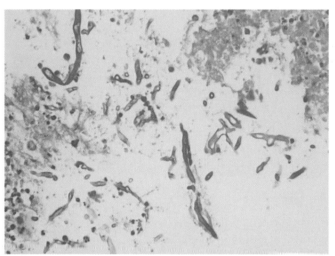

Fig. 77.13 Periodic Acid-Schiff (PAS) stain demonstrates broad aseptate hyphae in mucormycosis.

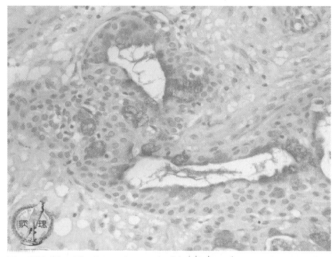

Fig. 77.14 Mucicarmine stain highlights the mucin-secreting cells in mucoepidermoid carcinoma (MEC).

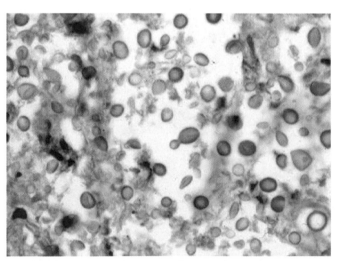

Fig. 77.15 Mucicarmine stains the capsule in cryptococcosis.

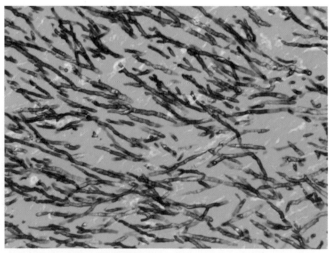

Fig. 77.16 Grocott methenamine silver (GMS) stains the fungal hyphae in aspergillosis.

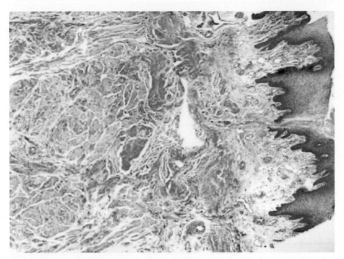

Fig. 77.17 Congo red stains the amyloid deposit in the subepithelial tissue of the buccal mucosa.

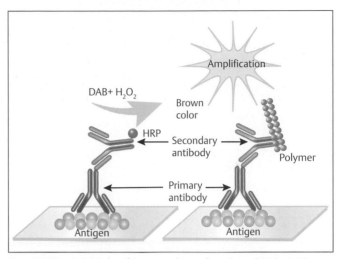

Fig. 77.18 Principle of immunohistochemistry (IHC): Antigen–antibody complexes demonstrated by a colored product.

Immunohistochemistry

- Immunohistochemistry (IHC) is an important ancillary method for pathologists as it specifically visualizes distribution and amount of a certain molecule in the tissue using a specific antigen–antibody reaction. The applications of IHC in head and neck lesions have gained momentum in the recent years, as more and more molecules involved in pathogenesis, diagnosis, and prognosis of the lesions are discovered. With the advent of therapeutic targets, this test has become indispensable in modern medicine and patient management.
- The unique feature that makes IHC stand out is that it is performed without destruction of histologic architecture, and thus the assessment of an expression pattern of the molecule is possible in the context of microenvironment.

■ Principle

IHC essentially detects antigens or haptens in cells of a tissue section by exploiting the principle of antibodies binding specifically to antigens in biological tissues. The antibody–antigen binding can be visualized using chromogens such as diaminobenzidine (DAB). The positivity of the colored product, its location, and intensity of staining are used as roadmaps for subtyping tumors (**Fig. 77.18**).

■ Steps in IHC Tests

1.	Fixation	10% neutral buffered formalin (NBF) for 24 h at room temperature
2.	Embedding and sectioning	Paraffin embedding: Mostly 4 μm Frozen sections: Between 4 and 6 μm in thickness
3.	Antigen (or epitope) retrieval	Heat-induced epitope retrieval (HIER) is most widely used
4.	Add primary antibody	Antibody dilution by protein-blocking solution or premixed Ab diluents Appropriate antibody selection and titration is done Incubation for 30–60 min at room temperature
5.	Add secondary antibody	Incubation for 30–60 min at room temperature
6.	Add substrate	250 μL of 1% diaminobenzidine (DAB), and 250 μL of 0.3% hydrogen peroxide to 5 mL of phosphate buffer saline (PBS), 1–3 min, room temperature
7.	Counterstain	Hematoxylin, 1 min

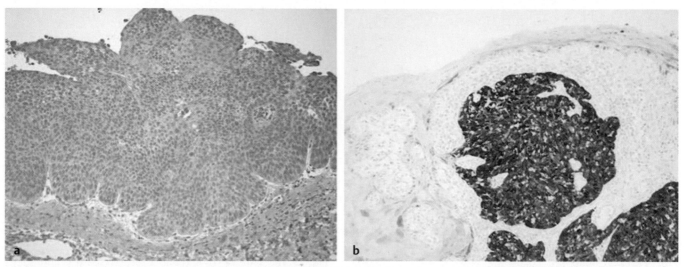

Fig. 77.19 Oropharyngeal squamous cell carcinoma **(a)** with p16 positivity on immunohistochemistry (IHC) analysis **(b)**.

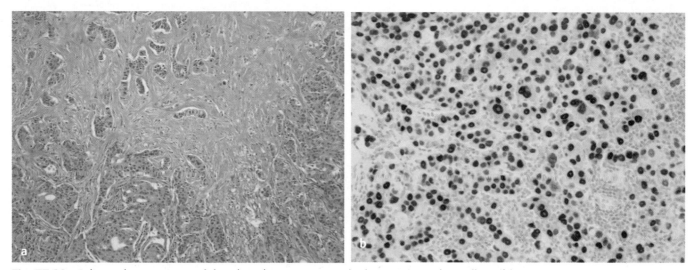

Fig. 77.20 Salivary duct carcinoma **(a)** with androgen receptor (AR) positivity in the nucleus **(b)**.

■ Applications

- p16 expression in oropharyngeal squamous cell carcinoma (**Fig. 77.19**). A strong and diffuse nuclear and cytoplasmic positivity in >70% tumor cells is considered as positive expression. It also is used as a substitute/surrogate marker for human papillomavirus (HPV)–associated lesions and portends a good prognosis.
- In salivary duct malignancies, IHC is useful in distinguishing morphologic mimickers. In adenocarcinomas of the major salivary gland, positive expression of IHC such as androgen receptor (AR) can differentiate it from other high-grade carcinomas (**Fig. 77.20**).

- In small, round, blue tumors of the nasal cavity, such as an olfactory neuroblastoma, the positive expression of neuroendocrine markers such as synaptophysin and negative expression of CD99 helps distinguish it from other malignancies such as Ewing sarcoma and lymphoblastic lymphomas (**Fig. 77.21**).
- In poorly differentiated malignancies, where the histomorphology is not certain in subtyping a neoplasm, IHC can help in improving precision of the diagnosis. For instance, in a metastatic carcinoma deposit in a cervical lymph node, nuclear p40 expression can unearth a squamous cell carcinoma (**Fig. 77.22**).

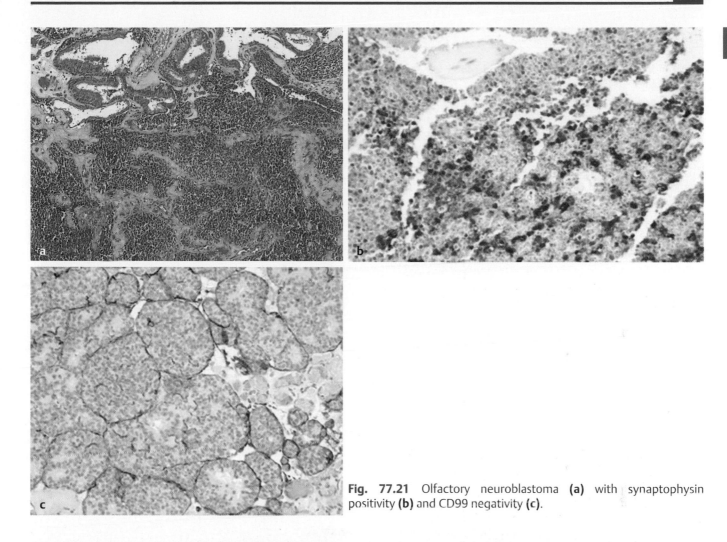

Fig. 77.21 Olfactory neuroblastoma **(a)** with synaptophysin positivity **(b)** and CD99 negativity **(c)**.

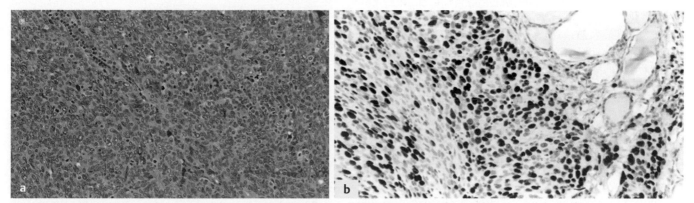

Fig. 77.22 Metastatic grade 3 squamous cell carcinoma in a node **(a)** with p40 positivity **(b)**.

Frozen Section

Intraoperative diagnosis is a major branch of modern patient care. It has evolved from being a niche skill set to an integral part of the patient management plan. The indications of an intraoperative diagnosis are manifold. But quintessentially it serves to provide a direct foundation for both the type and extent of surgery for appropriate management. Apart from diagnostic utility, there is an ever-increasing application of this technique in the field of research.

Although popularly referred to as intraoperative frozen section or simply as "frozen section," the technically accepted term is *cryosection*. The term "frozen" refers to a section of tissue that has been rapidly cooled using cryostat.

■ Principle

As the tissue of interest is frozen at temperatures of –20°C, the intracellular water crystallizes and hardens the tissue, making it firm enough for embedding and cutting for analysis.

■ Indications

- *Establish the presence of a lesion*: The surgeon may require a histologic corroboration when clinical and radiology profiling lead to more questions than answers.
- *Establish the nature of a lesion*: When the lesion has been identified but is not unequivocally identified as either benign or malignant, or even nonneoplastic, it necessitates a need for an intraoperative consultation.
- *Determine the presence of synchronous or co-incidental lesions*: During an intraoperative procedure, the identification of a separate lesion, hitherto not reported/recognized by the radiologist, may require additional probing.
- *Determine the adequacy of margins*: In the realm of modern-day oncosurgery, this aspect has been placed at the forefront of the indications for a frozen section. With an ever-expanding prevalence of conservative surgeries, the assessment of margin clearance has become a norm rather than an exception.
- *Determine the site of the lesion*: When the tissue plane is seen to overlap, especially with parathyroid lesions and thyroid lesions, the frozen section is beneficial to distinguish and identify the tissues, and by extension, the pathology.
- *Acquire fresh tissue for special studies*: The comprehensive cancer care mandates molecular analysis of the tissues for a "complete diagnosis." This aspect is more relevant in some malignancies over others. For instance, for breast and colon cancers, where the mRNA is the core material for ancillary studies (in-situ hybridization), the intraoperative frozen tissue section is the material

of choice. Same goes for additional tests, such as flow cytometry, culture, etc.
- *Demonstration of fat and enzymes (ATPase and NADPase in muscle biopsies).*
- *Nonenzyme histochemistry (carbohydrate, proteins).*
- *Demonstration of ganglion cells in Hirschsprung disease.*

■ Components

Preanalysis

- *Maintenance of the cold ischemia time during sample transport*: The sample should be deposited at the laboratory within 20 minutes, ideally. This aids to prevent tissue autolysis and unnecessary delays in report generation.
- *Prior intimation*: At least a 2-hour prior intimation is necessary.
- *Test request form*: Test request form should be duly filled with relevant clinical details, including notes on previous biopsy or cytology reports. Radiology profile is an additional useful data that may support a reasonable diagnosis. The margins for clearance should be mentioned with corresponding sutures and a labeled diagram, indicating the same.
- *Nature of sample submitted*: The tissue should be put directly into a suitable size, wide-mouthed container with labels (when necessary). Care should be exercised not to add fixative/saline/any liquid media into the container.

Analysis

Steps of the analysis are as follows:
- *Handling the specimen appropriately and gross examination*: In case of a composite resection specimen for oral cancers, orient the specimen appropriately and check that all tissues described are present.
- *Weight and dimensions of the sample*: This step is essential, especially with respect to cystic masses. The cyst fluid drained can be collected in a container for sediment analysis or cell block preparation, if necessary. Additionally, the nature of the cyst fluid is to be documented (serous, sero-sanguinous, or mucin).
- *Cytology preparations*: These techniques, apart from being simple, also provide extremely useful information to supplement the findings in a frozen section.
  The type of cytology preparation will vary with the type of tissue in question.
  - *Touch prep*: Suitable for lymph nodes and other very cellular tissues. This has the additional advantage of providing the surface details of the tissue such as architecture and borders.
  - *Scrape prep*: Suitable for firm or hard specimens. It is particularly useful in yielding cells in hard and poorly

cellular fibrotic tumors such as stromal tumors and sarcomas.

- *Crush preps*: Preparations can be made from tiny, soft specimens that are not amenable to scrape or can be manipulated for a touch prep. This method is particularly valuable in the interpretation of lesions of the brain and neural tumors, meningioma etc., where cytoplasmic processes and dyscohesive cells offer important clues.

- *Inking the specimen*: Traditionally, a single-color black ink is used to mark the resection margin, which is *less than or equal to 5 mm* from the advancing edge of the tumor. In cases where the margins may not have been tagged (e.g., salivary gland neoplasms), a circumferential inking is preferred with a specific reference in the report mentioning the distance of the nearest margin in millimeters.

- *Embedding of tissue for frozen section*: This step is performed using a microtome (**Figs. 77.23** and **77.24**). Hardening a tissue to a paraffin-like consistency allows effortless slicing of tissue in the desired micron range. In frozen section, the embedding step is substituted by simple process called "freezing." When exposed to a temperature of −20°C, the water in the tissue crystallizes. This renders the tissue to become firm and act as an embedding medium.

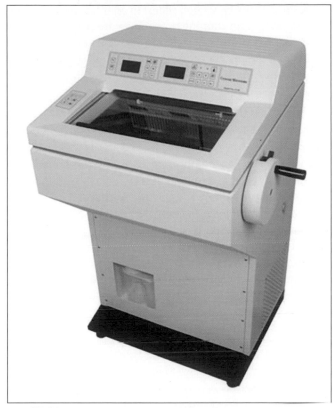

Fig. 77.23 Freezer microtome with stage.

Commercially available tissue freezing media (also referred to as embedding media) are composed of viscous aqueous solutions of polyvinyl alcohol and polyethylene glycol designed to both freeze and easily section at optimal cutting temperature (**Fig. 77.25**). These media adhere well to most tissues and provide a frame that adds stability to the section.

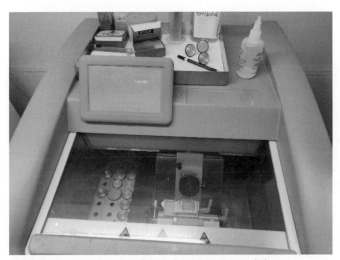

Fig. 77.24 Freezing media and sections on a slide.

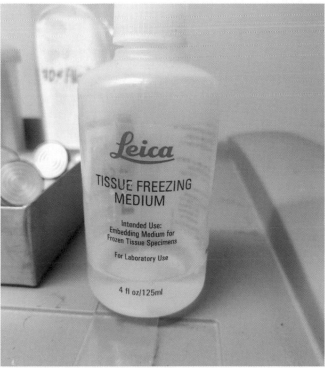

Fig. 77.25 Tissue freezing medium.

- *Staining of frozen section slides*: In an intraoperative consultation, rapid staining procedures are preferred due to the brevity of time. The stains most commonly used for intraoperative consultation are a rapid H&E stain and toluidine blue stain (**Figs. 77.26** and **77.27**).

■ Limitations

- *Poor sampling of tissue*: The tissue selected for analysis may not be representative.
- *Poor selection of appropriate tissue by the pathologist*: This may be due to inexperience, delays in the procedure, and potentially therapeutic mishaps.
- *Extensive tumor degeneration or necrosis*: The yield of diagnostic material is substantially reduced, leading to a lack of diagnosis.
- *Assessment of capsular or vascular invasion*: This is in context of follicular-patterned neoplasm of thyroid glands. This has a poor concordance with post paraffin fixed sections.

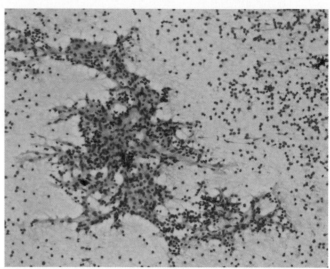

Fig. 77.26 Parathyroid adenoma (rapid hematoxylin and eosin [H&E], x200).

Points to Ponder

- Throat swabs are taken mainly for bacterial infection like *S. pyogenes*.
- Most viral infections do not need a swab test for confirmation.
- Swab should be taken prior to antibiotic use.
- Culture and sensitivity are important for persistent and recurrent infections like MRSA.
- FNAC is a minimally invasive procedure which can give a tissue diagnosis prior to further treatment.
- H&E is the commonest stain used.
- IHC is useful in differentiating certain malignancies, grading certain malignancies, and detecting HPV in oropharyngeal malignancy.
- Frozen section during surgery can help in determining the nature of the lesion and the possible further treatment.

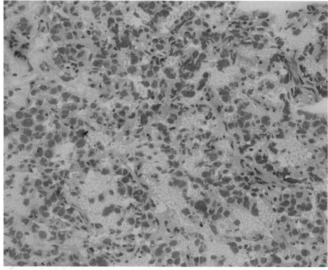

Fig. 77.27 Salivary gland tumor (rapid hematoxylin and eosin [H&E], x400).

Case-Based Questions

1. **A 14-year-old boy presented with history of fever, body ache, and sore throat of 2 days duration. On examination, there was generalized congestion of the oropharyngeal mucosa.**

   a. What test can be done?
   b. If the sore throat persists for more than 6 days and the boy has severe odynophagia with whitish spots on the tonsil and palpable, tender jugulodigastric lymph nodes, what test needs to be done?
   c. If a greyish-white membrane is seen on the tonsil and surrounding mucosa, which bleeds on attempt to remove, and the boy has toxic features with breathing difficulty and large jugulodigastric lymph nodes, what test needs to be done?

   Answers
   a. If a SARS-CoV-2 is suspected, a swab may be taken. Most viral infections are self-limiting, and a swab is not necessary. Only symptomatic treatment is required.
   b. Likely to be a bacterial infection. A throat swab is taken for Gram staining and for culture and sensitivity. For rapid antigen detection of *Streptococcal pyogenes*, kits like Alere are used.

c. Possibility of *Corynebacterium diphtheria* should be ruled out. A swab for Albert's stain is taken. Culture can be done, and toxigenicity test is important.

2. **A 47-year-old male presented with a solitary nodule of the right lobe of thyroid of 5 months duration.**

   a. What is the investigation test required for getting a possible tissue diagnosis?

   b. If the report comes as Bethesda III, that is, atypia/follicular cells of undetermined significance, what is to be done?

   c. If the report is follicular neoplasm of the thyroid, what needs to be done?

Answers

a. Fine-needle aspiration cytology by the nonaspiration technique, that is, without negative pressure.

b. As the patient is a male above the age of 45 years, there is a possibility of malignancy. Counsel the patient and proceed for a hemithyroidectomy with frozen section. If the frozen section comes as papillary carcinoma, a total thyroidectomy is done. If the frozen section is benign, no further treatment may be required.

c. In case of Bethesda IV, that is, follicular neoplasm, a hemithyroidectomy is done and the specimen is sent for histopathological examination. On frozen section a follicular adenoma cannot be differentiated from follicular carcinoma (i.e., detection of vascular and capsular invasion). The final histopathology will determine the further course of treatment.

Frequently Asked Questions

1. What is the organism commonly responsible for acute epiglottitis? What precautions should be taken when collecting a swab in such patients?

2. Describe the various transport media for bacteria.

3. What is FNAC?

4. Describe the technique of FNAC for a thyroid mass.

5. What are the stains that can be used for FNAC?

6. Describe some of the stains used in head and neck lesions.

7. What is frozen section? What are its limitations?

8. What is immunohistochemistry? Describe its application in head and neck tumors.

Endnote

Robert Koch (1843–1910) was a German physician and microbiologist. He was responsible for discovering the organisms behind deadly infectious diseases such as cholera, anthrax, and tuberculosis. He is regarded as the father of modern bacteriology. His contributions to microbiology include developing bacterial culture methods using agar kept in a petri dish and the application of oil immersion lens but he stands out for his Koch's postulates which describe the link between pathogen and disease. For his contribution to medicine, he was awarded the Nobel Prize in 1905.

78 National Programs in India Related to Ear, Nose, and Throat

Kirthinath Ballal and Afraz Jahan

The competency covered in this chapter is as follows:

EN2.15 Describe the national programs for prevention of deafness, cancer, and noise and environmental pollution.

Deafness

A person who is not able to hear as well as someone with normal hearing (normal hearing has hearing thresholds of 20 dB or better in both ears) is said to have hearing loss. Hearing loss may be conductive, sensorineural, or mixed, and the severity of deafness is classified as mild, moderate, severe, or profound. It can affect one ear or both ears and leads to difficulty in hearing conversational speech or loud sounds.

Hard of hearing refers to people with hearing loss ranging from mild to severe. People who are hard of hearing usually communicate through spoken language and can benefit from hearing aids, cochlear implants, and other assistive devices as well as captioning.

Deaf people mostly have profound hearing loss, which implies very little or no hearing. They often use sign language for communication. The other option is a cochlear implant.

Epidemiology

The World Health Organization (WHO) reports an estimated 360 million individuals worldwide suffer from disabling hearing loss, of which 91% are adults and 9% children. Hearing loss is the second most common cause of years lived with disability (YLD), accounting for 4.7% of the total YLD due to all causes.

The prevalence of deafness in Southeast Asia ranges from 4.6 to 8.8%. In India, 63 million people (6.3%) suffer from significant auditory loss. The National Sample Survey Organization (NSSO) in 1981 carried out the first country-wide comprehensive survey of physically disabled persons. The 58th round of NSSO reported 291 persons per 100,000 population suffered from severe to profound hearing loss.

Impact of Unaddressed Hearing Loss

- **At individual level:**
  - Communication and speech.
  - Cognition.
  - *Education and employment*: In developing countries, children with hearing loss and deafness often do not receive schooling. Adults with hearing loss also have a much higher unemployment rate.
  - Social isolation, loneliness, and stigma.
- **Impact on society and economy:**
  - WHO estimates that unaddressed hearing loss poses an annual global cost of US$ 980 billion. This includes health sector costs (excluding the cost of hearing devices), costs of educational support, loss of productivity, and societal costs. Of this, 57% is attributed to low- and middle-income countries.

> **Pearl**
>
> Damage to the cochlea sets in when the ear is exposed to sounds greater than 90 dB over a prolonged period. The threshold of discomfort is 110 dB. The threshold of pain is when the sound is above 130 dB. An example of sound above the threshold of pain is the sound of a jet engine, which is 140 dB.

Prevention

Many of the causes that lead to hearing loss can be avoided through public health strategies and clinical interventions implemented across the life course. Prevention of hearing loss is essential throughout the life course—from prenatal and perinatal periods to older age. In children, nearly 60% of hearing loss is due to avoidable causes that can be prevented through implementation of public health measures. Likewise, in adults, most common causes of hearing loss, such as exposure to loud sounds and ototoxic medicines, are preventable.

Effective strategies for reducing hearing loss at different stages of the life course include the following:
- Immunization.
- Good maternal and childcare practices.
- Genetic counselling.
- Identification and management of common ear diseases.
- Occupational hearing conservation programs for noise and chemical exposure.
- Safe listening strategies for the reduction of exposure to loud sounds in recreational settings.
- Rational use of medicines to prevent ototoxic hearing loss.

Identification and Management

- Early identification of hearing loss and ear diseases is key to effective management.
- This requires systematic screening for detection of hearing loss and related ear diseases in those who are most at risk. This includes the following:
  - Newborn babies and infants.
  - Preschool and school-age children.
  - People exposed to noise or chemicals at work.
  - People receiving ototoxic medicines.
  - Older adults.
- Hearing assessment and ear examination can be conducted in clinical and community settings. Tools such as the WHO "hearWHO" app and other technology-based solutions make it possible to screen for ear diseases and hearing loss with limited training and resources.
- Once hearing loss is identified, it is essential that it is addressed as early as possible and in an appropriate manner to mitigate any adverse impact.
- Measures available to rehabilitate people with hearing loss include the following:
  - The use of hearing technologies, such as hearing aids, cochlear implants, and middle ear implants.
  - The use of sign language and other means of sensory substitution, such as speech reading, use of print on palm or Tadoma, and signed communication.
  - Rehabilitative therapy to enhance perceptive skills and develop communication and linguistic abilities.
- The use of hearing assistive technology, and services such as frequency modulation and loop systems, alerting devices, telecommunication devices, captioning services, and sign language interpretation, can further

improve access to communication and education for people with hearing loss.

National Programme for Prevention and Control of Deafness

The Ministry of Health Family Welfare, Government of India, launched the National Programme for Prevention and Control of Deafness (NPPCD) on the pilot phase basis in the year 2006 to 2007 (January 2007) covering 25 districts. At present, the program is being implemented in 558 districts of 36 states and union territories.

◼ Objectives

- To prevent the avoidable hearing loss on account of disease or injury.
- Early identification, diagnosis, and treatment of ear problems responsible for hearing loss and deafness.
- To medically rehabilitate persons of all age groups, suffering from deafness.
- To strengthen the existing inter-sectoral linkages for continuity of the rehabilitation program, for persons with deafness.
- To develop institutional capacity for ear care services by providing support for equipment and material and training personnel.

◼ Strategies

- To strengthen the service delivery for ear care.
- To develop human resource for ear care services.
- To promote public awareness through appropriate and effective information education communication (IEC) strategies with special emphasis on prevention of deafness.
- To develop institutional capacity of the district hospitals, community health centers, and primary health centers selected under the program.

◼ Components of the Program

- *Manpower training and development*: For prevention, early identification, and management of hearing impaired and deafness cases, training would be provided from medical college–level specialists (ear, nose, and throat [ENT] and audiology) to grassroots-level workers.
- *Capacity building* for the district hospital, community health center (CHC), and primary health center (PHC) in respect of ENT/audiology infrastructure.
- *Service provision including rehabilitation*: Screening camps for early detection of hearing impairment and deafness, management of hearing- and speech-impaired cases, and rehabilitation (including provision of hearing aids), at different levels of health care delivery system.

- *Awareness generation through IEC activities* for early identification of hearing impairment, especially children, so that timely management of such cases is possible and to remove the stigma attached to deafness.
- Monitoring and evaluation.

Universal Newborn Hearing Screening

Newborns are categorized into "no-risk" and "high-risk" groups. All newborns are assessed by the otoacoustic emission (OAE) test:

- If a baby "passes" the OAE test, that is, the outer hair cell function is normal on OAE, no further intervention is required.
- If a baby "fails" the OAE test, reassessment by OAE is done at 4 to 6 weeks.

The two-stage OAE test reduces the false-positive rate. If a baby "passes" the test, no further intervention is required. If a baby "fails" the test, then brainstem evoked response audiometry (BERA) is done. The BERA is done at 3 to 6 months of age for all infants who had failed the OAE and infants who are in the high-risk group, that is, maternal infection (like cytomegalovirus, rubella, and toxoplasmosis), head injury, meningitis, and and those suffering from various syndromes like Alport syndrome, Treacher Collins syndrome, and Waardenburg syndrome.

In India, institution- and community-based infant screening programs have been implemented in some districts. The advantage is early detection and intervention including fitting of hearing aids and cochlear implantation. This is important for speech and language development.

Assistance to Disabled Persons Scheme for Cochlear Implantation

This is a Government of India scheme with the objective to assist the needy disabled persons in procuring durable, sophisticated and scientifically manufactured, modern, standard aids and appliances to promote physical, social, and psychological rehabilitation of *persons with disabilities* by reducing the effects of disabilities and at the same time enhance their economic potential. The Ministry of Social Justice and Empowerment will recognize an institute of national stature from each zone to recommend children eligible under the scheme for cochlear implant with a ceiling of Rs. 6 lakhs per unit to be borne by the government.

The ministry will identify suitable agencies for providing cochlear implant under the scheme. The scheme is meant for individuals whose family is below the poverty line. Based on the monthly income, the implant may be free (for persons whose income is below Rs. 15,000/-) or provided at 50% of the cost if the income ranges from Rs. 15,000 to 20,000. The profiling and sanctioning of the implant to the individual is done at the Ali Yavar Jung National Institute of Speech and Hearing Disabilities (Divyangjan), Mumbai.

Noise Pollution

Sound waves are vibrations of air molecules carried from a noise source to the ear. Sound is typically described in terms of the loudness (amplitude) and the pitch (frequency) of the wave. Loudness (also called sound pressure level or SPL) is measured in logarithmic units called decibels (dB). The normal human ear can detect sounds that range between 0 dB (hearing threshold) and about 140 dB, with sounds between 120 and 140 dB causing pain (pain threshold).

Any sound that is undesired or interferes with one's hearing of something is considered as noise. Any unwanted or disturbing sound that affects the health and well-being of humans and other organisms is considered noise pollution.

■ WHO Noise Quality Guidelines

WHO has guidelines for community noise in specific environments (**Table 78.1**).

■ Causes

Environmental Causes

The common causes are lightning, thunderstorm, cyclones, tornadoes, earthquakes, and volcanic eruptions.

Man-Made Causes

These are vehicular noise, industrial noise, construction activities, noise related to public events, fireworks, etc. Ships, oil drills, sonar devices, seismic tests, and naval sonar devices give rise to loud underwater noise.

■ Effects of Noise Pollution

Noise pollution can cause health problems for people and wildlife, both on land and in the sea.

Effect on Human Life

Noise pollution impacts millions of people on a daily basis. *Auditory effects* include tinnitus, auditory fatigue, deafness, and noise-induced hearing loss (NIHL). *Nonauditory effects* include high blood pressure, heart disease, sleep disturbances, and stress. These health problems can affect all age groups, including children. Many children who live near noisy airports or streets have been found to suffer from stress and other problems, such as memory impairments, and poor attention level and reading skill.

Table 78.1 Guideline values for community noise in specific environments

Specific environment	Critical health effect(s)	L_{Aeq} (dB(A))	Time base (h)	L_{Amax} fast (dB)
Outdoor living area	Serious annoyance, daytime and evening	55	16	–
	Moderate annoyance, daytime and evening	50	16	
Dwelling, indoors	Speech intelligibility and moderate annoyance, daytime and evening	35	16	45
Inside bedrooms	Sleep disturbance, nighttime	30	8	
Outside bedrooms	Sleep disturbance, window open (outdoor values)	45	8	60
School classrooms and preschools, indoors	Speech intelligibility, disturbance of information extraction, and message communication	35	During class	–
School, playground outdoor	Annoyance (external source)	55	During play	–
Hospital, ward rooms, indoors	Sleep disturbance, nighttime	30	8	40
	Sleep disturbance, daytime and evenings	30	16	–
Hospitals, treatment rooms, indoors	Interference with rest and recovery	#1		
Industrial, commercial shopping, and traffic areas, indoors and outdoors	Hearing impairment	70	24	110
Ceremonies, festivals, and entertainment events	Hearing impairment (patrons: <5 times/y)	100	4	110
Public address, indoors and outdoors	Hearing impairment	85	1	110
Music and other sounds through headphones/earphones	Hearing impairment (free-field value)	85 #4	1	110
Impulse sounds from toys, fireworks and firearms	Hearing impairment (adults)	–	–	140 #2
	Hearing impairment (children)	–	–	120 #2
Outdoors in parkland and conservation areas	Disruption of tranquility	#3		

Note: #1: As low as possible.
#2: Peak sound pressure (not LAF, max) measured 100 mm from the ear.
#3: Existing quiet outdoor areas should be preserved and the ratio of intruding noise to natural background sound should be kept low.
#4: Under headphones, adapted to free-field values.

Environmental Effects

Animals use sound to navigate, find food, attract mates, and avoid predators. Noise pollution affects their ability to survive by interfering with these tasks. Marine mammals such as whales and dolphins rely on echolocation to communicate, navigate, feed, and find mates, and excess noise interferes with their ability to effectively echolocate.

Prevention and Control

The Central Pollution Control Board advises the central government on any matter concerning the prevention, control, and abatement of noise pollution, and provide technical assistance and guidance to the State Pollution Control Board (SPCB). The SPCB inspects noise pollution areas, assesses quality of noise, and takes steps for the prevention, control, and abatement of noise pollution in such areas.

For regulation of noise pollution, the *Noise Pollution (Regulation and Control) Rules, 2000* was promulgated under the Environment (Protection) Act, 1986 (**Table 78.2**). The rules lay restrictions on the use of loudspeakers/public address system and sound-producing instruments and on the use of horns, sound-emitting construction equipment, and bursting of firecrackers.

■ Consequences of Any Violation in Silence Zone/Area

Whoever, in any place covered under the silence zone/area, commits any of the following offence shall be liable for penalty under the provisions of the act:
• Whoever plays any music or uses any sound amplifiers.

Table 78.2 Ambient air-quality standards in respect of noise as per the Noise Pollution (Regulation and Control) Rules, 2000

Ambient air quality standards in respect of noise			
Area code	Category of area/zone	Limits in dB(A) Leq[a]	
(A)	Industrial area	75	70
(B)	Commercial area	65	55
(C)	Residential area	55	45
(D)	Silence zone	50	40

[a]dB (A)Leq denotes the time-weighted average of the level of sound in decibels on scale A, which is relatable to human hearing.

- Whoever beats a drum or tom-tom or blows a horn either musical or pressure, or trumpet or beats or sounds any instrument.
- Whoever exhibits any mimetic, musical, or other performances of a nature to attract crowds.
- Whoever bursts sound emitting firecrackers.
- Whoever uses a loudspeaker or a public address system.

Noise Management

To avoid noise pollution, measures must be taken to manage indoor noise levels with policies and legislation and ensure the enforcement of regulatory standards.
- Monitoring human exposures to noise.
- Mitigation of noise emissions and noise source emissions.
- Consider the noise consequences when planning transport systems and land use.
- Introduce surveillance systems for noise-related adverse health effects.
- Assess the effectiveness of noise policies in reducing adverse health effects and exposure, and in improving supportive "soundscapes."
- Adopt precautionary actions for a sustainable development of the acoustical environments.

Cancer

■ Epidemiology

According to the WHO Global Cancer Observatory 2020, the most common cancers globally in decreasing order were breast cancer, followed by lung cancer, prostate cancer, colon cancer, and stomach cancer.

The National Cancer Registry Programme under the Indian council of Medical Research (ICMR) gives information on the incidence, mortality, and distribution of cancer in India. As per the Global Cancer Consortium, India, the 5-year prevalence of cancer was 2,720,251, the number of new cases was 1,324,413, and the number of deaths was 851,678.

In India, the five most common cancers among men were the following:
- Cancer of the lip and oral cavity.
- Lung.
- Stomach.
- Colorectum.
- Esophagus.

The most common cancers among women were the following:
- Cancer of the breast.
- Cervix.
- Uterus.
- Ovary.
- Lip and oral cavity.
- Colorectum.

■ Causes

- Environmental factors:
  - Tobacco (smoking and chewing).
  - Betel nut chewing.
  - Alcohol.
  - Dietary factors: Smoked fish, food additives, and contaminants.
  - Occupational exposures to benzene, arsenic, asbestos, etc.
  - *Viruses*: Hepatitis B and C—hepatocellular carcinoma and HPV—cervical cancer.
- *Genetic factors*: They are nonmodifiable and difficult to identify, for example, retinoblastoma and leukemia.

■ Prevention and Control

Primary Prevention

With growing knowledge on the causative factors for cancers, measures to prevent it can be applied at a large scale:
- Regulation on the use of tobacco and alcohol.
- Use of personal protective equipment to reduce occupational exposure to carcinogens.
- Legislations and measures to address environmental causes such as radiation and environmental pollution.
- Improvement in personal hygiene.
- Testing of food, drugs, and cosmetics for carcinogens.

- Cancer education to the general public especially high-risk groups to motivate them to seek early diagnosis and treatment.

Secondary Prevention

- Early detection of cases through cancer screening. Screening programs can be of two types:
  - *Mass screening*: This is screening of large number of people for the presence of precancerous lesions. It may be a comprehensive cancer detection examination where one or more body sites are examined or single site screening, for example, screening for cervical cancer among a large group of women.
  - *Selective screening*: This is screening of a high-risk group more prone to the risk of cancer, for example, screening for cervical cancer among parous women of lower socioeconomic group of ≥35 years of age.
- *Treatment*: Modalities available include surgical removal, radiation, and chemotherapy.

Tertiary Prevention

It is palliative care and management of cancer pain.

■ National Program

The National Cancer Control Programme was launched in 1975–1976. In view of the magnitude of the problem and gaps in the availability of cancer treatment facilities across the country, the program was revised in 1984–1985 and subsequently in December 2004. During 2010, the program was integrated with the National Programme for Prevention and Control of Cancer, Diabetes, Cardiovascular Diseases and Stroke (NPCDCS).

Objectives

- *Primary prevention* of cancers by health education.
- *Secondary prevention*, that is, early detection and diagnosis of common cancer such as cancer of the cervix, mouth, breast, and tobacco-related cancer by screening/self-examination method.
- *Tertiary prevention*, that is, strengthening of the existing institutions of comprehensive therapy including palliative care.

Schemes under the Revised Program

- *Regional Cancer Center Scheme*: Strengthening the existing regional cancer centers to act as referral centers for complicated and difficult cases at the tertiary level.

- *Oncology Wing Development Scheme*: To reduce the geographic gaps in the availability of cancer treatment facilities in the country, central assistance is provided for purchase of equipment for management of cancer. Assistance of Rs. 3 crore per institution is provided under the scheme.
- *Decentralized nongovernmental organization (NGO) scheme*: The scheme is operated by the nodal agencies and the NGOs and are given financial assistance for undertaking health education, IEC, and early detection of cancer activities.
- *IEC activities at the central level*: IEC activities to publicize the anti-tobacco legislation and discourage the consumption of cigarettes and other tobacco-related products. Create awareness about the ill effects of consumption of tobacco and tobacco-related products.
- *Research and training*: Training programs, monitoring, and research activities are organized at the central level.

Cancer Services under the NPCDCS

- Common diagnostic services, basic surgery, chemotherapy, and palliative care for cancer cases are being made available at 100 district hospitals.
- Each district is being supported with Rs. 1.66 crore per annum for the following:
  - Chemotherapy drugs are provided for 100 patients at each district hospital.
  - Day care chemotherapy facilities is being established at 100 district hospitals.
  - Facility for laboratory investigations including mammography is being provided at 100 district hospitals. If not available, this can be outsourced at government rates.
- Home-based palliative care is being provided for chronic, debilitating, and progressive cancer patients at 100 districts.
- Support is being provided for contractual manpower through a medical oncologist, one cytopathologist, one cytopathology technician, and two nurses for day care.
- State cancer institutes (SCIs) will provide comprehensive cancer diagnosis, treatment, and care services. SCIs will be the apex institution in the state for cancer treatment activities.
- A total of 45 centers were to be strengthened as tertiary cancer centers (TCCs) to provide comprehensive cancer care services at a cost of Rs. 6 crore each, during 2011–2012.

Points to Ponder

- In children, 60% of hearing loss is due to avoidable causes.
- One of the objectives of the NPPCD is early identification, diagnosis, and treatment of ear problems responsible for hearing loss and deafness.
- In the universal newborn screening program, infants are categorized into "pass or fail" after administering the OAE.
- The assistance to disabled persons (ADIP) scheme is available for the purchase of cochlear implants for families with an income of less than Rs. 15,000 per month.
- Any sound that is undesired or interferes with hearing is considered as "noise."
- Causes of noise pollution can be divided into environmental causes and man-made causes.
- National Cancer Registry Programme under the ICMR gives information on the incidence, mortality, and distribution of cancer in India.
- The commonest cancer among men is cancer of the lip and oral cavity.
- The commonest cancer among women is cancer of the breast.

Case-Based Questions

1. **A mother brings a 1-month-old infant to the hospital because she was referred for hearing assessment for the infant. History revealed that the infant had failed the OAE immediately after birth.**

   a. What is OAE?
   b. When is the first one administered?
   c. If the first OAE is failed, then what is the next step?

   Answers
   a. The OAE test is part of a newborn hearing screening program. It is an objective test.
   b. The first one is administered before the baby is discharged from the hospital after birth. It can be performed as early as the first day after birth.
   c. If the baby fails the first OAE test, then the mother and infant are asked to come to the hospital for a repeat OAE 1 month later. If this is also "fail," then a BERA is performed.

2. **A 2-week-old neonate with a history of premature birth had developed meningitis. The neonate was treated for the same and had recovered. The parents are below the poverty line with an income of Rs. 14,000.**

   a. What is the program for hearing assessment in this age group?
   b. If found to have a possible hearing loss, how can it be confirmed?
   c. If the child has profound hearing loss, how can the rehabilitation be done?
   d. What is the scheme the family can avail for the treatment?

   Answers
   a. Universal newborn screening program.
   b. BERA.
   c. Cochlear implant
   d. The ADIP scheme

Frequently Asked Questions

1. Which board advises the Indian government on noise pollution?
2. What are the objectives of the NPPCD?
3. What are the methods of prevention and control of cancer?
4. What are the objectives of the National Cancer Control Programme?
5. What are the schemes under the National Cancer Control Programme?
6. What are the problems with untreated hearing loss?
7. What is the universal newborn screening program?

Endnote

Noise pollution can cause sleep disturbance. This can affect health in the short term in the form of sleepiness and tiredness the next day or it can have long-term consequences, affecting mental health and cardiovascular disease. In Europe, 20% of the population are exposed to high noise levels that can affect their health. According to WHO, the average noise exposure at night, during sleep, should not exceed 40 dB. If a person is exposed to higher levels over a year, it can impact their health in the form of insomnia, high blood pressure, and even cardiac arrests. Forty decibels is equivalent to the sound in a quiet street in a residential neighborhood.

79 Radiology in ENT

Ajay Bhandarkar

The competencies covered in this chapter are as follows:

EN2.9 Choose correctly and interpret radiological investigations relevant to ENT disorders.

PE28.17 Interpret X-ray of the paranasal sinuses and mastoid, and/or use written report in case of management. Interpret chest X-ray in foreign body aspiration and lower respiratory tract infection; understand the significance of thymic shadow in pediatric chest X-rays.

Introduction

Radiology forms an important investigative modality in diagnosis of disorders in otorhinolaryngology. A wide range of radiological investigations are used to detect pathologies in otorhinolaryngology and head and neck surgery. The objective of this chapter is to familiarize the student with certain basic principles of ENT radiology, role of various radiological investigations, and the differential diagnosis of various findings in common conditions in ENT. Adequate description will be given for plain and contrast radiographs in order to understand the anatomy which forms an important section of undergraduate curriculum.

The reading of any radiological investigation involves four components:
- Plain or contrast.
- The part and the view on the film.
- Identification of normal structures.
- Identification of possible pathology and extent.

Based on the findings, a diagnosis or a differential diagnosis can be made.

Paranasal Sinuses

The following views are used for pathologies of the paranasal sinuses:
- Waters' view or occipitomental view.
- Modified Waters' view or Pier's view.
- Caldwell's view or occipitofrontal view.
- Lateral view.
- Submentovertical view or basal view.
- Optic canal view or Rhese view.

Waters' view or occipitomental view, modified Waters' view or Pier's view, and Caldwell's view or occipitofrontal view are commonly used in the current era. The other three views are seldom used.

Pier's view (modified Waters' view): This view is obtained with the mouth open. It helps in the visualization of the sphenoid sinus (**Fig. 79.1**).

Waters' view (inclined posteroanterior view or nose–chin position): This view depicts the best visualization of the sinuses in the following order: Maxillary sinus > ethmoid sinus > frontal sinus > sphenoid sinus. These structures are visualized in **Fig. 79.2**.

Caldwell's view (occipitofrontal view): This view depicts the best visualization of the sinuses in the following order: Frontal sinus > ethmoid sinus > maxillary sinus > sphenoid sinus. Maxillary sinus view is obscured by the overlap of the petrous temporal bone. Hence, it is not used to visualize the maxillary sinus pathologies.

Lateral view: It helps to visualize the pterygopalatine fossa and nasopharynx.

Submentovertical view: This view helps to depict the visualization of the sinuses in the following order: Sphenoid sinus > posterior ethmoid sinus > maxillary sinus. It also shows the zygoma and mandible.

Optic canal view (Rhese view): It helps in visualization of optic canal.

■ Pathologies of Paranasal Sinuses

Note: Always compare opacity within the sinuses to that of the orbit to determine whether it is normal. If the

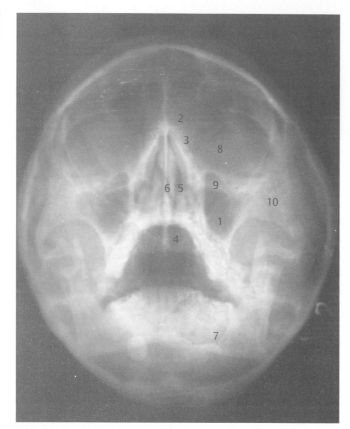

Fig. 79.1 Structures visualized in Pier's view of paranasal sinuses (normal): 1 to 10. 1, maxillary sinus; 2, frontal sinus; 3; ethmoid sinus; 4, sphenoid sinus; 5, nasal cavity; 6, nasal septum; 7, mandible; 8, orbit; 9, infraorbital foramen; 10, zygoma.

radiograph has a technical issue (over-exposure), it may depict a wrong interpretation of the radiograph.

Six important imaging findings in paranasal sinuses may be noted on radiography:

- Opacity with concavity upwards: It indicates air-fluid level or fluid within the sinus (blood, pus, or cerebrospinal fluid [CSF]). Blood (haemantrum) and pus are common in the maxillary sinus whereas CSF is rarely seen in the sinuses unless there is a breach in the skull base. This is commonly seen in the sphenoid sinus. Differential diagnoses are acute sinusitis, hemosinus, and CSF rhinorrhea (**Figs. 79.2** and **79.3**).
- Opacity with convexity upward (dome-shaped opacity): This indicates a cyst, polyp, or mucocele. Early stages of malignancy may sometimes be masqueraded by the former (**Fig. 79.4**).
- Diffuse opacity along the margins of the sinuses: This indicates a mucosal thickening along the sinus walls (**Fig. 79.5**).
- Erosion of bony confines of the paranasal sinuses: Differential diagnoses for erosion of bone include a granulomatous disease, invasive fungal infection, and malignancy. Loss of scalloping of frontal sinus margins

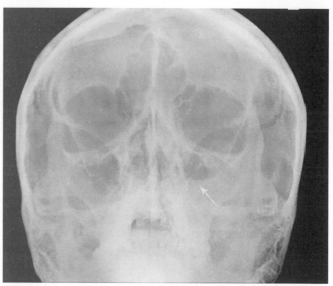

Fig. 79.2 Waters' view of paranasal sinuses showing concavity in the left maxillary sinus (air–fluid level).

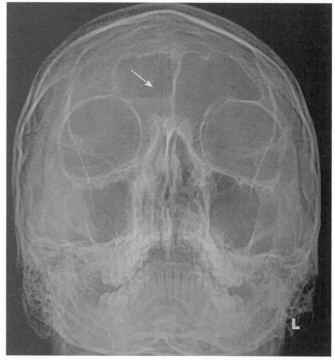

Fig. 79.3 Waters' view of paranasal sinuses showing concavity in the right frontal sinus (air–fluid level).

with opacity within the frontal sinus may indicate a mucocele in the frontal sinus. Complete opacification of the sinuses with intact bony margins indicates a differential diagnosis of polyp, mucocele, or cyst (**Fig. 79.6**).

- Opacity in the sinus with hyperattenuation: This indicates allergic fungal rhinosinusitis.
- Tear drop sign: Localized prolapse of orbital contents through the floor of the orbit (blow-out fracture) may be visualized in the maxillary sinus.

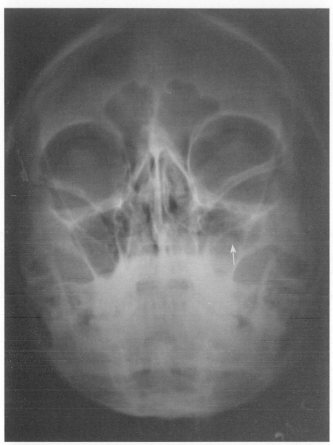

Fig. 79.4 Waters' view of paranasal sinus showing convexity (dome-shaped opacity) in left maxillary sinus. Sign of a maxillary polyp.

Nasal bone: Lateral views of both sides are used for nasal bone injuries. Displaced/undisplaced fracture lines can be visualized on radiography. The other view is the superior–inferior (sky) view. It is important for documentation and medicolegal purposes.

> **Pearl**
>
> Differential diagnosis of unilateral opacity of the maxillary sinus include:
>
> Acute sinusitis, fungal ball (mycetoma), haemantrum, early malignancy, and benign tumors.

Temporal Bone/Mastoid

The following views are used to diagnose pathologies of the temporal bone:
- Law's view.
- Schuller's view.
- Stenver's view.
- Towne's view.
- Owen's view.

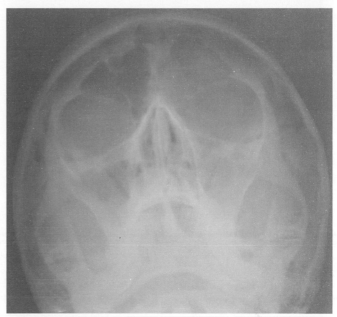

Fig. 79.5 Waters' view of paranasal sinus showing mucosal thickening in the walls of left maxillary sinus.

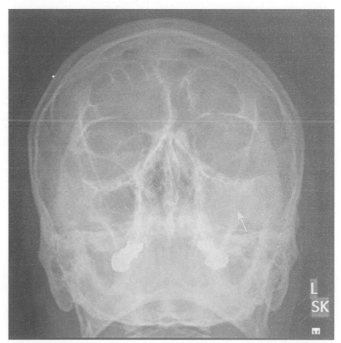

Fig. 79.6 Waters' view of paranasal sinus showing unilateral left maxillary sinus opacity.

- Transorbital view.
- Basal view.

Law's view, Schuller's view, and Stenver's view are commonly used in the current era. The other three views are seldom used due to the advent of high-resolution computed tomography (CT) imaging. Law's view, Schuller's view (**Fig. 79.7**), Owen's view, and Towne's view provide visualization of the middle ear and mastoid. Stenver's view,

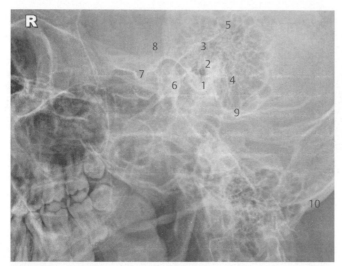

Fig. 79.7 Structures visualized on Schuller's view of left mastoid (normal). 1, External auditory canal; 2, mastoid antrum; 3, dural plate; 4, sinus plate; 5, sinodural angle; 6, temporomandibular joint; 7, zygoma; 8, squamous temporal bone; 9, mastoid air cells; 10, occipital bone.

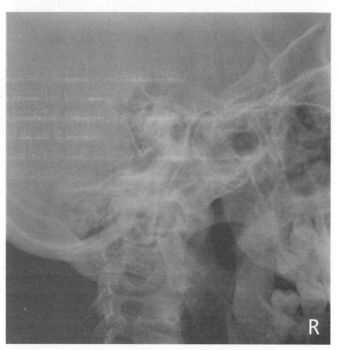

Fig. 79.8 Schuller's view of right mastoid showing diploeic pneumatization.

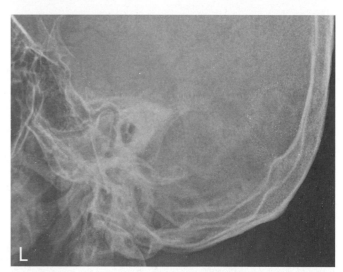

Fig. 79.9 Schuller's view of left mastoid showing secondary sclerosis.

transorbital view, and basal view provide visualization of the petrous temporal bone by conventional use. Stenver's view is used for confirming the proper placement of cochlear implant post implantation surgery.

Law's view and Schuller's view should give us the following normal anatomical details of the mastoid and middle ear as shown in **Fig. 79.7**:

- Temporomandibular joint—first landmark noted.
- External auditory canal—posterior to the temporomandibular joint.
- Degree of pneumatization of mastoid: Whether pneumatized, diploeic, or sclerosed. If sclerosed, whether it is primary or secondary sclerosis (**Figs. 79.8** and **79.9**). In primary sclerosis, the dural plate lies low, the sinus plate is more anterior, and the sinodural angle is more acute.
- Location of the dural plate.
- Location of the sinus plate.
- Sinodural angle.
- Zygoma.
- Occipital bone.

X-ray is taken of both sides for comparison.

Law's view: Conventionally known as lateral oblique view (15 degrees X-ray beam angulation to horizontal). Aditus, antrum, and attic are not visualized clearly in this view, which may be seen better in Schuller's view.

Schuller's view: Conventionally known as lateral oblique view (30 degrees X-ray beam angulation to horizontal). Although similar to the Law's view except for the angulation, it helps visualize the aditus, antrum, and attic. The lateral oblique view avoids superimposition of one mastoid over the other.

Stenver's view: The petrous temporal bone long axis is parallel to the X-ray film. Structures visualized are the inner ear, internal auditory meatus, petrous temporal bone, and arcuate eminence.

Towne's view: By convention it is an anteroposterior view with a 30 degrees craniofrontal tilt. Structures visualized are the superior semicircular canal and arcuate eminence, internal auditory meatus, cochlea, mastoid, tympanic cavity, and external auditory canal. It was clinically used in diagnosis of acoustic neuroma and petrous pathologies before the advent of CT imaging.

Owen's view, transorbital view, and basal view are rarely used.

■ Pathologies of Temporal Bone

Note: It is best to identify the temporomandibular joint and external auditory canal relation before proceeding to identify the various structures and pathologies.

The following pathologies may be noted in the plain radiograph:

- Cavity in the mastoid (**Fig. 79.10**): The differential diagnoses for a cavity in the mastoid are cholesteatoma, post mastoidectomy surgery, large mastoid antrum, malignancy, eosinophilic granuloma, gunshot injury, and multiple myeloma. The following will help to differentiate a post mastoidectomy cavity from a cholesteatoma cavity:
  - Cavity wall: Smooth in cholesteatoma whereas irregular in post mastoidectomy.
  - Location: Cholesteatoma cavity is commonly localized to epitympanum and mastoid antrum.
  - Soft tissue in cavity (cotton-wool appearance), with surrounding peripheral zone of sclerosis with an intervening translucent area, is seen in cholesteatoma whereas it is not present in post mastoidectomy.
- Haziness/cloudiness in mastoid is seen in acute mastoiditis.
- Secondary sclerosis of mastoid: This is commonly seen in chronic otitis media due to chronic inflammation of the middle ear cleft. It has to be differentiated from primary sclerosis, which occurs due to impaired development of mastoid. The sinodural angle is extremely acute, the dural plate is extremely low lying, and the sinus plate appears to be merged with the posterior wall of the external auditory canal (more anterior) in primary sclerosis.
- Erosion of bone: It is seen in cholesteatoma, granulomatous diseases, and malignancy.

Pharynx, Larynx and Neck, Nasal Bones

The following views are used to visualize the pharynx and larynx and neck:

- Lateral view.
- Anteroposterior view.

Lateral view: It is used to visualize the nasopharynx, supraglottic region, glottis region, subglottic region and trachea, hypopharynx, and the bony and cartilaginous architecture of the following structures: Epiglottis, thyroid cartilage, cricoid cartilage, trachea, hyoid bone, and cervical spine. It is also used to detect fractures of the nasal bones (**Fig. 79.11**).

Anteroposterior view: It is used to visualize the airway and the tracheal displacement.

> ### Pearl
>
> Both the lateral and anteroposterior views are mandatory in a suspected history of foreign body of the pharynx and larynx in order to diagnose the anatomical site of the foreign body (airway or digestive tract).

The conditions which can be diagnosed by plain radiograph are:

- Adenoid enlargement and antrochoanal polyp (soft tissue causing nasopharyngeal airway narrowing) in

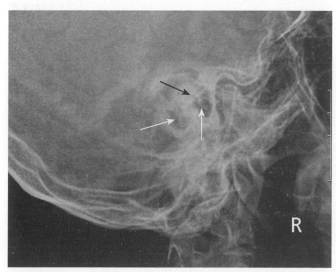

Fig. 79.10 Schuller's view of right mastoid showing cavity within the mastoid (*yellow arrow*). Presence of opacity within the cavity (cholesteatoma—cotton wool appearance) is noted (*red arrow*).

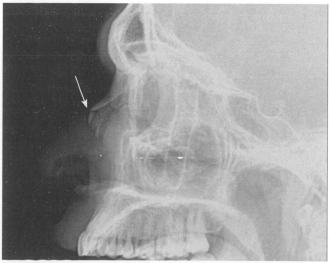

Fig. 79.11 Plain radiograph: Lateral view of the left nasal bone demonstrating a displaced left nasal bone fracture (*white arrow*).

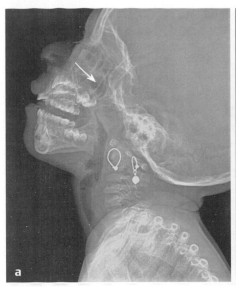
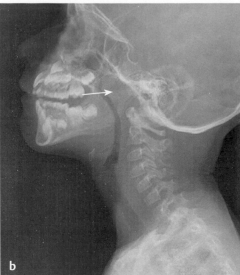

Fig. 79.12 (a, b) Plain radiograph: Lateral view of soft tissue of the nasopharynx demonstrating an opacity filling the nasopharynx located in the basisphenoid and basiocciput region (*white arrow*) which may be adenoids.

nasopharynx. X-ray is taken with extension of the head and in inspiration. This is done to avoid overlap and for better contrast of air and soft tissue (**Figs. 79.12a, b** and **79.13**).

- Foreign body of airway/digestive tract: The largest diameter of the airway is in the sagittal plane, and the largest diameter of the cricopharynx and esophagus is in the coronal plane. Circular foreign bodies tend to lodge in the airway/digestive tract along the greatest dimensions as noted in the image. Foreign bodies with irregular margins do not behave the same way (**Figs. 79.14–79.17**).
- Acute epiglottitis: A characteristic thumb sign is seen on lateral view.
- Acute laryngotracheobronchitis: A characteristic steeple sign (resembles church steeple) is seen on anteroposterior view.
- Fractures of laryngeal skeleton.
- Laryngeal stenosis.
- Cervical spine pathologies.
- Retropharyngeal abscess: This can be diagnosed on a lateral view.
  - Presence of an air-fluid level.
  - Soft tissue widening of prevertebral space along the entire length of the neck. More than two-thirds the diameter of the vertebral body in adults (or >21 mm at C6, >7 mm at C1/C2) and three-fourths in children (or >14 mm at C6) are considered as prevertebral widening. Bamboo spine appearance, that is, loss of cervical lordosis due to spasm of prevertebral muscles, is also noted (**Fig. 79.18a, b**).

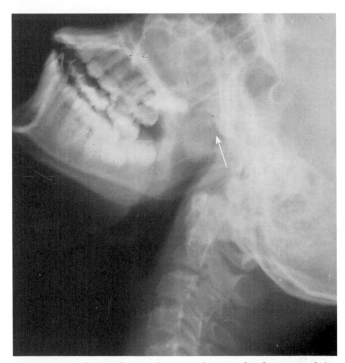

Fig. 79.13 Plain radiograph: Lateral view of soft tissue of the nasopharynx demonstrating crescent sign characteristically seen in antrochoanal polyp (*yellow arrow*).

  - Loss of intervertebral disc space and vertebral body erosion are seen only in chronic retropharyngeal abscess caused by tuberculosis .
- Localization of the position of the tracheostomy tube.

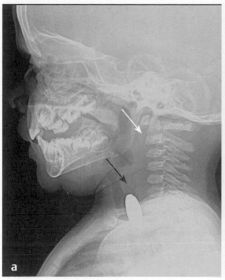

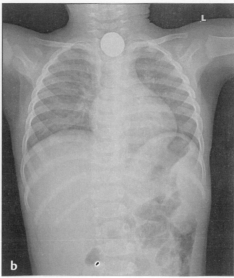

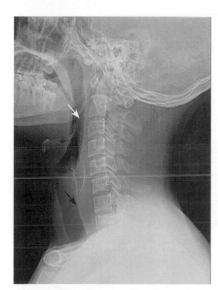

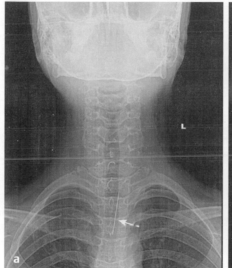

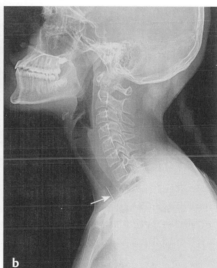

Fig. 79.14 Plain radiograph of soft tissue of the neck and chest: **(a)** Lateral and **(b)** anteroposterior views showing a radiopaque foreign body (double rim appearance—commonly seen in button batteries) located in the region of the cricopharynx (C6–C7). White arrow shows loss of normal cervical lordosis (due to paraspinal muscle spasm). *Black arrow* shows prevertebral widening (more than two-third the body of the vertebra).

Fig. 79.15 Plain radiograph of soft tissue of the neck and mediastinum: Lateral view showing a radiopaque, linear foreign body (*blue arrow*) located in the region of the cricopharynx (C5–C6). *White arrow* shows loss of normal cervical lordosis (due to paraspinal muscle spasm). *Black arrow* shows prevertebral widening (more than two-third the body of the vertebra) which is suggestive of acute retropharyngeal abscess.

Fig. 79.16 Plain radiograph of soft tissue of the neck and chest: **(a)** Anteroposterior and **(b)** lateral views showing a linear radiopaque foreign body in the airway (trachea) opposite the C7–T1 vertebra.

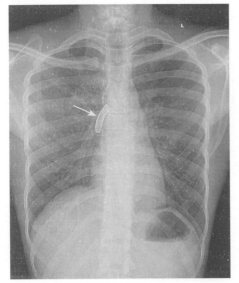

Fig. 79.17 Plain radiograph of soft tissue of the neck and chest: Anteroposterior view showing a linear radiopaque foreign body in the airway (right mainstem bronchus).

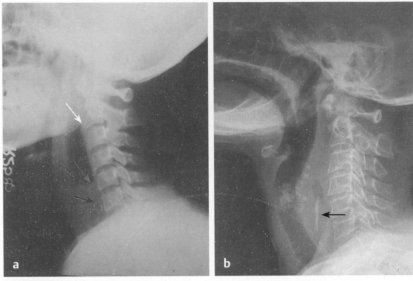

Fig. 79.18 Plain radiograph of soft tissue of the neck and chest: **(a)** Lateral and **(b)** anteroposterior views showing an air–fluid level (air due to gas-producing organisms) (*blue arrow*). *White arrow* shows loss of normal cervical lordosis (due to paraspinal muscle spasm). *Orange arrow* shows prevertebral widening (more than two-third the body of the vertebra) leading to diagnosis of acute retropharyngeal abscess. Foreign body with acute retropharyngeal abscess noted in the second image (*red arrow*).

Contrast Radiograph

It is used to detect esophageal pathologies. The various contrast materials used are barium sulphate (water insoluble) and Gastrografin (water soluble).

Barium sulphate is an inert, nondegradable, nonabsorbable substance in the gastrointestinal tract and can be suspended in water. It acts as a lethal foreign agent outside the gastrointestinal tract causing an uncontrollable inflammatory response. Hence, it should not be used in suspected perforation of the gastrointestinal tract and in aspiration. It should be replaced with Gastrografin in such circumstances. In the airway, barium sulphate can cause a foreign body reaction and can also get inspissated causing obstruction of the bronchi.

Note: The contrast agent is semisolid and bitter. Hence, it is mixed with a flavoring agent like lime to make it palatable. *Right anterior oblique view* is ideal for a contrast radiograph. The pathologies which can be identified on contrast radiograph are:

- Esophageal motility disorders like "corkscrew esophagus," which shows simultaneous multiple contractions which are nonperistaltic (**Fig. 79.19**).
- Malignancy: The following findings are noted in contrast radiograph:
  - Irregular filling defect which is also known as apple core appearance and is seen in malignancy of middle one-third of esophagus. On contrast X-ray, there is

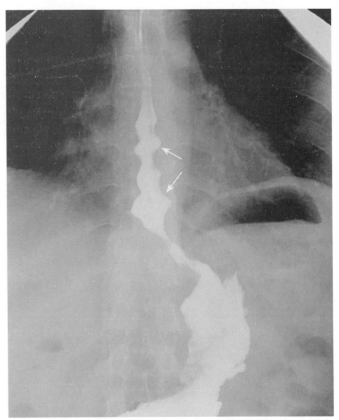

Fig. 79.19 Contrast radiograph (barium swallow) of soft tissue of the neck and chest: Anteroposterior view showing the appearance of a corkscrew (corkscrew esophagus).

irregularity and narrowing in between the upper and lower contrast filling zones.

- Rat tail appearance in malignancy of the lower one-third of esophagus which appears as irregularity with narrowing in lower end of esophagus.
- Shouldering sign in which the contrast agent appears to flow over the lesion into the irregular filling defect site (**Fig. 79.20**).
- Achalasia cardia: Contrast radiograph shows proximal dilation with beaking or sudden narrowing at the lower gastro-esophageal junction (bird beak appearance) (**Fig. 79.21**).
- Post-cricoid web: Shelf-like projection is identified at the level of post-cricoid region (C5–C6 region) on the anterior aspect (**Fig. 79.22**).

Other Imaging Investigations Used in ENT

■ Computed Tomography (CT)

This imaging modality has replaced plain radiography as the baseline investigation in otorhinolaryngology and head and neck surgery. It gives in-depth information of the bony architectural anatomy and disease pattern and spread. Water is taken as attenuation value of 0 Hounsfield units (HU). Bone and air are the at the extreme values of +1000 HU and −1000 HU, respectively. Reduced slice thickness on CT scan gives an accurate information of the various structures and gives an opportunity to reconstruct a three-dimensional architecture of the pattern as recognized by CT imaging. Contrast-enhanced CT gives an in-depth information about tumor spread, involvement of lymph nodes, abscesses, and a multitude of other ENT disorders (**Figs. 79.23** and **79.24**).

■ Magnetic Resonance Imaging (MRI)

This imaging modality gives accurate information about the soft tissue architecture and soft tissue pathology demarcation but poor information on the bony architecture. It does not have radiation hazards in contrast to a CT scan. Various sequences are present in MRI like T1-weighted, T2-weighted, spin, contrast (gadolinium) enhanced, fat suppression, gradient echo imaging, and angiography which are used in various disorders. MRI is contraindicated in patients using pacemakers for the heart or with metallic implants.

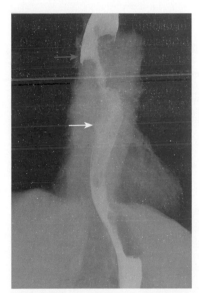

Fig. 79.20 Contrast radiograph (barium swallow) of soft tissue of the neck and chest: Right anterior oblique view showing irregular filling defect with apple core appearance (*white arrow*) and shouldering sign (*blue arrow*) in the middle one-third of the esophagus suggestive of malignancy of the middle one-third of the esophagus.

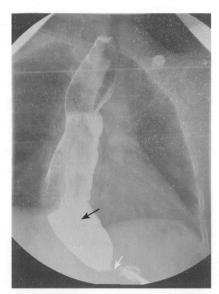

Fig. 79.21 Contrast radiograph (barium swallow) of soft tissue of the neck and chest: Right anterior oblique view showing narrowing at the lower end of esophagus (*yellow arrow* shows bird beak appearance) with proximal dilation (*red arrow*) which is suggestive of achalasia cardia.

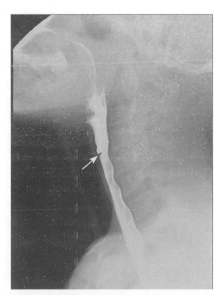

Fig. 79.22 Contrast radiograph (barium swallow) of soft tissue of the neck and chest: Lateral view showing a shelf-like projection anteriorly at C5 level suggestive of post-cricoid web (*yellow arrow*).

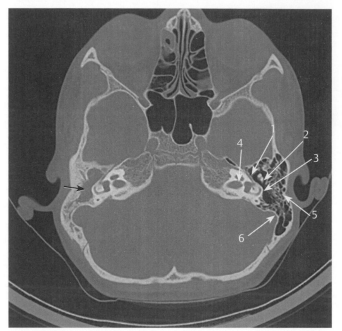

Fig. 79.23 High-resolution computed tomography (HRCT) of the temporal bone showing a cavity with soft tissue in the right mastoid (*red*). Other structures visualized in this slice: 1, horizontal segment of facial nerve; 2, head of malleus and body and short process of incus (ice cream cone appearance); 3, lateral semicircular canal (bucket handle appearance); 4, cochlea; 5, mastoid cellularity; 6 sigmoid sinus.

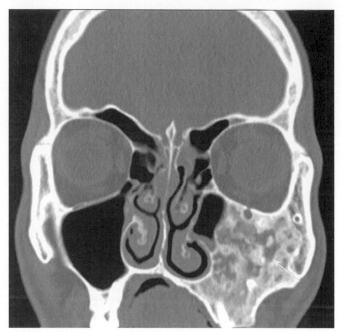

Fig. 79.24 Computed tomography of the left maxillary sinus showing fibrous dysplasia (*yellow arrow*).

Positron Emission Tomography or PET Scan

This can be PET–CT or PET–MRI. This imaging modality is based on the principle that cancer cells which are metabolically active take up more glucose compared to normal tissues. A radiotracer is combined to glucose to identify and demarcate the malignant tissue. This modality is mainly used in carcinoma of unknown primary to detect metastasis and postradiotherapy for detection of residual or recurrent disease.

Angiography

Digital subtraction angiography (DSA) is an investigative modality which gives accurate information about the feeding vessels to vascular tumors. It is used for vascular tumors like juvenile nasopharyngeal angiofibroma (JNA) and paragangliomas.

Ultrasound

This noninvasive imaging modality is used in thyroid and parotid disorders and for evaluation of neck node disease and other neck swellings. An ultrasound-guided FNAC is more precise.

80 Instruments in ENT

R. Archana Pillai

The competency covered in this chapter is as follows:

EN2.10 Identify and describe the use of common instruments in ENT.

Otology Instruments

Hartmann Aural Speculum

It is used to examine the external ear canal and tympanic membrane. The largest speculum that will fit into the ear canal comfortably is selected. It should not be too big (as the skin of the canal may fold into the lumen of the speculum and cause pain) nor too small (as the vision will be

narrow). The speculum is inserted up to the cartilaginous canal (**Fig. 80.1**).

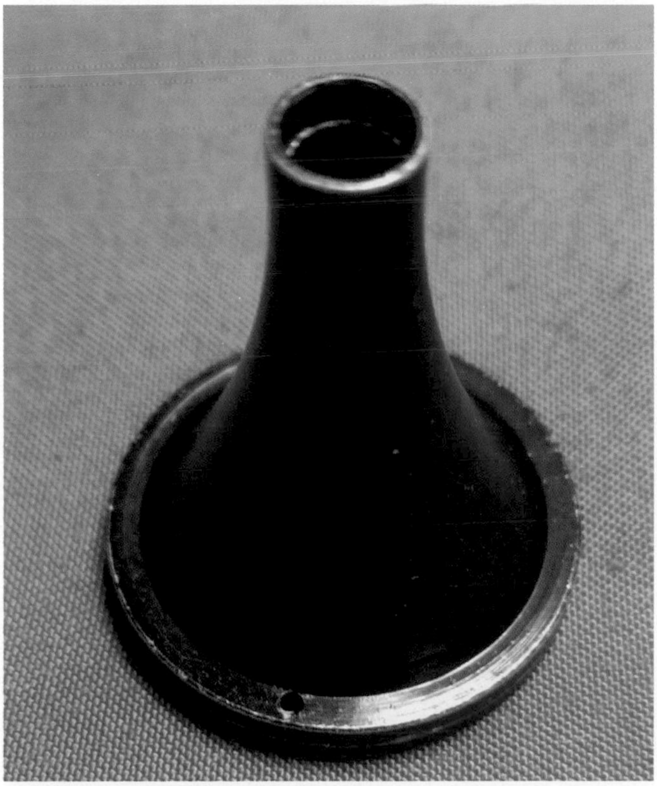

Jobson Horne Ear Probe with Ring Curette

One end is a serrated probe, and the other end has a ring. The curette end is used for removal of wax or foreign body from ear and nose, and removal of granulations in the ear. The probe end is used to probe polyp or mass in the nose and ear, and as a cotton swab carrier to clean the ear canal and to use chemical cautery in the ear and nose for granulation tissue (**Fig. 80.2**).

Mollison's Self-Retaining, Hemostatic, Mastoid Retractor

It has four prongs on either side which help in retraction of the tissues and provide hemostasis by compressing the vessels. It is used for exposure during harvesting of temporalis fascia, in mastoidectomy, in tympanoplasty, and in head and neck surgeries like tracheostomy and laryngofissure surgery and thyroplasty (**Fig. 80.3**).

Simpson Aural Syringe

It is a metallic syringe with a nozzle. There is a piston inside a cylindrical body and a handle. It is used for syringing. The procedure is described in Chapter 3 "History Taking and Examination of the Ear" (**Fig. 80.4**).

Rose Eustachian Tube Catheter

It is a 12- to 15-cm long metallic catheter with curved proximal end and a ring toward the opposite end which indicates the side of the curvature after it is inserted into the nose. Earlier, it was used to test the patency of the Eustachian tube and to inflate the middle ear. It can be used (instead of a curved suction cannula) to remove foreign body from the nose (**Fig. 80.5**).

Fig. 80.1 Hartmann aural speculum.

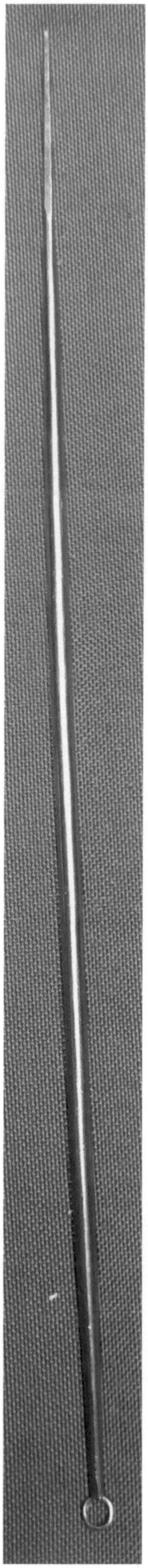

Fig. 80.2 Jobson Horne ear probe with ring curette.

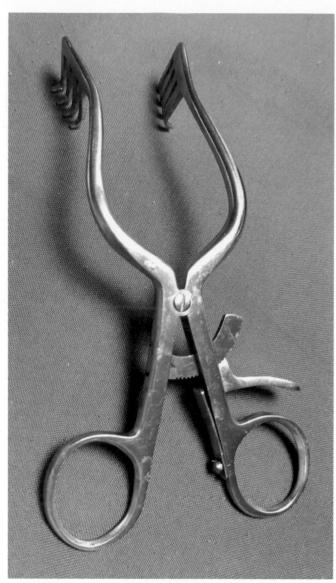

Fig. 80.3 Mollison's self-retaining, hemostatic, mastoid retractor.

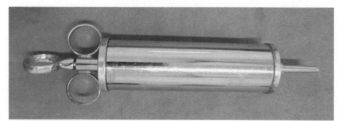

Fig. 80.4 Simpson aural syringe.

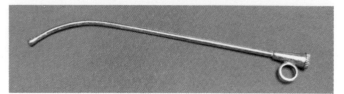

Fig. 80.5 Eustachian tube catheter.

■ Myringotomy Knife

It is used to make a myringotomy incision on the tympanic membrane (**Fig. 80.6**).

■ MacEwen's Cell Seeker

One end is a curved probe. It is used to determine the direction of aditus, antrum, and other mastoid cells. The other end can be used as a curette (**Fig. 80.7**).

■ Farabeuf's Mastoid Periosteal Elevator with Thumb Rest

It is used to elevate the mastoid periosteum, which exposes the outer mastoid cortex during mastoid surgeries. It can also be used in raising the periosteum in Caldwell-Luc procedure (**Fig. 80.8**).

■ Tuning Fork

The parts of a tuning fork include: two prongs (or tines), shoulder, stem/handle, and foot piece (**Fig. 80.9**).

There are two types of tuning forks—Hartmann and Gardiner Brown. Frequencies commonly used in otology are 256, 512, and 1,024 Hz.

The most commonly used frequency is 512 Hz because it lies in the mid speech frequency range, and has minimal overtones, more auditory than tactile vibration, and optimal tone decay.

Rhinology Instruments

■ Killian Long Bladed Self-Retaining Nasal Speculum

This is a self-retaining nasal speculum and is available with blades of different sizes. The distance between the blades can be adjusted and fixed with a screw.

It is used for following purposes:
- *Diagnostic*: Anterior rhinoscopy for examination of the nasal cavities.
- *Therapeutic*: For removal of foreign bodies, antral puncture, nasal packing, surgical procedures inside the nose like polypectomy, submucosal resection, septoplasty, and turbinectomy/turbinoplasty (**Fig. 80.10a, b**).

■ Thudicum Nasal Speculum

This is a self-retaining nasal speculum commonly used in the ENT outpatient clinic. It is held over the hooked index finger of the nondominant hand with the thumb on top for support. The blades are then closed by pressing between the middle and ring fingers.

It is used for following purposes:
- *Diagnostic*: Anterior rhinoscopy.

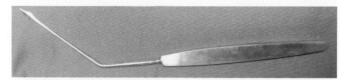

Fig. 80.6 Myringotomy knife.

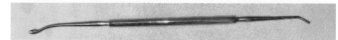

Fig. 80.7 MacEwen's cell seeker.

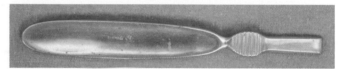

Fig. 80.8 Farabeuf's mastoid periosteal elevator with thumb rest.

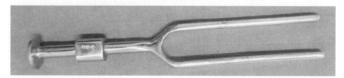

Fig. 80.9 Tuning fork.

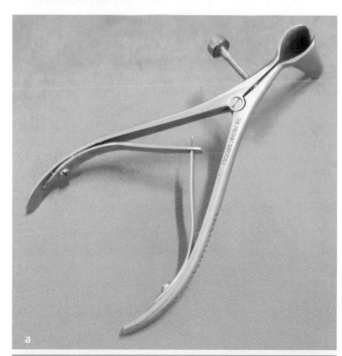

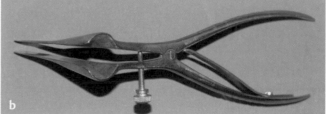

Fig. 80.10 (a, b) Killian long bladed self-retaining nasal speculum.

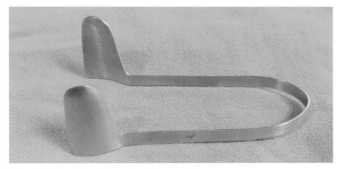

Fig. 80.11 Thudicum nasal speculum.

- *Therapeutic*: Removal of foreign bodies, antral wash, nasal packing, and surgical procedures inside the nose (**Fig. 80.11**).

St Clair Thompson Postnasal Mirror

It has a bayonet-shaped handle. It is available in different sizes starting from 0 to 5. It is used to examine roof of nasopharynx, choana, posterior end of septum and turbinates, Eustachian tube opening, and posterior nasopharyngeal wall (**Fig. 80.12**).

Freer Double Ended Mucoperichondrial Elevator

It is used to elevate mucoperichondrial and periosteal flap in septal surgeries. It is useful for displacement of inferior turbinate in antrostomy operation, for elevating posterior canal skin in tympanomastoid surgeries, for elevation of mucosa in Caldwell-Luc operation, for spreading and teasing temporalis fascia graft, for displacement of structures like middle and inferior turbinates during guiding of the nasal endoscope, and for performing uncinectomy (**Fig. 80.13**).

Ballenger Swivel Knife

This is a knife that can rotate 360 degrees within its two prongs. Hence, it can be positioned without rotating the instrument and the direction can be changed. This instrument is used in correction of a deviated nasal septum by submucosal resection of septum and to harvest cartilage for rhinoplasty and tympanoplasty (**Fig. 80.14a, b**).

Tilley Forceps

It is used for placing an anterior nasal pack (**Fig. 80.15**).

Luc's Forceps

It is used to take biopsies in the oral cavity, oropharynx, and nose. It is used in septoplasty and submucosal resection. It is useful in polypectomy and in tumor removal. It can be used as a tonsil holding forceps but the edges are sharp and can cut the tonsil (**Fig. 80.16**).

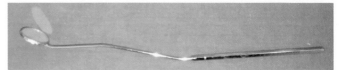

Fig. 80.12 St Clair Thompson postnasal mirror.

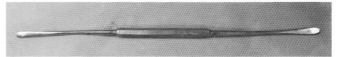

Fig. 80.13 Freer double ended mucoperichondrial elevator.

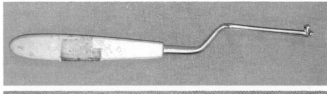

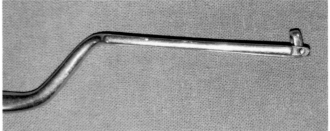

Fig. 80.14 Ballenger swivel knife.

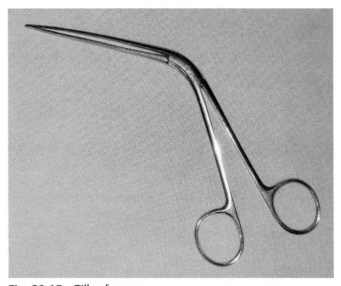

Fig. 80.15 Tilley forceps.

Tilley Lichtwitz Trocar and Canula

Tilley Lichtwitz trocar and canula consists of a handle with long pointed end (trocar) and cannula with connecting end for irrigation (**Fig. 80.17a, b**).

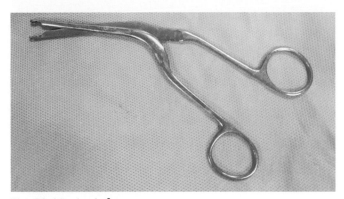

Fig. 80.16 Luc's forceps.

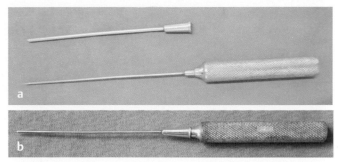

Fig. 80.17 Tilley Lichtwitz trocar and canula. **(a)** The trocar is on the left and the canula is on the right. **(b)** The trocar is placed inside the canula.

It is used for following purposes:
- Diagnostic proof puncture to obtain aspirate from the maxillary sinus for analysis like culture and sensitivity, fungal culture, and cytology.
- To drain pus in maxillary sinusitis.
- For instillation of medicine into maxillary antrum.
- To detect site of oro-antral fistula.

Procedure of Antral Puncture

After administering a topical anesthetic with decongestant in the inferior and middle meati, the trocar and cannula are directed into the inferior meatus, the cannula covering the tip of trocar so as not to traumatize the inferior turbinate. Approximately 1 cm from the anterior end of the inferior turbinate, the trocar is directed toward the ipsilateral outer canthus of the eye or tragus and the puncture is made (after exposing the trocar tip) into the maxillary sinus. The index finger is used as a guard to avoid over-inserting the trocar. The trocar is then withdrawn, and the cannula is retained temporarily for diagnostic or therapeutic purpose.

Complications

Complications include bleeding from the turbinate, entry into the orbit, entry into pterygopalatine fossa, injury to the root of the ipsilateral maxillary teeth, and entry into the subcutaneous tissue of the cheek.

■ Tilley's Antral Harpoon and Myle's Naso-Antral Perforator

These instruments are used for intranasal antrostomy. The Tilley's antral harpoon is used to make opening in the inferior meatus into the maxillary sinus (**Fig. 80.18a**). (The technique for making the opening in the inferior meatus is similar to antral puncture.) The *Myle's naso-antral perforator* is used to enlarge or widen the opening (**Fig. 80.18b**). The *Tilley's antral bur* is used to smoothen the edges.

The intranasal antrostomy can be done when the mucociliary clearance is not functioning and dependent drainage is required as in Kartagener's syndrome and cystic fibrosis.

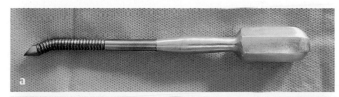

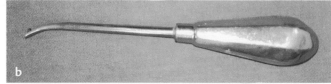

Fig. 80.18 **(a)** Tilley's antral harpoon. **(b)** Myle's naso-antral perforator.

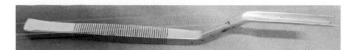

Fig. 80.19 Tilley's nasal gouge.

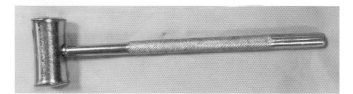

Fig. 80.20 Heath mallet.

The antrostomy is also useful following a Caldwell-Luc procedure when a pack is kept in the antrum and can be removed at a later date through the intranasal antrostomy.

■ Tilley's Nasal Gouge

It is bayonet shaped and the tip has a "v"-shaped slot for better anchorage of the maxillary crest. It is used for removal of a prominent maxillary crest (**Fig. 80.19**).

■ Heath Mallet

It is used along with a gouge, chisel, or osteotome. The gouge is to be hit by a mallet with movement at the wrist during septal surgery (**Fig. 80.20**).

◾ Walsham Forceps

It is used for nasal bone fracture reduction (**Fig. 80.21**).

◾ Ash Forceps

It is used for nasal septal fracture reduction (**Fig. 80.22**).

◾ Common Instruments for Endoscopic Sinus Surgery (Fig. 80.23)

- Sickle knife is used in uncinectomy and other mucosal incisions.

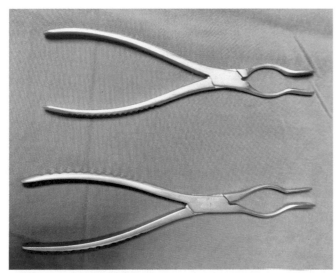

Fig. 80.21 Walsham forceps.

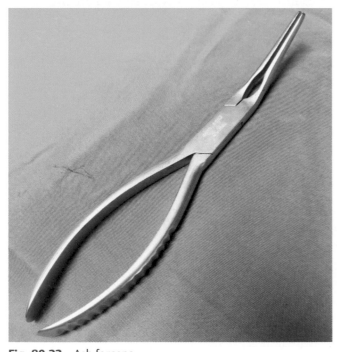

Fig. 80.22 Ash forceps.

- "J" curette is used in opening the cells, especially in the frontal recess.
- Ball probe is useful in palpating deeper structures and for detecting openings especially in the frontal recess.
- Curved suction cannula is used for clearing secretions and blood, and for clearing disease like mycetoma in the maxillary sinus.

◾ Common Instruments in Endoscopic Sinus Surgery (Fig. 80.24)

- Endoscopic scissors are used in resecting concha bullosa.
- Blakesley thru-cut forceps are used to cut and remove without shearing the mucosa.
- Ostrum's back-biting forceps are used in uncinectomy and middle meatal antrostomy.
- Blakesley-Weil 45 degrees upturned forceps are more suitable for reaching the structures that are higher up in the nasal cavity and the lateral wall of the nose.
- Blakesley straight forceps is used for removal of diseased tissue/cells and polypi in endoscopic sinus surgery. It can also be used for taking biopsy from the nose, oral cavity, and oropharynx.

Throat Instruments

◾ Lac Tongue Depressor

It has a flat end and a slightly curved end. The flat end is placed over the anterior two-thirds of the tongue to depress it. The posterior one-third should not be touched in order to prevent gag reflex. The following are its uses: Examination of oral cavity and oropharynx, to retract lips and cheek, to express pus out of the tonsil (septic squeeze test), to test

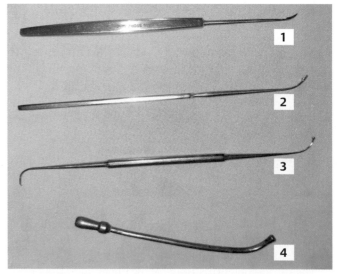

Fig. 80.23 Common instruments for endoscopic sinus surgery. 1, Sickle knife; 2, "J" curette; 3, ball probe; 4, curved suction cannula.

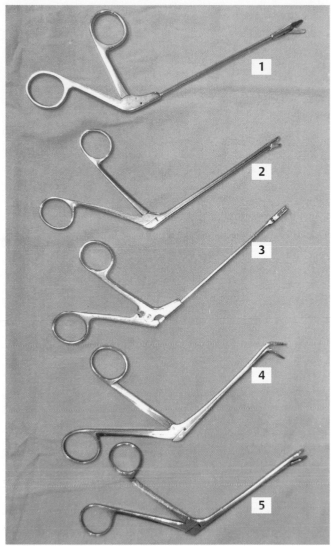

Fig. 80.24 Common instruments in endoscopic sinus surgery. 1, Endoscopic scissors; 2, Blakesley thru-cut forceps; 3, Ostrum's back-biting forceps; 4, Blakesley-Weil 45 degrees upturned forceps; 5, Blakesley straight forceps.

gag reflex, for cold spatula test to check patency of the nasal airway, for posterior rhinoscopy, and for oral cavity procedures like injection of steroids, biopsy, and excision of cysts (**Fig. 80.25**).

Indirect Laryngoscopy Mirror

This instrument has a handle, a shaft, and a plain mirror at an angle. The focal length of this mirror is at infinity. The mirror is available in various sizes ranging from 8 to 30 mm (**Fig. 80.26**).

It is used for examination of tongue base, valleculae, glossoepiglottic fold, pharyngoepiglottic fold, arytenoids, aryepiglottic folds, ventricular bands, vocal cords, interarytenoid region, pyriform fossae, and posterior pharyngeal wall. These regions can be examined for foreign body and

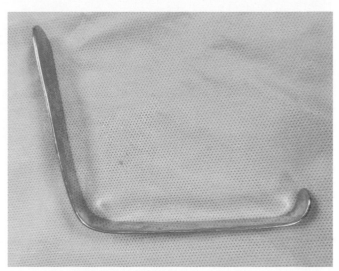

Fig. 80.25 Lac tongue depressor.

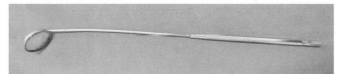

Fig. 80.26 Indirect laryngoscopy mirror.

for inflammatory, traumatic, or neoplastic lesions. It can be used to visualize the oropharynx and hypopharynx while removing small foreign bodies like fish bone and while taking a biopsy.

Boyle Davis Mouth Gag with Tongue Blade

It has two components, the blade and the gag, that are used simultaneously. It helps to keep the mouth open and push the tongue away from the operation site. The upper tooth plate has small holes to which a rubber tube is sutured to prevent trauma to the incisor tooth. The mouth gag is introduced in the closed position after opening the mouth with the head extended. The mouth gag is gradually opened, and the ratchet lock makes it self-retaining. The whole assembly can be lifted up and maintained in that position using Draffin's bipod with stand. Some blades like the Daughty blade has a groove or gap in the middle for the endotracheal tube. Indications of the mouth gag and blade include tonsillectomy, adenoidectomy, surgeries of the palate and nasopharynx, and excision of choanal polyp (**Fig. 80.27a–c**).

Draffin's Bipod with Stand (Maguaran's Plate)

It has two rods with multiple rings in a row. It is used to anchor and fix the Boyle Davis mouth gag. The plate helps to maintain the position of the stand (**Fig. 80.28**).

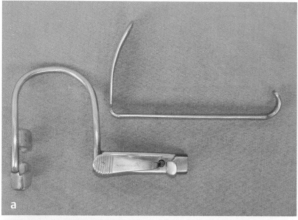

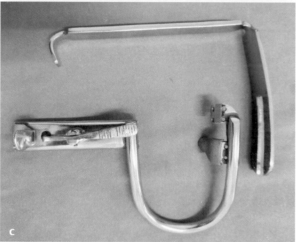

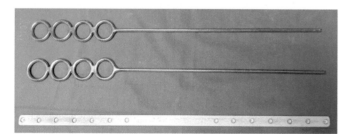

Fig. 80.27 **(a–c)** Boyle Davis mouth gag with tongue blade.

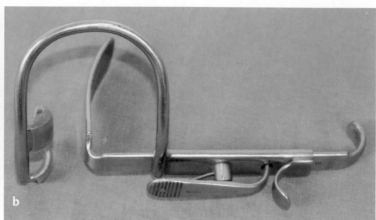

Fig. 80.28 Draffin's bipod with stand (Maguaran's plate).

■ Dennis Browne Tonsil Holding Forceps

It is used to hold the tonsil and pull it medially during the process of dissection. This instrument resembles Luc's forceps but differs from it as the edges of the jaw are blunt and do not cut tissue, the upper jaw is smaller than the lower jaw, and the tip has a box mechanism (**Fig. 80.29**).

■ Mollison Tonsillar Dissector and Anterior Pillar Retractor

It has a blunt end used for initial atraumatic dissection of the tonsil. The pillar retractor is used after removal of the

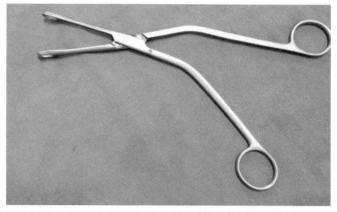

Fig. 80.29 Dennis Browne tonsil holding forceps.

tonsil to look for bleeding points and tags (remnants) of tonsillar tissue left behind. The retractor can also be used to visualize a small fibrotic tonsil (**Fig. 80.30**).

■ Eve's Tonsillar Snare

The snare has a stainless-steel wire which is usually 3 inches long and a thickness of 28 gauge. It is used to snare

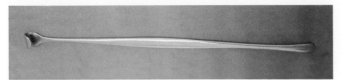

Fig. 80.30 Mollison tonsillar dissector and anterior pillar retractor.

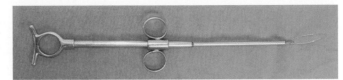

Fig. 80.31 Eve's tonsillar snare.

the lower pole of the tonsil after dissection. The lower pole is crushed on snaring and thromboplastin is released which is a powerful vasoconstrictor (**Fig. 80.31**).

■ Yankauer Pharyngeal Suction Tube

It is a long, bent instrument with a stout handle. The tip of the tube has a rounded blunt cap with small holes. This prevents trauma to the dissection field. The bent tube enables the surgeon to visualize the dissection field better. The multiple openings in the tip of suction tube will facilitate suction even if the main opening is blocked. This instrument is used for all oral and oropharyngeal surgeries including adenotonsillectomy (**Fig. 80.32**).

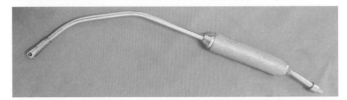

Fig. 80.32 Yankauer pharyngeal suction tube.

■ Straight Artery Forceps

It is used to hold tissues and clamp vessels in head and neck surgeries and to catch bleeding points in the tonsillar fossa after tonsillectomy. It is replaced by Negus second artery forceps underneath the first artery forceps before ligation (**Fig. 80.33**).

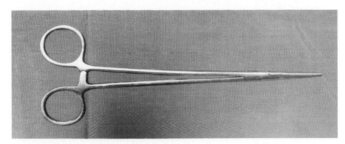

Fig. 80.33 Straight artery forceps.

■ Negus Second/Replacement Artery Forceps

It has a curved tip and is used after the first artery forceps for ligating blood vessels in a deeper site. The curve may be "L" shaped or "J" shaped (**Fig. 80.34**).

■ Negus Knot Tier and Ligature Pusher

It is used to push the ligature loop on the Negus second artery forceps to ligate the bleeding point (**Fig. 80.35**).

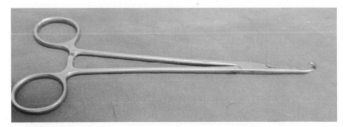

Fig. 80.34 Negus second/replacement artery forceps.

■ Quincy Forceps

It is used for drainage of peritonsillar abscess. It is a bayonet-shaped instrument with a sharp trocar tip. It has a guard at some distance from tip to prevent deep entry. For draining quinsy, the sharp tip is used to pierce the tissues with the forceps closed. The instrument is then opened like a sinus forceps to drain the abscess (**Fig. 80.36a, b**).

■ St Clair Thompson Adenoid Curette with Cage (Fig. 80.37)

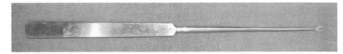

Fig. 80.35 Negus knot tier and ligature pusher.

■ St Clair Thompson Adenoid Curette without Cage

This instrument is used to curette the adenoids by a blind technique. The curette is introduced behind the soft palate with the blade facing down. It is held like a dagger and the adenoid is curetted from the nasopharyngeal wall in the midline by sweeping movement. The cage is used to prevent slipping of the excised tissue into the throat.

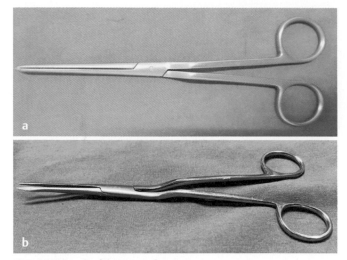

Fig. 80.36 **(a, b)** Quincy forceps.

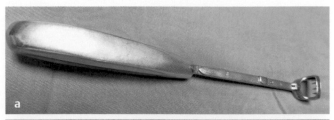

Fig. 80.37 **(a, b)** St Clair Thompson adenoid curette with cage.

During the procedure, the neck of the patient should not be in too much extension as it might injure the atlanto-occipital joint (**Fig. 80.38**).

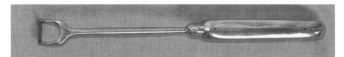

Fig. 80.38 St Clair Thompson adenoid curette without cage.

■ Doyen's Mouth Gag

It is used to keep the mouth open during procedures in the oral cavity (**Fig. 80.39**).

■ Cheek Retractor

It is used to retract the cheek/angle of the mouth during procedures in the oral cavity (**Fig. 80.40**).

Instruments for the Neck

■ Bard Parker Handle

It is used for attaching the blade (**Fig. 80.41**).

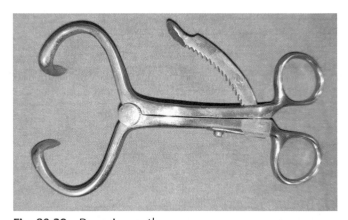

Fig. 80.39 Doyen's mouth gag.

■ Needle Holder

It is used to hold the needle while suturing. It comes in different sizes and shapes (**Fig. 80.42a, b**).

■ Cricoid Hook—Blunt

During tracheostomy it is used to retract the isthmus of thyroid and other tissues (**Fig. 80.43**).

■ Cricoid Hook—Sharp

It helps to retract the cricoid cartilage superiorly and stabilize it prior to dilatation of trachea while doing tracheostomy (**Fig. 80.44**).

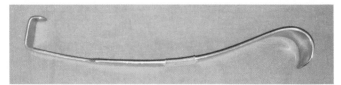

Fig. 80.40 Cheek retractor.

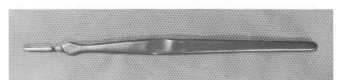

Fig. 80.41 Bard Parker handle.

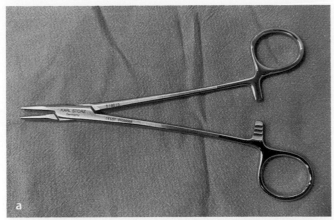

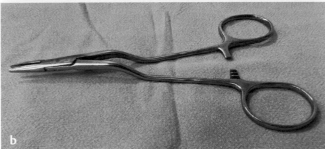

Fig. 80.42 (a, b) Needle holder.

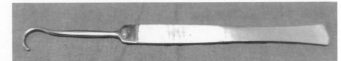

Fig. 80.43 Cricoid hook—blunt.

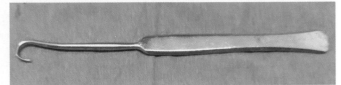

Fig. 80.44 Cricoid hook—sharp.

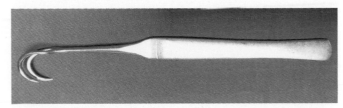

Fig. 80.45 Double hook.

Double Hook

It is used to retract the soft tissues, like strap muscles, in neck surgery including tracheostomy (**Fig. 80.45**).

Trousseau Tracheal Dilator

It is an instrument used to dilate the tracheostoma during or after the tracheostomy to insert the tracheostomy tube. It allows easier introduction of the tracheostomy tube and prevents formation of a false passage (**Fig. 80.46**).

Fuller's Biflanged Metallic Tracheostomy Tube

The tracheostomy tube is made of German silver. It comprises of an inner and an outer tube. The outer tube is biflanged. The tube can be inserted into the trachea by compressing the flanges. The inner tube is longer than the outer tube. If the inner tube gets blocked due to thick secretions or crusts, it can be removed, cleaned, and reinserted without removing the outer tube. The inner tube has a small opening. When the tube is blocked with a finger from the outside the patient can attempt phonation. The other use of the opening is for decannulation. The tube is blocked at its outer opening in the neck for 24 to 48 hours and the patency of the airway above the tube is assessed prior to removal of the tube which is called decannulation (**Fig. 80.47a, b**).

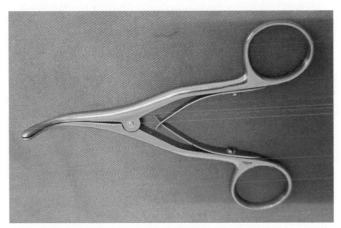

Fig. 80.46 Trousseau tracheal dilator.

The disadvantage of the tube is that it can cause a skin/soft tissue reaction, it can erode the anterior tracheal wall (trachea–innominate artery fistula has been reported), and the flange can break and present as a foreign body in the bronchus. The tube cannot be used during radiotherapy.

Jackson Metallic Tracheostomy Tube

The parts of Jackson metallic tracheostomy tube are outer tube, inner tube, and pilot or obturator.

The inner tube is longer than the outer tube which facilitates cleaning when blocked. The obturator is used for inserting the tube into the trachea. There is a lock on the upper part of the outer tube which prevents dislodgement of the inner tube especially during bouts of coughing (**Fig. 80.48**).

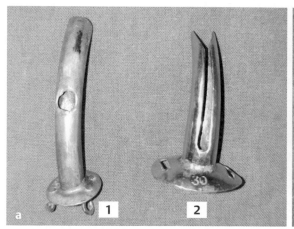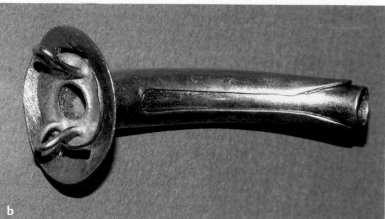

Fig. 80.47 Fuller's biflanged metallic tracheostomy tube. **(a)** Inner tube (1) and outer tube (2). **(b)** Inner tube inserted into the outer tube.

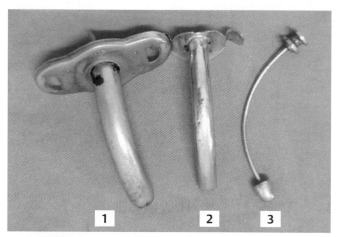

Fig. 80.48 Jackson metallic tracheostomy tube. 1, Outer tube; 2, inner tube; 3, pilot or obturator.

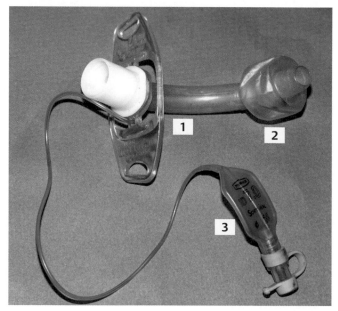

Fig. 80.49 Portex cuffed tracheostomy tube. 1, Single tube with collar; 2, cuff; 3, balloon with valve for air.

The disadvantages are: phonation is not possible, patency of the natural air passage cannot be checked by blocking the tube, risk of granulation tissue formation, and soft tissue/skin reaction. The tube cannot be used during radiotherapy.

■ Portex Cuffed Tracheostomy Tube

The parts of Portex cuffed tracheostomy tube are a single tube with collar, cuff, balloon with valve for air, and a pilot or obturator (not shown).

It is made up of soft material so as to cause less trauma to the tracheal wall. The cuff may help prevent aspiration and is useful in giving intermittent positive pressure ventilation especially in an intensive care unit (ICU) setting. There is a blue radio-opaque line for visualization during imaging. The advantages over an endotracheal tube is that the dead space is less, bronchial toilet is easier, and the incidence of subglottic or tracheal stenosis is less (**Fig. 80.49**).

The disadvantages are that it is difficult to clean, phonation is not possible, and cuff might cause tracheal mucosal necrosis and lead to stenosis if inflated for a long time.

Tubes with double cannula are available. The outer cannula has fenestra. There are two types of inner cannula: a nonfenestrated cannula which is useful during intermittent positive pressure ventilation and a fenestrated cannula which can facilitate phonation and decannulation.

Upper Aerodigestive Tract Endoscopic Instruments

■ Rigid Nasal Endoscopes

Types:
- **Adult:** Outer diameter is 4 mm.
- **Pediatric:** Outer diameter is 2.7 mm.
- **Angles:** 0, 30, 45, 70, 90, and 120 degrees.

Each endoscope is 18-cm long. The 0-degree endoscope is the most commonly used as it gives an end-on view. The 30-degree endoscope is preferred for diagnostic nasal endoscopy. It allows better visualization of the structures in the lateral wall of nose. The 70- and 90-degree endoscopes are useful to visualize and work in the frontal recess and in the maxillary antrum. They are also useful in visualizing the laryngeal and hypopharyngeal structures, as an alternative to indirect laryngoscopy. The 120-degree endoscope is used to inspect the anterior wall of the maxillary sinus through the antrostomy opening. Color code for endoscopes are as follows: 0 degree, *green*; 30 degrees, *red*; 45 degrees, *black*; 70 degrees, *yellow*; and 90 degrees, *blue* (**Fig. 80.50**).

■ Macintosh Laryngoscope

The various parts of Macintosh laryngoscope are as follows (**Fig. 80.51**):
- *Handle*: It has a rough surface for proper grip. It contains batteries inside for illumination of the blade tip.
- *Mouth*: This has a pin that accepts blades of various sizes. When properly fitted and closed, the electrical circuit is completed, and the bulb is switched on.

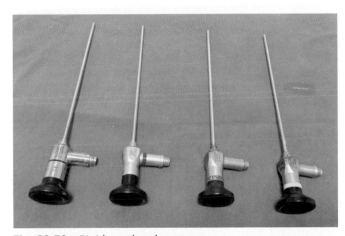

Fig. 80.50 Rigid nasal endoscopes.

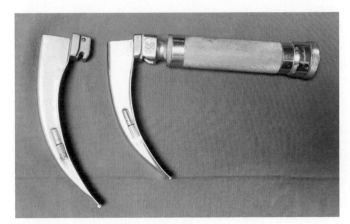

Fig. 80.51 Macintosh laryngoscope.

- *Blade*: The blade is curved and has a bulb at its tip for illumination. The straight blade is referred to as the Miller blade.

Macintosh laryngoscope is used:
- For endotracheal intubation.
- For inserting bronchoscope.
- To take biopsy from the base of tongue, pharynx, or larynx.
- For removal of foreign bodies in the oropharynx and hypopharynx.
- For guided insertion of Ryle's tube.

■ Direct Laryngoscope

Based on the type of illumination, there are two types of scopes—*Negus* (proximal illumination) and *Jackson* (distal illumination). The disadvantage of the light source being close to the distal tip is that it gets frequently smudged with secretions or blood (**Fig. 80.52**).

It is used for examination of larynx, pharynx, and upper esophagus, biopsy from these areas, foreign body removal, and excision of mass from glottis or supraglottis.

The details are described in Chapter 59 "Direct Laryngoscopy."

■ Rigid Bronchoscope

This is a rigid hollow metallic tube with a beveled end. It comes in various sizes for adult and pediatric use. The adult scope is 40 to 45 cm long. It has vents on the side for ventilation of the contralateral bronchus when inserted into

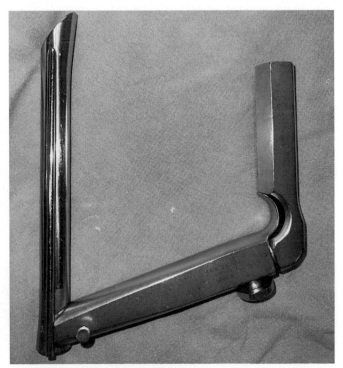

Fig. 80.52 Direct laryngoscope.

a major bronchus. It differs from esophagoscope as it has these vents and the esophagoscope is wider especially at its beveled end. The rigid bronchoscope can be used as an esophagoscope but an esophagoscope cannot be used as a bronchoscope (**Fig. 80.53a–c**).

Uses:
- *Diagnostic*:
  - For examination of the tracheobronchial tree for pathology like growth, ulcer, and stricture.
  - Biopsy from a suspicious growth or ulcer.
  - Bronchial lavage from secretions.
  - Bronchography.
  - Autofluorescence and photodynamic diagnosis.
- *Therapeutic*:
  - Foreign body removal.
  - Tracheobronchial stenting.
  - Aspiration of secretions.
  - Removal of tumors.

The details are elaborated in Chapter 62 "Bronchoscopy."

Hypopharyngoscope

This instrument is similar to an esophagoscope, but it is shorter in length, around 29 cm, and referred to as a cervical esophagoscope or esophageal speculum. The distal end of the scope is wider than its proximal end, like in a typical esophagoscope (**Fig. 80.54**).

Hypopharyngoscope is used:
- To remove foreign bodies from the hypopharynx or cricopharynx.
- To take biopsy from the above regions.
- For cricopharyngeal dilatation.
- Excision or dilatation of cricopharyngeal web.

Rigid Esophagoscope

It consists of a rigid hollow tube of 40 to 45 cm length and 16 to 20 mm diameter. There are two types, namely, Negus and Jackson, depending on the type of illumination (**Fig. 80.55**).

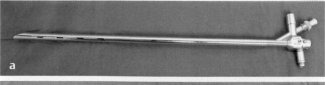
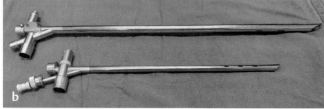
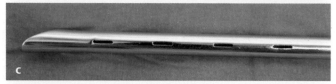

Fig. 80.53 (a–c) Rigid bronchoscope.

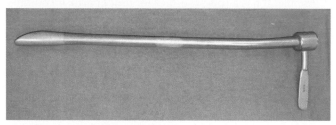

Fig. 80.54 Hypopharyngoscope.

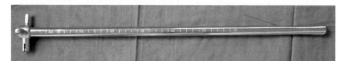

Fig. 80.55 Rigid esophagoscope.

The parts of a rigid esophagoscope are handle, eyepiece (proximal end), body or shaft, light carrier, and distal opening.

The description of esophagoscopes and esophagoscopy is covered in Chapter 67.

Appendix

Communication Etiquette and Bioethics for Medical Students in Training

Mary Kurien

"Listen to your patient, he is telling you the diagnosis. Care more for the individual patient than for the special features of the disease. Put yourself in his/her place... The kindly word, the cheerful greeting, the sympathetic look—these the patient understands" (**Sir William Osler,**[1] 1849–1919)

Known as the "father of modern medicine," he revolutionized medical education, establishing internship and residency system, was the first to bring medical students out of the lecture hall for bedside clinical training, and he is well known for his humanist approach to medical practice.[1]

Over the years, with the development of better diagnostic techniques and improved therapies, although changes in medical practice have occurred, it still remains a *"human endeavor,"* and human nature does not change! When patients visit the doctor, they may be anxious or in fear. The doctor has the responsibility to calm their fears and provide hope as well. An accomplished doctor is humane and compassionate, empathetic and supportive.[2]

Medical ethics (bioethics) refer to a set of moral principles that relates to good and bad conduct in medical practice while etiquette is a customary code which indicates the proper and polite way to behave in society. The key strategies of etiquette-based communication in medical practice are (1) greeting the patient as he/she enters the doctor's room or knocking/asking to enter the patient's room, (2) introducing oneself, (3) explaining one's role in the patient's care, (4) asking open-ended questions, and (5) sitting down with the patient. Improved patient satisfaction using these communication etiquettes have been reported.[3]

Good medical practice is "professionalism in action" with respect for patient-centered care. It has four domains:
- Be competent and keep professional knowledge and skills up to date.
- Take prompt action if patient safety is being compromised.
- Maintain good communication with patients and work with colleagues in patients' interests.
- Maintain trust—be honest, open, and act with integrity. Never abuse your patients' trust in you or the public's trust in the profession.

This patient-centered care has also been shown to improve patient's experience and clinical outcomes.[4] Good medical practice which is patient-centered with communication etiquette are essential to achieve the objectives of "the four pillars" of bioethics:
- *Autonomy*: Respect patient's dignity and give full information so that he/she is able to come to the treatment decision.
- *Beneficence*: "Do what is best" for the patient. Recognize one's professional limitation and seek help from seniors when needed.
- *Nonmaleficence*: "Do no harm." Involve colleagues/seniors if need arises.
- *Justice*: Protect/promote health of individual and public.

"It is unsettling how little it takes to defeat success in medicine. ... In this work against sickness, we begin not with genetic or cellular interactions but with human one" (**Gawande A**[5])

"We are here to add what we can to life, not to get what we can from life" (**Sir William Osler**[1])

A Clinical Scenario Based on a True Incident

A 27-year-old patient came to the ENT outpatient department along with his elder brother with chief complaints of neck pain for 2 days, following slipping and falling on a rope. However, he was reluctant to give details of the injury. The attending resident doctor also noted that the patient was avoiding eye contact while giving history. The patient was not in distress, and he had a ligature mark which was superficial on the left and deep on the right side on his neck.

As the doctor was concerned regarding the history about the injury, he approached his senior colleague for help. They then reassured the patient, requesting his elder brother to

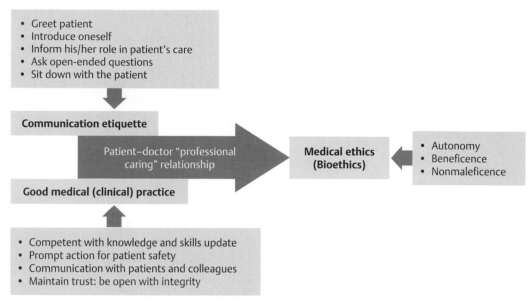

- Greet patient
- Introduce oneself
- Inform his/her role in patient's care
- Ask open-ended questions
- Sit down with the patient

Communication etiquette

Patient–doctor "professional caring" relationship

Medical ethics (Bioethics)

- Autonomy
- Beneficence
- Nonmaleficence

Good medical (clinical) practice

- Competent with knowledge and skills update
- Prompt action for patient safety
- Communication with patients and colleagues
- Maintain trust: be open with integrity

Patient–doctor "professional caring" relationship

wait outside so that the patient could give details of his injury. They also explained to the patient that a complete disclosure of mode of his injury is essential so that he can be given the best possible treatment. The patient then volunteered that 2 days ago he had a quarrel with his friends after they consumed alcohol. Following this, he attempted suicide by hanging himself. Fortunately, he was rescued immediately. He was sent to his home the next day. The following day, he was brought to our hospital. In addition to attending his neck wound, these doctors realized that the incident of "attempted suicide" was indeed a "sentinel sign" of underlying life-threatening suicidal risk factors, be it individual, relationship, cultural, or societal. This was way beyond the capacity of the attending doctors' ENT specialty and required urgent psychiatric opinion with management. This concern was shared with the patient and his brother as well (with the patient's permission). Psychiatric opinion and management were urgently sought following which the patient underwent de-addiction therapy as well.

Analysis of Patient–Doctor Relationship: Interrelated Good Medical Practice and Medical Ethics

The attending doctor was concerned about the history not correlating with the examination findings. He, however, recognized the limits of his competence and took the help of his senior colleague. The compassionate approach along with the patient concern developed trust in the patient–doctor relationship. These are domains of good medical practice.

These doctors requested for detailed history to be taken in the absence of his elder brother because they respected the dignity and privacy of their patient (*autonomy*). They communicated in detail regarding the mode of injury, explaining that this was necessary to give the best possible treatment for their patient (*beneficence*). They realized that their patient's "attempted suicide" was "red flag" for imminent risk to his life. The urgent need to "do no harm" (*nonmaleficence*) warranted an additional urgent psychiatric intervention, thus protecting as well as promoting his health (*justice*). These are the pillars of medical ethics.

Patients, after all, really make a doctor a doctor!!

References

1. Silverman ME, Murray TJ, Bryan CS. eds. The Quotable Osler. Philadelphia: American College of Physicians; 2003:283

2. Silverman BD. Physician behavior and bedside manners: the influence of William Osler and The Johns Hopkins School of Medicine. Proc Bayl Univ Med Cent 2012;25(1):58–61

3. Tackett S, Tad-y D, Rios R, Kisuule F, Wright S. Appraising the practice of etiquette-based medicine in the inpatient setting. J Gen Intern Med 2013;28(7):908–913

4. Street RL Jr, Makoul G, Arora NK, Epstein RM. How does communication heal? Pathways linking clinician-patient communication to health outcomes. Patient Educ Couns 2009;74(3):295–301

5. Gawande A. Better: A Surgeon's Notes on Performance. New York: Metropolitan Books; 2007:81–82

Index